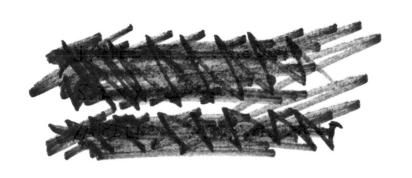

c/o Dept. of Chemistry
NEW YORK UNIV.
WASHINGTON SQUARE
NEW YORK   N.Y 10003

AGING, CARCINOGENESIS, AND RADIATION BIOLOGY

The Role of Nucleic Acid Addition Reactions

AGING, CARCINOGENESIS, AND RADIATION BIOLOGY

The Role of Nucleic Acid Addition Reactions

Edited by

Kendric C. Smith

Stanford University School of Medicine

PLENUM PRESS · NEW YORK AND LONDON

Library of Congress Cataloging in Publication Data

Main entry under title:

Aging, carcinogenesis, and radiation biology.

"The symposium . . . was sponsored by the American Society for Photobiology."
Includes bibliographies and index.
1. Proteins—Congresses. 2. Deoxyribonucleic acid—Congresses. 3. Aging—Congresses. 4. Carcinogenesis—Congresses. 5. Radiobiology—Congresses. I. Smith, Kendric
C., 1926-   II. American Society for Photobiology. [DNLM: 1. DNA—Congresses.
2. Aging—Congresses. 3. Carcinogens—Congresses. 4. Radiobiology Congresses. 5.
Proteins—Congresses. QU58 A267 1975]
QP551.A33 1976   574.8'732   75-42528
ISBN 0-306-30911-4

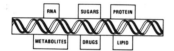

Proceedings of an International Conference entitled "Proteins and Other Adducts
to DNA: Their Significance to Aging, Carcinogenesis, and Radiation Biology" held
in Williamsburg, Virginia on May 2-6, 1975

©1976 Plenum Press, New York
A Division of Plenum Publishing Corporation
227 West 17th Street, New York, N.Y. 10011

United Kingdom edition published by Plenum Press, London
A Division of Plenum Publishing Company, Ltd.
Davis House (4th Floor), 8 Scrubs Lane, Harlesden, London, NW10 6SE, England

Printed in the United States of America

Preface

The covalent attachment to deoxyribonucleic acid *in vivo* of a large number of different types of chemical compounds (both normal cellular constituents such as proteins and amino acids, and also exogenous compounds such as drugs, carcinogens, etc.) have been shown to exert profound effects upon cells. Four research activities, formerly considered to be totally independent, relate to this problem of nucleic acid adducts--(1) *normal* covalent attachment of DNA to membranes, protein linkers in chromosomes, etc.; (2) the roles of radiation and chemical enhancement of DNA adduct formation in cell killing and mutagenesis. (A related field is the use of known cross-linking reactions to gain information on structural associations in macromolecular complexes.); (3) the relevance of DNA adducts to chemical and radiation carcinogenesis; (4) the relevance of DNA adducts to the cross-linking theory of cellular aging.

(1) There are numerous examples of normal linkages between DNA and protein, e.g., DNA-membrane attachment sites, protein linkers in chromosomes, amino acids covalently linked to DNA as a function of growth conditions, and gene regulation by non-covalently bound proteins. A summary of data on natural adducts to DNA thus serves to introduce the subject of the radiation and chemical enhancement of DNA adduct formation.

(2) In the past, radiation biology has been concerned mainly with trying to understand the radiation chemistry of purified DNA, and the biological effects and repair of these radiation-induced alterations when produced in cellular DNA. Great progress has been made with this approach, but the biological effects of radiation cannot be wholly explained by the radiation products produced in purified DNA. This is not at all surprising since DNA does not exist in pure form within cells, but is surrounded by proteins, lipids, carbohydrates, RNA and small molecular precursors and metabolites. Many compounds have been shown to combine covalently with DNA when irradiated *in vitro* and *in vivo*. Profound biological effects have been observed for these addition products when produced *in vivo*, especially the cross-linking of DNA and protein. Since many of the known radiation-induced adducts to DNA appear to

be mediated by radical reactions whether X- or UV-radiation is used, the subject of DNA adducts offers a unique common ground for a useful dialogue between radiation chemists and photochemists.

Most of our current insights concerning the mechanism of mutagenesis come from radiation studies. It now appears certain that mutagenesis occurs as a consequence of the inaccurate repair of DNA damage.

Perhaps the best evidence that a field has achieved a certain maturity is when fundamental observations are converted into methods to solve specific problems. For example, cross-linking techniques are now being used to investigate the packing arrangement of the DNA in phage, the association sites between specific aminoacyl-t-RNA synthetases and their specific t-RNAs, and the active sites of enzymes.

(3) Most chemical carcinogens have been shown to bind covalently to DNA, either directly, after metabolic activation, or after radiation-induced activation. Therefore, addition reactions to DNA appear to play a central role in chemical carcinogenesis. Since all ultimate carcinogens have been shown to be mutagens, another close tie with radiation biology is apparent.

(4) One theory of aging suggests that DNA becomes cross-linked with proteins and other compounds such that the template activity to DNA is impaired. In support of this hypothesis, the DNA from the tissues of older animals has been shown to be more difficult to deproteinate. It is also known that radiation can modify the aging process.

DNA adducts appear to arise frequently through radical-type reactions. While radicals and/or activated compounds are formed *in vivo* through normal metabolic processes, the most convenient way of generating radicals is with radiation. A considerable wealth of information is available from radiation biology that is relevant to the field of chemical carcinogenesis and to the cross-linking theory of aging. It thus seems most appropriate and timely to review these fields--fields which may at first seem philosophically divergent but which, in fact, have a strong convergence at the level of molecular mechanisms.

It is hoped that these proceedings will stimulate research on the chemistry and biological effects of DNA adducts, and will improve the dialogue among workers in the fields of Aging, Carcinogenesis and Radiation Biology.

Stanford, California   Kendric C. Smith
October 1975

Acknowledgments

The Symposium from which these Proceedings are derived was sponsored by the American Society for Photobiology and supported in part by the Energy Research and Development Administration, the National Cancer Institute, and the National Science Foundation.

I wish to express my sincere thanks to Mrs. Terry Marshall for retyping the manuscripts.

Contents

ATTACHMENT OF CHROMOSOMES TO MEMBRANES IN BACTERIA AND ANIMAL CELLS

Moselio Schaechter

Department of Molecular Biology and Microbiology, Tufts University School of Medicine, Boston, Massachusetts 02111

1. INTRODUCTION

It has been proposed that in bacteria the attachment of DNA to the cytoplasmic membrane serves to ensure proper chromosome segregation (Jacob *et al.*, 1963). The lack of a mitotic apparatus has made this an appealing suggestion and the subject of considerable study. The methodology available--electron microscopy and cell fractionation--is not sufficiently developed to allow definitive conclusions about the nature and physiological importance of the connection between the two structures. Nevertheless, there are indications that DNA-membrane complexes may play a role in other functions than chromosome segregation, namely, replication, transcription, or the maintenance of the physical configuration of the DNA. We have recently reviewed these subjects in some detail (Leibowitz and Schaechter, 1975). In addition, the suggestion has been made that changes in the membrane provide the signal for initiation of DNA replication (Marvin, 1967; Helmstetter, 1974). The cell membrane appears to be directly involved in the replication and maturation of bacteriophages and other viruses. In these systems, the physiological role of the membrane is even less understood (for a review, see Siegel and Schaechter, 1973).

In the higher cells, the attachment of interphase chromosomes to the nuclear membrane has also been the subject of many reports. There is considerable controversy on several points, principally whether or not the membrane is the site of DNA replication (for reviews, see Barlow, 1972; Huberman, 1973). It should be noted that attachment of chromosomes to the membrane through interphase may preserve their topological relationship.

2.   METHODOLOGICAL CONSIDERATION OF CELL FRACTIONATION

A DNA-membrane complex is not a precisely defined subcellular fraction, and its physical or chemical properties can only be defined operationally. Thus, it is possible to obtain fractions containing virtually all the membrane and all the DNA, intermediate amounts of each, or a small proportion of both membrane and DNA. Each of these types of preparations lends itself to a particular study. At present none of the methods used can be assumed to be free of artifacts that may arise during preparation, either at the time of cell breakage or thereafter. In general, these studies are constrained by technical problems and represent an early stage of penetration into the subject. Nonetheless, interesting and highly suggestive information on several points has become available.

The techniques used for obtaining DNA-membrane complexes require gentle mechanical manipulations to avoid shearing the DNA. In the case of bacteria, this is done by converting them into spheroplasts, usually by the action of lysozyme. Spheroplasts can then be lysed with detergents, osmotic shock, or relatively weak mechanical forces. DNA-membrane complexes can then be isolated in a variety of ways. There are three types of techniques in current use:

i)   In certain cell lysates these complexes are the heaviest fraction and can be obtained by *velocity* centrifugation through a sucrose gradient (e.g., Sueoka and Quinn, 1965). Similarly, one can utilize the unique density or change of these complexes and retrieve them by *equilibrium* centrifugation through renografin gradients (Ivarie and Pene, 1970), or sucrose gradients (Daniels, 1971), or by free electrophoresis (Olsen *et al.*, 1974).

ii) The hydrophobic properties of the membrane have also been utilized, taking advantage of their binding to the surface of crystals of Mg^{++}-sarkosyl. The crystal-membrane-DNA complex, after isopycnic banding, forms a so-called M-band (Tremblay *et al.*, 1969; Earhart *et al.*, 1968).

Apparently different portions of the membrane vary in their affinity for the surface of the crystals, with the DNA-bearing portion having very high affinity (Ballesta *et al.*, 1972). Of the methods originally developed for use with bacteria, velocity centrifugation and the M-band method have been used extensively with animal cells (cf., Comings, 1972).

iii) The nucleoids of bacteria can be isolated in a folded, compact state which probably resembles the intracellular condition (Stonington and Pettijohn, 1971). These isolated nucleoids contain various amounts of membrane material, depending on the conditions used in their isolation (Worcel and Burgi, 1972). They promise to be particularly useful in studies on the specificity of attachment of DNA to the membrane because they constitute relatively purified material.

3. IS DNA ATTACHED TO A SPECIAL PORTION OF THE MEMBRANE?

In addition to the cytoplasmic membrane, gram-negative bacteria possess an outer membrane, located outside their cell wall. When these two membranes are separated isopycnically on sucrose gradients, the DNA of *Escherichia coli* is found mainly in the cytoplasmic membrane (Holland and Darby, 1973). The membrane component of isolated nucleoids includes some of the outer membrane proteins (Worcel and Burgi, 1974). It seems likely that this is due to the adherence of the outer and cytoplasmic membrane at defined sites (Bayer, 1968a, b) which conceivably play a special role in the attachment of the DNA.

The portions of the membrane retrieved by the M-band technique have been shown to differ from the rest of the membrane in their affinity for Mg^{++}-sarkosyl crystals and in being enriched for phosphatidylethanolamine (Daniels, 1971; Ballesta *et al.*, 1972). DNA-membrane preparations from *Bacillus subtilis* contain special bands when analyzed by SDS-polyacrylamide gel electrophoresis (Sueoka and Hammers, 1974).

Morphological studies on ultrathin sections suggest that DNA of bacteria is not attached to the cytoplasmic membrane directly but to its invagination, the mesosome (Ryter, 1968). The connection between the DNA and the mesosome became apparent in the following experiment, performed by Ryter and others (cf., Ryter and Landman, 1967): when *B. subtilis* is placed in hypertonic media, mesosomes evaginate and are extruded into the medium. Sections through these cells show that the nucleoids are no longer centrally located but are now in contact with the cell's periphery at the site of mesosome extrusion. Similar results are seen when mesosomes are evaginated during spheroplast formation. Despite these findings, our knowledge on the role of mesosomes in DNA segregation is uncertain because considerable controversy surrounds their biochemistry and morphology (cf., Reusch and Berger, 1973).

In animal cells correspondingly little is known about the specificity of the region of the nuclear membrane to which chromosomes may be attached. There are morphological indications that the attachment takes place at the annuli of the nuclear membranes (cf., Barlow, 1972; Engelhardt and Pusa, 1972). I am not aware of relevant studies on the biochemical level.

4. THE POSSIBLE ROLE OF THE MEMBRANE IN CHROMOSOME SEGREGATION

At a first glance, this problem is most relevant to bacteria because they lack a mitotic apparatus. The question may actually be more general because mitosis in certain eucaryotes such as yeast cells involves the nuclear membrane.

The original suggestion for the replicon specified that segregation of sister chromosomes takes place by their binding to both sides of an equatorial band of membrane growth (Jacob *et al.*, 1963). The disposition of new membrane material at this band would by itself lead to a separation of the sister DNA molecules because of lateral displacement of the attachment points. By and large, evidence for such semiconservative membrane segregation is inconclusive. Mindich and Dales (1972) reported that, in pulse labeled *B. subtilis* examined by autoradiography, newly made lipids are not found at specific sites. However, lipids are mobile in membranes and one cannot equate their location with their site of synthesis. This complication makes it difficult to interpret the finding that segregation of membrane constituents follows a dispersive, rather than a semiconservative mode (Lin *et al.*, 1971; Wilson and Fox, 1971; Green and Schaechter, 1972). The only report of semiconservative membrane growth is that of Kepes and Autissieres (1972) who, using indirect measurements, found that permease molecules segregated semiconservatively. Clearly, more work is necessary to establish the mode of membrane growth and, consequently, its role in chromosome segregation. It may be noted that the segregation apparatus may only have a passive requirement for a surface. In this case, membrane attachment may be relevant to this process regardless of how the membrane itself is partitioned.

5. IS THE ORIGIN OF REPLICATION BOUND TO THE MEMBRANE?

It is well established that chromosome replication in bacteria starts at a genetically defined locus, the origin. This site appears to be attached to the membrane in *B. subtilis* because, in

transformation assays, DNA proximal to the membrane is enriched in
genetic markers known to be close to the origin of replication
(Sueoka and Quinn, 1968; O'Sullivan and Sueoka, 1969; Ivarie and
Pene, 1970; Yamaguchi *et al.*, 1971). Similar conclusions were
reached in *E. coli* where the origin was located by radioactive
labeling (Fielding and Fox, 1970; Parker and Glaser, 1974). Recent
work has shown that the membrane attachment of the origin of replication in *E. coli* is resistant to the action of single-strand
specific endonuclease S1, whereas other sites of DNA attachment
are sensitive to this enzyme. This suggests that attachment of the
origin is chemically different from that of other sites of the DNA
(Abe, Boyd, Brown, Cote and Schaechter, unpublished data).

There are no reasons to believe that this attachment is tempo-
rary or cyclic during the division cycle. An earlier report that
the chromosome of *E. coli* detaches at the end of its replication
(Worcel and Burgi, 1974) has been shown to be due to artifacts of
preparation (Ryder and Smith, 1974, 1975). Bacterial DNA detaches
from the membrane only under conditions that can be expected to
cause extensive structural damage to the membrane (e.g., the addition of phenethyl alcohol, as reported by Masker and Eberle, 1972).
In view of the spatial difficulties that can be expected if a
specific region of the DNA had to find a specific region of the
membrane at the start of each replication cycle, it would be
surprising if their connection were not permanent. An indication of this permanence is suggested by the findings of Chao and
Lark (1967) and Pierucci and Zuchowski (1973) that chromosomes of
E. coli do not segregate randomly.

There is no evidence that the origins of DNA replication in
animal cell chromosomes are attached to the membrane. When cells
labeled with [^{3}H]thymidine early in the S period are examined by
autoradiography, newly made DNA is not preferentially associated
with the nuclear membrane (Comings and Okada, 1973; Huberman *et
al.*, 1972). These experiments do not deal with initiations that
take place later in the S period. Chromosomes of higher cells
consist of many replicating units which do not initiate synchro-
nously (Huberman, 1973). This makes it very difficult to determine
if the origins of some of the units of replication in some of the
chromosomes are indeed attached to the nuclear membrane. Actually,
this problem appears formidable in the light of the available
methodology.

6. THE MEMBRANE AS THE SITE OF DNA REPLICATION

In both bacteria and higher cells, the first reports in this
field indicated that DNA replication takes place on or near the
membrane (cf., Leibowitz and Schaechter, 1975; Comings, 1972). At
the present time, this question has not been settled either for

procaryotes or eucaryotes. In bacteria, when cells are pulse-labeled
with radioactive thymidine and this DNA is subjected to mild shearing,
the specific activity of the DNA remaining on the membrane is 2-4
times higher than that which is removed. While this suggests that
the replication point is proximal to the membrane, several complications make this interpretation difficult. Newly made DNA has
special properties (e.g., it can be more easily denatured, as shown
by Kidson, 1960), which may allow spurious attachment. Conversely,
small fragments of DNA formed during replication are spuriously
detached during M-band formation (Leibowitz and Schaechter, unpublished data). In view of uncertainties in our knowledge of DNA
replication, it is not surprising that this question has not yet
been settled.

Several early studies in animal cells reported that newly made
DNA is associated with the nuclear membrane, both by cell fractionation and by autoradiography (cf., Comings, 1972). It was shown by
Fakan *et al.* (1972) and Huberman *et al.* (1972) that these results
are due either to the drastic regime used to synchronize DNA replication, or to the fact that heterochromatin is preferentially
located near the periphery of the nuclei. When the synthesis of
euchromatin is studied in relatively healthy cells, newly made DNA
is localized throughout the nucleus and not just on the membrane.
It is not clear if the location of newly made heterochromatin at or
near the membrane simply reflects the higher concentration of this
condensed DNA at the peripheral site, or if it is in fact replicated
at the membrane. As in bacteria, enrichment for newly made DNA on
the membrane may be due to spurious attachment of denatured DNA
(Fakan *et al.*, 1972).

7. THE INVOLVEMENT OF THE MEMBRANE IN OTHER DNA FUNCTIONS

The number of attachment points of bacterial DNA to the membrane has been estimated to be 20 to 30 in *E. coli* (Rosenberg and
Cavalieri, 1968; Dworsky and Schaechter, 1973) and 70 to 90 in *B.
subtilis* (Ivarie and Péne, 1973). While these numbers are probably imprecise, they are larger than expected if bacterial chromosomes were attached solely at the origin and/or sites of replication. Dworsky and Schaechter (1973) showed that the points of
attachment fall into two classes. Some, 2-5 in number, are present after treatment of *E. coli* with rifampin, while the rest are
no longer detectable a short time after addition of the drug.
Since rifampin binds free RNA polymerase and inhibits initiation
of RNA synthesis, this suggests that this enzyme may play a
special role in attaching DNA to the membrane.

A hint on the chemical nature of some of these attachment
points comes from the finding that single-stranded DNA tends to
stick to membranes (Fakan *et al.*, 1972; Dworsky and Schaechter,

1973). This suggests that *in vivo* attachment may be at regions of
DNA denaturation. In a series of experiments currently in progress
we have observed that the single-strand specific endonuclease S1
detaches about 90% of the DNA of *E. coli* (Abe, M., Boyd, D., Brown,
C., Cote, R. and Schaechter, M., unpublished data). The detached
DNA is very large, representing, on the average, pieces whose size
is 1/20 of the chromosome. A comparison of this enzyme with pancreatic deoxyribonuclease indicates that S1 nuclease acts at or
near the site of membrane attachment. These results do not
definitely show that S1 nuclease acts on single-stranded regions
because other activities may be present at low levels even in
highly purified preparations. However, control experiments show
that no double-strand nuclease activity is detectable under the
conditions used in these experiments.

Multiple attachment of animal cell chromosomes have been
reported by Ormerod and Lehmann (1971), spaced at intervals of
about 1000 μm along the DNA.

The nucleoid of bacteria consists of folded, highly compact
DNA. It has been proposed by Worcel and Burgi (1972) that the
compactness of isolated nucleoids is due to supercoiling of the
DNA. They showed that the intact chromosome acts as if separated
into 10 to 80 individual supercoils. They proposed that these
units are separated by a special class of RNA or proteins. An
alternative explanation suggests itself because this range of
figures is the same as that of membrane attachment sites. It
seems possible, therefore, that the separation of each supercoiled
loop may be due to its attachment to the membrane. The amount of
membrane material in isolated nucleoids can be as low as 0.1% of
the total. However, such nucleoids form M-bands (A. Wright and
S. Michaelis, personal communication) and their small amount of
membrane may suffice to retain the topological properties of
nucleoids *in vitro*.

8. CONCLUSION

The notion that the membrane may play a regulatory role in
chromosome physiology is singularly appealing although it cannot
yet be tested rigorously.

The available data suggests that chromosomes of both procaryotes and eucaryotes are attached to the membrane, probably throughout the division cycle. In bacteria there is considerable evidence
that one of the points of attachment is the origin of DNA replication. As yet, there are indications, but no assurance, that attachment of DNA to the membrane may play a role in segregation, replication, transcription, or maintaining the compactness of the
bacterial chromosome.

References

Ballesta, J.P., Cundliffe, E., Daniels, M.J., Silverstein, J.L., Susskind, M.M., and Schaechter, M., 1972, Some unique properties of the deoxyribonucleic acid-bearing portion of the bacterial chromosome, *J. Bacteriol.* 112:195-199.

Barlow, P.W., 1972, The ordered replication of chromosomal DNA: A review and a proposal for its control, *Cytobios* 6:55-80.

Bayer, M.E., 1968a, Areas of adhesion between wall and membrane of *Escherichia coli, J. Gen. Microbiol.* 53:395-404.

Bayer, M.E., 1968b, Adsorption of bacteriophages to adhesions between wall and membrane of *Escherichia coli, J. Virol.* 2:346-356.

Comings, D.E., 1972, The structure and function of chromosomes, *Annu. Human Gen.* 3:237-431.

Comings, D.E., and Okada, T.A., 1973, DNA replication and the nuclear membrane, *J. Mol. Biol.* 75:609-618.

Daniels, M.J., 1971, Some features of the bacterial membrane studied with the aid of a new fractionation technique, *Biochem. J.* 122:197-207.

Dworsky, P., and Schaechter, M., 1973, Effect of rifampin on the structure and membrane attachment of the nucleoid of *Escherichia coli, J. Bacteriol.* 116:1364-1374.

Earhart, C.F., Tremblay, G.Y., Daniels, M.J., and Schaechter, M., 1968, DNA replication studied by a new method for the isolation of cell membrane-DNA complexes, *Cold Spring Harbor Symp. Quant. Biol.* 33:707-710.

Engelhardt, P., and Pusa, K., 1972, Nuclearpore complex: "Press-Stud" elements of chromosomes in pairing and control, *Nature New Biol.* 240:163-166.

Fakan, S., Turner, G.N., Pagano, J.S., and Hancock, R., 1972, Sites of replication of chromosomal DNA in a eukaryotic cell, *Proc. Nat. Acad. Sci. USA* 69:2300-2305.

Fielding, P., and Fox, C.F., 1970, Evidence for stable attachment of DNA to membrane at the replication origin of *Escherichia coli, Biochim. Biophys. Res. Commun.* 41:157-162.

Green, E.W., and Schaechter, M., 1972, The mode of segregation of the bacterial cell membrane, *Proc. Nat. Acad. Sci. USA* 69:2312-2316.

Helmstetter, C.E., 1974, Initiation of chromosome replication in *Escherichia coli.* II. Analysis of control mechanism, *J. Mol. Biol.* 84:21-36.

Holland, I.B., and Darby, V., 1973, Detection of a specific DNA-cytoplasmic membrane complex in *Escherichia coli* by equilibrium density centrifugation on sucrose gradients, *FEBS Lett.* 33:106-108.

Huberman, J.A., 1973, Structure of chromosome fibers and chromosomes, *Annu. Rev. Biochem.* 42:355-378.

Huberman, J.A., Tsai, A., and Deich, R.E., 1973, DNA replication sites within nuclei of mammalian cells, *Nature* 241:32-36.

Ivarie, R.D., and Péne, J.J., 1970, Association of the *Bacillus subtilis* chromosome with the cell membrane: Resolution of free and bound deoxyribonucleic acid on renografin gradients, *J. Bacteriol.* 104:839-850.

Ivarie, R.D., and Péne, J.J., 1973, Association of many regions of the *Bacillus subtilis* chromosome with the cell membrane, *J. Bacteriol.* 114:571-576.

Jacob, F., Ryter, A., and Cuzin, F., 1966, On the association between DNA and membrane in bacteria, *Proc. Royal Soc.* B 164:267-278.

Kepes, A., and Autissier, F., 1972, Topology of membrane growth in bacteria, *Biochim. Biophys. Acta* 265:443-469.

Kidson, C., 1966, Deoxyribonucleic acid secondary structure in the region of the replication point, *J. Mol. Biol.* 17:1-9.

Leibowitz, P.J., and Schaechter, M., 1975, The attachment of the bacterial chromosome to the cell membrane, *Int. Rev. Cytol.* 41:1-28.

Lin, E.C.C., Hirota, Y., and Jacob, F., 1971, On the process of cellular division in *Escherichia coli*. VI. Use of a methyl cellulose autoradiographic method for the study of cellular division in *Escherichia coli*, *J. Bacteriol.* 108:375-385.

Marvin, D.A., 1969, Control of DNA replication by membrane, *Nature* 219:485.

Masker, W.E., and Eberle, H., 1972, Effects of phenethylalcohol on deoxyribonucleic acid-membrane association in *Escherichia coli*, *J. Bacteriol.* 109:1170-1174.

Mindich, L., and Dales, C., 1972, Membrane synthesis in *Bacillus subtilis*. III. The morphological localization of the sites of membrane synthesis, *J. Cell Biol.* 55:32-41.

Olsen, W.L., Heidrich, H.-G., Hefechneider, P.H., and Hanning, K., 1974, Deoxyribonucleic acid-envelope complexes isolated from *Escherichia coli* by free-flow electrophoresis: Biochemical and electron microscope characterization, *J. Bacteriol.* 118: 646-653.

Ormerod, M.G., and Lehmann, A.R., 1971, The release of high molecular weight DNA from a mammalian cell (L5178Y). Attachment of the DNA to the nuclear membrane, *Biochim. Biophys. Acta* 228:331-343.

O'Sullivan, M.A., and Sueoka, N., 1972, Membrane attachment of the replication origin of a multifork (dichotomous) chromosome in *Bacillus subtilis*, *J. Mol. Biol.* 69:237-248.

Parker, D.L., and Glaser, D.A., 1974, Chromosomal sites of DNA-membrane attachment in *Escherichia coli*, *J. Mol. Biol.* 87: 153-168.

Rosenberg, B.H., and Cavalieri, L.F., 1968, Shear sensitivity of the *E. coli* genome: multiple membrane attachment points of the *E. coli* DNA, *Cold Spring Harbor Symp. Quant. Biol.* 33: 65-72.

Ryder, O.A., and Smith, D.W., 1974, Isolation of membrane-associated folded chromosomes from *Escherichia coli*: Effect of protein synthesis inhibition, *J. Bacteriol.* 120:1356-1363.

Ryder, O.A., and Smith, D.W., 1975, Properties of membrane-associated
     folded chromosomes of *E. coli* related to initiation and termina-
     tion of DNA replication, *Cell* 4:337-345.
Ryter, A., 1968, Association of the nucleus and the membrane of
     bacteria: a morphological study, *Bacteriol. Rev.* 32:39-54.
Ryter, A., and Landman, O.E., 1964, Electron microscope study of
     the relationship between mesosome loss and the stable L state
     (or protoplast state) in *Bacillus subtilis, J. Bacteriol.* 88:
     457-467.
Siegel, P.J., and Schaechter, M., 1973, The role of the host cell
     membrane in the replication and morphogenesis of bacterio-
     phages, *Annu. Rev. Microbiol.* 27:261-282.
Stonington, O.G., and Pettijohn, D.E., 1971, The folded genome of
     Escherichia coli isolated in a protein-DNA-RNA complex, *Proc.
     Nat. Acad. Sci. USA* 68:6-9.
Sueoka, N., and Quinn, W.G., 1965, Membrane attachment of the
     chromosome replication origin in *Bacillus subtilis, Cold
     Spring Harbor Symp. Quant. Biol.* 33:695-705.
Sueoka, N., and Hammers, J.M., 1974, Isolation of DNA-membrane
     complexes in *Bacillus subtilis, Proc. Nat. Acad. Sci. USA*
     71:4787-4791.
Tremblay, G.Y., Daniels, M.J., and Schaechter, M., 1969, Isolation
     of a cell membrane-DNA-nascent RNA complex from bacteria, *J.
     Mol. Biol.* 40:65-76.
Wilson, G., and Fox, C.F., 1971, Membrane assembly in *Escherichia
     coli*. II. Segregation of preformed and newly formed membrane
     proteins into cells and minicells, *Biochem. Biophys. Res.
     Commun.* 44:503-509.
Worcel, A., and Burgi, E., 1972, On the structure of the folded
     chromosome of *Escherichia coli, J. Mol. Biol.* 71:127-147.
Worcel, A., and Burgi, E., 1974, Properties of a membrane-attached
     form of the folded chromosome of *Escherichia coli, J. Mol.
     Biol.* 82:91-105.
Yamaguchi, K., Murakawi, S., and Yoshikawa, H., 1971, Chromosome-
     membrane association in *Bacillus subtilis*. I. DNA release
     from membrane fraction, *Biochem. Biophys. Res. Commun.*
     44:1559-1565.

LINKERS IN MAMMALIAN CHROMOSOMAL DNA

John T. Lett

Department of Radiology and Radiation Biology and

Committee on Cellular and Molecular Biology, Colorado

State University, Fort Collins, Colorado 80523

1. INTRODUCTION

Ever since the helical model for DNA was proposed by Watson and Crick, the possibility that it does not provide a complete description of the architecture of eukaryotic chromosomal DNA has been the subject of sporadic, but increasing, experimentation and hypothesis. The arguments have generally centered on the proposition that eukaryotic DNA is discontinuous in the Watson-Crick sense, and it is in that sense that I will consider DNA continuity for the remainder of this article. The rationale behind the questioning has been based upon criteria ranging from experimental evidence to such innate feelings as: "All that DNA just cannot be packed into

11

the nucleus or the chromosome without folding points!" Conversely, proponents of the concept that eukaryotic chromosomal DNA is continuous have based their arguments on experimental data or on the feeling: "The DNA in the eukaryotic chromosome must be continuous, therefore experimental evidence to the contrary must be artifactual!" Unfortunately, in certain areas, the latter feeling has been elevated to the rank of religious dogma.

Because emotion has frequently subordinated objectivity in this field, I shall attempt to present the evidence favoring eukaryotic DNA discontinuity as objectively as possible. However, in order that the reader shall be able to judge that objectivity, I must state my personal predilections in the matter. Over the past 20 years my feelings have fluctuated, for reasons which will become clear, but now I believe that the accumulation of evidence, from a variety of different sources, is such that the concept of eukaryotic DNA discontinuity deserves careful consideration. As it happens, a description of the chronological accumulation of that evidence provides the most satisfactory mode for its evaluation, and that is the course which I will follow here.

2. THE PROPHETS IN THE WILDERNESS

2.1. Residual Protein

Following the revolution created by the Watson-Crick helical structure for DNA, concerted efforts were made to improve the techniques for DNA isolation so that "pure" DNA preparations could be studied experimentally. Principal among the scientists involved in that endeavor was K.S. Kirby. Working in England at the Chester Beatty Research Institute, Royal Cancer Hospital, London, Kirby (1957, 1958, 1959) attempted to optimize the efficiency of the phenol-extraction method for the preparation of eukaryotic DNA. Kirby's studies showed: that ∿99.5% of the protein could be removed from deoxynucleoproteins from a variety of sources by improved phenol-extraction; but that the remaining ∿0.5% could not be removed despite recycling of the extraction procedures. The non-extractable protein was termed residual protein, and analysis of its amino-acid composition indicated that it was probably not histone. The questions which now arose were: why is it not possible to remove residual protein from DNA preparations despite repeated phenol-extraction and, if residual protein is not histone, what is it?

The nature and function of residual protein taxed Kirby's imagination and he proposed a number of explanations for its mode of binding to DNA, e.g., as metal-ion complexes (Kirby, 1957, 1958). It was my privilege during that period, as a graduate student at

the Chester Beatty Research Institute, to discuss these ideas with
Kirby in detail. Shortly before his untimely death, Kirby had
reached the conclusion that the best explanation for the presence
of residual protein was that it was covalently bound between
sequences of DNA; in other words, residual protein might represent
protein linkers between DNA molecules. I have not been able, as
yet, to find a statement to this effect in Kirby's papers and can
only assume that his death curtailed its formal presentation. I
was skeptical of the concept of protein linkers at the time mainly
because, as part of my doctoral research, I had isolated DNA preparations from salmon and trout sperm (using sodium dodecyesulfate)
which contained less than 0.02% of residual protein (e.g., Lett
and Stacey, 1960). In fact, protein could not be detected in those
DNA preparations even when they were analyzed by Kirby himself;
and the level given for residual protein in the fish sperm DNA
preparations (Lett and Stacey, 1960), was the limit of sensitivity
of the chromatographic method used for amino acid analysis by
Kirby. There was no question about the highly polymeric nature
of the fish sperm DNA preparations because their molecular weights,
circa 1-2 × 10^7 daltons, were as high as any other DNA preparations
isolated at, or before, that time.

With Kirby's death the matter rested until Bendich and his
colleagues applied themselves to the nature of residual protein
and the continuity of the DNA structure in eukaryotic cells.

In a brief review article in 1963, Bendich and Rosenkranz
considered the then currently available evidence to the effect
that DNA was not continuous. Of particular interest in the
present context was the finding that hydroxylamine cleaved DNA
preparations of size ∿6 × 10^6 daltons into DNA molecules of size
∿5 × 10^5 daltons but no further. From this and other evidence,
Bendich and Rosenkranz (1963) proposed that linked DNA structures,
such as that shown in Fig. 1, exist *in situ*. The concept that
amino acid (or peptide) ester linkages might join DNA subunits of
size ∿5 × 10^5 daltons was proposed independently by Welsh (1962).
He found that DNA preparations were cleaved into molecules of size
∿5 × 10^5 daltons under conditions expected to reduce the level of
metal ions. Furthermore, that cleavage was accompanied by the
release of acid-soluble phosphate-containing peptides.

Bendich and his collaborators appeared to leave this field
after their studies of *circa* 1965, but Welsh has persisted. With
Vyska (Welsh and Vyska, 1971), he described specific sites in
mammalian DNA preparations which were sensitive to the actions of
chelating agents, especially EDTA; and very recently Welsh and
Vyska (1975a, b) have presented the results obtained from extensive studies of those specific sites. Cleavage at EDTA-sensitive
sites seems to yield the same (∿5 × 10^5 molecular weight) DNA
subunits that Welsh, and Bendich and Rosenkranz, described

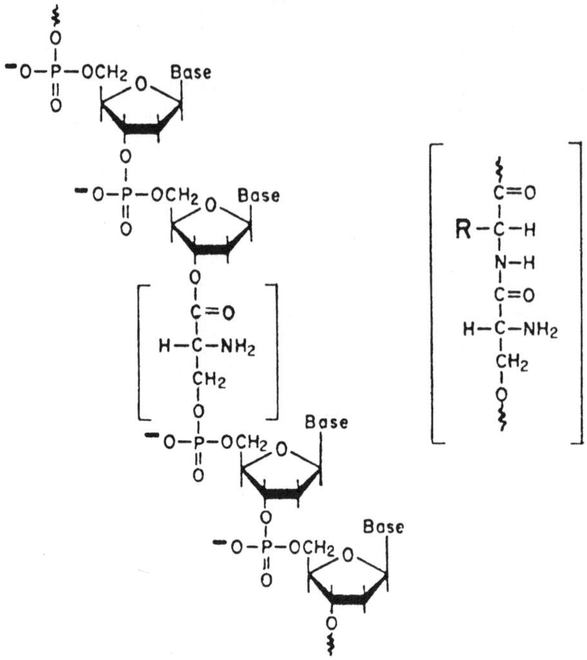

Fig. 1. A hypothetical linkage of serine (or a serylpeptide) in the main polynucleotide chain of deoxyribonucleic acid (From Benedich and Rosenkranz, 1963).

originally. The following summary is taken directly from a pre-print of the recent paper by Welsh and Vyska (1975b).

"A new form of high molecular weight DNA has been pre-pared from purified calf thymus nuclei under conditions designed to maintain the properties of the DNA as close as possible to those existing *in vivo*. The DNA thus obtained has a mean molecular weight of approximately 20 million and can be cleaved as a result of EDTA treat-ment into subunits having a mean molecular weight of about 500,000. This cleavage is shown to be an ordered process, which involves no enzymatic or shear degrada-tion. The process of cleavage consists of an initial 5-day EDTA treatment and 14 subsequent dialyses of 5 days each. The cleavage was considered to have reached an end state when no further change in DNA mean mole-cular weight for two successive dialyses was observ-able. The material released into the dialysates during the cleavage was collected and determined to

be a mixture of phosphopeptides, containing phosphoserine, glycine, alanine, glutamic and aspartic
acids, and having molecular weights of between 900
and 1400 daltons. In a kinetic study it was shown
that the amount of peptide material firmly bound in
the DNA as well as the amount of phosphopeptides collected in the dialysates could be correlated to the
extent of cleavage."

Clearly amino acid linkers, or links mediated by peptides,
would go a long way towards explaining the low "residual protein"
contents in certain DNA preparations.

2.2. Nuclear Gels

Throughout the period in which the residual protein of DNA
preparations was studied, the potential involvement of proteins
in chromosomal DNA architecture was attacked in quite another way.
Over a period of more than 20 years, Dounce and his colleagues
investigated the nature of the gels which are formed when cell
nuclei are swollen in aqueous solution; and Dounce (1971) has
reviewed the trials and tribulations experienced during those
studies. Those workers also concluded that residual protein
was present in nuclear gels and that it constituted linkers between
DNA molecules. Moreover, they found evidence that S-S bonds were
the crucial components in those linkers. Dounce's basic model for
chromosomal DNA structure (Dounce, 1971) is shown in Fig. 2, and
one of the later extrapolations of that model (Dounce *et al.*, 1973)
to the more formal, looped, structures of overall chromosomal
architecture is given in Fig. 3.

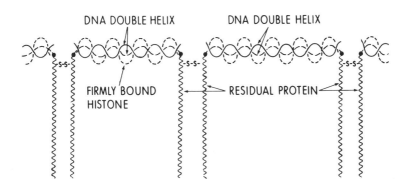

Fig. 2. The schematic diagram of the model proposed for the
structure of chromosomal fibers by Dounce (1971).

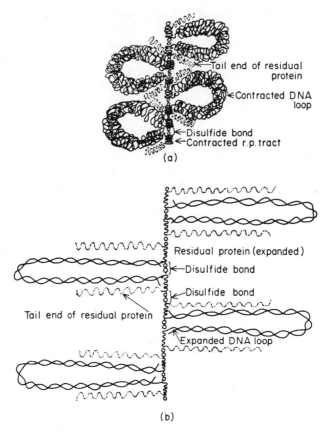

Fig. 3. Schematic diagrams of models (a) metaphase and (b) interphase type chromosomes. 0-0, Disulfide bond (From Dounce *et al.*, 1973).

It is fair to say that the data and ideas of Dounce and his colleagues have never been generally accepted; but is equally fair to say that they have usually been rejected on the grounds: "I believe the DNA in the eukaryotic chromosome is continuous; therefore, Dounce must be wrong!"

2.3. ν Bodies

An explanation for the presence of residual protein in eukaryotic DNA may reside in the entities observed in chromatin fibers by electron microscopy which are known as ν bodies (Olins and Olins, 1974). ν Bodies contain protein and seem to occur at fairly regular intervals along chromatin fibers like "particles on a string" (Olins and Olins, 1974).

3. ALKALI-LABILE BONDS

3.1. Chromosomal DNA and the "Subunit Hypothesis"

Until the mid 1960's studies of the size and shape of nuclear DNA, except for experiments like those of Dounce, required that the DNA be extracted from the nucleus (chromosome) before it could be analyzed. The extraction procedures had one very serious draw-back--they subjected DNA solutions to hydrodynamic shearing. The very size of DNA molecules, and their configurations in solution (as worm-like chains), makes them extremely susceptible to hydro-dynamic shearing. At one time, around 1960, it was believed that the size of all mammalian DNA was about 6×10^6 daltons; but it turned out that the extents of hydrodynamic shearing involved in the standard isolation methods were similar, and that the shearing had simply reduced the DNA molecules to similar sizes. The specter of hydrodynamic shearing is ever present in DNA studies. For example, if bacteriophage T4 DNA, MW = 1.2×10^8 daltons and length 60 μm, can be sheared in solution by simply tilting the container back and forth, what chance do we have of handling eukaryotic DNA? If the DNA in the average mammalian chromosome is all in one piece, it will have a MW $\simeq 10^{11}$ daltons and a length of some 5 cm. Further-more, some chromosomes could contain uninterrupted DNA molecules which are meters long.

A weapon with which to approach the problem posed by very long DNA molecules was provided by McGrath and Williams (1966); it was an adaption of sucrose gradient sedimentation to cellular systems. McGrath and Williams lysed bacterial spheroplasts in alkaline lytic zones upon alkaline sucrose gradients in centrifuge tubes. Since the liberated DNA could then be sedimented without further distur-bance, other than from gentle handling of the centrifuge tubes and the Coriolis forces experienced during rotor acceleration, hydro-dynamic shearing was reduced--hopefully to a minimum. However, the hydrodynamic shearing which occurred during cell lysis still represented an unknown quantity. With this experimental technique, now identified by their names, McGrath and Williams (1966) were able to demonstrate that certain bacteria possess the capacity to rejoin radiation-induced DNA strand breaks. Extension of the McGrath-Williams technique to mammalian systems by Lett *et al.* (1967) soon followed, but serious centrifugation and lysis arti-facts were encountered with mammalian DNA. I must treat these artifacts in detail here because some authors have brought the McGrath and Williams technique into disrepute, either by paying insufficient attention to the true nature of the artifacts and the problems they cause, or by waxing enthusiastic about their

biological significance. Considerable confusion has resulted and
it is necessary that I attempt to dispel that confusion here.

When mammalian cells were lysed on alkaline sucrose gradients
(Lett *et al.*, 1967) gels were formed which quite naturally exhibited abnormal sedimentation characteristics--that is, they did not
behave as freely-sedimenting DNA molecules would have been expected
to behave. Freely-sedimenting single-stranded DNA molecules were
only liberated after lengthy exposure to alkali or moderate doses
of ionizing radiation; but in each case the upper limit of molecular
size of the freely-sedimenting DNA molecules was only $\sim 2 \times 10^8$ daltons. Although microscopic gels formed from individual nuclei
would have been useful for correlation with Dounce's investigations, it was soon obvious that the gel formation observed in the
alkaline sucrose gradients was a simple, but extremely annoying,
artifact. The gels themselves were clearly visible to the naked
eye when the centrifuge tubes were illuminated through their bases;
they appeared in the gradients as approximately spherical, macroscopic entities, which often had streamers attaching them to the
bases of the tubes. Assuredly they were not sedimenting in zones.
Much of the time the gels appeared to sediment to approximately
isopycnic density positions; but when, after centrifugation, the
centrifuge tubes were stored under unit gravity, the gels slowly
collapsed and sank through the gradients. This latter behavior
was especially vexing, because it meant that the sedimentation
properties of the gels would vary with sedimentation time. Thus
it eliminated the experimental flexibility afforded by a fixed
value of $\omega^2 t$ [(rotor speed)^2 × time] at different rotor speeds.
Under those circumstances the sedimentation properties of the gels
would appear to depend on rotor speed whereas actually they would
depend primarily on centrifugation time.

The macroscopic gels distorted the DNA sedimentation profiles
in another, more serious, fashion. If freely-sedimenting DNA
molecules were also present when gelation occurred they often
became entangled or trapped within the gels. This feature can
easily be demonstrated with marker DNA molecules or the simultaneous lysis of heavily-irradiated cell populations. Many other subcellular components suffered the fate of the smaller DNA molecules,
so that the gels were composed of an essentially random collection
of proteins, lipids, nucleic acid molecules of varying sizes, and
the larger degradation products of subcellular components. Clearly,
biologically significant macromolecular architecture, such as
structures of the Dounce type or attachment points to membranes,
could not meaningfully be studied in such a morass.

The difficulties with macroscopic gels were resolved, or at
least substantially reduced, by introducing the chelating agent,
ethylenediamine tetraacetic acid, EDTA, into the alkaline lytic
zone (Lett *et al.*, 1970). In the presence of this compound, the

degradation of mammalian DNA seems to be relatively specific and to proceed via species of defined sizes (Lett *et al.*, 1970); and an important degradation product appears to be a single-stranded molecule (or narrow distribution of closely related molecules) of size $\sim5 \times 10^8$ daltons (165S). From the degradation pathways it was possible to formulate a working hypothesis (Lett *et al.*, 1970, 1972):

i)   That the overall DNA structure was related to the 165S molecule as multicomponent arrays of its double-stranded equivalent.

ii) That the 165S molecule, or structural subunit, was itself composed of subsidiary arrays of smaller molecules which are important in the replication process.

iii) That in the cell types studied [Chinese hamster ovary (CHO); human (HeLa); murine (L5178Y)] these two features pertained to all stages of the cell cycle.

Fundamental to this hypothesis, which has become known as the subunit hypothesis, e.g., (Cleaver, 1974), is the postulate that the DNA molecules are connected by alkali-labile bonds or alkali-labile regions, and that those bonds or regions are also specially susceptible to damage by low doses of ionizing radiation because they occur at exposed regions in the nucleohistone structure (Lett and Sun, 1970; Lett *et al.*, 1970, 1972). The working model has been developed in detail elsewhere (Lett *et al.*, 1972; Lett, 1975), but I reproduce its heuristic formulation here, as Fig. 4, because of the remarkable similarity of that formulation to the Dounce models in Fig. 2 and 3. The two general models shown in Fig. 2 and 4 resulted from investigations of entirely different types, and in my case, to my chagrin, the model was proposed in complete ignorance of the other. I have given the molecular weight of the supposed 165S molecule(s) as $\sim5 \times 10^8$ daltons but evaluation of all the available data (Lett, 1975) suggests that its (their) size(s) is $5 \pm 1 \times 10^8$ daltons. That error range also defines the accuracy with which the size and/or location of the alkali-labile bonds and/or regions can be identified. I must emphasize that the above studies revealed nothing about the chemical nature of the alkali-labile bonds (regions) except that in cell lysates they were labile to alkaline-EDTA (pH >12.5) at 20°C.

These ideas have been challenged on the grounds that the "molecules" which seem to be present in the sedimentation profiles are artifacts of one type or another. The authors of most of these challenges have confused a phenomenon called speed-dependence with centrifugation artifacts, such as the "anomalous" sedimentation behavior of the gels described previously. Zimm (1974) has evolved a theory, based on differential viscous drag at different

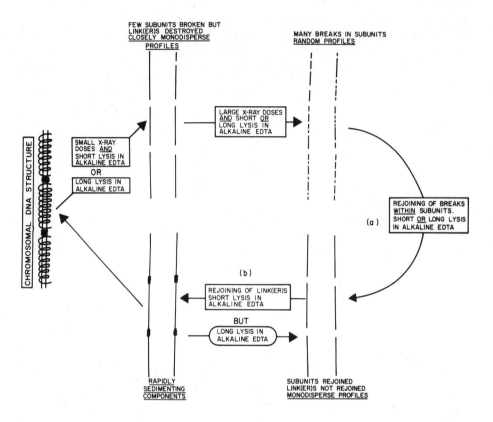

Fig. 4. A diagrammatic representation of a possible breakdown
scheme for eukaryotic chromatin (From Lett *et al.*, 1972).

positions on a sedimenting macromolecule at high centrifugal fields,
which prescribes: that the sedimentation coefficient of a very
large linear macromolecule will be a function of rotor speed; and
that the true sedimentation coefficient of that macromolecule will
only be revealed when the rotor speed is reduced below a certain
critical value. We have investigated the sedimentation profiles
which we believe to consist of partially degraded distributions of
165S molecules by fractionation and resedimentation (Lett, 1975),
see Fig. 5. The results of these studies are consistent with our
interpretation of the sedimentation profiles and they indicate that
the critical rotor speed for a 165S molecule sedimenting at an
average radial distance through a 5-20% sucrose gradient (containing 0.9 M NaCl, 0.1 M NaOH, 0.01 M EDTA) at 20°C in a Beckman SW
25.1 rotor is ∿18,000 rpm. These resedimentation studies also
indicate that, while the expression of the Zimm (1974) equation

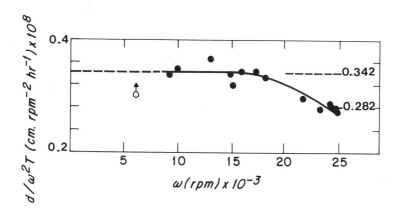

Fig. 5. The resedimentation of fractionated single-stranded eukaryotic DNA of size 165S as a function of rotor speed. For a description of the experimental details, see Lett (1975). ω, rotor speed; T, centrifugation time; d, sedimentation distance (From Lett, 1975).

may be formally correct, its numerical constants do not apply to single-stranded DNA of size $\sim$165S sedimenting through solutions of high ionic strengths. The most likely explanation for this finding is that single-stranded DNA molecules are not random coils in those gradients--a necessary assumption in the Zimm theory. Moreover, the resedimentation studies also indicate that many, if not all, of the claims in literature that the shapes of DNA sedimentation profiles may change with rotor speed, are indeed true; but the causes of those shape changes can, in most cases, be traced to simple centrifugation artifacts related to zone instability caused by convection-diffusion difficulties at, or near, the gradient-lytic zone interface.

The resedimentation data given in Fig. 5 put the sedimentation coefficient of the supposed subunit molecule at 170S rather than 165S, but since these two figures lie within the experimental error of the measurements, I will retain the latter figure here.

Recently, Hozier and Taylor (1975) have investigated the DNA structure of Chinese hamster ovary cells in the G_1 position of the cell cycle. Because of the confusion that exists about the alkaline sucrose gradient experiments, which, as we have seen above, is primarily due to a lack of understanding of the true origins of certain centrifugation phenomena, Hozier and Taylor (1975) resorted to a self-generating NaI gradient. They also observed band-spreading artifacts in that system, but ironically, the effects occurred at high speeds--the converse of the situation in preformed sucrose gradients. The reasons for this are probably quite simple: if insufficient time (i.e., high rotor speeds) elapses in a self-generating system, an inadequate gradient will be generated which will be unstable because its loading capacity will be exceeded; conversely, if too long a time is allowed to elapse (i.e., low rotor speeds) in experiments with preformed gradients, then extensive diffusion occurs at the lytic zone-gradient interface, gradient capacity is lost, and instability and droplet sedimentation occur.

The experiments of Hozier and Taylor (1975) suggest the presence of two classes of single-stranded DNA subunits in mammalian DNA. The first of these has a size of 170 μm and is released from the bulk of the DNA by exposure to alkali. The second component, which has a size of 60 μm, is released following *extensive* exposure (days) to pronase at pH 9.3. I have deliberately emphasized the word extensive here for later reference. Hozier and Taylor have reached the reasonable conclusion that the 170 μm subunit is probably composed of three 60 μm subunits. The latter component, of course, is tantalizingly similar in size to the replication distances detected by Huberman and Riggs (1968) in autoradiographic experiments. But what is the chemical nature of the alkali-labile bonds? Segments of RNA are plausible candidates, but also: "One possibility is an acyl linkage, if DNA chains terminate in a ribonucleoside at the 3'-end as with transfer RNA. A covalently linked protein dimer might couple the two 2' or 3'-OH groups by two acyl bonds at the carboxyl termini of the two polypeptide chains, thereby linking two polynucleotide chains of opposite polarity..." (Hozier and Taylor, 1975). Have we come full circle to Kirby, Bendich, Welsh and Dounce?

3.2. Mitochondrial DNA

Before we leave the subject of alkali-labile bonds in eukaryotic DNA we must consider another DNA-containing system of the eukaryotic cell, namely, the mitochondrion.

Recently, three independent studies of the lability of mitochondrial DNA have appeared. The investigations of Grossman *et al.* (1973), Porcher and Koch (1973), and Wong-Staal *et al.* (1973) have shown that alkali-labile and ribonuclease-sensitive sites are involved in the supercoiled and circular configurations of mitochondrial DNA. Although the experiments conducted, and the specific conclusions reached, differ among the three research groups, the general conclusions are very similar: alkali-labile and ribonuclease-labile sites occur in each DNA strand of the mitochondrial duplex, and these sites probably involve ribonucleotide or RNA linkers which maintain the supercoiled (and circular) structures of mitochondrial DNA. At least one of the sites seems to be DNA strand specific.

So it would seem that chromosomal DNA is not the only eukaryotic DNA to contain alkali-labile sites.

4. DOUBLE-STRANDED SUBUNITS

If we consider the hypothetical structure shown in Fig. 4 we must ask the question, is there evidence to support the speculation of a double-stranded subunit of size $\sim 10^9$ daltons? Less effort has been spent on studies of possible double-stranded components of eukaryotic DNA than their alkali-degraded counterparts, and there is a compelling reason: the difficulties encountered in alkaline sucrose gradients are compounded in neutral sucrose gradients. Not the least of the complications in the latter systems is the fact that the nucleases in the cell lysates have not been destroyed (inhibited) by exposure to high pH. Two research groups have perservered under those conditions of extreme difficulty; they are Cole, Corry, and their colleagues in Houston, and Lange and his colleagues in Rochester.

Because of the experimental difficulties the impetus in this field was achieved once again (as in the case of single-stranded DNA) with radiation studies. We shall consider those studies later, but for now it is sufficient to say that both groups of workers claim to have observed that double-stranded DNA molecules of size $\sim 10^9$ daltons are liberated from larger DNA structures by a variety of treatments. The speed-dependent characteristics of these molecules have been studied by A. Cole *et al.* (personal communication) and are recorded as the lower curve in Fig. 6. Those data, which indicate that the sedimentation coefficients of the molecules are about 130S, were sent to Zimm for comparison with his theoretical treatment, *viz.* (Zimm, 1974). Zimm analyzed the empirical relationship between the sedimentation coefficient and rotor speed and deduced that molecules of size $\sim 8 \times 10^8$ daltons were involved. Cole *et al.* (personal communication) have also seen indications of larger molecules during experiments involving strand-break rejoining. The sedimentation behavior of those molecules is also shown in Fig. 6.

In Lange's case the molecules of size $\sim 10^9$ daltons were liberated from larger DNA structures of size $1-2 \times 10^{10}$ daltons by treatments which break S-S bonds. When Lange first suggested this possibility he was heavily criticized, for the following reasons. Klotz and Zimm (1972) developed a viscoelastometer which can be used to determine molecular parameters of very large DNA molecules. For example, with this technique Kavenoff and Zimm (1973) have claimed to have measured DNA molecules of the sizes of the total DNA

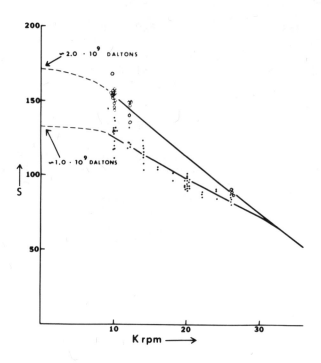

Fig. 6. The sedimentation characteristics of double-stranded eukaryotic DNA molecules of sizes ∿1.0 and 2.0 × 10⁹ daltons as functions of rotor speed. Zimm's (1974) theory indicates that the solid lines should plateau in the fashion indicated by the broken lines (A. Cole, personal communication).

complements of *drosophila* chromosomes; and Uhlenhopp and Zimm (1975) have registered sizes of single-stranded and double-stranded DNA from *E. coli* which correspond to the complete genome. Now double-stranded molecules of the size claimed by Lange, *viz.* 1.7 × 10¹⁰ daltons, should be so highly speed-dependent that they could only be detected in sedimentation profiles at very low rotor speeds (e.g., Fig. 6). This was not so in Lange's experiments--hence the criticisms. Lange has silenced the criticisms, at least temporarily, by an interesting *coup de main*. He went to Zimm's laboratory, measured the size of the larger DNA component with the viscoelastometer, and obtained the sizes of 1.3-1.7 × 10¹⁰ daltons! So now what? If the measurements in the viscoelasto-meter are correct, then are the sedimentation measurements also correct? And if the sedimentation measurements are wrong, then are the viscoelastic measurements also wrong? It is clear that *all* claims about the sizes of large eukaryotic DNA molecules must be viewed with *similar* caution.

Interestingly enough, when the viscoelastometer was used in attempts to measure the size of mammalian DNA in the presence of alkali (Uhlenhopp, 1975), the results showed that the single-stranded molecules (if such were actually measured) were smaller than the equivalent size of the DNA in the average mammalian chromosome. Furthermore, the molecules obtained from exponentially growing cells differed in size from those of plateau phase cells by a factor of 4. These latter results may be especially important, because by its very intrinsic properties the viscoelastometer measures only the largest molecules present in the lysate, and with all the studies reported using that instrument so far, only some 5-10% of the molecules present are of the sizes claimed. The instrument is extremely sensitive to molecular aggregations. The lesson is clear: If you want to believe in continuous DNA you should not accept claims for chromosomal-sized DNA without due circumspection. Conversely, if you want to believe in subunits you should not accept claims for subunit-sized molecules uncritically.

5. RADIATION STUDIES

Most of the studies of eukaryotic DNA structure reported to date have involved the concomitant, or prior, investigation of DNA damage produced by ionizing radiation. In such cases emphasis has been placed on the use of ionizing radiation as a research tool for probing the structure of eukaryotic nucleochromatin. And information about that structure can be gleaned not only from the damage introduced by the radiation but also from the behavior of the repair mechanisms during restoration of the broken structure. Since I have recently reviewed that type of approach in detail (Lett, 1975), I will only provide a summary of its efficacy here.

The radiation studies of this reviewer and his colleagues, of Cole and his colleagues, and of Lange and his colleagues, suggest that radiation damages the eukaryotic chromosomal DNA structure in two basic ways. Low doses of radiation induce damage at specific sites, or in specific regions, which are analogous to those of the alkali-labile bonds or regions. Larger doses induce further damage in an approximately random fashion, although this damage is probably a mixture of truly randomly-situated damage and specific damage at the "linker-sites" in the subsidiary arrays of subunits [i.e., molecules of the sizes seen by Hozier and Taylor (1975)] which would comprise the larger, "structural," subunits. All three research groups, *viz.* Lett *et al.* (1970), Cole *et al.* (1975), and Lange (1975)--and see also the review by Lett (1975)-- claim to see architectural order at a level above that of the "structural" subunits. Cole and his colleagues have gone one step further and investigated the possible correlation of the "link(er)s" between the $\sim 10^9$ daltons subunits with attachment sites at the nuclear membrane. Of course, the macroscopic gelatinous masses which complicate the sedimentation profiles (see Section 3.1) are quite unsuitable for that task. Clearly, such gels can contain DNA which is attached, or bound, or adhered, to nuclear membranes (or practically any other combination of the mixture of components present in the cell lysate); but just as clearly, the presence of DNA-membrane combinations in those gels does not constitute proof of the existence of biologically-meaningful DNA-membrane attachment sites *in situ*. Because Cole and his colleagues were acutely aware of this riposte they tackled the problem in an ingenious way. By using ionizing particles of limiting penetration, they found that disruption of the eukaryotic DNA structure into subunits occurred when those particles just penetrated the nuclear membrane--note that by its very nature, the particle penetration will follow the curvature or irregularities of the nuclear membrane.

So we may tentatively extend the subunit hypothesis to the statement that: link(er)s between single-stranded, $\sim 5 \times 10^8$ dalton, DNA molecules, which are sensitive to radiation because they are at exposed sites in the chromatin (Lett and Sun, 1970; Lett *et al.*, 1972), and link(er)s between the double-stranded, $\sim 10^9$ dalton DNA molecules, which are near the nuclear membrane (Cole *et al.*, 1975), are the same, and may also be DNA-membrane attachment sites. From both sets of data it also follows that, as far as the DNA is concerned, the potential for these sites also exists in metaphase chromosomes, i.e., when the nuclear membrane as such does not exist. Indeed, Cole and his colleagues (1975) have adduced evidence from three-dimensional electronmicrographs that mitotic chromatids "contain about 64 DNA molecules of about 10^9 daltons arranged in a quasi-parallel array which is collapsed when in a condensed configuration." Those authors also believe that many other radiation-sensitive sites of association between the DNA and the nuclear membrane occur along the $\sim 10^9$ dalton segments (Cole *et al.*, 1975); but these sites are of a secondary type. The heuristic model which is currently in favor with Cole and his colleagues (personal communication) is shown as Fig. 7.

6. DISCUSSION

Let us consider the status of the concept of eukaryotic DNA discontinuity in the light of the foregoing evidence. To the reviewer it appears that things are beginning to fall into place. And yet, I have a feeling of unease: Are we generating a myth akin to that of the emperor's new clothes? Since I cannot give definitive answers to these considerations I will attempt instead: a.) To rebut arguments which are usually invoked against the

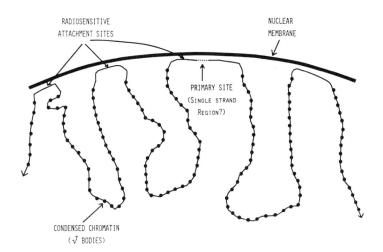

Fig. 7. A model for interphase chromatin. A primary site is strongly attached and is very radiosensitive. Radiation damage at that site allows the release of DNA subunits of about 10^9 daltons from the membrane (A. Cole, personal communication).

hypothesis of DNA discontinuity; b.) To offer alternative explanations of the evidence presented above which allow the DNA to be continuous.

6.1. Rebuttal of Arguments Against DNA Discontinuity

One of the ironies of this whole field is that claims for DNA continuity are frequently made from observations of cytologically "intact" chromosome preparations. Yet, when cytologically "intact" chromosome preparations are made by standard techniques, and are then subjected to DNA analysis by sucrose gradient sedimentation, it is found that the DNA is very heavily degraded. Indeed, a major problem for molecular studies of chromosomal DNA structure is to obtain chromosome preparations in which the DNA is still even relatively intact!

Proponents of eukaryotic DNA continuity usually evoke evidence that chromosomal DNA is resistant to attack by ribonucleases and proteolytic enzymes. Yet the experiments of Welsh and Vyska (1975) required repeated cycles of dialyses (some in the presence of mild alkali); the experiments of Hozier and Taylor (1975) utilized *extensive* (see Section 3.1) treatment with alkali, or pronase at pH 9.3, to release the 170 μm and 60 μm subunits; and the

experiments of Lett *et al.* (1970) utilized high pHs in the lytic
zones of the alkaline sucrose gradients. Is it not possible,
therefore, that the frequently cited results of treatments which
did not cause DNA degradation, were simply results from experiments
which were not drastic enough? Or was it that, when DNA degradation finally did occur after extended treatments, the assumption
was naturally inferred that the effects of traces of endogenous
DNases were being registered?

What about the loops in chromosomes? We find on p. 269 of
the book by Dupraw (1970) the statement with regard to lampbrush
chromosomes "...and since each loop is roughly 100 μm long...
Since the loops can be stretched up to five times their usual
length before they break, the DNA axis may be packed as a type A
fibril with a 5:1 DNA packing ratio." If this information
actually means that the length of the DNA in a chromosome loop
is 500 μm, or 10^9 daltons, then we have an interesting situation
for further investigation. The reviewer is grateful to Dr. W.C.
Dewey for this observation.

6.2. Rebuttal of Evidence Supporting DNA Discontinuity

Can the evidence adduced in support of DNA discontinuity be
reasonably explained in other ways? The answer is yes. In the
first place, molecules of the size of the "structural" subunit,
and even the molecules described by Hozier and Taylor (1975),
could result from hydrodynamic shearing. However, I do not
believe this to be true for 165S molecules, because in this
laboratory we have also studied single-stranded molecules with
sedimentation coefficients as large as 220S under seemingly identical shearing conditions. Similar considerations apply to the
molecules studied by Cole *et al.* (1975), see Fig. 6. Nevertheless,
objections based upon hydrodynamic shearing cannot be refuted
unambiguously at this time.

More serious objections can be leveled at the experimental
conditions employed by Welsh and Vyska (1975), Hozier and Taylor
(1975), Lett *et al.* (1970), and Cole *et al.* (1975) because all
of them could cause breaks in continuous DNA. One of the contro-
versies over the past 15 years has been whether alkylating agents
esterify the phosphate groups of DNA (e.g., Lett *et al.*, 1962).
Phosphate esterification by alkylating agents was disputed by
Brookes and Lawley (1961) who claimed initially that only base
alkylation occurred, primarily at the 7-position in guanine.
This and subsequent challenges are now irrelevant because
extensive DNA phosphate esterification by alkylating agents,
even *in situ*, is now established beyond doubt. Let us now consider the consequences of both types of reaction to the behavior
of alkylated DNA under hydrolytic conditions.

Suppose, for example, a chromosomal loop in continuous DNA is maintained by a link formed by a bifunctional alkylation between bases. Alkylated bases are eliminated from DNA under mild conditions with subsequent hydrolysis of the adjacent sugar-phosphate bonds and the formation of strand breaks (Lett *et al.*, 1962). Thus, (alkali) labile bonds can be introduced into continuous DNA, and one can visualize a number of molecular combinations where a protein linker between bases could be eliminated from continuous DNA with strand breakage.

Another type of base elimination mechanism, the well-known depurination reaction, does not even require alkylation. This reaction will also result in scission of the sugar-phosphate backbone, but presumably the production of subunits (of any size) by this mechanism would require the specific location of special base sequences or clusters.

The hydrolytic pathways of phosphate tri-esters will be determined by the chemical structures of the ester groups, so it is plausible that certain DNA tri-esters will hydrolyse by cleaving the sugar-phosphate backbone. Thus two distant parts of a continuous DNA molecule could be linked through two tri-ester bonds by a non-DNA component. Such linkers could also be the sites of (alkali) labile bonds in continuous DNA.

The origins of the chromosomal loops could also be found in S-S bonds, metal-ion linkages, etc., between sections of continuous molecules of DNA. Let us consider the experiments of Andoh and Ide (1972). They have described a DNA-protein complex with a sedimentation coefficient of 340S which, on treatment with pronase or 2-mercaptoethanol, is reduced to a DNA component with a sedimentation coefficient of 130S. Initially, Andoh and Ide (1972) considered that this change could involve protein linkers between segments of DNA. More recently, however, (Andoh *et al.*, 1975) they have preferred the idea that the non-histone proteins in the complex are involved in maintaining supercoiled configurations in chromosomal DNA. That explanation does not preclude the involvement of other linkers between DNA segments. I much prefer their current explanation, because according to speed-dependence theory (Zimm, 1974), neither the 340S nor the 130S component can be linear DNA molecules if they have those sedimentation coefficients at the rotor speeds employed by Andoh and Ide (1972)--see also Fig. 6. This contention is supported by the fact that both components exist in supercoiled configurations when examined by electronmicroscopy (Andoh and Ide, 1972). Of course, a similar explanation can be offered for the data of Lange (1975) and Dounce *et al.* (1973). But if that explanation is true for the experiments of the former group, then all the results obtained on large DNA molecules by viscoelastometry must be viewed with great caution.

Finally, we must consider specific degradation by nucleases. One of the anticipated functions of the alkaline lytic zone in the experiments of Lett *et al.* (1970) is the inactivation of nucleases. But suppose that traces of specific nuclease activity can still occur even under such extremes of pH--for release of a 165S molecule an enzyme need only attack one in 2×10^6 nucleotides--then, once again breaks could arise at specific sites in continuous DNA.

So all the evidence that I have presented in support of DNA discontinuity can also be explained at this time in other ways. However, if *any* of the claims for DNA discontinuity are correct, then from the standpoint of chromosomal DNA structure the situation is best expressed in the American idiom by the phrase "It's a whole new ball game."

Acknowledgment. Supported by the Department of Health, Education and Welfare with NIH Grant No. CA10714 from the National Cancer Institute.

References

Andoh, T., and Ide, T., 1972, A novel DNA-protein complex in cultured mouse fibroblasts, strain L-P3, *Exp. Cell Res.* 73:122-128.

Andoh, T., Nakane, M., and Ide, T., 1975, Supercoiled DNA folded by non-histone proteins in mammalian cells. Abstr. Int. Symp. "Protein and Other Adducts to DNA: Their Significance to Aging, Carcinogenesis and Radiation Biology," Williamsburg, Virginia, May 2-6, 1975.

Bendich, A., and Rosenkranz, H.S., 1963, Some thoughts on the double-strand model of deoxyribonucleic acid, *Prog. Nucleic Acid Res.* 1:219-230.

Brookes, P., and Lawley, P.D., 1961, The reaction of mono- and difunctional alkylating agents with nucleic acids, *Biochem. J.* 80:496-503.

Cleaver, J.E., 1974, Confirmation of DNA in alkaline sucrose: the subunit hypothesis in mammalian cells, *Biochem. Biophys. Res. Commun.* 59:92-99.

Cole, A., Robinson, S., Shonka, F., Datta, R., and Chen, R., 1975, Organization of mammalian chromosomes interpreted from radiation and other studies, *Biophys. J.* 15:207a.

Dounce, A.L., 1971, Nuclear gels and chromosomal structure, *Amer. Sci.* 59:74-83.

Dounce, A.L., Chandra, S.K., and Townes, P.L., 1973, The structure of higher eukaryotic chromosomes, *J. Theor. Biol.* 42:274-285.

Dupraw, E.J., 1970, "DNA and Chromosomes," Holt, Rinehart and Winston, Inc., New York.

Grossman, L.I., Watson, R., and Vinograd, J., 1973, The presence of ribonucleotides in mature closed-circular mitochondrial DNA, *Proc. Nat. Acad. Sci. USA* 70:3339-3343.

Hozier, J.C., and Taylor, J.H., 1975, Length distributions of single-stranded DNA in Chinese hamster ovary cells, *J. Mol. Biol.* 93:181-201.

Huberman, J.A., and Riggs, A.D., 1968, On the mechanism of DNA replication in mammalian chromosomes, *J. Mol. Biol.* 32:327-341.

Kavenoff, R., and Zimm, B.H., 1973, Chromosome-sized DNA molecules from *drosophila*, *Chromosoma (Berl)* 41:1-27.

Kirby, K.S., 1957, A new method for the isolation of deoxyribonucleic acids: evidence on the nature of bonds between deoxyribonucleic acid and protein, *Biochem. J.* 66:495-504.

Kirby, K.S., 1958, Preparation of some deoxyribonucleic acid-protein complexes from rat-liver homogenates, *Biochem. J.* 70:260-265.

Kirby, K.S., 1959, The preparation of deoxyribonucleic acid by the p-aminosalicylate-phenol method, *Biochim. Biophys. Acta* 36:117-124.

Klotz, L.C., and Zimm, B.H., 1972, Size of DNA determined by visco-elastic measurements: results on bacteriophages, *Bacillus subtilis* and *Escherichia coli*, *J. Mol. Biol.* 72:779-800.

Lange, C.S., 1975, Size and structure of a mammalian DNA determined by sedimentation and confirmed by viscoelastometry, *Biophys. J.* 15:205a.

Lett., J.T., 1975, Formation and rejoining of DNA strand breaks in X(γ)-irradiated cells in relation to the structure of mammalian chromatin, *in* "Molecular Mechanisms for the Repair of DNA" (P.C. Hanawalt and R.B. Setlow, eds.), Plenum Press, New York (in press).

Lett, J.T., Caldwell, I., Dean, C.J., and Alexander, P., 1967, Rejoining of X-ray induced breaks in the DNA of leukaemia cells, *Nature (London)* 214:790-792.

Lett, J.T., Klucis, E.S., and Sun, C., 1970, On the size of the DNA in the mammalian chromosome: structural subunits, *Biophys. J.* 10:277-292.

Lett, J.T., Parkins, G.M., and Alexander, P., 1962, Physicochemical changes produced in DNA after alkylation, *Arch. Biochem. Biophys.* 97:80-93.

Lett, J.T., and Stacey, K.A., 1960, The relationship between molecular weight and viscosity as a criterion of damage in DNA, *Makromol. Chem.* 38:204-211.

Lett, J.T., and Sun, C., 1970, The production of strand breaks in mammalian DNA by X-rays: at different stages in the cell cycle, *Radiat. Res.* 44:771-787.

Lett, J.T., Sun, C., and Wheeler, K.T., 1972, Restoration of the DNA structure in X-irradiated eucaryotic cells *in vitro* and *in vivo*, in *Proc. Fifth Int. Symp. on Mol. Biol., Johns Hopkins Med. J.*, Suppl. 1:147-158.

McGrath, R.A., and Williams, R.W., 1966, Reconstruction *in vivo* of irradiated *Escherichia coli* deoxyribonucleic acid; the rejoining of broken pieces, *Nature (London)* 212:534-535.

Olins, A.D., and Olins, D.E., 1974, Spheroid chromatin units (ν bodies), *Science* 183:330-332.

Porcher, H., and Koch, J., 1973, The anatomy of mitochondrial DNA: the localisation of the heat-induced and RNAse-induced scissions in the phosphodiester backbones, *Eur. J. Biochem.* 40: 329-336.

Uhlenhopp, E.L., 1975, Viscoelastic analysis of high molecular weight, alkali-denatured DNA from mouse 3T3 cell, *Biophys. J.* 15:233-237.

Uhlenhopp, E.L., and Zimm, B.H., 1975, Viscoelastic characterization of single-stranded DNA from *Escherichia coli*, *Biophys. J.* 15:223-232.

Welsh, R.S., 1962, Nondegradative isolation of deoxyribonucleic acid in subunit form from calf thymus nuclei, *Proc. Nat. Acad. Sci. USA* 48:887-893.

Welsh, R.S., and Vyska, K., 1971, Properties of a new form of DNA from whole calf thymus nuclei: evidence for reactive, special sites in DNA, *Arch. Biochem. Biophys.* 142:132-143.

Welsh, R.S., and Vyska, K., 1975a, Characterization of special sites in high molecular weight calf thymus DNA at which non-random cleavage occurs, *Biophys. Soc. Abstr.* 97a.

Welsh, R.S., and Vyska, K., 1975b, Release of phosphopeptides from highly purified calf thymus DNA during its cleavage into subunits, *J. Mol. Biol.* (in press).

Wong-Staal, F., Mendelson, J., and Goulian, M., 1973, Ribonucleotides in closed circular DNA from HeLa cells, *Biochem. Biophys. Res. Commun.* 53:140-148.

Zimm, B.H., 1974, Anomalies in sedimentation. IV. Decrease in sedimentation coefficients of chains at high fields, *Biophys. Chem.* 1:279-291.

AMINO ACIDS BOUND TO DNA

M. Earl Balis

Sloan Kettering Institute for Cancer Research

1275 York Avenue, New York, New York 10021

The purest preparations of DNA from many laboratories and many tissues have always been reported to contain small amounts of amino acids (Bendich and Rosenkrantz, 1963). Recently a number of investigators have attempted to verify this observation. Using a variety of techniques and several different sources, they, too, were unable to prepare samples completely free of amino acids (Bendich and Rosenkrantz, 1963; Champagne *et al.*, 1964; Sarfert and Venner, 1965; Olenick and Hahan, 1964; Berns and Thomas, 1965). Some, despite the consistency of this observation, feel that the amino acids are simply impurities difficult to remove and refer to their DNA preparations as having "less than" a certain arbitrary amount of amino acids. Nevertheless, the most striking aspect of these observations is the fact that no matter which solvents or precipitants are used, even when completely new procedures are introduced such as biphasic liquid-liquid extraction in which no opportunities for coprecipitation of impurities is given, a limiting value is reached; the same amount of amino acids are found (Rudin and Albertsson, 1967; Favre and Pettijohn, 1967). Not only do all DNAs have amino acids associated with them but the amounts and kinds bound to the DNA from a given source are reproducible. These amino acids are tissue and species specific and vary with the age and sex of the source (Salser and Balis, 1967, 1972).

An early observation that the amount and kind of amino acids associated with bacterial DNA were influenced by the medium in which the bacteria were grown was suggestive of a possible function of these DNA-bound amino acids. The DNA extracted from bacteria grown in a minimal medium contains larger amounts of amino acid residues than that obtained from cells grown in enriched media (Balis *et al.*, 1964; Webb, 1967). Despite the fact that the

33

DNA-bound amino acids found in cells grown under the same conditions are completely reproducible, altering the growth medium can
produce about a ten-fold change. Table 1 shows data that illustrate
the findings from replicate isolations. Table 2 demonstrates the
effects of growth media on DNA-bound amino acids.

Considerable skepticism existed and still does exist regarding
the possible role of these amino acids and as to whether they are
artifacts of isolation or simply impurities. Many proteins bind
DNA. The highly acidic nature of the phosphate groups makes it
quite reasonable to believe that salt bonds would be formed, and
this possibility has been investigated (Roewekamp and Sekeris,
1974). In one study, DNA that had been highly purified and freed
of amino acids as far as possible was mixed with rat liver homogenate and reextracted under conditions which normally yielded
DNA with somewhat higher amounts of amino acids; no reassociation
of the liver protein with the DNA was found (Kirby, 1958). Similarly, DNA was precipitated from a solution containing large amounts
of ribonuclease, the structure of which suggests it might be bound
to DNA, and repurified in conventional ways; no change in bound
amino acids was noted (Salser and Balis, 1967). *E. Coli* strain

Table 1. Amino Acid Content of DNAs Isolated Independently from
Same Batches of Bacteria (Salser and Balis, 1969)

Amino acid	*E. coli* B		Strain 835A	
	1	2	1	2
Lysine	1.57	1.49	0.402	0.395
Histidine	0.43	0.41	0.027	0.028
Arginine	1.04	1.09	0.348	0.312
Aspartic acid	1.86	1.73	1.067	1.036
Glutamic acid	1.57	1.60	1.116	1.068
Threonine	0.77	0.79	1.079	0.929
Serine	0.93	0.93	0.736	0.920
Proline	0.61	0.54	0.064	0.076
Alanine	1.83	1.88	0.558	0.655
Half cystine	+	0.02	+	+
Valine	1.17	1.20	0.473	0.423
Methionine	0.28	0.28	0.030	0.049
Isoleucine	0.73	0.73	0.291	0.244
Leucine	1.21	1.24	0.540	0.530
Tyrosine	0.52	0.53	0.180	0.173
Phenylalanine	0.52	0.53	0.228	0.226
Total	15.04	14.99	7.139	7.064

Table 2. Amino Acid Residues in Several *E. coli* DNA's Grown in Different Media

(μg amino-acid residue/100 mg DNA)

	Minimal media				Enriched media		
	No. 1*	No. 2+	No. 3+	No. 4*	No. 5+	No. 6*	No. 7+
Aspartic acid	212	116	150	27	27	32	31
Threonine	77	129	76	13	8	20	17
Serine	80	123	110	24	27	44	28
Glutamic acid	201	91	177	52	40	36	43
Proline	58	-	57	15	-	7	6
Alanine	129	73	56	19	19	16	13
Valine	115	54	86	13	-	20	22
Methionine	37	16	109	13	8	5	5
Isoleucine	82	44	111	9	7	13	12
Leucine	136	58	40	22	2	20	21
Tyrosine	85	37	46	13	4	14	15
Phenylalanine	77	38	38	12	4	13	12
Lysine	169			76			
Histidine	49			11			
Arginine	138			47			
Basic amino-acids	356			134			
Neutral and acidic amino-acids	1,288	779	1,056	230	146	241	225

* DNA was extracted from washed log phase *E. coli* B cells by the procedure of Kirby (1957). An extra deproteinizing step was carried out just prior to dialysis. The DNA was dissolved in 10% NaCl, and deproteined twice with chloroform-isoamyl alcohol, and reprecipitated with cold EtOH. Samples of bacteria, 1-5, were kindly supplied by Dr. L. Kaplan, of this Institute. Samples 6 and 7 were purchased from General Biochemicals, Chagrin Falls, Ohio, and were in late log phase; all others were in mid-log.

+ DNA was extracted as described by Marmur (1961).

No. 1: grown in an American Sterilizer Co. Biogen, Davis (1950) salt medium without citrate and 1% glucose. Nos. 2 and 3: grown in Davis salt medium and 1% glucose in two independent batches. No. 4: grown in a Biogen as No. 1 but with addition of 0.6% yeast extract. No. 5: grown in 2.5% Difco heart infusion broth. Nos. 6 and 7: batch grown with 4% yeast extract, 2% dextrose, 0.3% KH_2PO_4, 0.1% K_2HPO_4. No. 7 was treated with 50 mg/l proflavine and irradiated with a 750-W lamp at 8 in. for 60 min. No. 6 was an untreated control for No. 7. Based upon data published by Balis, Salser and Elder (1964).

15T⁻ was incubated in thymine-free medium. This organism has an
obligate requirement for thymine and incubation in thymine-free
media leads to cell death. Under these conditions of thymine
starvation little net synthesis of DNA but considerable synthesis
of protein can occur (Fig. 1). Amino acids labeled with [¹⁴C] were
added and after 45 min cells were harvested and the DNA and total
protein were each isolated. The radioactivity of the DNA-bound and
general protein amino acids was determined (Fig. 2). The activity
of the general protein was 300 times as great as was that of the
amino acids associated with the DNA. At a time when protein activity reached 97,000 cpm/mg the DNA contained amino acids equal to
1% protein but it had <3 cpm/mg. Thus, under the conditions of
limited DNA synthesis amino acids associated with DNA were not
exchanged or added. Thus, these amino acids are under a different
metabolic control than is general protein synthesis. Furthermore,
this experiment shows that DNA can be isolated from the milieu of
labeled amino acids, peptides and proteins without artifactually
picking up any of these amino acid derivatives (Salser and Balis,
1968). This is one of the strongest bits of evidence that these
amino acids are a true functional entity.

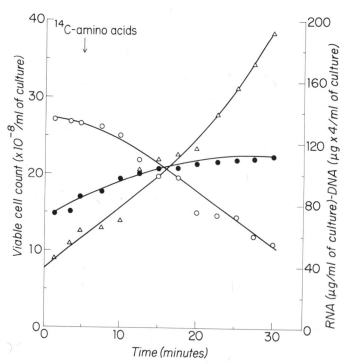

Fig. 1. Time course of viability and nucleic acid changes in
E. coli strain 15T⁻. o——o, viable cell count; △——△, RNA content;
●——●, DNA content (4 times the actual experimental values). Cells

(Fig. 1, cont.) Cells were grown and harvested at the end of mid-
log phase. Washed cells were resuspended in minimal salts containing glucose and added with stirring and aeration to equilibrated
medium. At 5 min after introduction of the inoculum, mixed [^{14}C]-
amino acids from a Chlorella protein hydrolysate were added. Samples
were taken at various time intervals for viable cell count and
fractionation into nucleic acid and protein components. For viable
cell count, serial dilutions were plated in medium containing 1.5%
agar in addition to glucose and thymidine. The packed cells from
15 ml aliquots of the samples were washed twice. RNA was determined by the orcinol reaction with highly polymerized yeast RNA
as standard; and DNA, by the diphenylamine reaction. Based upon
data of Salser and Balis (1969).

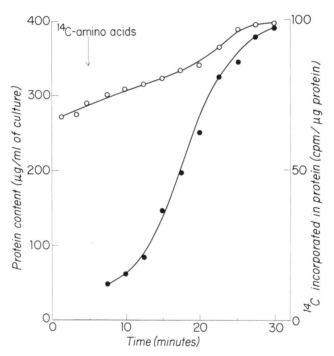

Fig. 2. Protein content and specific activity of *E. coli*
15T⁻. o——o, protein content; ●——●, specific activity. Cells
were grown as in Fig. 1. The protein-content was determined by
the method of Lowry *et al.* with bovine serum albumin as standard.
The [^{14}C] content of the various protein samples as well as that
of the purified DNA isolated from the bulk of the cells was assayed
in a liquid scintillation counter. Based upon data of Salser and
Balis (1969).

It is unfortunate that other time points were not examined in view of the unusual changes in UV response seen by Smith *et al.* (1966) with *E. coli* 15 TAU, a strain derived from 15T⁻. They found that the fraction of cells surviving UV radiation decreases with length of time the cells were incubated under conditions of thymine starvation for about 50 min. This is about the time when cell death becomes rapid. The amount of DNA extractable after radiation is minimal at about the same time. With longer incubation time there is a rapid decrease in viability but the remaining cells are less UV sensitive and the fraction of DNA that is recovered returns to normal. The question of whether a change in DNA-bound amino acids occurs or whether this represents the outgrowth of a thymine independent revertant needs exploration.

A strong source of support for the concept that the amino acids are covalently linked to the DNA are the experiments by Sonnenbichler and Bornkamm (1967) who demonstrated that fragments are formed by enzymatic digestion of DNA by DNase and venom phosphodiesterase that contain these proteins but are highly acidic due to the presence of associated nucleotides. These amino acid-nucleotide complexes could not be dissociated by Sephadex chromatography or by ultracentrifugation.

The DNA-bound amino acids of tumors seem to be quite different from those of normal host tissues. There are more amino acids bound to the DNAs from malignant sources (Table 3) but there is no apparent correlation between the amount of bound amino acids and the growth rate of the tumors. On the other hand, DNA from regenerating liver had more amino acid bound than that from normal liver (Salser and Balis, 1968) (Table 4). Furthermore, tumor DNA's contain less of the basic amino acids than normal tissue DNA's (Table 3).

An unusual amino acid that appeared on ion-exchange chromatography between phenylalanine and tyrosine occurs in many tumors. This same material had also been noted in bacteria in early log phase (Salser and Balis, 1969) (Table 5). The DNA of amino acids found in primary tumors almost always contains this unusual amino acid. As tumors are carried through several transplant generations in animals of the strain of origin the unusual amino acid gradually disappears from their DNA (Table 6). Interestingly, there are often rather sudden changes in the amounts and kinds of amino acids bound in DNA. These changes seem to coincide with morphologic changes found in various transplant generations, a fact that suggests an interrelationship between the two (Salser *et al.*, 1969).

If the peptides are functional entities closely bound to the DNA the question naturally arises as to what their function is. Even before evidence for the existence of closely bound amino acids was presented there had been speculation that protein linkers did, in fact, exist and play a role in the structure of the chromosomes.

Table 3. Amino Acids Bound to DNA of Animal Tumors*

Amino acid	Mouse S180	Hamster thyroid tumor	Rat thyroid tumor	Rat fibrosarcoma	
				KS 17	KS 12
Lysine	1.157	0.465	0.368	1.635	0.926
Histidine	0.160	0.114	0.537	0.564	0.281
Arginine	0.541	0.195	0.215	0.932	0.441
Aspartic acid	1.286	0.564	0.527	2.479	1.079
Glutamic acid	1.646	0.698	0.660	2.886	1.212
Threonine	0.581	0.282	0.279	1.336	0.561
Serine	0.705	0.350	0.375	1.430	0.672
Proline	0.573	0.289	0.364	1.364	0.558
Alanine	0.888	0.688	0.419	1.574	0.643
Half cystine	0.050	0.056	0.052	0.264	0.112
Valine	0.714	0.425	0.430	1.525	0.624
Methionine	0.167	0.062	0.042	0.307	0.110
Isoleucine	0.406	0.213	0.186	0.917	0.387
Leucine	0.967	0.538	0.408	1.942	0.725
Tyrosine	0.243	0.209	0.268		
				10.807^{+}	3.204^{+}
Phenylalanine	0.392	0.235	0.334		
Total	10.476	5.383	5.464	29.964	11.535
Amino acids (μg)‡	1203	606	640	2130	1433
Mole fraction					
Basic	0.177	0.144	0.205	0.105	0.143
Acidic	0.280	0.234	0.217	0.179	0.199
Neutral	0.543	0.622	0.578	0.716	0.658

* Values, unless otherwise specified, are μmole(s)/100 mg DNA.
+ Value represents single unresolved aromatic peak.
‡ μg of total amino acids/100 mg DNA, calculated on the assumption that all these residues are involved in peptide linkages (From Salser and Balis, 1968).

It was postulated that there are proteins or peptides covalently linked to termini of stretches of DNA and that these peptides serve as connectors and permit bending and folding and formation of the quaternary structure of chromosomes. It was suggested that these covalently attached proteins are cross-linked by disulfide bonds. Working on these hypotheses, chromosomal gels were analyzed and evidence accumulated suggesting that this was a valid structure. Breaking the postulated disulfide bond resulted in a loss of viscosity of chromosomal gels. Enzymatic degradation of the postulated junction-point material yielded residual fragments containing both DNA and peptides. Treatment of chromosomal gels with proteases

Table 4. Amino Acids Bound to Rat Liver and Hepatoma DNA*

Amino acid	Normal liver	Regenerating liver	Hepatoma
Lysine	0.256	0.416	1.053
Histidine	0.004	0.358	0.605
Arginine	0.019	0.091	0.511
Aspartic acid	0.210	0.221	1.410
Glutamic acid	0.293	0.275	1.619
Threonine	0.055	0.135	0.701
Serine	0.103	0.196	0.827
Proline	+[†]	0.144	0.659
Alanine	0.071	0.169	1.002
Half cystine	0.064	0.157	0.082
Valine	0.040	0.202	0.895
Methionine	0.012	0.202	0.194
Isoleucine	0.029	0.069	0.523
Leucine	0.056	0.160	1.482
Tyrosine	0.024	0.070	0.399
Phenylalanine	0.025	0.082	0.498
Total	1.261	2.947	12.460
Amino acids (μg)[‡]	144	346	1435
Mole fraction			
Basic	0.221	0.294	0.174
Acidic	0.399	0.168	0.243
Neutral	0.380	0.538	0.583

* Values, unless otherwise specified, are μmole/100 mg DNA.
[†] +, Present but too small to calculate.
[‡] μg of total amino acids/100 mg DNA, calculated on the assumption that all these residues are involved in peptide linkages (Based upon data by Salser and Balis, 1968).

caused them to lose some of their structural integrity as evidenced by loss of viscosity, changes in solubility properties, and large changes in sedimentation coefficients (Hilgartner, 1968; Mackay et al., 1968). The objection to these presentations lies in the weakness of the evidence of extensive deproteinization. It may be that the proteins that are destroyed by the protease and whose disulfide bonds are reduced by the reagents employed play a role in DNA-protein structures which is real and vital to the cell but in no way involves covalent linkage or even extremely tightly bound linkage of the protein. In another series of studies Andoh and Ide (1972a, b) presented data that is even more convincing that the protein is an integral part of the DNA. They grew mouse fibroblasts in the presence of ^{3}H-thymidine and isolated the labeled

Table 5. Amino Acid Residues in DNA Isolated From Different
Growth Phases of *Escherichia coli* B Grown in Enriched Media*

Amino acid	Early log	Mid-log	Late log	Late late log
Lysine	0.55	0.47	0.37	0.11
Histidine	0.05	0.07	0.04	0.06
Arginine	0.05	0.05	0.04	0.05
Aspartic acid	0.51	0.46	0.36	0.16
Glutamic acid	0.64	0.46	0.39	0.13
Threonine	0.15	0.20	0.21	0.16
Serine	0.18	0.22	0.22	0.13
Proline	0.13	0.13	0.10	0.07
Alanine	1.01	0.73	0.48	0.18
Half cystine	+	+	+	+
Valine	0.18	0.17	0.17	0.17
Methionine	0.02	0.01	0.01	0.01
Isoleucine	0.08	0.07	0.07	0.07
Leucine	0.11	0.10	0.10	0.09
Tyrosine	0.42[†]	0.28[†]	0.15	0.04
Phenylalanine			0.05	0.05
Total	4.08	3.42	2.76	1.48
Amino acids (μg)	450	374	304	164
Mole fraction				
Basic	0.16	0.17	0.16	0.15
Acidic	0.28	0.27	0.27	0.19
Neutral	0.56	0.56	0.56	0.66

* All of the cultures were grown in high peptone, except late
log which was grown in a medium containing 4% yeast extract. All
values, unless otherwise specified, are expressed as micromole(s)
per 100 mg of DNA. The total, expressed as micrograms per 100 mg
of DNA, has been calculated on the assumption that all these
residues are involved in peptide linkages. +, designates presence in amounts too small to calculate and [†], a single unresolv-
able peak (From Salser and Balis, 1969).

DNA after cell lysis. The sedimentation in neutral sucrose gradients and the density in cesium chloride was the same as that of
highly purified DNA. This material yielded DNA with sharply
lowered sedimentation coefficients after treatment with reducing
agents and proteases (Andoh and Ide, 1972a, b). Of further
interest was the finding that the treatment of the cells in culture resulted in changes in sedimentation quite similar to those
seen with reducing agents and proteases. These changes were
reversed in less than 3 h by growth of the cells in fresh medium

Table 6.   DNA-Bound Amino Acids: Changes in Successive Transplants of Rat Fibrosarcoma, MT 1*

Amino acid	Tumor								Mean mean value+	Standard deviation (%)
	P	F-1	F-5	F-6	F-8	F-11	F-16	F-25		
Lysine	7.8	8.6	8.3	8.4	8.4	8.3	9.4	6.6	8.0	12.5
Histidine	2.9	3.4	2.7	2.9	3.0	3.2	2.6	1.8	2.6	23.1
Arginine	5.7	5.9	5.0	5.3	5.6	5.9	8.2	6.3	6.2	12.9
Aspartic acid	11.0	10.8	10.2	10.0	9.7	9.3	10.0	14.2	11.3	15.9
Glutamic acid	13.5	12.9	13.1	12.5	12.3	12.4	11.9	15.0	13.2	9.8
Threonine	5.6	5.3	5.2	5.2	5.0	4.3	4.8	6.0	5.3	9.4
Serine	7.5	7.2	7.5	7.8	8.2	12.4	8.5	6.1	8.0	21.3
Proline	6.1	6.6	4.3	4.5	4.7	5.8	4.8	4.1	5.0	16.0
Alanine	8.9	7.1	8.0	7.8	7.5	6.7	9.9	8.2	8.0	12.5
Half cystine	0.7	1.2	1.0	1.0	1.0	1.1	1.2	0.9	1.0	10.0
Valine	7.3	8.1	8.3	8.1	8.0	6.5	6.9	7.8	7.5	6.7
Methionine	1.0	0.8	1.8	1.8	1.9	2.0	1.1	2.0	1.6	31.2
Isoleucine	3.6	3.5	3.6	3.5	3.3	3.0	2.9	4.7	3.8	18.4
Leucine	8.2	7.7	8.2	8.0	7.9	7.0	7.9	9.0	8.2	8.5
Tyrosine	10.1‡	10.9‡	12.8‡	5.1	5.5	4.9	4.0	3.1	4.1	26.8
Phenylalanine				8.1	8.0	7.2	5.9	4.2	5.9	27.1
Basics	16.4	17.9	16.0	16.6	17.0	17.4	20.2	14.7		
Acidics	24.5	23.7	23.3	22.5	22.0	21.7	21.9	29.2		
Neutrals	59.1	58.4	60.7	60.9	61.0	60.9	57.9	56.1		
Total (µmol/100 mg DNA)	9.7	3.9	3.4	3.4	3.3	3.1	4.2	13.4		

*Unless otherwise specified values are mole percent, calculated from the total amino acids determined. P is primary tumor. Fn represents the nth transplant generation.
+Calculated on the assumption that all these transplants are replicates of a single sample. Values for F-10, F-15, F-18, F-20, F-22 and F-24 though not listed are included in the calculated mean values. The percent standard deviation for actual replicate isolations average less than 10%.
‡Value represents single unresolved aromatic peak (From Salser, Teller, and Balis, 1969).

(Andoh and Ide, 1972c). The rapid reversible changes are similar
in some ways to the rapid changes seen in bacteria following enrichment of media (Webb, 1967). These offer considerable support to
an *in vivo* linkage of peptides and DNA.

More recently, many investigators have shown interest in more
tightly bound protein DNA complexes, for example, Robinson *et al.*
(1973) have published a paper on a circular DNA-protein from
adenoviruses. These investigators, and others like him, however,
have very much shied away from the implication that there is a
covalent linkage (Robinson *et al.*, 1973; Helinski and Clewell,
1971). The arguments that associated peptides are not covalently
linked because they can in some systems be released by procedures,
such as relatively mild heating in certain salts, that do not
normally cleave covalent bonds has always seemed a little bizarre
when applied to a molecule that can be broken into smaller pieces
on being poured from one vessel to another or by sonication. The
chemical properties of DNA are not simply those of fragments of
double-stranded oligodeoxynucleotides. Many investigators in
this field have, nevertheless, felt that DNA may form circular
entities and that the closing of the ring is brought about in some
way by proteins or peptides. More recently, Helinski has proposed
the existence of a covalently linked swivel protein in the coli-
cinogenic factor E1 (Helinski, 1975).

There is considerable evidence to indicate a relationship be
between certain kinds of DNA and protein moieties that can be
interpreted, in view of our current thought about DNA synthesis,
to mean that the protein is bound to DNA in such a way as to serve
as a connector to cell membranes. Goldstein and Brown (1961) showed
that after growing bacteria in the presence of ^{32}P-phosphates they
could separate recently labeled DNA from previously synthesized
DNA of *E. coli* protoplasts or cells on the basis of differential
sensitivity to sonic disintegration. Ben-Porat *et al.* (1962) found
what appeared to be a nascent DNA which was separable from the bulk
of mammalian cellular DNA by the fact that it remained in the
interphase after extraction with chloroform and isoamyl alcohol, a
procedure that releases 90% of the cellular DNA. Jacob *et al.*
(1963) proposed a model in which replicating DNA is closely associated with the cell membrane. Ryter and Jacob (1963) showed electron microscopically that in *B. subtilis* much of the DNA is physically associated with cell membranes. Hanawalt and Ray (1964)
then showed that nascent DNA that was difficult to extract could
be released by prior treatment with proteolytic enzymes. Ganesan
and Lederberg (1965) by the use of [^{3}H]thymidine demonstrated that
a nascent DNA which was the first labeled fraction formed had a
lower density than the rest of the DNA and that this DNA could be
released by protease treatment. Their data led to the postulate
that DNA synthesis occurs at the cell membrane and that there is
an attachment of the DNA by a protein-like linkage. The postulate

that the DNA is attached to the membrane by a protein has been
supported by considerable evidence (Schaechter, This Volume).
Some of it implicates a role for RNA as well (Porter and Fraser,
1968).

It is noteworthy that the amount of DNA bound to a material
that behaves like cell membrane in extraction procedures has been
shown to vary as a function of the growth cycle of *E. coli* (Salser
and Balis, 1975). When the growth rate of the cells was maximal,
i.e., at mid-log phase, approximately 50% of the bacterial DNA was
associated with interphase material. Earlier studies have shown
that the total amount of amino acid residues bound to DNA was also
a function of the growth rate (Salser and Balis, 1969). Furthermore, pronase treatment released DNA that contained more amino
acids bound to it than did the extractable DNA. However, the relative distribution of amino acids was essentially the same in
extractable DNA and interphase bound DNA. This seems to suggest
that some of the amino acids, at least, are involved in linkages
which are made and broken during the attachment and release of DNA
from membrane.

An alternate suggestion for a role of the amino acids in DNA
proposes that they are attached in such a way that they terminate
the transcription of DNA and thus serve as punctuation marks or
initiator points in the reading of the genetic code (Bendich *et al.*,
1964). A somewhat related interpretation follows from the observations that there is a considerable difference in the amount of
amino acids bound to DNA of bacteria that have been grown in media
with varying degrees of enrichment. This led to the proposal that
the amino acids could serve as derepressors of DNA transcription
(Balis *et al.*, 1964; Webb, 1967). These differences were dramati-
cally demonstrated by the work of Webb (1967) who showed that the
transfer of washed cells from a fully enriched medium to a minimal
one resulted in a more than a ten-fold increase in the amount of
amino acids bound within 10 min after the transfer. The speed of
the change is evidence of a fundamental biochemical event. In 5
min there was a seven-fold increase and after 10 min a maximal
increase in the amount of amino acids bound to the DNA (Table 7).
In an attempt to extend this interpretation of the role of the
peptides to abnormal growth the amino acid content of tumor DNA
was examined and it was found that there were considerably more
amino acids bound than to DNA of non-malignant sources. However,
it has not been possible to interpret this finding in the context
of repression and derepression (Salser and Balis, 1968).

Thus there are data that give some support for four hypothetical functions for amino acids bound to DNA. They are: (1) part
of the overall chromosomal structure providing a mechanism by
which the straight DNA rods can be folded along side others and
which by cross-linkage could yield the viscous gels found *in vivo*;

Table 7.   The Influence of Incubation Time in Minimal Medium After
Transfer From Enriched Medium on the Residual Proteins Attached
to the DNA of *E. coli* B (From Webb, 1967)

Amino acid	Time after transfer, min			
	0	3	5	10
Aspartic	22	28	103	244
Glutamic	19	34	124	204
Histidine	0	0	22	51
Arginine	16	54	92	173
Lysine	18	33	88	184
Alanine	4	10	51	116
Isoleucine	3	6	56	83
Leucine	4	5	71	146
Methionine	0	0	4	26
Proline	0	6	11	46
Phenylalanine	3	4	31	68
Serine	15	10	58	92
Tyrosine	4	8	33	68
Threonine	10	4	48	84
Valine	2	18	62	126
Total	120	220	854	1711

2) a swivel point by which DNA could be formed into circles in
certain specific kinds of DNA and as a pivot site in replication;
3) linkers to attach DNA to cell membrane providing a rigid firm
structure yet one which could be released quickly when DNA synthesis was proceeding and 4) as derepressors of DNA function or
as indicators of points for commencing and terminating transcrip-
tions.   It may be that all of these roles are actually played by
amino acids at various times.

If the DNA and amino acids are covalently linked, the next
question is what is the molecular nature of this attachment? Well
before the data were available to substantiate the hypothesis,
several Russian investigators had proposed that there was in fact
covalent linkage of amino acids or peptides to DNA. Manoilov *et al.*
(1948) proposed that amino acids or peptides could be attached to
DNA by formation of amides between the carboxyl group of a terminal
amino acid and 6-amino group of adenine. This group felt that the
aromatic amino acids were involved in the direct attachment to the
nucleic acid purine. They had analytical evidence to suggest that
there were more amino acid residues attached to DNA of rapidly
growing tissues than that of resting cells. This was particularly
true of sarcomas. Interestingly, they suggested that in cells in

which growth was rapid the nucleic acid would be renewed more rapidly than were the amino acids or peptides attached thereto.

In an effort to determine the nature or the site of the attachment of peptides in DNA, Dr. Salser in our laboratory prepared a sample of DNA from beef spleen and determined the amino acid contents as shown in Table 8. A sample of this DNA was then degraded to apurinic acid (Petersen and Burton, 1964). Under the conditions of this degradation something in the order of 6 or less percent of the DNA guanine but no adenine remained attached to the deoxyribosephosphate backbone. As can be seen in Table 8 some 85% of the DNA-bound amino acid residues have been removed together with the purines. It must be remembered, however, that the molecular weight of DNA is reduced extensively by this procedure. This experiment demonstrates not that the amino acids are necessarily associated with purines but that they are associated either to purines and/or to points in the polydeoxyribose phosphate chain that are susceptible to acid hydrolysis. I might point out in passing that milder treatment with acid does not liberate the purines from DNA. The other obvious experiment was to prepare apyrimidinic acid. This was carried out by direct hydrazinolysis (Chargaff *et al.*, 1963). This is a somewhat more drastic treatment than that involved in the production of apurinic acid in that the deoxyribophosphates are converted to derivatives, most probably hydrazones, and there is extensive internucleotide cleavage. Therefore, the fact that there was a reduction in amino acid content of the apyrimidinic acid by about 1/3 could well be attributed to artifact. A more logical interpretation would be that the relative small loss of amino acids following this treatment would indicate that a small fraction if any, of the amino acids were pyrimidine-bound.

This last finding is most discouraging since a number of examples have been found of compounds with amino acids linked to pyrimidines that could serve as models for the attachment of amino acids or peptides to DNA. For example, a 1-alanyl-uracil and a 3-alanyl-uracil have been isolated from pea seedlings. Structures of these are shown in Fig. 3 (Lambein and Van Parijs, 1968). Another compound that could be used as a model for amino acid attachment to DNA was also isolated from pea seedlings. It consists of a peptide attached to the pyrimidine β-(2,6-dihydroxypyrimidine-5-yl)-alanine (Fig. 3) (Brown and Mangat, 1969). This compound could obviously serve as a model for the attachment site.

Two purine peptides have been reported from RNA. In one of these a rat liver complex of peptide AMP-CMP has been demonstrated (Ondarza, 1962). No definite structure of this compound has been established nor has a structure been established for the other derivative which was obtained from yeast RNA. In this last case it was shown that the peptide is attached to guanosine (Akashi *et al.*, 1965). Furthermore, degradation of the guanosine to

Table 8. Amino Acid Content of Beef Spleen DNA, Apyrimidinic and
Apurinic Acid*

	DNA	μmol/100 mg APu	APy
Lysine	0.315	0.106	0.287
Histidine	0.179	0.066	0.173
Arginine	0.295	0.040	0.154
Aspartic acid	0.616	0.155	0.467
Glutamic acid	0.840	0.151	0.706
Threonine	0.326	0.056	0.222
Serine	0.420	0.092	0.273
Proline	0.399	-	0.140
Alanine	0.991	0.139	0.742
Half cystine	0.023	-	0.020
Valine	0.421	0.056	0.313
Methionine	0.072	-	0.018
Isoleucine	0.204	0.015	0.165
Leucine	0.484	0.041	0.328
Tyrosine	0.161	0.014	0.112
Phenylalanine	0.284	0.031	0.146
Total	6.030	0.962	4.266

* DNA was isolated by a modified p-aminosalicylate-phenol
method (Kirby, 1957, 1959). The modification consisted primarily
of extra deproteinizing steps before and after incubation with
ribonuclease. Apurinic acid was prepared by formic acid hydrolysis
(Petersen and Burton, 1964) and apyrimidinic acid by hydrazinolysis
(Chargaff *et al.*, 1963). Unpublished data of Salser and Balis.

guanine and ribose showed the peptides are attached to the sugar.
The sugar peptide attachment is somewhat labile. Thus it is possible by analogy that the peptides that were released from the DNA
on the formation of apurinic may have been produced by hydrolysis
of a 3' or 5' bond. Several workers have postulated structures of
intrachain amino acid linkers (Fig. 4).

It is not possible to discuss the role of cross-linked peptides
or amino acids in DNA without considering the interactions of DNA
with membranes that we have referred to earlier, and without dis-
cussing interaction of DNA in peptides or amino acids as influenced
by drugs and by radiation. It is most fortunate that this conference will include discussions of these other influences on the peptide or amino acid-bound DNA. The DNA samples that have been
analyzed in the supposed absence of mutagens in general, or carcinogens or radiation always contain some amino acids that cannot be

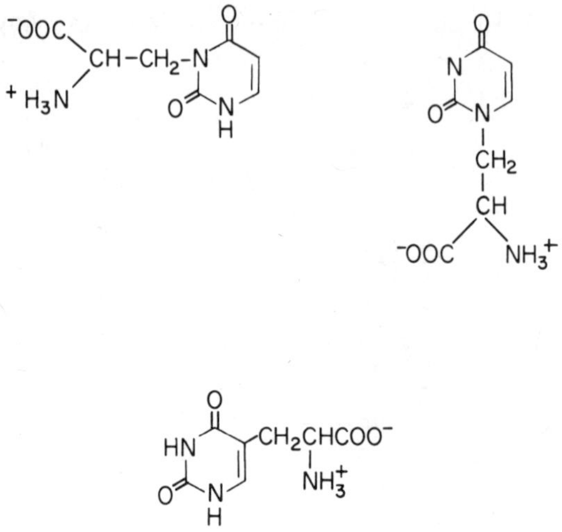

Fig. 3. Three compounds serve as models for attachments of amino acids that could be termini of peptides to pyrimidines. They were extracted from germinating pea seeds. (There is no evidence to identify them with DNA *per se*.) The upper left compound is 3-alanyl-uracil (isowillardine), upper right is 1-alanyl-uracil (willardine). The lower compound is 3-alanyl-6-amino-uracil. It was isolated as a 5-ribosyl derivative (Lambein and Van Parijs, 1969).

removed without extensive degradation of the DNA. It is, of course, impossible to say that these are not always due to some inadvertent exposure of the living cell to agents that cause this. I think this is merely a philosophical argument since all samples which have been obtained from living cells contain these bound materials. Complete and final proof requires, of course, that the exact structure of the adducts be determined.

This conference is concerned with the effects of aging and cancer on adducts to DNA. Certainly there are profound changes due to both of these factors. To yield to the temptation to link these parallel changes causally would be unwise but it would be still more unwise to ignore them.

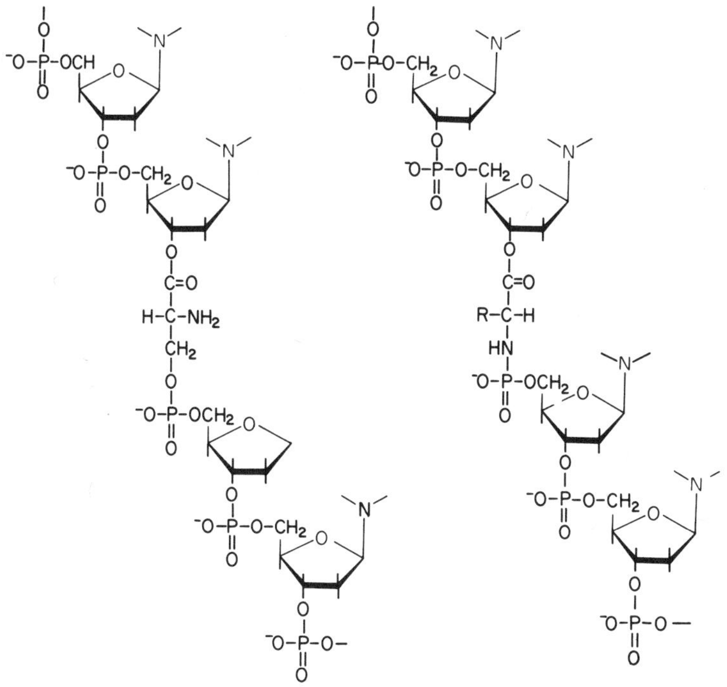

Fig. 4. The compound on the left contains an internucleotide phosphoserine linker. The primary amino group could be joined by an amide linkage to a peptide residue (Bendich *et al.*, 1964). The compound on the right contains a phosphamide that could be joined via the R group to other proteins or peptides either by disulfide bonds or through secondary carboxyl or amino groups as would be found in asparagine, glutamic or lysine or arginine. These kinds of linkers would create spacing between bases of the DNA as well as points of attachment for peptides.

References

Akashi, S., Murachi, T., Ishihara, H., and Goto, H., 1965, Studies on the amino acids in yeast RNA in bound form. V. The amino acids bound to guanosine, *J. Biochem.* 58:162-167.

Andoh, T., and Ide, T., 1972a, A novel DNA-protein complex in cultured mouse fibroblasts, Strain L-P3, *Exp. Cell Res.* 73:122-128.

Andoh, T., and Ide, T., 1972b, Disulfide bridges in proteins linking DNA in cultured mouse fibroblasts, Strain L-P3, *Exp. Cell Res.* 74:525-531.

Andoh, T., and Ide, T., 1972c, Scission of proteins linking DNA in cultured mammalian cells induced by 4-nitroquinoline 1-oxide (4NQO) and their repair, *Saibo Seibutsugaku Shimpojiumu* 23: 69-74.

Balis, M.E., Salser, J.S., and Elder, A., 1964, A suggested role of amino-acids in deoxyribonucleic acid, *Nature* 203:1170-1171.

Bendich, A., Borenfreund, E., Korngold, G.C., Krim, M., and Balis, M.E., 1964, Amino acids or small peptides as punctuation in the genetic code of DNA, *in* "Symposium on Nucleic Acids and their Role in Biology," pp. 214-237, Pavia, Tipografia Successori Fusi.

Bendich, A., and Rosenkrantz, H.S., 1963, "Progress in Nucleic Acid Research" (J.N. Davidson and W.E. Cohn, eds.), Vol. 1, p. 219, Academic Press, New York.

Ben-Porat, T., Stere, A., and Kaplan, A.S., 1962, The separation of nascent deoxyribonucleic acid from the remainder of the cellular deoxyribonucleic acid, *Biochim. Biophys. Acta* 61: 150-152.

Berns, K.I., and Thomas, C.A., Jr., 1965, Isolation of high molecular weight DNA from Hemophilus influenzae, *J. Mol. Biol.* 11:476-490.

Brown, E.G., and Mangat, B.S., 1969, Structure of a pyrimidine amino acid from pea seedlings, *Biochim. Biophys. Acta* 177:427-433.

Champagne, M., Mazen, A., and Pouyet, T., 1964, Amino acid residues in deoxyribonucleic acids, *Biochim. Biophys. Acta* 87:682-684.

Chargaff, E., Rust, P., Temperli, A., Morisawa, S., and Danon, A., 1963, Investigation of the purine sequences in deoxyribonucleic acids, *Biochim. Biophys. Acta* 76:149-151.

Comings, D.E., and Kakefuda, T., 1968, Initiation of deoxyribonucleic acid replication at the nuclear membrane in human cells, *J. Mol. Biol.* 33:225-229.

Davis, D.B., and Mingioli, E.S., 1950, Mutants of *Escherichia coli* requiring methionine or Vitamin B_{12}, *J. Bacteriol.* 60:17-28.

Dounce, A.L., and Hilgartney, 1964, A study of DNA nucleoprotein gels and the residual protein of isolated cell nuclei, *Exp. Cell Res.* 36:228-241.

Favre, J., and Pettijohn, D.E., 1967, A method for extracting purified DNA or protein-DNA complex, *Eur. J. Biochem.* 3:33-41.

Ganesan, A.T., and Lederberg, J., 1965, A cell-membrane bound fraction of bacterial DNA, *Biochem. Biophys. Res. Commun.* 18:824-835.

Goldstein, A., and Brown, B.J., 1961, Effect of sonic oscillation upon "Old" and "New" nucleic acids in *Escherichia coli, Biochim. Biophys. Acta* 53:19-28.

Hanawalt, P.C., and Ray, D.S., 1964, Isolation of the growing point in the bacterial chromosome, *Proc. Nat. Acad. Sci. USA* 52:125-132.

Helinski, D., 1974, Characteristic of plasmid DNA replication *in vitro*. ICN-UCLA Winter Conference on DNA Synthesis and its Regulation, Abstr., p. 33.

Hilgartner, C.A., 1968, The binding of DNA to residual protein in mammalian nuclei, *Exp. Cell Res.* 49:520-532.

Jacob, F., Brenner, S., and Cuzin, F., 1963, On the regulation of DNA replication in bacteria, Cold Spring Harbor Symp. Quant. Biol. 28:329-348.

Kirby, D.S., 1957, A new method for the isolation of deoxyribonucleic acids: Evidence on the nature of bonds between deoxyribonucleic acid and protein, *Biochem. J.* 66:495-504.

Kirby, K.S., 1958, Preparation of some deoxyribonucleic acid-protein complexes from rat-liver homogenates, *Biochem. J.* 70:260.

Kirby, K.S., 1959, The preparation of deoxyribonucleic acids by the p-amino-salicylate-phenol method, *Biochim. Biophys. Acta* 36: 117-124.

Lambein, F., and Van Parijs, R., 1968, Isolation and characterization of 1-alanyl-uracil (Willardiine) and 3-alanyl-uracil (*Iso*-Willardiine) from *Pisum Sativum*, *Biochem. Biophys. Res. Commun.* 32:474-479.

Mackay, M., Hilgartner, C.A., and Dounce, A.L., 1968, Further studies of DNA-nucleoprotein gels and residual protein of isolated cell nuclei, *Exp. Cell Res.* 49:533-557.

Manoilov, S.E., Setkina, O.L., and Orlov, B.A., 1948, Preparative extraction, fractionation and spectroscopic study of nucleo-proteins of rat sarcoma, *Biokhimiia* 13:337-345.

Marmur, J., 1961, A procedure for the isolation of deoxyribonucleic acid from micro-organisms, *J. Mol. Biol.* 3:208-218.

Olenick, J.G., and Hahan, F.E., 1964, Amino acids in hydrolysates of deoxyribonucleic acid of *Escherichia coli*, *Biochim. Biophys. Acta* 87:535-537.

Ondarza, R.N., 1962, A new dinucleotide peptide from rat liver, *Biochim. Biophys. Acta* 59:728-730.

Petersen, G.B., and Burton, K., 1964, Sequences of consecutive cytosine deoxynucleotides in deoxyribonucleic acid, *Biochem. J.* 92:666-672.

Porter, B., and Fraser, D.K., 1968, Involvement of protein and ribo-nucleic acid in the association of deoxyribonucleic acid with other cell components of *Escherichia coli*, *J. Bacteriol.* 96: 98-104.

Robinson, A.J., Younghusband, H.B., and Bellett, A.J.D., 1973, A circular DNA-protein complex from adenoviruses, *Virology* 56: 54-69.

Roewekamp, W., and Sekeris, C.E., 1974, Binding of nuclear proteins to DNA, *Arch. Biochem. Biophys.* 160:156-161.

Rudin, L., and Albertsson, P.-A., 1967, A new method for the isola-tion of deoxyribonucleic acid from microorganisms, *Biochim. Biophys. Acta* 134:37-44.

Ryter, A., and Jacob, F., 1963, Electron microscopic study of the relations between mesosomes and nucleic of *Bacillus subtilis*, *Acad. des Sci.* 13:3060-3063.

Salser, J.S., and Balis, M.E., 1967, Investigations on amino acids bound to DNA, *Biochim. Biophys. Acta* 149:220-227.

Salser, J.S., and Balis, M.E., 1968, Amino acids associated with
    DNA of tumors, *Cancer Res.* 28:595-600.
Salser, J.S., and Balis, M.E., 1969, Effect of growth conditions
    on amino acids bound to deoxyribonucleic acid, *J. Biol. Chem.*
    244:822-828.
Salser, J.S., and Balis, M.E., 1972, Alterations in deoxyribonucleic
    acid bound amino acids with age and sex, *J. Gerontol.* 27:1-9.
Salser, J.S., and Balis, M.E., 1975, Relationships between non-
    extractable DNA and the bacterial growth cycle, *Biochim. Biophys.*
    Acta 378:22-34.
Salser, J.S., Teller, M.N., and Balis, M.E., 1969, Changes in DNA-
    bound amino acids in experimental tumor transplants, *Cancer*
    Res. 29:1002-1007.
Sarfert, E., and Venner, H., 1965, Isolation of deoxyribonucleic
    acid from microorganism in pure, high molecular form, *Hoppe-*
    Seyler's Z. Physiol. Chem. 340:157-173.
Schwartz, D.J., 1955, Studies on crossing over in maize and droso-
    phila, *J. Cell Comp. Physiol.* 45:Suppl. 2:171-188.
Smith, K.C., Hodgkins, B., and O'Leary, M.E., 1966, The biological
    importance of ultraviolet light induced DNA-protein cross-
    links in *Escherichia coli* 15 TAU, *Biochim. Biophys. Acta*
    114:1-15.
Sonnenbichler, Von J., and Bornkamm, G.W., 1967, Fractionation of
    calf thymus-chromatin and characterization of a specific DNA-
    protein-complex, *Hoppe-Seyler's Z. Physiol. Chem.* 348:1579-1588.
Taylor, J.H., 1963, DNA synthesis in relation to chromosome repro-
    duction and the reunion of breaks, *J. Cell Comp. Physiol.*
    62:Suppl. 1:73-86.
Webb, S.J., 1967, The influence of growth media on proteins bound
    to DNA and their possible role in the response of *Escherichia*
    coli B to ultraviolet light, *Can. J. Microbiol.* 13:57-68.

GENE REGULATION: SELECTIVE CONTROL OF DNA HELIX OPENINGS*

John H. Frenster

Department of Medicine, Stanford University School of

Medicine, Stanford, California 94305

1. INTRODUCTION

Gene regulation implies differential activity of DNA molecules within an individual cell. Such differential activity is observed during both gene transcription and gene replication (Frenster, 1966), and is a feature of DNA molecules within both prokaryotes (Chamberlin, 1974) and eukaryotes (Frenster and Herstein, 1973). Because gene replication appears to be secondary to gene transcription (Klevecz and Hsu, 1964; Champoux and McConaughy, 1975), the critical feature of the regulatory event appears to lie in the molecular details of selective gene transcription (Frenster, 1965d; Chamberlin, 1974). Such selectivity involves both the choice of a particular gene locus and the choice of a particular DNA strand on which to effect messenger RNA synthesis (Frenster, 1966).

*Supported in part by Research Grants CA-10174 and CA-13524 from the National Cancer Institute, by Research Grant IC-45 from the American Cancer Society, and by a Research Scholar Award from the Leukemia Society.

2. SELECTIVE TRANSCRIPTION

Each normal diploid cell of an individual animal contains a
full and identical complement of all DNA molecular species characterizing that individual (McCarthy and Hoyer, 1964; Kohne and
Byers, 1973). Only a limited number of DNA molecules are transcribed to RNA within any one cell or tissue (Frenster et al.,
1963), and these are characteristic of the particular tissue type
(McCarthy and Hoyer, 1964; Paul and Gilmour, 1968).

Stable epigenetic mechanisms select specific portions of the
genome for transcription (Grumbach et al., 1963; Davidson et al.,
1963), and these mechanisms can be defined within isolated native
complexes of repressed heterochromatin and de-repressed euchromatin
prepared in parallel from a single tissue sample (Frenster et al.,
1963). By these analyses, polycationic histone proteins (Fig. 1)
are found to combine non-specifically with the phosphate groups on
the exterior of the DNA helix (Frenster, 1965b; Oliver and Chalkley,
1974). The effect of such histone molecules is to stabilize the
DNA helix against the helix openings that follow localized separations of the DNA strands (Frenster, 1965b, d), and concurrently to
markedly decrease the template activity of the DNA molecule
(Frenster et al., 1961; Huang and Bonner, 1962). This concordance
of effects in fact provided the first evidence that DNA helix openings via localized strand separations are a necessary molecular
feature of DNA molecules during the RNA synthesis of selective gene
transcription (Frenster, 1965c, d).

2.1. DNA Helix Openings

Recently, many additional examples of localized DNA helix openings have been recognized in both bacterial (Chan and Wells, 1974;
Dickson et al., 1975) and mammalian (Suzuki et al., 1974; Chetsanga
et al., 1975) cells. Nuclear ligands other than histones which share
with histones the ability to bind preferentially to double-stranded
DNA (Table 1) and are thereby capable of stabilizing the DNA helix
against helix openings, have similarly been found to decrease the
template activity of DNA molecules (Frenster, 1965e), thus further
confirming the requirement for helix openings in DNA template molecules during the RNA synthesis of selective gene transcription
(Frenster, 1965d, e).

Conversely, nuclear ligands capable of binding preferentially
to single-stranded DNA (Table 1) and are thereby capable of inducing
DNA helix openings (Frenster, 1965e) have been found to be capable
also of increasing the activity of DNA templates for RNA synthesis,
again indicating the crucial role of helix openings for DNA template
activity in selective transcription (Frenster, 1965e). It is now
possible to separately analyze both the equilibrium and kinetic

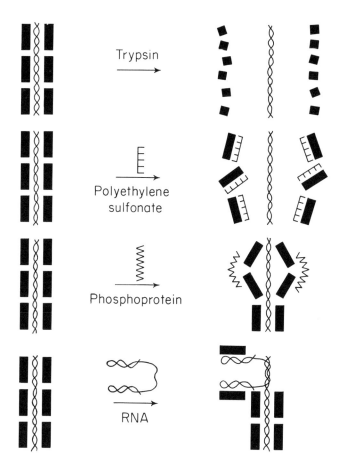

Fig. 1. Polycationic histone proteins bind non-specifically to
the phosphate groups on the exterior of the DNA helix, thereby stabilizing the DNA helix against any localized strand separations or
openings in the helix, and consequently repressing the helix against
RNA or DNA synthesis (Frenster, 1965b). Trypsin digestion of such
histones or polyethylene sulfonate reaction with such histones result
in physical removal of the histones from the underlying DNA templates
under experimental conditions, thereby permitting localized DNA
strand separations and openings of the DNA helix, with increased
rates of RNA or DNA synthesis (Frenster, 1965b). Nuclear acidic
proteins, phosphoproteins, lipoproteins, and RNA are capable of
partially displacing histones from underlying DNA templates, and
nuclear de-repressor RNA has the added capability of selecting particular gene loci for such histone displacements, resulting in spontaneous or induced localized DNA strand separations and helix openings, with increased rates of RNA synthesis at particular gene
loci (Frenster, 1965b).

Table 1. Correlations of Nuclear Ligand Binding and Effects on RNA
                                    Synthesis

     A great variety of molecules with biological activity penetrate
into the cell nucleus and bind to DNA. These nuclear ligands can
be classified as to their preference for binding to DNA in the
double-stranded state or in the single-stranded state (Frenster,
1965e). Those ligands binding preferentially to DNA in the double-
stranded state are all found to decrease the rate of RNA synthesis
by DNA after such binding. Conversely, those ligands binding preferentially to DNA in the single-stranded state are all found to
increase the rate of RNA synthesis by such DNA after binding
(Frenster, 1965e). These data are consistent with a ligand-induced
closing or opening of DNA helices, respectively, and indicate the
central role played by such DNA helix openings in the molecular
control of selective transcription (Frenster, 1965e).

Nuclear ligand	Preferred form of DNA	Effect on RNA synthesis
Histones	Double-stranded	Decreased
Protamines	Double-stranded	Decreased
Actinomycin D	Double-stranded	Decreased
Acridine orange	Double-stranded	Decreased
Chloroquine	Double-stranded	Decreased
Lac repressor	Double-stranded	Decreased
Testosterone	Single-stranded	Increased
Estradiol	Single-stranded	Increased
Methylcholanthrene	Single-stranded	Increased
RNA polymerase	Single-stranded	Increased
De-repressor RNA	Single-stranded	Increased
Polyoma viral DNA	Single-stranded	Increased

aspects of the interaction of such DNA ligands with the DNA molecule (McGhee and von Hippel, 1975).

     The recent findings concerning the quartenary structure of
chromatin (Bram *et al.*, 1975) suggest that superhelical coils of
DNA helices may favor DNA helix openings in DNA segments from which
covering histones have been displaced (Fig. 1, 2), in a manner
similar to the effects of such superhelical twisting on DNA helix
openings in covalently-closed circular bacterial and viral DNA
(Chamberlin, 1974; Champoux and McConaughy, 1975). In this instance,

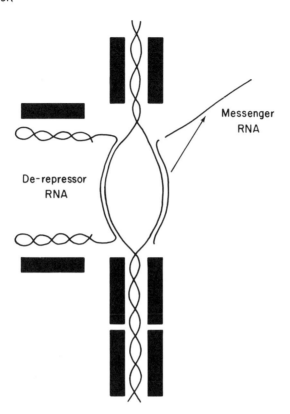

Fig. 2. De-repressor RNA (chromosomal RNA, activator RNA) has
the structural capability for selecting particular gene loci by
combining with the complementary sequences on the anti-coding strand
of the DNA helix opening. This frees the remaining strand for
single-strand specific messenger RNA synthesis (Frenster, 1965c).
The rigidity imposed by the histones along the length of the DNA
helix serves to concentrate any torsional influences on the helix
to the area of histone displacement, where such torsion can result
in induced DNA strand separations and the formation of a DNA helix
opening.

the presence of histones on intervening segments of DNA may accen-
tuate the degree of local DNA helix opening at the target site by
preventing it at any other site.

2.2. Histone Displacement

In animal cells, histones are usually in close apposition with
underlying DNA templates (Fig. 1), and therefore must be displaced

from such templates before gene transcription can occur (Frenster, 1965c, d). Many examples of such displacement of histones from active DNA template sites have now been demonstrated, including histone displacement within isolated de-repressed euchromatin complexes (Frenster, 1965b), within lymphocytes undergoing activation (Killander and Rigler, 1969), within activated cell hybrids (Bolund *et al.*, 1969), within the atypical lymphocytes of infectious mononucleosis (Bolund *et al.*, 1970), and with the entrance of inactive mitotic cells into active interphase (Nakatsu *et al.*, 1974).

Conversely, evidence for the re-positioning of displaced histones during inactivation of the DNA template has also been found within a variety of animal systems, including within the cells progressing through spermatogenesis (Gledhill *et al.*, 1966), within cells inactivated by high-density culture (Zetterberg and Auer, 1970), and within cells progressing through normal bone marrow cell differentiation and early mitosis (Nakatsu *et al.*, 1974). In each of these cell systems, histone displacement is correlated with DNA template activity for RNA synthesis, while histone re-positioning is correlated with DNA template inactivity for RNA synthesis (Frenster *et al.*, 1974).

2.3. Acidic Chromatin Macromolecules

The molecular mechanisms mediating histone displacement and de-repression are complex, and usually involve a variety of acidic macromolecules found in association with DNA in de-repressed euchromatin complexes (Frenster, 1965b). These acidic macromolecules include acidic non-histone residual proteins, phosphoproteins, lipoproteins, and RNA, all of which are capable of displacing histones from DNA templates (Fig. 1), thereby converting repressed heterochromatin to de-repressed euchromatin, with a resultant marked increase in the rate of RNA synthesis (Frenster, 1965b; Gilmour and Paul, 1969). The tissue-specific and gene-selective properties of gene transcription are mediated by macromolecular species contained in these acidic chromatin supernates (Bekhor *et al.*, 1969; Huang and Huang, 1969; Gilmour and Paul, 1970; Barrett *et al.*, 1974). The preparative methods for obtaining these acidic macromolecules all include significant amounts of nuclear RNA (Frenster, 1965b; Gilmour and Paul, 1969; Levy *et al.*, 1972; van den Broek *et al.*, 1973; Chae, 1975; Umansky *et al.*, 1975; Doenecke and McCarthy, 1975), and it has been shown that such nuclear RNA can de-repress previously-repressed heterochromatin, markedly increasing the rate of RNA synthesis (Frenster, 1965b), and conferring both tissue and gene selectivity upon the transcription process (Bekhor *et al.*, 1969; Huang and Huang, 1969; Dahmus and Bonner, 1970).

2.4. De-Repressor RNA

These species of nuclear RNA, variously referred to as de-repressor RNA (Frenster, 1965c), chromosomal RNA (Bekhor *et al.*, 1969a, b; Holmes *et al.*, 1974b), or activator RNA (Britten and Davidson, 1969), is capable of hybridizing to double-stranded DNA in 5 M urea solutions (Bekhor *et al.*, 1969a, b; Huang and Huang, 1969), apparently binding to the non-coding strand of DNA at a particular gene locus, thereby forming a DNA helix opening (Fig. 2), and freeing the remaining coding strand of DNA for messenger RNA synthesis (Frenster, 1965c; Britten and Davidson, 1969).

As RNA synthesis proceeds, the immediate transcription product consists of both repeated and unique sequences (Holmes *et al.*, 1974b), and appears capable of forming partially double-stranded heterometric duplex RNA (Fig. 3), or fully double-stranded homo-metric duplex RNA (Stern and Friedman, 1971; Montagnier and Harel, 1971; Kronenberg and Humphreys, 1972) with the 5' end of the RNA molecule (Jelinek and Darnell, 1972) probably representing hybrids between de-repressor RNA and the operator RNA of the immediate transcription product (Frenster and Herstein, 1973). Such de-repressor or chromosomal RNA has been shown to be of moderately-repetitive sequence composition (Holmes *et al.*, 1974b; Sevall *et al.*, 1975), and may be bound by the operator RNA sequences of the immediate transcription product when transcription rates at a parti-cular gene locus are excessive (Fig. 3), resulting in removal of de-repressor RNA from the DNA template, closure of the DNA helix opening, and an effective feed-back inhibition of gene transcription specific for individual gene loci (Frenster and Herstein, 1973). De-repressor RNA may also represent that nuclear RNA which migrates to the cytoplasm during early mitosis, and which returns to the nucleus early in interphase when RNA synthesis is resuming (Gold-stein, 1974).

The acidic chromatin macromolecules remain in the supernatant phase after sedimentation of DNA in 2 M NaCl and may also de-repress previously-repressed heterochromatin and increase the rate of RNA synthesis (Frenster, 1965b; Gilmour and Paul, 1969), but these are thought not to be the active molecules in selective gene transcrip-tion but rather consequences of such transcription (Pederson, 1974; Doenecke and McCarthy, 1975).

2.5. De-Repression by Exogenous DNA

A variety of DNA molecules can also interact with specific portions of the cellular genome, thereby inducing DNA helix open-ings, and increasing the rate of RNA synthesis at the particular gene locus (Fig. 4). Transformation by bacterial DNA of competent target bacterial cells involves interactions of single-stranded

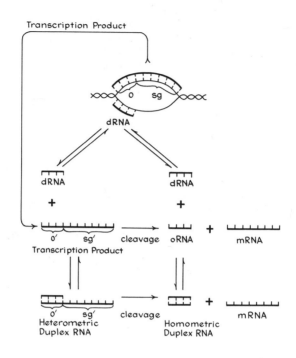

Fig. 3. The immediate transcription product RNA consists of both repetitive and single-copy sequences on the same high molecular weight molecule (Holmes and Bonner, 1974a), corresponding to operator gene (o) and structural gene (sg) sequences (Britten and Davidson, 1969; Frenster and Herstein, 1973). Operator RNA (oRNA) is complementary in base composition to de-repressor RNA (dRNA), and is capable of forming heterometric or homometric RNA-RNA duplexes with dRNA after excessive rates of gene transcription, thereby inducing the removal of dRNA from the DNA helix opening, and providing a gene-specific mechanism for feedback inhibition of RNA synthesis (Frenster and Herstein, 1973).

transforming DNA with the DNA of the host genome (Eisenstadt *et al.*, 1975). Similarly, transformation by exogenous DNA in eukaryotic systems is thought to involve a single-stranded interaction with the host genome (Fox *et al.*, 1970; Ledoux *et al.*, 1974).

Finally, oncogenic viral DNA undergoes single-stranded integration with the host genome (Frenster, 1973, 1975; Tanaka and Nonoyama, 1974), thereby forming a DNA helix opening, and allowing both messenger RNA synthesis on the remaining free host DNA strand, and anti-messenger RNA synthesis on the remaining free viral DNA

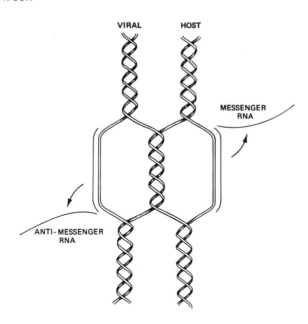

Fig. 4.   Oncogenic viral genomes contain base sequences complementary to sequences in the host genome DNA.   Such viral DNA is
capable of binding the anti-coding strand of the host DNA, freeing
the coding strand of DNA for messenger RNA synthesis.   Concurrently,
the remaining strand of viral DNA is freed for anti-messenger RNA
synthesis, and such RNA products are capable of forming RNA-RNA
duplexes (Aloni and Locker, 1973).   Single-strand scissions of an
unpaired DNA strand (IUDR, BUDR, radiation) result in liberation of
the viral genome from the integrated state (Lowy *et al.*, 1971;
Teich *et al.*, 1973), and allow the previously-transformed cells to
revert to normal phenotypic behaviour (Nomura *et al.*, 1973; Tanaka
et al., 1975).   Portions of the viral and host genomes not involved
in DNA helix openings are not involved in RNA synthesis (Frenster,
1975).

strand (Fig. 4).   Messenger RNA and anti-messenger RNA may then
form double-stranded RNA duplexes in viral-transformed cells (Aloni
and Locker, 1973), while single-strand breaks in the integrated DNA
sequences can free the viral genome (Lowy *et al.*, 1971; Teich *et al.*,
1973) and result in reversion of the transformed cell to normal
phenotypic behaviour (Nomura *et al.*, 1973).   A similar reversion
can be observed after removal of the viral genome by a variety of
polar compounds (Tanaka *et al.*, 1975).

3. IMPLICATIONS AND SUMMARY

As detailed above, DNA helices must undergo openings in the form of localized strand separations in order to permit the onset of RNA synthesis during gene transcription and the onset of DNA synthesis during gene replication. The selective control of such DNA helix openings at particular gene loci is the central molecular feature of gene regulation in both prokaryotes and eukaryotes.

Such DNA helix openings are mediated by a variety of associated chromatin macromolecules, including nuclear RNA, acidic non-histone proteins, saline-soluble proteins, lipoproteins, and even non-integrated exogenous DNA.

It is now necessary to explore the molecular details of such DNA helix openings and their control during such vital cellular processes as aging (Chetsanga *et al.*, 1975), oncogenesis (Fig. 4, 5; Huang *et al.*, 1975); response to radiation (Kaplan and Howsden, 1964); as well as in the finer details of chromatin fibril ultra-structure (Frenster, 1965a).

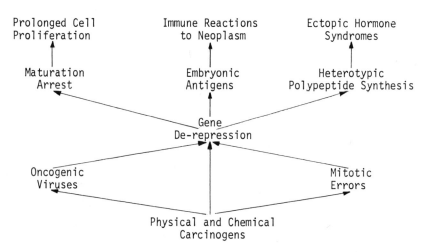

Fig. 5. Gene de-repression, whether induced by oncogenic viruses, physical or chemical carcinogens, or mitotic errors, plays a central role in human neoplastic diseases (Frenster and Herstein, 1973). By virtue of persistent gene de-repression within neoplastic cells, an arrest in the normal maturation process occurs, allowing a continued high growth fraction of proliferating cells and a prolonged individual cell life span with decreased death rates of individual cells. Such gene de-repression may also allow re-expression of fetal antigens in the neoplastic cells, with resultant immune responses in lymphocytes and macrophages (Frenster *et al.*, 1974). Neoplastic gene de-repression may also on occasion result in the ectopic synthesis by non-endocrine neoplasms of polypeptide hormones resulting in ectopic hormone syndromes (Frenster and Herstein, 1973).

References

Aloni, Y., and Locker, H., 1973, Symmetrical *in vivo* transcription of polyoma DNA and the separation of self-complementary viral and cell RNA, *Virology* 54:495-505.

Barrett, T., Maryanka, D., Harrlyn, P.H., and Gould, H.J., 1974, Non-histone proteins control gene expression in reconstituted chromatin, *Proc. Nat. Acad. Sci. USA* 71:5057-5061.

Bekhor, I., Bonner, J., and Dahmus, G.H., 1969, Hybridization of chromosomal RNA to native DNA, *Proc. Nat. Acad. Sci. USA* 62: 271-277.

Bekhor, I., Kung, G.M., and Bonner, J., 1969, Sequence-specific interaction of DNA and chromosomal proteins, *J. Mol. Biol.* 39:351-364.

Bolund, L., Gahrton, G., Killander, D., Rigler, R., and Wahren, B., 1970, Structural changes in the deoxyribonucleoprotein complex of leukocytes from patients with infectious mononucleosis, *Blood* 35:322-332.

Bolund, L., Ringertz, N.R., and Harris, H., 1969, Changes in the cytochemical properties of erythrocyte nuclei reactivated by cell fusion, *J. Cell Sci.* 4:71-87.

Bram, S., Butler-Browne, G., Boudy, P., and Ibel, K., 1975, Quartenary structure of chromatin, *Proc. Nat. Acad. Sci. USA* 72:1043-1045.

Britten, R.J., and Davidson, E.H., 1969, Gene regulation in higher cells: a theory, *Science* 165:349-357.

Chae, C.B., 1975, Reconstitution of chromatin: mode of reassociation of chromosomal proteins, *Biochemistry* 14:900-906.

Chamberlin, M.J., 1974, The selectivity of transcription, *Annu. Rev. Biochem.* 43:721-775.

Champoux, J.J., and McConaughy, B.C., 1975, Priming of superhelical SV40 DNA by *E. coli* RNA polymerase for *in vitro* DNA synthesis, *Biochemistry* 14:307-316.

Chan, H.W., and Wells, R.D., 1974, Structural uniqueness of the lactose operator, *Nature* 252:205-209.

Chetsanga, C.J., Boyd, V., Peterson, L., and Rushlan, K., 1975, Single-stranded regions in DNA of old mice, *Nature* 253:130-131.

Dahmus, M.E., and Bonner, J., 1970, Nucleoproteins as regulators of gene function, *Fed. Proc.* 29:1255-1260.

Davidson, R.G., Nitowsky, H.M., and Childs, B., 1963, Demonstration of two populations of cells in the human female heterozygous for glucose-6-phosphate dehydrogenase variants, *Proc. Nat. Acad. Sci. USA* 50:481-485.

Dickson, R.C., Abelson, J., Barnes, W.M., and Reznikoff, W.S., 1975, Genetic regulation: the lac control region, *Science* 187:27-35.

Doenecke, D., and McCarthy, B.J., 1975, The nature of proteins associated with chromatin, *Biochemistry* 14:1373-1378.

Eisenstadt, E., Lange, R., and Willecke, K., 1975, Competent *Bacillus subtilis* synthesize a denatured DNA binding activity,

Proc. Nat. Acad. Sci. USA 72:323-327.

Fox, A.S., Duggleby, W.F., Gelbert, W.M., and Yoon, S.B., 1970, DNA-induced transformations in Drosophila: evidence for transmission without integration, Proc. Nat. Acad. Sci. USA 67:1834-1838.

Frenster, J.H., 1965a, Ultrastructural continuity between active and repressed chromatin, Nature 205:1341-1342.

Frenster, J.H., 1965b, Nuclear polyanions as de-repressors of synthesis of RNA, Nature 206:680-683.

Frenster, J.H., 1965c, A model of specific de-repression within interphase chromatin, Nature 206:1269-1270.

Frenster, J.H., 1965d, Localized strand separations within DNA during selective transcription, Nature 208:894-896.

Frenster, J.H., 1965e, Correlation of the binding to DNA loops or to DNA helices with the effect on RNA synthesis, Nature 208:1093-1094.

Frenster, J.H., 1966, Control of DNA strand separations during selective transcription and asynchronous replication, Information Exchange Group Number 7, March, 1966, and in "The Cell Nucleus-Metabolism and Radiosensitivity" (H.M. Klouwen, ed.), pp. 27-46, Taylor and Francis Ltd., London.

Frenster, J.H., 1973, Molecular aspects of the integration and de-repression of oncogenic viral genomes, U.S. Atomic Energy Commission, "Third Conference on Embryonic and Fetal Antigens in Cancer," Report CONF-731141 (Nov. 4-7, 1973), pp. 19-20.

Frenster, J.H., 1975, Model of single-stranded integration of oncogenic viral genomes, Biophys. J. 15:137a-138a.

Frenster, J.H., Allfrey, V.G., and Mirsky, A.E., 1961, In vivo incoration of amino acids into the proteins of isolated nuclear ribosomes, Biochim. Biophys. Acta 47:130-137.

Frenster, J.H., Allfrey, V.G., and Mirsky, A.E., 1963, Repressed and active chromatin isolated from interphase lymphocytes, Proc. Nat. Acad. Sci. USA 50:1026-1032.

Frenster, J.H., and Herstein, P.R., 1973, Gene de-repression, New England J. Med. 288:1224-1229.

Fresnter, J.H., Nakatsu, S.L., and Masek, M.A., 1974, Ultrastructural probes of DNA templates within human bone marrow and lymph node cells, in "Advances in Cell and Molecular Biology," (E. DuPraw, ed.), Vol. 3, pp. 1-19, Academic Press, New York.

Gilmour, R.S., and Paul, J., 1969, RNA transcribed from reconstituted nucleoprotein is similar to natural RNA, J. Mol. Biol. 40:137-140.

Gilmour, R.S., and Paul, J., 1970, Role of non-histone components in determining organ specificity of rabbit chromatin, FEBS Lett. 9:242-245.

Gledhill, B.L., Gledhill, M.P., Rigler, R., and Ringertz, N.R., 1966, Changes in deoxyribonucleoprotein during spermiogenesis in the bull, Exp. Cell Res. 41:652-665.

Goldstein, L., 1974, Stable nuclear RNA returns to post-division nuclei following release to the cytoplasm during mitosis,

Exp. Cell Res. 89:421-425.

Grumbach, M.M., Morishima, A., and Taylor, J.H., 1963, Human sex chromosome abnormalities in relation to DNA replication and heterochromatinization, *Proc. Nat. Acad. Sci. USA* 49:581-589.

Holmes, D.S., and Bonner, J., 1974a, Interspersion of repetitive and single-copy sequences in nuclear RNA of high molecular weight, *Proc. Nat. Acad. Sci. USA* 71:1108-1112.

Holmes, D.S., Mayfield, J.E., and Bonner, J., 1974b, Sequence composition of rat ascites chromosomal RNA, *Biochemistry* 13: 849-855.

Huang, A.T., Riddle, M.M., and Koons, L.S., 1975, Some properties of a DNA-unwinding protein unique to lymphocytes from chronic lymphocytic leukemia, *Cancer Res.* 35:981-986.

Huang, R.C.C., and Bonner, J., 1962, Histone a suppressor of chromosomal RNA synthesis, *Proc. Nat. Acad. Sci. USA* 48:1216-1222.

Huang, R.C.C., and Huang, P.C., 1969, Effect of protein-bound RNA associated with chick embryo chromatin on template specificity of chromatin, *J. Mol. Biol.* 39:365-378.

Jelinek, W., and Darnell, J.E., 1972, Double-stranded regions in heterogenous nuclear RNA from Hela cells, *Proc. Nat. Acad. Sci. USA* 69:2537-2541.

Kaplan, H.S., and Howsden, F.L., 1964, Sensitization of purine-starved bacteria to X rays, *Proc. Nat. Acad. Sci. USA* 51:181-188.

Killander, D., and Rigler, F., 1969, Activation of deoxyribonucleo-protein in human leukocytes stimulated with phytohemagglutinin, *Exp. Cell Res.* 54:163-170.

Klevecz, R., and Hsu, T.C., 1964, The differential capacity for RNA synthesis: a cytological approach, *Proc. Nat. Acad. Sci. USA* 52:811-817.

Kohne, D.E., and Byers, M.J., 1973, Amplification and evolution of DNA sequences expressed as RNA, *Biochemistry* 12:2373-2378.

Kronenberg, L.H., and Humphreys, T., 1972, Double-stranded RNA in sea urchin embryos, *Biochemistry* 11:2020-2026.

Ledoux, L., Huart, R., and Jacobs, M., 1974, DNA-mediated genetic correction of thiamineless arabidopsis thaliana, *Nature* 249: 17-21.

Levy, S., Simpson, R.T., and Sober, H.A., 1972, Fractionation of chromatin components, *Biochemistry* 11:1547-1554.

Lowy, D.R., Rowe, W.P., Teich, N., and Hartley, J.W., 1971, Murine leukemia virus: high frequency activation *in vitro* by 5-IUDR and 5-BUDR, *Science* 174:155-156.

McCarthy, B.J., and Hoyer, B.H., 1964, Identity of DNA and diversity of messenger RNA molecules in normal mouse tissues, *Proc. Nat. Acad. Sci. USA* 52:915-922.

McGhee, J.D., and von Hippel, P.H., 1975, Formaldehyde as a probe of DNA structure. I. Reaction with exocyclic amino groups of DNA bases, *Biochemistry* 14:1281-1296.

Montagnier, L., and Harel, L., 1971, Homology of double-stranded

RNA from rat liver cells with the cellular genome, *Nature New Biol.* 229:106-108.

Nakatsu, S.L., Masek, M.A., Landrum, S., and Frenster, J.H., 1974, Activity of DNA templates during cell division and cell differentiation, *Nature* 248:334-335.

Nomura, S., Fischinger, P.J., Mattern, C.F.T., Gerwin, B.I., and Dunn, K.J., 1973, Revertants of mouse cells transformed by murine sarcoma virus: flat variants induced by FUDR and colcemide, *Virology* 56:152-163.

Oliver, D., and Chalkley, R., 1974, Assymmetric distribution of histones on DNA: a model for nucleohistone primary structure, *Biochemistry* 13:5093-5098.

Paul, J., and Gilmour, R.S., 1968, Organ-specific restriction of transcription in mammalian chromatin, *J. Mol. Biol.* 34:305-316.

Pederson, T., 1974, Gene activation in eukaryotes: are nuclear acidic proteins the cause or the effect? *Proc. Nat. Acad. Sci. USA* 71:617-621.

Sevall, J.S., Cockburn, A., Savage, M., and Bonner, J., 1975, DNA-protein interactions of rat liver non-histone chromosomal protein, *Biochemistry* 14:782-789.

Stern, R., and Friedman, R., 1971, RNA synthesis in animal cells in the presence of actinomycin, *Biochemistry* 10:3635-3645.

Suzuki, T., Tsutsui, Y., and Takahashi, T., 1974, Ultrastructural detection of single-stranded DNA in rat liver nucleus by the electronmicroscopic immuno-peroxidase method, *Exp. Cell Res.* 89:306-310.

Tanaka, A., and Nonoyama, M., 1974, Latent DNA of Epstein-Barr virus: separation from high molecular weight cell DNA in neutral glycerol gradients, *Proc. Nat. Acad. Sci. USA* 71: 4658-4661.

Tanaka, M., Levy, J., Terode, M., Breshon, R., Rifkind, R.A., and Marks, P.A., 1975, Induction of erythroid differentiation in murine virus infected erythroleukemia cells by highly polar compounds, *Proc. Nat. Acad. Sci. USA* 72:1003-1006.

Teich, N., Lowy, D., Hartley, J.W., and Rowe, W.P., 1973, Studies of the mechanism of induction of infectious murine leukemia virus from AKR mouse embryo cells by 5-IUDR and 5-BUDR, *Virology* 51:163-173.

Umansky, S.R., Kovalev, Y.I., and Tokarskaya, V.I., 1975, Specific interaction of chromatin non-histone proteins with DNA, *Biochim. Biophys. Acta* 383:242-254.

van den Broek, W.K., Nooden, L.D., Sevall, J.S., and Bonner, J., 1973, Isolation, purification, and fractionation of non-histone chromosomal proteins, *Biochemistry* 12:229-236.

Zetterberg, A., and Auer, G., 1970, Proliferative activity and cyto-chemical properties of nuclear chromatin related to local density of epithelial cells, *Exp. Cell Res.* 62:262-270.

RADIATION-INDUCED CROSS-LINKING OF DNA AND PROTEIN IN BACTERIA

Kendric C. Smith

Department of Radiology, Stanford University School of

Medicine, Stanford, California 94305

1. INTRODUCTION

The cross-linking of DNA and protein was the first *in vivo* photochemical hetero-addition reaction to be reported (Smith, 1962; Alexander and Moroson, 1962). It was observed that with increasing fluences of UV radiation, decreasing amounts of DNA free of protein could be extracted from the irradiated cells (Fig. 1). The DNA that was unextractable was found in the insoluble protein fraction (Smith, 1962). This phenomenon of decreased extractability of DNA has been observed after the UV irradiation of bacteria (Smith, 1962; Smith *et al.*, 1966; Smith and O'Leary, 1967; Alexander and Moroson, 1962; Bridges *et al.*, 1967; Thomas *et al.*, 1972; Bücker *et al.*, 1975),

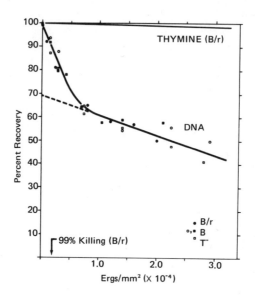

Fig. 1. The extractability of DNA from *E. coli* following
irradiation with increasing fluences of UV radiation. *E. coli* were
grown overnight in medium containing thymine-2-^{14}C, irradiated with
increasing fluences of UV radiation and treated with sodium lauryl
sulfate to isolate their DNA. The graph represents the recovery of
free DNA. The DNA not isolated remained associated with the denatured
proteins. For comparison, data of Smith (1961) are included on the
rate of formation of thymine dimers in *E. coli* B/r with increasing
fluences of UV radiation (plotted here as the loss of recovery of
thymine) (From Smith, 1962).

mammalian cells (Todd and Han, This Volume), salmon sperm heads
(Alexander and Moroson, 1962), and of mixtures of DNA and protein
and RNA and protein (Schimmel *et al.*, This Volume).

2.   BIOLOGICAL IMPORTANCE

One way to assess the biological importance of a given photoproduct in DNA is to determine if its yield varies with radiation
fluence in the same manner as the efficiency for killing, when cells
are pretreated under various experimental conditions that affect
their sensitivity to UV radiation. For the enhanced yield of a
given photoproduct to have an enhanced effect on the killing of
cells, one must postulate that the photoproduct is not always
repaired efficiently and/or accurately. That the cross-linking of
DNA and protein plays a significant role in the killing of UV-

irradiated cells has been shown by such correlations for several
experimental conditions.

2.1. Thymine Starvation

When *E. coli* 15 TAU cells are starved for thymine required for
their growth, their sensitivity to UV radiation changes (Fig. 2).
The cells become progressively more sensitive to killing by UV
radiation over the first 40 min of thymine starvation and then
become progressively more resistant. The amount of DNA cross-linked
to protein in these cells by a fixed fluence of UV radiation changed
with the time of thymine starvation in the same manner as cell killing, i.e., the greater the amount of UV-induced DNA-protein cross-
linking the greater the amount of UV-induced killing (Smith *et al.*,
1966). These results suggest that the cross-linking of DNA and
protein by UV radiation must play an important role in the loss of
viability of UV-irradiated cells and that the magnitude of this
role can be altered by prior starvation for thymine. Presumably

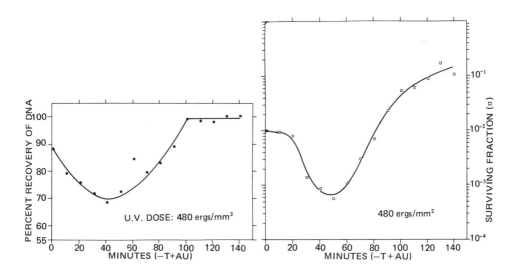

Fig. 2. The susceptibility of *E. coli* 15 TAU to killing and to
the cross-linking of their DNA and protein by UV radiation at various
times of growth under conditions of (-T+AU). A logarithmic culture
of *E. coli* 15 TAU was rapidly switched to a medium devoid of thymine
by filtration and resuspension. At various times thereafter, two
aliquots were withdrawn from the culture. One of these aliquots
was irradiated with 48.0 J m^{-2} (254 nm) and then both aliquots were
assayed for viable cells and for the amount of DNA that could be
extracted free of protein (Adapted from Smith *et al.*, 1966).

the juxtaposition of DNA and protein is changed in these cells when
their metabolism is altered by thymine starvation, leading to a more
efficient photochemical reaction between the two polymers.

2.2. Frozen Cells

When cells of *E. coli* are frozen they show an increased efficiency for killing by UV radiation that varies as a function of the
temperature at which they are irradiated (Ashwood-Smith *et al.*,
1965). Table 1 lists bacterial strains that are sensitized to UV
radiation while frozen, strains that are moderately sensitized, and

Table 1. Sensitivity of Cells to UV Radiation while Frozen vs Non-
Frozen

Strain	Reference
Sensitized at -79°C	
Escherichia coli B/r	Smith and O'Leary, 1967
Escherichia coli B/r WP2	Ashwood-Smith *et al.*, 1965
	Ashwood-Smith and Bridges, 1967
	Bridges *et al.*, 1967
Escherichia coli K-12 (AB1157)	Bridges *et al.*, 1967
Escherichia coli B (when plated with pantoyl lactone)	Bridges *et al.*, 1967
Moderately Sensitized at -79°C	
Escherichia coli WP2 *hcr*⁻	Ashwood-Smith *et al.*, 1965
Escherichia coli K-12 (*uvrA6*) (AB1886)	Bridges *et al.*, 1967
Escherichia coli K-12 (*recA13*) (AB2463)	Bridges *et al.*, 1967
Escherichia coli B_{s-1} (when plated on minimal medium)	Bridges *et al.*, 1967
Escherichia coli B (when plated on complex medium)	Bridges *et al.*, 1967
Not Sensitized at -79°C	
Escherichia coli B_{s-1} (when plated on complex medium)	Bridges *et al.*, 1967
Micrococcus radiodurans	Ashwood-Smith and Bridges, 1967

some strains that are not sensitized by freezing. There is no simple explanation to account for this varied response by the several
strains, rather it will probably require specific studies on the
production and repair of different photoproducts by each strain in
order to clarify this situation.

Since the sensitivity of *E. coli* B/r to killing by UV radiation
varies in a non-progressive manner as a function of the temperature
at which the cells are irradiated (Fig. 3), one may ask if there is
a photoproduct in DNA that varies in yield as a function of temperature in the same manner as cell killing (Smith and O'Leary, 1967).
The rate of formation of cyclobutane-type thymine dimers, however,
decreased progressively when the temperature of the cells during
irradiation was varied from +21° to -79°, and to -196°C. Therefore, the yields of thymine dimers at the different temperatures
do *not* correlate with the relative differences in the survival
curves in Fig. 3.

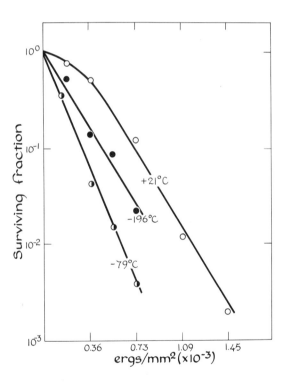

Fig. 3. Survival of *E. coli* B/r *thy* as a function of the
fluence of UV radiation (254 nm) at different temperatures (From
Smith and O'Leary, 1967).

Concomitant with the decrease in yield of thymine dimers as the temperature at which the cells were UV irradiated was decreased, there was a decrease in the amount of photoreactivation shown by these cells (see also Hieda and Ito, 1968). Since the photoreactivating enzyme is known to be specific for the *in situ* repair of cyclobutane-type pyrimidine dimers (J.K. Setlow, 1966), the reduced amount of photoreactivation observed in cells that were UV irradiated while frozen is consistent with the observed decrease in the production of cyclobutane-type thymine dimers under these conditions (Smith and O'Leary, 1967).

Since there is no correlation between the production of thymine dimers and the increased killing of *E. coli* B/r by UV irradiation at -79° and -196°C, it suggests that cyclobutane-type thymine dimers do not play as significant a role in the events leading to the death of cells irradiated while frozen as they appear to play at room temperature (R.B. Setlow, 1966). These results provide further evidence that the relative biological importance of a given photoproduct can change markedly, depending upon growth or irradiation conditions (for a review see Smith, 1967).

The photochemical event that does correlate with the loss of viability under these conditions is the cross-linking of DNA with protein. A larger percentage of DNA was cross-linked to protein by a given fluence of UV radiation when the cells were irradiated at -79° or at -196°C as compared to +21°C (Fig. 4). There is clearly a correlation in rank between the several cross-linking curves in Fig. 4 and the survival curves in Fig. 3. The configuration or the proximity of the protein and DNA may be altered by the freezing of the cells so that the probability of forming DNA-protein cross-links by UV radiation is greatly enhanced, thus leading to the greater lethality observed under these conditions (Smith and O'Leary, 1967).

2.3. Dry Cells

A decrease in yield of thymine dimers, an increase in sensitivity to killing by UV radiation, and an increase in yield of DNA-protein cross-links were all observed when cells of *E. coli* B/r were UV irradiated (254 nm) under vacuum as compared to irradiation in solution (Thomas *et al.*, 1972).

These results are consistent with the observation that the formation of thymine dimers is greatly depressed if DNA is irradiated while dry (Riklis, 1965; Smith and Yoshikawa, 1966). Since bacteriophage T1 cannot be photoreactivated if UV irradiated dry (Hill and Rossi, 1952; Riklis, 1965), it implies that pyrimidine dimers are not formed in phage DNA under these conditions. Other types of lesions must therefore explain the lethal effects of UV radiation when phage are irradiated while dry.

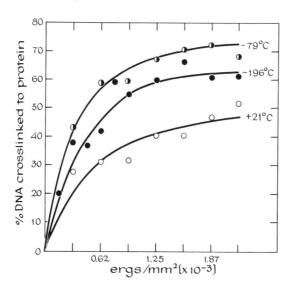

Fig. 4. Cross-linking of DNA and protein in *E. coli* B/r *thy* as a function of the fluence of UV radiation (254 nm) at different temperatures (From Smith and O'Leary, 1967).

2.4. Bromouracil Substitution

When cells of *E. coli* B/r were grown under conditions such that about 70% of their DNA thymine was replaced by 5-bromouracil, they were markedly sensitized to killing by UV radiation (Kaplan *et al.*, 1962), and were sensitized to the formation of UV-induced DNA-protein cross-links (Smith, 1964a). This enhancement in the rate of production of DNA-protein cross-links in cells containing 5-bromouracil suggests yet another mechanism to explain how 5-bromouracil sensitizes cells to killing by UV radiation (Smith, 1961).

2.5. Action Spectra

While the action spectrum for the killing of *E. coli* has a maximum at about 260 nm, that for the killing of *M. radiodurans* has a broad peak with maxima at both 260 and 280 nm (Fig. 5). Classically, a peak at 280 nm has indicated the involvement of protein while a peak at 260 nm has indicated the involvement of nucleic acid. It has therefore been suggested (J.K. Setlow and Boling, 1965) that while *M. radiodurans* appears to be extremely efficient in its ability to repair thymine dimers, what ultimately kills this organism is some sort of damage to DNA and to protein.

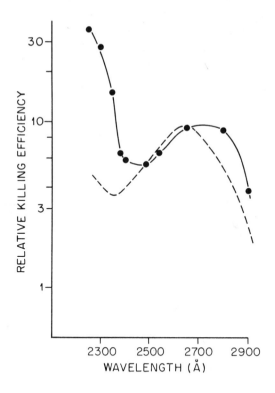

Fig. 5.   Action spectra for the killing of *Escherichia coli*
H/r 30R and *Micrococcus radiodurans*.   Data for *E. coli* are given
by the dotted line; data for *M. radiodurans* are given by the solid
line (Adapted from Setlow and Boling, 1965).

One such type of damage may be the cross-linking of DNA and protein.

It is interesting that while *E. coli* has an action spectrum for
killing at room temperature that suggests only the involvement of
DNA, it is markedly sensitized to killing by freezing and, as discussed above, the lesion of importance in this enhanced killing is
the UV-induced cross-linking of DNA and protein.   On the other hand,
M. radiodurans has an action spectrum that implicates the alteration
of both DNA and protein in UV-induced killing at room temperature
and it is not sensitized to UV radiation by freezing (Table 1).
These results may possibly be explained by the assumption that,
in *E. coli*, the DNA and protein are not optimally juxtaposed for
photochemical interaction at room temperature but they are when
the cells are frozen.   On the other hand, in *M. radiodurans* the DNA
and protein may be maximally juxtaposed at room temperature and

freezing does not appear to affect this juxtaposition. This hypothesis could be tested by running cross-linking experiments on *M.
radiodurans* and/or by running action spectra for killing on both
bacteria at -79°C.

3.   THE PORTION OF THE DNA OF *E. coli* THAT IS ACTIVELY BEING REPLICATED IS THE MOST SENSITIVE TO UV-INDUCED CROSS-LINKING WITH PROTEIN

The sensitivity of a given segment of DNA to cross-linking with
protein depends upon its position in the DNA replication cycle of
the cell (Smith, 1964b). It was observed that the portion of the
DNA that was most recently replicated was the most sensitive to
cross-linking with protein and that the cyclicity of this phenomenon
was tied to the generation cycle of the cells (Fig. 6). Thus, the
state of the DNA within the cell has a profound effect on its sensitivity to UV-induced cross-linking with protein (Smith, 1975).

4.   PHOTODYNAMIC ACTION AND CROSS-LINKING

When bacterial cells that had been pretreated with either
acridine orange or methylene blue were exposed to intense visible
light they were rapidly killed (Fig. 7). In addition, this treatment was very efficient in producing DNA-protein cross-links (Fig.
7, insert). In fact, there appears to be a correlation between the
relative killing efficiency of the two dyes and the relative production of DNA-protein cross-links (Smith and Hanawalt, 1969,
p. 188).

Petrusek (1971) demonstrated that when cells of *E. coli* B/r
were irradiated with visible light in the presence of acridine
orange, their DNA became cross-linked both to membrane material
and to proteins within the cells. The amount of cross-linking
increased with the time of exposure to visible light. The post-
irradiation incubation of the cells did not reduce the amount of
cross-linking, suggesting that this lesion may not be reparable.

After treatment of *E. coli* B with proflavine and light under
conditions such that only 15% of the DNA was extractable (i.e.,
85% was cross-linked with protein), the extracted DNA contained
similar amounts of bound amino acids as the DNA isolated from
unirradiated cells (Balis *et al.*, 1964). While there were some
small differences in the amounts of specific amino acids to the
control and irradiated samples, more assays would be required to
determine if these differences are significant. For a further
discussion of photosensitized cross-linking reactions, see Helene
(This Volume).

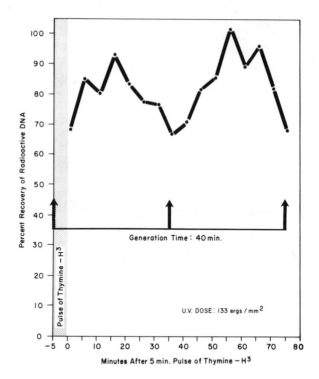

Fig. 6. Sensitivity of a pulse labeled section of bacterial
DNA to be cross-linked to protein by a constant fluence of UV
radiation as a function of the time after the pulse. A log phase
culture of *E. coli* 15 TAU was pulsed with thymine-³H for 5 min,
the radioactive thymine was removed by filtration, the cells
returned to a medium containing non-radioactive thymine, and then
allowed to continue logarithmic growth. At various times two
aliquots were removed from the culture. One of these was irradiated
with 13.3 J m⁻² (254 nm) and then both were treated with deter-
gent for the isolation of their DNA. The percent recovery of DNA
(vs the unirradiated control aliquots) is plotted against the time
following the pulse of thymine-³H. Only the radioactive DNA is
assayed in this experiment (From Smith, 1964b).

5.   X-RAYS AND CROSS-LINKING

After an X-ray dose of 1 krad there was about a 5% loss in the
extractability of DNA from *E. coli* B but doses up to 40 krads did
not alter this value (Smith, 1962). Since the addition of amino
acids to DNA by X irradiation has been observed *in vitro* (Yamamoto,
This Volume), and since the radicals implicated in the production
of UV-induced amino acid-pyrimidine adducts are also produced by

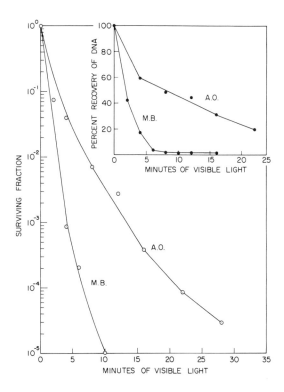

Fig. 7. The killing of *E. coli* B/r *thy* and the cross-linking of DNA and protein by visible light in the presence of acridine orange (3.4 µg/ml) or methylene blue (4 µg/ml). Stationary phase cells were washed and suspended in 0.1 M phosphate buffer (pH 6.8) and dye was added to the final concentrations indicated. Solutions were irradiated with a 150 W General Electric floodlight (PAR-38) through 2.5 cm of water in a heavy Pyrex dish. Viability was determined on nutrient agar plates. The DNA was isolated after lysing the cells with sodium lauryl sulfate (From Smith and Hanawalt, 1969, p. 188).

X irradiation (Elad, This Volume; Myers, This Volume), it is surprising that a larger amount of DNA was not cross-linked with protein in X-irradiated *E. coli*. The answer may reside, however, in the fact that the assay procedure (Smith, 1962) depends upon the selective precipitation of cross-linked molecules of DNA and protein. The chain breaks produced in macromolecules by X-rays could interfere with the selective precipitation procedure. Thus, the question of whether or not the cross-linking of DNA and protein by X-rays occurs in bacteria should be reevaluated by analytical procedures less dependent upon the molecular weight of DNA and protein

When the residual protein content of DNA isolated from the tissues of γ-irradiated animals was measured, a statistically significant increase in the bonding of protein to DNA was observed (Ivannik and Ryabchenko, 1969; Strazhevskaya *et al.*, 1969, 1972). No cross-linking was observed when phage T2 was γ-irradiated with 20 kR (Strazhevskaya *et al.*, 1972). DNA-protein cross-links have been implicated in γ-irradiated phage T1 (Bohne *et al.*, 1970) and T7 (Hawkins, 1975), however.

6. CHEMICAL NATURE OF DNA-PROTEIN CROSS-LINKS

The precise chemical mechanisms by which nucleic acids and protein are cross-linked *in vivo* are not yet known, however, the isolation of a mixed photoproduct of thymine and cysteine (5-S-cysteine, 6-hydrothymine) from the *in vitro* UV irradiation of a solution of thymine and cysteine may serve as a possible model for the cross-linking phenomenon. Cysteine also adds photochemically to poly-rU, poly-dC, poly-dT, and to RNA and DNA (Smith, 1975).

In addition to cysteine the following amino acids add photochemically to thymine: arginine, lysine, tyrosine, tryptophan, and cystine (Schott and Shetlar, 1974). The following amino acids add photochemically to uracil: glycine, serine, cysteine, cystine, methionine, lysine, arginine, histidine, tryptophan, phenylalanine, and tyrosine (Smith, 1969). The other common amino acids were unreactive under the conditions tested. For reviews on the mechanisms by which amino acids combine photochemically with the nucleic acids see Smith (1975), Varghese (This Volume), and Shapiro (This Volume).

7. REPAIR OF DNA-PROTEIN CROSS-LINKS

Mechanisms for the repair of damaged DNA have been reviewed recently (Hanawalt and Setlow, 1975); however, data on the repair of DNA-protein cross-links are fragmentary. It has been reported that this lesion is not photoreactivated (Smith, 1962). This is not surprising in view of the known specificity of the photoreactivating enzyme for cyclobutane-type pyrimidine dimers (J.K. Setlow, 1966).

Since the *uvr⁻* (deficient in excision repair) and *rec⁻* (deficient in postreplication repair) mutants of *E. coli* are only partially sensitized to UV radiation by freezing when compared to wild-type *E. coli* (Table 1), one may infer that DNA-protein cross-links can be repaired, at least partially, by the repair systems controlled by the *rec* and *uvr* genes. Preliminary studies indicate that DNA-protein cross-links are amenable to postreplication repair (Smith, 1974). The possible mechanisms by which DNA-protein cross-links are repaired need to be further explored.

It is of interest that another type of cross-link, an inter-strand cross-link produced in DNA by psoralen plus light, has been shown to be repaired by a complex mechanism that involves the sequential action of excision repair (*uvr* genes) and recombinational repair (*rec* genes) (Cole, 1973).

8. CONCLUSIONS

Protein and DNA become cross-linked when bacteria are exposed to UV radiation, photodynamic action, and probably also to X radiation. Under certain experimental conditions, DNA-protein cross-links appear to be the major lethal lesion produced by UV irradiation. The portion of the bacterial genome undergoing replication is the most sensitive to UV radiation induced cross-linking with proteins.

These results dramatize three important points. 1.) DNA does not exist in pure solution within a cell but is surrounded by other organic molecules that can be caused to combine with the DNA. 2.) Hetero-addition reactions with DNA are biologically important lesions. 3.) The relative production and biological importance of a given radiation-induced lesion can vary markedly under different experimental conditions.

Further studies are needed, however, to elucidate the chemical nature of DNA-protein cross-links *in vivo*, and to gain further insight as to the biological consequences and repairability of these lesions.

References

Alexander, P., and Moroson, H., 1962, Cross-linking of deoxyribonucleic acid to protein following ultraviolet irradiation of different cells, *Nature* 194:882-883.

Ashwood-Smith, M.J., and Bridges, B.A., 1967, On the sensitivity of frozen micro-organisms to ultraviolet radiation, *Proc. Royal Soc.*, B 168:194-202.

Ashwood-Smith, M.J., Bridges, B.A., and Munson, R.J., 1965, Ultraviolet damage to bacteria and bacteriophage at low temperatures, *Science* 149:1103-1105.

Balis, M.E., Salser, J.S., and Elder, A., 1964, A suggested role of amino acids in deoxyribonucleic acid, *Nature* 203:1170-1171.

Bohne, L., Coquerelle, T., and Hagen, U., 1970, Radiation sensitivity of bacteriophage DNA. II. Breaks and cross-links after irradiation *in vivo, Int. J. Radiat. Biol.* 17:205-215.

Bridges, B.A., Ashwood-Smith, M.J., and Munson, R.J., 1967, On the nature of the lethal and mutagenic action of ultraviolet light on frozen bacteria, *Proc. Royal Soc.,* B 168:203-215.

Bücker, H., Dose, K., Thomas, C., and Toth, B., 1975, Photoinduced DNA-protein cross-links: A study on model compounds *in vitro* and on *E. coli* B/r *in vivo.* Abstr. Int. Symp. "Protein and Other Adducts to DNA: Their Significance to Aging, Carcinogenesis and Radiation Biology," Williamsburg, Virginia, May 2-6, 1975.

Cole, R.S., 1973, Repair of DNA containing interstrand crosslinks in *Escherichia coli:* Sequential excision and recombination, *Proc. Nat. Acad. Sci. USA* 70:1064-1068.

Hanawalt, P.C., and Setlow, R.B. (eds.), 1975, "Molecular Mechanisms for the Repair of DNA," Plenum Press, New York (in press).

Hawkins, R.B., 1975, Ionizing radiation induced covalent protein to DNA cross-links in coliphage T7. Abstr. Int. Symp. "Protein and Other Adducts to DNA: Their Significance to Aging, Carcinogenesis and Radiation Biology," Williamsburg, Virginia, May 2-6, 1975.

Hieda, K., and Ito, T., 1968, The enhancement of UV sensitivity of yeast in frozen state, *Mutat. Res.* 6:325-327.

Hill, R.F., and Rossi, H.H., 1952, Absence of photoreactivation in T1 bacteriophage irradiated with ultraviolet in the dry state, *Science* 116:424-425.

Ivannik, B.P., and Ryabchenko, N.I., 1969, Some physicochemical changes in DNA isolated from the organs of irradiated rats, *Radiobiology* 9, No. 1:7-17 (English translation by U.S. A.E.C.).

Kaplan, H.S., Smith, K.C., and Tomlin, P.A., 1962, Effect of halogenated pyrimidines on radiosensitivity of *E. coli, Radiat. Res.* 16:98-113.

Petrusek, R.L., 1971, Photodynamic lesions in DNA, Ph.D. Thesis No. T22500, University of Chicago.

Riklis, E., 1965, Studies on mechanism of repair of ultraviolet-irradiated viral and bacterial DNA *in vivo* and *in vitro, Can. J. Biochem.* 43:1207-1219.

Schott, H.N., and Shetlar, M.D., 1974, Photochemical addition of amino acids to thymine, *Biochem. Biophys. Res. Commun.* 59:1112-1116.

Setlow, J.K., 1966, Photoreactivation, *Radiat. Res.* Suppl. 6:141-155.

Setlow, J.K., and Boling, M.E., 1965, The resistance of *Micrococcus radiodurans* to ultraviolet radiation. II. Action spectra for killing, delay in DNA synthesis, and thymine dimerization, *Biochim. Biophys. Acta* 108:259-265.

Setlow, R.B., 1966, Cyclobutane-type pyrimidine dimers in polynucleotides, *Science* 153:379-386.

Smith, K.C., 1961, A chemical basis for the sensitization of bacteria to ultraviolet light by incorporated bromouracil, *Biochem. Biophys. Res. Commun.* 6:458-463.

Smith, K.C., 1962, Dose dependent decrease in extractability of DNA from bacteria following irradiation with ultraviolet light or with visible light plus dye, *Biochem. Biophys. Res. Commun.* 8:157-163.

Smith, K.C., 1964a, Photochemistry of the nucleic acids, *Photophysiology* 3:329-388.

Smith, K.C., 1964b, The photochemical interaction of deoxyribonucleic acid and protein *in vivo* and its biological importance, *Photochem. Photobiol.* 3:415-427.

Smith, K.C., 1967, Biologically important damage to DNA by photoproducts other than cyclobutane-type thymine dimers, *in* "Radiation Research" (G. Silini, ed.), pp. 756-770, North-Holland Publishing Co., Amsterdam.

Smith, K.C., 1969, Photochemical addition of amino acids to ^{14}C-uracil, *Biochem. Biophys. Res. Commun.* 34:354-357.

Smith, K.C., 1974, Post-replicational repair after UV irradiation of frozen cells of *E. coli* B/r, Abstr. TPM-C4, American Society for Photobiology.

Smith, K.C., 1975, The radiation-induced addition of proteins and other molecules to nucleic acids, *in* "Photochemistry and Photobiology of Nucleic Acids" (S.Y. Wang, ed.), Academic Press, New York (in press).

Smith, K.C., and Hanawalt, P.C., 1969, "Molecular Photobiology," Academic Press, New York.

Smith, K.C., Hodgkins, B., and O'Leary, M.E., 1966, The biological importance of ultraviolet induced DNA-protein crosslinks in *Escherichia coli* 15TAU, *Biochim. Biophys. Acta* 114:1-15.

Smith, K.C., and O'Leary, M.E., 1967, Photoinduced DNA-protein cross-links and bacterial killing: A correlation at low temperatures, *Science* 155:1024-1026.

Smith, K.C., and Yoshikawa, H., 1966, Variation in the photochemical reactivity of thymine in the DNA of *B. subtilis* spores, vegative cells and spores germinated in chloramphenicol, *Photochem. Photobiol.* 5:777-786.

Strazhevskaya, N.B., Troyanovskaya, M.L., Struchkov, V.A., and Krasichkova, Z.I., 1969, Disturbance of the state of the DNA-protein complex of chromatin in the cell nucleus under the influence of ionizing radiation, *Radiobiology* 9, No. 6:165-168 (English translation by U.S. A.E.C.).

Strazhevskaya, N.B., Krivtsov, G.G., Krasichkova, Z.I., and Struchkov, V.A., 1972, Change in the complex of supermolecular DNA--Residual protein in the thymus and liver of γ-irradiated rats, *Radiobiology* 12, No. 1:24-33 (English translation by U.S. A.E.C.) A.E.C.).

Thomas, C., Schwager, M., and Bücker, H., 1972, Photoproducts in *E. coli* cells produced by UV-irradiation in vacuum, Abstr. No. 130, 6th Int. Cong. Photobiol., Bochum, Germany.

UV-INDUCED DNA TO PROTEIN CROSS-LINKING IN MAMMALIAN CELLS

Paul Todd

Department of Biophysics, The Pennsylvania State

University, University Park, Pennsylvania 16802

Antun Han

Division of Biological and Medical Research

Argonne National Laboratory, Argonne, Illinois 60439

1. INTRODUCTION

Evidence for the cross-linking of DNA to protein was discovered almost simultaneously in UV-irradiated microorganisms and mammalian cells (Smith, 1962; Alexander and Moroson, 1962). Subsequent experiments in which DNA to protein adducts were sought in mixtures of protein and DNA exposed to ultraviolet light clearly indicated that such a reaction is possible (Smith, 1962; 1964a, b; 1967; Sklobovskaya and Ryabchenko, 1970a, b). This report has two aims: first, to summarize the information indicating that DNA-protein cross-links are induced in mammalian cells by ultraviolet light, and second, to review experimental studies that attempt to correlate cross-link induction and biological damage. The demonstration of cross-linking has been done in two ways: (1) the detection of unextractable DNA in irradiated cells, and (2) the isolation and identification of specific photoproducts from irradiated cells. Correlations concerning the involvement of protein in UV-induced lethality have been made utilizing (1) action and absorption spectra, (2) the investigation of biological damage not attributable to pyrimidine dimers, (3) correlations of cross-link induction with biological effect under various experimental conditions, and (4) a search for repair processes associated with DNA-protein cross-linking.

This review is organized around the above six categories of experiments that have been done and will first discuss the materials and methods used and then review the results. It will attempt to integrate the findings in terms of present day understanding of the cross-linking process, dimer induction, and molecular repair.

2. MATERIALS AND METHODS

2.1. Extractable DNA

The most popular method for demonstrating DNA to protein cross linkage is based on the DNA extraction procedure of Marmur (1961). For example, Habazin and Han (1970) treated cultured mammalian cells at 60°C for 30 min in 3.3% sodium dodecyl sulfate in a solution of EDTA and 1/3 isotonic saline. The so-called protein fraction is precipitated from this solution by the addition of two volumes of cold 95% ethanol and chilling rapidly. The fraction of DNA extractable can be determined by radioactive counting of DNA from previously labeled cells or by chemical determination of the amount of DNA dissolved in the extract, and the amount in a similar extract after the ethanol-precipitated residue has been treated with a proteolytic enzyme such as trypsin (Alexander and Moroson, 1962). A modification of the method described by Smith (1962b) was used in the recent work of Han *et al.* (1975).

2.2. Photoproduct Detection

Several avenues of approach are available in the search for a nucleoprotein photoproduct. Most work in this area is preliminary, and Varghese and Rauth (1974) sought cysteine-thymine adducts in 6 N HCl-hydrolysed material extracted from irradiated (150-500 J/m^2) mouse L cells, HeLa cells, and Chinese hamster ovary cells. Chromatography of hydrolysates was performed for the purpose of detecting one of the many possible adducts previously identified by Varghese (1973) and Fisher *et al.* (1975). Macromolecular photoproducts have also been sought in mammalian cells exposed to ultraviolet light, and most of the studies are incomplete. Pathak (1972) and his colleagues (Kornhauser *et al.*, 1975) used combined methods of Sepharose 4B chromatography and density gradient ultracentrifugation of chromatin extracts of heavily irradiated (8 × 10^4 J/m^2, λ = 290-360 nm) Guinea pig epidermal cells. Elution profiles and optical density ratios at 260/230 nm were used to identify the fractions. Todd *et al.* (1974) also used Sepharose 4B chromatography as described by Loeb (1968) to examine chromatin prepared by the method of Johns (1971) from irradiated (100-1000 J/m^2) cultured Chinese hamster M3-1F3 cells prelabeled with radioactive thymidine and amino acids. In some experiments a pronase digestion preceded extraction in 2 M NaCl and Sepharose chromatography. This procedure had the paradoxical effect of producing lower molecular weight DNA molecules and intact chromatin proteins. It should be pointed out that a 2 M NaCl extract of chromatin prepared by the method of Johns contains less than 10% of the cells' DNA (Hardin and Todd, unpublished).

Attempts were also made to identify histone-thymine adducts in UV-irradiated culture Chinese hamster cells (Todd *et al.*, 1974). The general experimental schemes involved homogenizing irradiated (and control) cell populations prelabeled with [^{3}H]thymidine, incubating them exhaustively with bovine pancreatic DNAse, and extracting the incubation mixture with cold 0.25% HCl, which would presumably dissolve all of the histones from these cells (Todd, 1968) in addition to the radioactive mononucleotides released by the nuclease. The acid-soluble material was tested in various ways for the presence of thymine covalently bound to protein: thin layer chromatography, polyacrylamide gel electrophoresis of histones, and nitrocellulose filter adsorption.

2.3. Action Spectroscopy

Chu (1965) irradiated cultured Chinese hamster cells and scored various chromosome aberrations as a function of time after irradiation with various fluences at various wavelengths. The results were reported as aberration frequency per unit UV fluence, so that, at low fluence, the numerical values should be proportional

to the action cross section. Todd *et al.* (1968) and Johns and
Rauth (1970) scored colony-forming ability in cultured Chinese
hamster cells and mouse L cells, respectively, after graded exposures to monochromatic light.

2.4. Methods of Observing Non-Dimer Damage

Although their work was not deliberately designed to reveal
non-dimer type damage in the DNA of cultured mammalian cells, Buhl
et al. (1974) performed experiments including those in which endonuclease-sensitive sites were sought by the 5-bromodeoxyuridine
(BrdUrd)-DNA photolysis method, in which repair replication is
allowed to occur in the presence of BrdUrd, the cells are exposed
to 313 nm light, and the extracted DNA is analyzed for the resulting
single-strand breaks by alkaline sucrose gradient centrifugation
(Regan *et al.*, 1971).

Non-photoreactivable lethal damage was estimated using colony-
forming ability as the end-point. By using cells of the marsupial
mammal *Potorous tridactylus* exposed to various fluences of 254 nm
light and various times of "blacklight," Todd *et al.* (1973) were
able to determine photoreactivation kinetics and photoreactivable
sector of lethal damage in this mammalian cell type.

2.5. Cross-Links and Lethality

Cultured human HeLa cells were allowed to incorporate BrdUrd
at a concentration of 5×10^{-7} M prior to exposure to UV light in
order to evaluate the effects of BrdUrd-DNA on the production of
unextractable DNA (assay described in Section 2.1) (Han, 1973).
HeLa-F cells were synchronized by shaking mitotic cells selectively
from culture vessel surfaces and incubating for various periods of
time to establish various positions in the cell cycle at which UV
light was administered. Unextractable DNA assays were made immediately afterward. It was not possible to obtain enough cells in any
single experiment to study a whole cell cycle in this way, so the
results reported were pooled from several experiments with over-
lapping cycle time points (Han *et al.*, 1975).

3. EVIDENCE FOR DNA TO PROTEIN CROSS-LINKS

The direct chemical evidence for the occurrence of cross-links
in UV-irradiated mammalian cells exists in three forms: measurement
of unextractable DNA, identification of chemical photoproducts, and
detection of macromolecular adducts.

3.1. Unextractable DNA

In the first study of unextractable DNA in UV-irradiated mammalian cells (Alexander and Moroson, 1962), a similar method to that
described in Section 2.1. was used, but additional data were obtained
by comparing the unextractable precipitates from salmon sperm heads
and from mouse lymphoma cells. Specifically, it was found that
trypsin treatment released DNA from the lymphoma-cell precipitate
but not from the sperm-head precipitate, because the UV light
apparently caused DNA-DNA links in sperm heads, whereas DNA-protein
links were evident in lymphoma cells.

Figure 1 illustrates the linearity of the loss of extractable
DNA with increasing UV exposure (Habazin and Han, 1970). These
data led to the consideration that 50 J/m^2 of UV fluence rendered
5% of the cells' DNA unextractable. If all of this DNA is assumed
to be linked to an equal mass of proteins of about 15,000 molecular
weight (MW) (Phillips, 1971) then between 10^6 and 10^7 such molecules
would be linked. This corresponds to about the same number of
pyrimidine dimers if 0.1% of the cells' thymine appears in dimers
after the same UV exposure. In terms of cell lethality, exposure
equal to one D_0 (exposure required to reduce survival by a factor of 0.37, measured on the exponential region of survival plots)
would produce between 10^5 and 10^6 cross-links and dimers. The
assumptions used in making these estimations are not necessarily
correct, and the conclusions are relatively insensitive to the nucleohistone structure model chosen (Kornberg, 1974) but very sensitive
to the assumed minimum molecular weight of cross-linked DNA molecules. Lett (This Volume) and Lange *et al*. (1975) have summarized
recent evidence for various sizes of mammalian DNA subunits, and
Table 1 uses these sizes and the data of Habazin and Han (1970) to
estimate the number of cross-links per cell after exposure to
5 J/m^2, a biologically significant UV fluence. The table indicates
that this type of experiment leads to very broad limits on the estimated number of cross-links per cell.

3.2. Photoproducts

Of the thymine adducts identified by Varghese (1974) in UV-
irradiated aqueous solutions of glutathione and thymine, cysteine-
thymine appeared to be the most favorable product to seek after
acid hydrolysis. Experiments designed to seek this adduct chro-
matographically indicated that a compound with the expected chromatographic behavior is produced with 1/2 to 1/3 the efficiency
with which thymine-containing dimers are produced (Varghese and
Rauth, 1974). It was produced with similar efficiencies in mouse
L cells, human HeLa cells, and Chinese hamster ovary cells.
Administration of N-ethylmaleimide might be expected to block the
reactive participating sulfhydryl groups and hence prevent the

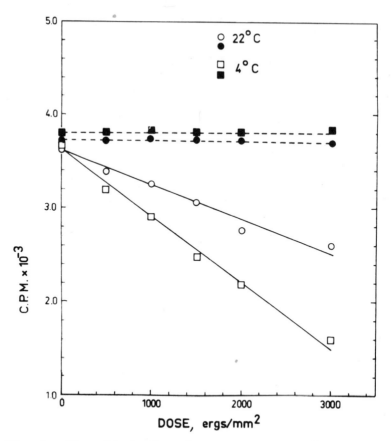

Fig. 1. The effect of various exposures on the amount of [^{14}C]DNA recovered from UV irradiated HeLa cells at 22°C (open circles) and at 4°C (open squares). Closed circles and squares show the amount of radioactivity obtained after trypsin action; closed circles for 22°C exposure and closed squares for 4°C exposure (From Habazin and Han, 1970).

production of the cysteine-thymine product. This treatment reduced the efficiency of production by about one-third (Varghese and Rauth, 1974).

Quantitative measurements indicated that 0.2% of the cells' thymine occurred in this photoproduct following 500 J/m^2 exposure and that this percent was a linear function of exposure. Rough calculations indicate that exposure to 5 J/m^2 would produce 10^5 such products per cell--numerically a little less than the number of pyrimidine dimers expected.

Table 1. Number of DNA to Protein Cross-Links Estimated on the Basis of Different DNA Subunit Sizes (Lett, 1975; Lange *et al.*, 1975) and the Observation that 5 J/m^2 Renders 0.5% of Mammalian Cell DNA Unextractable (Habazin and Han, 1970)

Assumed MW of linked DNA unit	Number of links/cell after 5 J/m^2
5×10^5	6×10^4
6×10^6	5×10^3
1×10^9	30
1.6×10^{10}	2

Other interesting photoproducts have been identified in irradiated relevant model systems. When thymine-labeled DNA and lysine were irradiated together in aqueous solution with light $\lambda > 260$ nm, acid hydrolysates were found to contain a photoproduct that behaved like thymine-lysine adduct (Shetlar and Lin, 1975). This photoadduct was identical in chromatographic behavior to the product of irradiated thymine-lysine mixtures (Schott and Shetlar, 1974). Arginine, cysteine, and cystine also form photoadducts when irradiated with thymine, and, in addition to these amino acids, the aromatic amino acids also form photoadducts with uracil (Schott and Shetlar, 1974; Varghese, 1974; Fisher *et al.*, 1974).

These findings are extremely pertinent to conditions in mammalian (and other eukaryotic) cells for two reasons: first, they suggest that the high concentrations of basic amino acids in histones might facilitate the occurrence of UV-induced histone-DNA covalent bonds, and second, they have implications concerning the possible early evolutionary selection of cells with no uracil in their DNA and no tryptophan in their histones. One might wish, in future research, to seek the presence of repair systems capable of dealing with arginine, lysine, and cysteine adducts to DNA but not capable of dealing with adducts of the aromatic amino acids.

Because the chemical cross-linking of histones to DNA is a known experimental procedure (Kornberg and Thomas, 1974; Hyde and Walker, 1975), it is reasonable to expect histones to be among the adducts to DNA in UV-irradiated mammalian cells. When nuclei of cultured cells are prepared in hypotonic medium (Robbins and Borun, 1963) it is possible to dissolve all of the histones, and possibly some additional nuclear proteins, in a simple 0.25 M HCl extract

(Todd, 1968). In a search for a histone-related photoproduct (Todd
et al., 1974) three analytical procedures were applied to such
extracts of Chinese hamster cells that had been prelabeled with
[^{3}H]thymidine, exposed to UV light, and subsequently treated
exhaustively with DNAse. Thin layer chromatography revealed a
fluence-dependent increase in the amount of HC1-soluble radioactive material that would not migrate in a system designed to
chromatograph nucleotides (Fig. 2). Adsorption of macromolecules
from such extracts on nitrocellulose filters revealed a fluence-
dependent increase in the amount of radioactive material retained
by the filters (Fig. 3). The chromatographic and filter methods
indicated that 2-5% of the thymine in the extract was immobilized
per 50 J/m^2 increment of exposure. These data would suggest that
up to 10^7 thymines per cell would be cross-linked per 5 J/m^2.
This induction rate is higher than those reported in Sections 3.1
and 3.2, and this may be due to the specialized nature of the HC1
extract of the DNAse-treated cells. Subsequent experiments indicated that only 5-10% of the total cellular thymine may be in such
extracts.

Pathak (1972) and coworkers (Kornhauser *et al.*, 1975) used

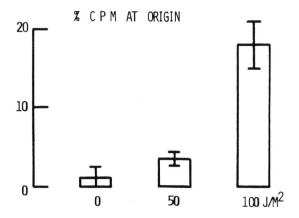

Fig. 2. The effect of UV light exposure on the amount of
acid soluble material from DNAse treated cells that will not
migrate on thin-layer chromatography (Allen and Todd, unpublished).

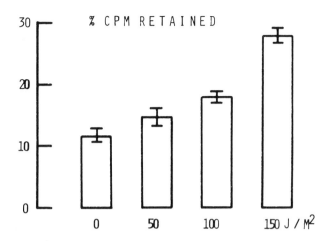

Fig. 3. The effect of UV light exposure on the amount of acid soluble material from DNAse treated cells that will adsorb to nitrocellulose filters (Allen and Todd, unpublished).

chromatography on Sepharose to reveal both low-MW DNA and DNA protein cross-links in Guinea pig epidermis. This method normally separates DNA and chromatin proteins completely (Loeb, 1968), but when chromatin is treated with pronase DNA does not elute early (fraction 38, Fig. 4, left panel) as it does in untreated chromatin extracts, but it elutes at the position of much lower molecular weight molecules, and the highest molecular weight (fraction 80) is found to contain lysine (triangles). There is a large peak of labeled lysine and protein eluting at the normal position (fraction 120). The right hand panel of Fig. 4 illustrates what happens when chromatin is prepared from UV-irradiated cells (100 J/m^2) and treated with pronase before the 2 M NaCl extract is applied to the Sepharose column. The DNA is in a higher molecular weight configuration than in the control cells and the lysine label elutes with much higher molecular weight material. Whether there is more lysine eluting with the DNA could not be determined quantitatively in such an experiment.

Possible interpretations of these observations include the UV cross-linking of postulated DNA peptide "linkers" (Lett, 1975) and the occurrence of protein molecules doubly cross-linked to DNA.

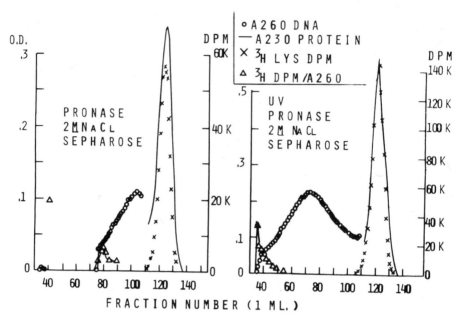

Fig. 4. Left Panel: Elution pattern on Sepharose 4B of 2 M
NaCl extract of chromatin. Cells were prelabeled with [³H]lysine.
Circles show elution profile of DNA, and solid curve shows elution
profile of protein. Right Panel: same as left panel, but chroma-
tin was prepared after cells were exposed to 100 J/m² UV light
(Hardin and Todd, unpublished).

4. DNA TO PROTEIN CROSS-LINKS AND LETHALITY

Events that influence lethality in UV-irradiated bacteria were
found to influence similarly the induction of DNA to protein cross-
links (Smith and O'Leary, 1967). Although correlations are not
demonstrations of cause and effect relationships, negative correlations can be sought to indicate the lack of a cause and effect
relationship. Available information suggests that cross-links and
lethality are related, and three such correlations were demonstrated:
photons absorbed by proteins would be expected to be damaging;
biological damage not attributable to pyrimidine dimers would be
expected; and conditions that modify lethality should also modify
the induction of cross-links.

4.1. Action Spectra

Action spectra have been determined for both chromosome aberrations and for lethality (based on colony-forming ability) of cells

in culture. Although the work was not done with mammalian cells,
it is useful to mention that Zirkle and Uretz (1963) determined the
action spectrum for "paling" of grasshopper neuroblast chromosomes
exposed to UV microbeams having different wavelengths. Paling meant
reduction in refractive index as seen in medium-dark phase contrast
microscopy. Attempts to match action spectra with absorption spectra
of molecules in solution yielded best agreement between the action
spectrum for paling and the absorption spectrum for histone solutions.

Chu (1965) scored aberrations in UV-irradiated cultured Chinese
hamster cells and reported an action spectrum with a broad peak
around 270-280 nm. Qualitative differences were also observed.
At $\lambda > 280$ nm a large fraction of the chromosomes suffered effects
originally called "chromosome demolition". At shorter wavelengths,
UV light induced conventional aberrations. Photons absorbed by
proteins evidently play a role in chromosome damage, and their
effects may differ from those of photons absorbed by nucleic acids.

This situation is repeated in experiments that measure cell
lethality on the basis of colony-forming ability by cultured Chinese
hamster cells (Todd *et al.*, 1968) and mouse L cells (Rauth, 1970).
Figure 5 shows the action spectrum for Chinese hamster cell inactivation, in which the per photon action cross section is derived
from the slopes of survival curves, which are approximately the
same shape at the different wavelengths investigated (Todd *et al.*,
1968). This spectrum has been subsequently corrected for cellular
absorption, which introduces almost no changes, and compared with
absorption spectra of cell components and solutions of macromolecules. The action spectrum best matches the absorption spectrum
of the cell nucleus and of a 2:1 mixture of histones with DNA
(Allen *et al.*, 1971).

4.2. Biological Damage not Attributable to Pyrimidine Dimers

In direct experiments that measure pyrimidine dimers and in
experiments that measure them indirectly by photoreactivation of
cell survival, it is possible to estimate the extent to which
dimers contribute to lethality.

Buhl *et al.* (1973) noticed that normal cultured human cells
and cells from patients with xeroderma pigmentosum were able to
close gaps in newly synthesized DNA after UV irradiation and later
to synthesize DNA in segments of normal length. This observation
means that full-size DNA segments could ultimately be synthesized
even when pyrimidine dimers were still present in the DNA, and it
was taken to imply that some non-dimer damage was responsible for
the early postirradiation interruptions in DNA synthesis. Later
work (Buhl *et al.*, 1974) in which photoreactivating *Potorous* cells

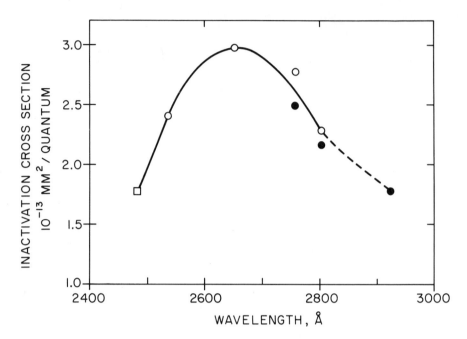

Fig. 5. Wavelength dependence of inactivation cross section calculated from the slopes of survival curves for cultured Chinese hamster cells (From Todd *et al.*, 1968).

were studied by the bromouracil photolysis method (Regan *et al.*, 1971) indicated that dimers do indeed interrupt postirradiation DNA synthesis, but a similar effect of non-dimer lesions could not be ruled out.

The cells of marsupial mammals, which possess photoreactivating enzyme (Cook and Regan, 1969), were tested for their ability to photoreactivate colony-forming ability (Todd *et al.*, 1973). Following a nearly saturating exposure to photoreactivating light, it was found that twice the 254 nm exposure was needed for equivalent cell killing of *Potorous tridactylus* cells in culture (Fig. 6). In these cells there is always some lethal damage not photoreactivated, and it is presumed, at least in part, that such damage is not in the form of pyrimidine dimers.

4.3.   Correlations with Cell Lethality

Two categories of experiments were designed to seek positive or negative correlations between DNA to protein cross-linking and cell lethality, namely, the effects of BrdUrd substitution and cell

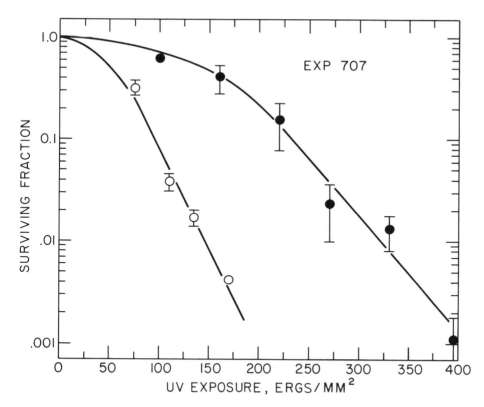

Fig. 6. Effect of 30 min of photoreactivating light on UV survival of PtK-2 rat kangaroo cells. Normal survival curve is plotted with open circles, and survival curve with photoreactivation is plotted with closed circles (From Todd *et al.*, 1973).

cycle age on cell lethality and DNA extractability.

On the basis of the observation that BrdUrd incorporated into DNA by cultured mammalian cells increases their sensitivity to UV radiation (Djordjevic and Szybalski, 1960; Djordjevic and Djordjevic, 1965), experiments were performed in which HeLa cells incorporated this drug into their DNA prior to UV irradiation and were subjected to cross-link assay (Han, 1973). The results, shown in Fig. 7, clearly indicate that cells with BrdUrd-DNA were more sensitive to cross-link induction.

In nearly all cells tested, maximum UV sensitivity occurs near the middle of S phase (Djordjevic and Djordjevic, 1965; Djordjevic and Tolmach, 1967; Domon and Rauth, 1969; Erikson and Szybalski, 1963; Han and Sinclair, 1968; Han, 1973; Rauth and

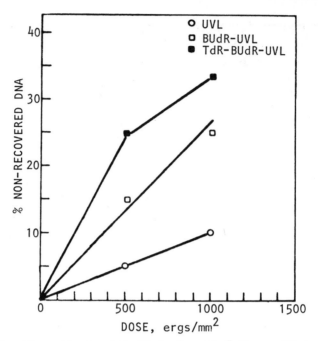

Fig. 7.   The effect of BrdUrd, 5×10^{-7} M, on UV-induced DNA to protein cross-linking in HeLa-F cells (From Han, 1973).

Whitmore, 1966; Sinclair and Morton, 1965; Williams and Little, 1971, 1972). Han *et al.* (1975) therefore studied possible varia- tions in the amount of extractable DNA of UV-irradiated synchronized HeLa cells and how they correlate with survival. Figure 8 summarizes the results of this study and shows that in these cells minimum extractability of DNA coincides with the same time that cell survi- val is at a minimum.

The cells were exposed to 300 J/m^2 at the times shown after synchronization and the DNA was extracted immediately after irradia- tion. For reasons mentioned previously, to obtain the age response, data from several experiments were collected and the different symbols in Fig. 7 indicate different experiments in which data were obtained. Each symbol on the graph represents the mean value for at least two, but not more than five, samples per point in a given experiment. These data show that cells are more sensitive to DNA-protein cross-linking between 12 and 15 h after synchroniza- tion, corresponding to the early and middle parts of the DNA syn- thetic phase. Cells are less sensitive to this damage at the beginning and at the end of the cycle. The general pattern of response indicates a similar UV sensitivity of G_1 and G_2 cells as measured by DNA-protein cross-linking (Han *et al.*, 1975).

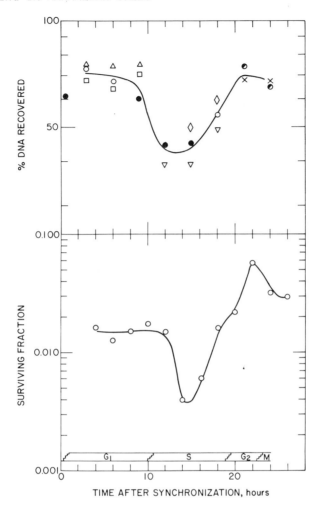

Fig. 8. Upper plot: Percent of DNA recovered after exposure
to 300 J/m^2 at different times after synchronization of HeLa-F
cells. Lower plot: Age response for survival based on colony
formation after exposure of HeLa-F cells to 21.6 J/m^2 (From Han
et al., 1975).

The fluence response curves determined at selected cell ages
(Fig. 9) show the highest sensitivity of S cells for DNA-protein
cross-linking, much higher than for cells of any other age. These
curves further suggest that production of DNA-protein cross-linking
is not very much different in G_1, G_2 and M cells and quite high
fluences have to be delivered to observe significant amounts of
cross-linking. For cells in the DNA synthetic phase, significant

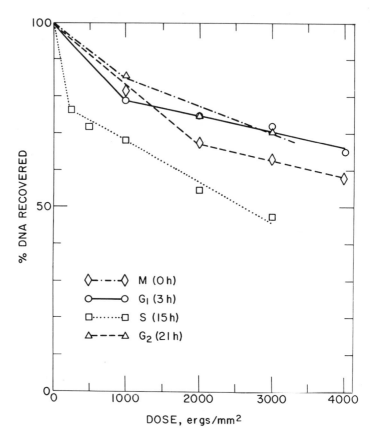

Fig. 9. Percent of DNA recovered as a function of UV light exposure at different times after synchronization of HeLa-F cells (From Han *et al.*, 1975).

amounts of cross-links are induced even after exposure to 25 J/m^2, which reduces the survival of mid-S cells to approximately 0.008. It is evident, therefore, that a significant decrease in the amount of DNA recovered is observed following exposure to fluences for which effective survival can be determined (Han *et al.*, 1975).

All the curves in Fig. 9 are biphasic; slopes decrease in all curves when 20-30% of the DNA becomes unextractable. It would be of considerable interest to obtain cross-linking kinetics at lower UV fluences than those represented in Fig. 9. It is possible that the low fluences first remove the DNA that is in the higher molecular weight aggregates (as discussed in Section 3.1 and Table 1) and that the aggregation states of DNA change with age in the cell cycle.

4.4. Repair of DNA to Protein Cross-Links

Despite a number of attempts to demonstrate the existence of repair of DNA to protein cross-links, it is not known whether they are repaired. Pathak (1972) reported briefly on evidence that the chromatographic behavior on Sepharose 4B columns of chromatin extracts from Guinea pig epidermis returns to normal 60 min after exposure to 8×10^4 J/m^2, whereas chromatin prepared immediately after irradiation behaved as if it contained DNA to protein cross-links. No other workers seeking evidence for repair of this lesion have reported positive results. An early split-fluence experiment (Todd *et al.*, 1969) showed no evidence for split-fluence recovery by cultured Chinese hamster cells between exposures to light of 280 nm. This result cannot be cited as absolute negative evidence, however, as it had previously been reported that asynchronous mouse cells did not recover between 254 nm light exposures (Han *et al.*, 1964), and it has since been shown (Domon and Rauth, 1973; Todd, 1973) that these experiments did not allow sufficient time for UV split-fluence recovery to occur.

Various attempts at macromolecular photoproduct quantitation (Todd *et al.*, 1974) did not reveal evidence for repair of cross-links, and studies of DNA extractability as a function of time after exposure to 254 nm light have not revealed any postirradiation increases for up to 10 h (Han *et al.*, 1975). This result is shown in Fig. 10. It was not possible to extend measurements to later times due to the loss of irradiated cells (Habazin and Han, 1970). That this damage is not repaired has also been reported by Smets and Cornelis (1971) for human kidney T cells. Thus, there is very little published evidence that DNA to protein cross-links are repaired.

5. CONCLUSIONS

Searches for photoproducts attributable to UV-induced DNA to protein cross-links have been partially successful (Varghese and Rauth, 1974; Todd *et al.*, 1974), but positive identifications of such photoproducts remain to be made. There is no proof that histones are linked to DNA.

There is sufficient evidence that proteins are involved in the UV response of mammalian cells. Todd and co-workers (1968) with Chinese hamster cells, and Rauth (1970) with L cells showed that exposures required to reduce survival to a given level are a firm function of wavelength, and the general patterns of the two action spectra are the same, both having a broad peak in the region of 270 nm, suggesting that DNA and protein are involved.

The incorporation of BrdUrd in the DNA of mammalian cells

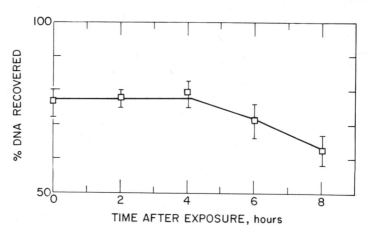

Fig. 10.   Percent of DNA recovered as a function of time after exposure from HeLa-F cells exposed to 50 J/m^2 15 h after synchronization (mid S phase).   Bars indicate standard error of the mean (From Han *et al.*, 1975).

significantly enhances the amount of DNA cross-linked to proteins (Smets and Cornelis, 1971; Han, 1973).   There is about a 3 to 5-fold increase in cross-linking when cells are grown for two generations in the presence of 5×10^{-7} M BrdUrd.   This drug is a very effective sensitizer of mammalian cells in the cases of both ionizing and UV irradiation (Djordjevic and Szybalski, 1960).

The cell cycle dependent fluctuations in the yield of DNA cross-linked to proteins are almost identical to the changes in cell survival throughout the cycle.   There are some other observations and results that indicate the importance of this damage in survival of UV-irradiated mammalian cells.

That formation of cross-links between DNA and proteins could contribute significantly to the killing of cells by UV radiation has been suggested by Alexander and Moroson (1962) as well as the possibility that in mammalian cells particular proteins may be involved in the expression of damage to DNA (Han and Sinclair, 1969).

The formation of cross-links between DNA and enzymes or other proteins (histones) in its vicinity could prevent normal DNA repair processes.   Consequently, damage would become irreparable and result in cell death.

Acknowledgments. We wish to acknowledge the many co-authors, co-workers and colleagues who participated in the performance of the research upon which this review is based, especially those who are sharing some previously unpublished data, Blair S. Allen, University of California; Carter B. Schroy, Alex Czeto, The Pennsylvania State University; Julia M. Hardin, George H. Shepherd, Phyllis C. Sanders, Los Alamos Scientific Laboratory; Vlasta Habazin, Institute for Medical Research, Zagreb; Mladen Korbelik and Jasna Ban, Central Institute for Tumors and Allied Diseases, Zagreb. In addition, helpful advice was provided by Drs. A.J. Varghese, A.M. Rauth, M.A. Pathak, and K.C. Smith. The authors wish to acknowledge partial support by the U.S. Energy Research and Development Administration.

References

Alexander, P., and Moroson, H., 1962, Cross-linking of deoxyribonucleic acid to protein following ultra-violet irradiation of different cells, *Nature* 194:882-883.

Allen, B.S., Czeto, A., and Todd, P., 1972, Comparison of ultraviolet light inactivation spectrum and absorption spectra of mammalian cells, *Biophys. Soc. Abstr.* 12:12a.

Buhl, S.N., Setlow, R.B., and Regan, J.D., 1973, Recovery of the ability to synthesize DNA in segments of normal size at long times after ultraviolet irradiation of human cells, *Biophys. J.* 13:1265-1275.

Buhl, S.N., Setlow, R.B., and Regan, J.D., 1974, DNA repair in *Potorous tridactylus*, *Biophys. J.* 14:791-803.

Chu, E.H.Y., 1965, Effects of ultraviolet radiation on mammalian cells. I. Induction of chromosome aberrations, *Mutat. Res.* 2:75-94.

Cook, J.S., and Regan, J.D., 1969, Photoreactivation and photoreactivating enzyme activity in an order of mammals (Marsupialia), *Nature* 223:1066-1067.

Djordjevic, B., and Djordjevic, O., 1965, Survival and chromosomal aberrations in a synchronized mammalian cell culture treated with 5-bromodeoxyuridine and irradiated by ultraviolet light, *in* "Progress in Biochemical Pharmacology" (R. Paoletti and R. Vertua, eds.), Vol. I, pp. 71-77, Butterworths, Washington.

Djordjevic, B., and Szybalski, W., 1960, Genetics of human cell lines. III. Incorporation of 5-bromo, 5-iododeoxyuridine into the deoxyribonucleic acid of human cells and its effect on radiation sensitivity, *J. Exp. Med.* 112:509-531.

Djordjevic, B., and Tolmach, L.J., 1967, Responses of synchronous populations of HeLa cells to ultraviolet irradiation at selected stages of the generation cycle, *Radiat. Res.* 32:327-346.

Domon, M., and Rauth, A.M., 1969, Ultraviolet irradiation of mouse L cells: Effects on cells in the DNA synthesis phase, *Radiat. Res.* 40:414-429.

Domon, M., and Rauth, A.M., 1973, Cell cycle specific recovery
    from fractionated exposures of ultraviolet light, *Radiat.*
    Res. 55:81-92.
Erikson, R.L., and Szybalski, W., 1963, Molecular radiobiology of
    human cell lines. IV. Variation in ultraviolet and X-ray
    sensitivity during the division cycle, *Radiat. Res.* 18:200-212.
Fisher, G.J., Varghese, A.J., and Johns, H.E., 1974, Ultraviolet-
    induced reactions of thymine and uracil in the presence of
    cysteine, *Photochem. Photobiol.* 20:109-120.
Habazin, V., and Han, A., 1970, Ultraviolet light-induced DNA-to-
    protein cross-linking in HeLa cells, *Int. J. Radiat. Biol.*
    17:569-575.
Han, A., 1973, Cell cycle dependent effects of ultraviolet light
    in mammalian cells, *Stud. Biophys.* 36/37:127-137.
Han, A., Korbelik, M., and Ban, J., 1975, DNA-to-protein cross-
    linking in synchronized HeLa cells exposed to ultraviolet
    light, *Int. J. Radiat. Biol.* 27:63-74.
Han, A., Miletic, B., and Petrovic, D., 1965, The action of ultra-
    violet light on repair of X-ray damage in L-cells grown in
    culture, *Int. J. Radiat. Biol.* 8:187-190.
Han, A., and Sinclair, W.K., 1969, Sensitivity of synchronized
    Chinese hamster cells to ultraviolet light, *Biophys. J.* 9:
    1171-1192.
Hyde, J.E., and Walker, I.O., 1975, Covalent cross-linking of
    histones in chromatin, *FEBS Lett.* 50:150-158.
Johns, E.W., 1971, The preparation and characterization of histones,
    in "Histones and Nucleohistones" (D.M.P. Phillips, ed.), pp.
    2-36, Plenum Press, London.
Kornberg, R.D., 1974, Chromatin structure: A repeating unit of
    histones and DNA, *Science* 184:868-871.
Kornberg, R.D., and Thomas, J.O., 1974, Chromatin structure: Oligo-
    mers of the histones, *Science* 184:865-868.
Kornhauser, A., Pathak, M.A., Zimmerman, E., and Szabo, G., 1975,
    The *in vivo* effect of UV irradiation on epidermal chromatin.
    Abstr. Int. Symp. "Protein and Other Adducts to DNA: Their
    Significance to Aging, Carcinogenesis, and Radiation Biology,"
    Williamsburg, Virginia, May 2-6, 1975.
Lange, C.S., Clark, R.W., and Mitchell, P., 1975, Demonstration of
    the protein linkages between DNA subunits and a model for the
    organization of DNA in the mammalian chromosome. Abstr. Int.
    Symp. "Protein and Other Adducts to DNA: Their Significance
    to Aging, Carcinogenesis, and Radiation Biology," Williams-
    burg, Virginia, May 2-6, 1975.
Loeb, J.E., 1968, Gel filtration of deoxyribonucleoprotein on
    agarose, *Biochim. Biophys. Acta* 157:424-426.
Marmur, J., 1961, A procedure for the isolation of deoxyribonucleic
    acid from micro-organisms, *J. Mol. Biol.* 3:208-218.
Pathak, M.A., and Zimmerman, E., 1972, Biochemical changes in
    epidermal nucleic acids following U.V. irradiation, VI Int.
    Congr. Photobiol. Abstr. No. 044.

Phillips, D.M.P. (ed.), 1971, "Histones and Nucleohistones," Plenum
    Press, New York.
Rauth, A.M., 1970, Effects of ultraviolet light on mammalian cells
    in culture, *Curr. Topics Radiat. Res.* 6:197-248.
Rauth, A.M., and Whitmore, G.F., 1966, The survival of synchronized
    L cells after ultraviolet irradiation, *Radiat. Res.* 28:84-95.
Regan, J.D., Setlow, R.B., and Ley, R.D., 1971, Normal and defective
    repair of damaged DNA in human cells: A sensitive assay
    utilizing the photolysis of bromodeoxyuridine, *Proc. Nat.
    Acad. Sci. USA* 68:708-712.
Robbins, E., and Borun, T.W., 1967, The cytoplasmic synthesis of
    histones in HeLa cells and its temporal relation to DNA repli-
    cation, *Proc. Nat. Acad. Sci. USA* 57:409-416.
Ryabchenko, N.I., Slobovskaya, M.V., Ivannik, B.P., and Yaskevich,
    A.G., 1965, UV cross-links DNA proteins, Tezisy Dokl. Nauchn,
    Sessi i, Inst. Med. Radiol. Akad. Nauk SSSR, ist Sb, Obninsk,
    pp. 24-26.
Schott, H.N., and Shetlar, M.D., 1974, Photochemical addition of
    amino acids to thymine, *Biochem. Biophys. Res. Commun.* 59:
    1112-1116.
Shetlar, M.D., and Lin, E.T., 1975, Formation of thymine-lysine
    adducts in irradiated DNA-lysine systems, Amer. Soc. Photobiol.,
    Abstr. p. 115.
Sinclair, W.K., and Morton, R.A., 1965, X-ray and ultraviolet sensi-
    tivity of synchronized Chinese hamster cells at various stages
    of the cell cycle, *Biophys. J.* 5:1-25.
Sklobovskaya, M.V., and Ryabchenko, N.I., 1970a, Snizheniye vykhoda
    DNK deproteinatziyi UF-ili gamma-obluchennykh rastvorov desoxy-
    nukleoproteida. Soobshchenie I. Zavisimost' velichiny effecta
    ot polnot' kompleksirovaniya DNK byelkom, *Radiobiologiya* 10:
    14-18.
Sklobovskaya, M.V., and Ryabchenko, N.I., 1970b, Snizheniye vykhoda
    DNK deproteinatziyi UF-ili gamma-obluchennykh rastvorov desoxy-
    nukleoproteida. II. Nekotorye voprosy formirovaniya povrezh-
    dyeniya, *Radiobiologiya* 10:332-337.
Smets, L.A., and Cornelis, J.J., 1971, Repairable and irrepairable
    damage in 5-bromouracil-substituted DNA exposed to ultraviolet
    radiation, *Int. J. Radiat. Biol.* 19:445-457.
Smith, K.C., 1962a, A chemical basis for the sensitization of
    bacteria to ultraviolet light by incorporated bromouracil,
    Biochem. Biophys. Res. Commun. 6:458-463.
Smith, K.C., 1962b, Dose dependent decrease in extractability of
    DNA from bacteria following irradiation with ultraviolet light
    or with visible light plus dye, *Biochem. Biophys. Res. Commun.*
    8:157-163.
Smith, K.C., 1964a, Photochemistry of the nucleic acids, *in* "Photo-
    physiology" (A.C. Giese, ed.), Vol. 2, pp. 329-388, Academic
    Press, New York.

Smith, K.C., 1964b, The photochemical interaction of deoxyribonu-
    cleic acid and protein *in vivo* and its biological importance,
    Photochem. Photobiol. 3:415-427.
Smith, K.C., 1967, Biologically important damage to DNA by photo-
    products other than cyclobutane-type thymine dimers, *in*
    "Radiation Research" (G. Silini, ed.), pp. 756-770, North-
    Holland Publishing Co., Amsterdam.
Smith, K.C., and O'Leary, M.E., 1967, Photoinduced DNA-protein
    cross-links and bacterial killing: A correlation at low
    temperatures, *Science* 155:1024-1026.
Steward, D.L., and Humphrey, R.M., 1966, Induction of thymine dimers
    in synchronous populations of Chinese hamster cells, *Nature*
    212:298-300.
Todd, P., 1968, Nuclear protein thiol in cultured mammalian cells,
    Biochem. J. 109:25P.
Todd, P., 1973, Fractionated ultraviolet light irradiation of
    cultured Chinese hamster cells, *Radiat. Res.* 55:93-100.
Todd, P., Allen, B.S., and Hardin, J.M., 1974, A search for a
    nucleoprotein photoproduct in mammalian cells exposed to
    ultraviolet light, Amer. Soc. Photobiol., Abstr. p. 66.
Todd, P., Allen, B.S., and Schroy, C.B., 1972, What ultraviolet-
    induced molecular lesions cause lethality in mammalian cells?
    VI Int. Congr. Photobiol. Abstr. No. 133.
Todd, P., Coohill, T.P., Hellewell, A.B., and Mahoney, J.A., 1969,
    Postirradiation properties of cultured Chinese hamster cells
    exposed to ultraviolet light, *Radiat. Res.* 38:321-339.
Todd, P., Coohill, T.P., and Mahoney, J.A., 1968, Response of
    cultured Chinese hamster cells to ultraviolet light of
    different wavelengths, *Radiat. Res.* 35:390-400.
Todd, P., Schroy, C.B., and Lebed, M.R., 1973, Post-irradiation
    effects of photoreactivating light and caffeine on cultured
    marsupial cells exposed to ultraviolet light, *Photochem.
    Photobiol.* 18:433-436.
Varghese, A.J., 1973, Properties of photoaddition products of thy-
    mine and cysteine, *Biochemistry* 12:2725-2730.
Varghese, A.J., 1974, Photochemical addition of glutathione to
    uracil and thymine, *Photochem. Photobiol.* 20:339-343.
Varghese, A.J., and Rauth, A.M., 1974, Evidence for the addition of
    sulfhydryl compounds to thymine in UV-irradiated mammalian
    cells. Amer. Soc. Photobiol., Abstr. p. 65.
Williams, J.R., and Little, J.B., 1971, Correlation of intracellular
    UV-dose absorption with survival in cultured human cells,
    Radiat. Res. 47:248-249.
Williams, J.R., and Little, J.B., 1972, Relationship of cell size
    and cell conformation to the UVL survival of synchronous
    cultures of human cells, *Radiat. Res.* 51:450.
Zirkle, R.E., and Uretz, R.B., 1963, Action spectrum for paling
    (decrease in refractive index) of ultraviolet-irradiated
    chromosome segments, *Proc. Nat. Acad. Sci. USA* 49:45-52.

ROLE OF PROTEIN IN THE INACTIVATION OF VIRUSES BY ULTRAVIOLET

RADIATION

Milton P. Gordon

Department of Biochemistry, University of Washington,

Seattle, Washington 98195

1. INTRODUCTION

The capsomers of viruses contain proteins, lipids, and carbo-hydrates. The components of the capsomer frequently participate in the initial stages of the infectious process and in some in-stances, furnish enzymatic activity vitally needed for viral repli-cation. The capsomers also serve to protect the viral nucleic acid from inactivation by a variety of enzymatic and physical agencies such as actinic radiation.

The purpose of this paper is to review the current knowledge of the action of light on viruses. The three areas which will be considered are: 1.) the introduction of protein-nucleic acid cross-links in viruses by light, 2.) the modification of the types of photochemical lesions introduced into nucleic acids by the presence of capsomer proteins, and 3.) the protection and sensi-tization of viral nucleic acids by proteins.

2. THE INTRODUCTION OF PROTEIN-NUCLEIC ACID CROSS-LINKS IN VIRUSES BY UV LIGHT

When tobacco mosaic virus (common strain, TMV-U1) is irradiated with 254 nm radiation in the range of from 1 to 14 lethal hits, the capsomer protein is altered in such a fashion that 1% sodium dodecyl sulfate at 50°C is not able to remove all of the protein subunits. A one-to-one correspondence was found between lethal hits and the bound subunits (Goddard *et al.*, 1966) (Fig. 1). However, a similar relationship between dose and bound subunits was found for the U2 strain of TMV in which the biological activity is destroyed at much lower UV doses (Streeter and Gordon, 1968) (Fig. 2). The exact nature of the protein-RNA linkage is still unknown. The subunits can be removed by 66% acetic acid, guanidine hydrochloride, or phenol so that if covalent bonds are present, they are readily broken. With larger doses of radiation, the particles become more heat labile (Oster and McLaren, 1950) and protein subunits are lost (McLaren and Kleczkowski, 1967). With continued irradiation, a complete breakdown of the structure occurs, the solution turns a dirty yellow, and a degraded nucleic acid is liberated (Zech, 1961). In contrast to the above reports, B. Singer (personal communication) had indications of the UV-induced covalent linkage of TMV capsomer protein to RNA in U1, U2, and HR strains of TMV. She used reconstituted virus containing [^{3}H]RNA and [^{14}C]protein. After UV irradiation, [^{14}C] label became associated with [^{3}H] label.

The *in vivo* uncoating of UV-irradiated TMV has been reported by Hayashi *et al.* (1969). When [^{35}S] labeled TMV or UV-irradiated [^{35}S] TMV irradiated to 0.01% residual infectivity was used to infect tobacco leaves, the sedimentation patterns of acid-precipitable [^{35}S] counts were identical. Since the authors estimated that about 25% of the protein was removed from the virus, the results indicate, with a good deal of uncertainty, no gross differences in the *in vivo* uncoating of the native and UV-treated viruses.

Polio virus also undergoes a loss of RNA upon UV irradiation (Katagiri *et al.*, 1967). As determined by sucrose density gradient centrifugation and electron microscopy, there are four stages in the morphological changes undergone by irradiated polio virus. The native 160S RNA-containing virus particles finally become 80S empty shells and the antigenicity of the protein changes. The native virions are RNase resistant, while intermediate stages are RNase sensitive.

In contrast to polio virus, mengovirus (another RNA picornavirus) does not form any empty capsids (Miller and Plagemann, 1974). During the initial stages of irradiation, 1.7 uracil dimers are formed per biological hit. With further irradiation, the

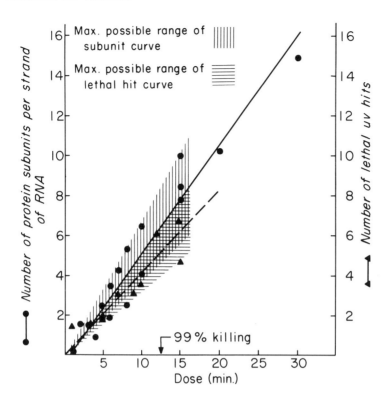

Fig. 1.   Protein subunits bound and lethal hits produced by
UV irradiation of TMV.   A one-to-one correspondence between lethal
hits and bound subunits is indicated (From Goddard *et al.*, 1966).

hemagglutination activity of the virus decreases and the appearance
of the particles in the electron microscope changes. The RNA also
becomes accessible to RNase and extractable by sodium dodecyl sulfate. With further irradiation, free protein particles appear,
some of which appear to be covalently cross-linked viral proteins.
The intact viral RNA and 30% of the capside proteins appeared as
80S ribonucleoprotein particles. Viral RNA prepared from the
extensively irradiated particles by sodium dodecyl sulfate treatment contained 1% of the viral protein in a form of heterogeneous
polypeptides probably covalently attached to the RNA. The RNA
containing the polypeptides had a greatly increased sedimentation
rate (41S versus 34S for native RNA). Nakashima and Konigsberg

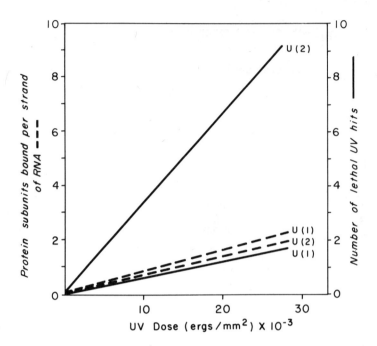

Fig. 2. Protein subunits bound and lethal hits produced by UV
irradiation at 254 nm of [^{35}S] labeled U1 TMV and [^{35}S] labeled U2
TMV. Both TMV strains were irradiated under the same conditions
and treated with 1% sodium dodecyl sulfate. Although the number of
subunits bound is identical in both strains of TMV, there is a gross
disparity between bound subunits and lethal hits in the U2 strain
(From Streeter and Gordon, 1968).

(1975) have found that 254 nm radiation causes the covalent attachment of the gene 5 protein of bacteriophage Fd to the single-stranded
circular DNA of this virus. The bond seems to consist of the reaction of cysteine 33 with a thymine residue.

Recently, Simukova and Budowsky (1974) have taken advantage
of the observation that saturation of the 5-6 double bond in cytosine increases the rate of reaction at carbon 4 so that the amino
group can be replaced by a variety of weak nucleophiles (Janion
and Shugar, 1967; Small and Gordon, 1968). Photochemical hydra-
tion of the 5-6 double bond would thus be expected to increase the
rate of reaction of "reactive" cytosine residues with nucleophilic
groups on proteins resulting in the formation of covalent

polynucleotide protein cross-links (Fig. 3). When the DNA-containing bacteriophage Sd was UV irradiated and DNA prepared by heat disruption, the viscosity of the liberated DNA was found to be decreased as a function of the absorbed energy. Protein was found to be associated with the DNA, as determined by the binding of [^{35}S]. Pronase treatment caused an increase in the viscosity of the DNA almost to control levels (dotted lines in Fig. 3). The results are interpreted as the UV-induced covalent linkage of protein to phage DNA resulting in the partial retention of the dense packing of DNA found within the phage head. Removal of the protein with pronase allows the DNA to express its native viscosity (Simukova and Budowsky, 1974). It has also been found that UV light and bisulfite can induce the formation of RNA-protein cross-links in MS2 bacteriophage (Turchinsky et al., 1974). Both of these treatments lead to the substitution of the amino group of a cytosine by a lysine as determined by the isolation of ε-N-(2-ketopyrimidyl-4)-lysine (Simukova et al., 1975; Turchinsky et al., 1975). Yamada et al. (1973) have found that with a dose that reduced the infectivity of MS2 to 0.01% of controls, the absorption to bacterial hosts was unaffected, while the penetration of viral RNA was reduced to 10% of controls. The possible covalent linkage of RNA to capsomer or A protein was not investigated in these experiments; indeed, such linkage has not been detected thus far in irradiated RNA coli phages. It appears that these procedures offer interesting possibilities for the exploration of nucleic acid-capsomer protein interactions in both DNA and RNA virions.

The formation of protein-DNA cross-links has been observed as a result of ^{60}Co gamma irradiation of T1 and T7 coliphages (Bohne et al., 1970; Hawkins and Ginsberg, 1971; Hawkins, 1975). In the case of T1, it was estimated that per inactivated phage 3.5 single-strand breaks, 0.17 double-strand breaks, 0.03 DNA-DNA cross-links, and 0.06 DNA-protein cross-links occurred.

3. THE MODIFICATION OF THE TYPES OF PHOTOCHEMICAL LESIONS INTRODUCED INTO NUCLEIC ACIDS BY THE PRESENCE OF CAPSOMER PROTEINS

In tobacco mosaic virus (U1 strain) the RNA is rigidly held in a hyperchromic configuration by the capsomer protein subunits (Bonhoffer and Schachman, 1960). In the depicted configuration, base-base interaction is minimal (Caspar, 1963) and the lack of base-base interaction is reflected by the lack of formation of photoreversible pyrimidine cyclobutane dimers upon UV irradiation of the intact virus (Tao et al., 1969; Carpenter and Kleczkowski, 1969; B. Singer, personal communication). The presence of the capsomer protein prevents the formation of photoreactivable lesions, and no photoreactivation is observed even if the RNA is subsequently freed of protein by phenol extraction (Goddard et al., 1966; Kleczkowski, 1971). Some ill defined types of dimeric materials

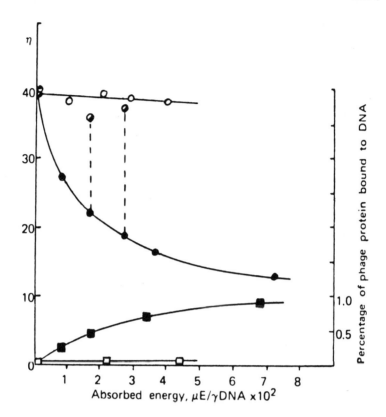

Fig. 3.   The effect of UV irradiation of bacteriophage Sd on
the viscosity of the solutions of heat-disrupted virions (circles)
and on the amount of [^{35}S]protein bound to DNA after phenol deproteinization of phages (squares). Open symbols, phage disrupted
before irradiation; closed symbols, phage disrupted after irradiation; half-closed symbols, phage disrupted after irradiation and
treated with pronase. The low viscosity of the DNA obtained from
irradiated intact phage is interpreted as the partial retention of
the dense packing of DNA within the phage head caused by DNA-
protein cross-links (From Simukova and Budowsky, 1974).

are formed, but their chemical nature has remained illusive. A
similar behavior has been observed in the case of the RNA of intact
coliphage R17 (Remsen *et al.*, 1970), where again only pyrimidine
photohydrates were formed upon UV irradiation. In both cases,
irradiation of the free viral RNAs in solution resulted in the
formation of both pyrimidine photohydrates and cyclobutane dimers.
It is expected that further investigations of this type will reveal

additional cases of the directive effect of capsomer-induced configurations on the course of photochemical alterations of viral nucleic
acids.

The geometric constraints imposed upon single-stranded circular
DNA molecules can influence the cross-links introduced into the
nucleic acid by UV irradiation. ΦX174 and M13 both contain single-
stranded circular DNA molecules. However, ΦX174 is a spherical
virion while M13 is filamentous. Upon irradiation of each of these
virus particles, cross-links are introduced into the constituent
DNAs. The cross-links in ΦX174 DNA hold the molecule in a condensed
structure, as would be expected from the tightly coiled packaging
of the DNA in a spherical virus (Fig. 4). The cross-links in M13
appear to be the result of side-to-side association of a circular
DNA as would be expected from the filamentous shape of the virion
(Fig. 5). The exact chemical nature of the cross-links could not
be determined, but they do not appear to be DNA-protein linkages.
The cross-links in ΦX174 account for about 5% of the lethal UV-
induced damage (Francke and Ray, 1972).

Another interesting example where the protein of a virus has
an effect on the nature of photoproducts is seen in raspberry
ringspot virus (Mayo *et al.*, 1973). This virus sediments as three
major components: T, M, and B. The M particle has one type of
RNA of molecular weight 1.4×10^6 daltons, while the B components
had RNAs of molecular weight 1.4×10^6 and 2.4×10^6 daltons. When
separated B components were irradiated, gel electrophoresis indicated that the RNA of 1.4×10^6 daltons had formed dimeric molecules.
The dimers of the RNA were only produced when the RNA was within
the B virion. Thus, these results indicated that two molecules of
the smaller RNA are present within one type of the B virion, and
that they become linked together by radiation. The cross-links
were pronase resistant and probably did not contain protein. These
results as well as those obtained by Francke and Ray (1972) for
ΦX174 and M13 indicate that the photochemical behavior of nucleic
acids can yield information concerning the composition as well as
the geometry of virus particles.

4.   THE PROTECTION AND SENSITIZATION OF VIRAL NUCLEIC ACIDS BY
CAPSOMER PROTEINS

The capsomer proteins of a number of viruses protect the viral
nucleic acid from inactivation by UV irradiation, in addition to
modifying the course of the introduction of photochemical lesions.
The quantum yield for inactivation of the biological activity of
the U1 strain of TMV is about two orders of magnitude smaller than
that for the free RNA using 254 nm radiation (McLaren and Moring-
Claesson, 1961; Rushizky *et al.*, 1960; McCleary and Gordon, 1973).

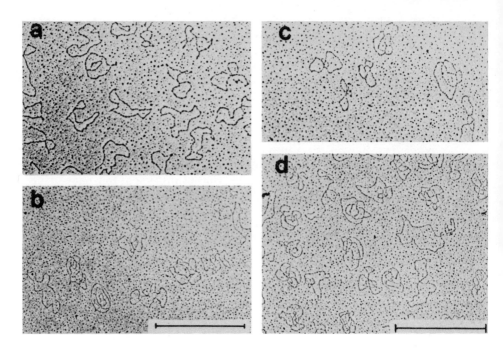

Fig. 4. Electron photomicrographs of DNA from UV irradiated
X174 phage. Frames (a) through (d) indicate fractions of DNA with
increasing sedimentation velocity in alkaline sucrose gradients.
The material in frame (a) sedimented at about the same rate as DNA
from unirradiated ⏀X174. The bar indicates 1 μm. The appearance
of cross-links reflects the packing of DNA in a spherical virion
(From Francke and Ray, 1972).

When the capsomer protein of the U1 strain aggregates around the
RNA of the UV-sensitive strain, TMV-U2 (Fig. 6), or around potato
virus X-RNA (Fig. 7), the UV sensitivities of the resulting pheno-
typically mixed particles are very similar to the sensitivity of
the U1 strain (Streeter and Gordon, 1967; Breck and Gordon, 1970;
McCleary and Gordon, 1973). The action spectrum of the U1 strain
deviates quite markedly from that of the free nucleic acid. The
protein appears to strongly protect the encapsulated RNA at 280
and 254 nm, but not at 230 nm (Kleczkowski and McLaren, 1967).
The protein of the U2 strain also protects encapsulated U1 or U2
RNA to the same extent, although the degree of protection is less
than afforded by U1 protein.

The quantum yields for the inactivation of PVX, a long filamentous virus, at a number of wavelengths have been determined,

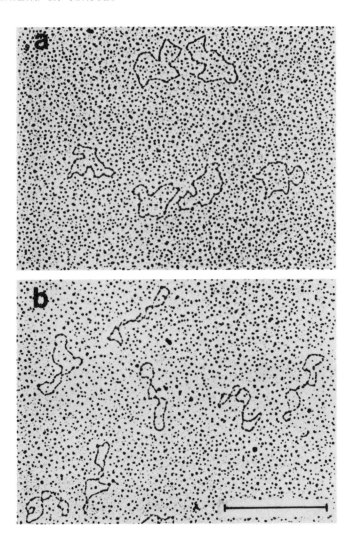

Fig. 5. Electron photomicrograph of (a) unirradiated M13 DNA and (b) DNA from phage irradiated to a survival of 0.13%. Bar indicates 1 μm. The cross-links reflect the packing of the DNA in a long filamentous virion (From Francke and Ray, 1972).

and they are about 5- to 20-times smaller than those found for free PVX-RNA, indicating some degree of protection, although less than in the case of TMV. In PVX, the RNA is apparently not held as rigidly as in TMV. Intraviral PVX-RNA forms dimers upon irradiation. The virus can undergo photoreactivation, and the intact

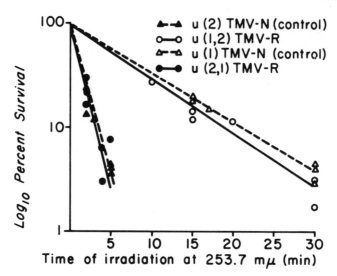

Fig. 6. Inactivation of native and cross-reconstituted TMV
strains at 253.7 nm. Irradiations were carried out in 0.1 M sodium
phosphate buffer, pH 7, at a virus concentration of 10 μg/ml using
a Mineralight V-41 mercury discharge lamp possessing an output
intensity of 985 ergs/mm^2 per min at a distance of 17 cm. Each
set of points represents three separate experiments and are plotted
by the method of least squares with the aid of an IBM 7040-7094
computer. The sensitivity of the reconstituted virions is thus
determined by the nature of the capsomer protein (From Streeter
and Gordon, 1967).

virus shows a kinetic isotope effect upon irradiation in H_2O and
D_2O, as does free RNA and in sharp contrast to TMV-U1 (McCleary
and Gordon, 1973; Huang and Gordon, 1974).

In the spherical virus, coliphage R17, the RNA is protected
to some extent as the formation of uridine photohydrates in the
virus is somewhat less than in the RNA after the same exposure to
280 nm radiation (55 residues in the virus as opposed to 77 in the
free RNA) (Remsen *et al.*, 1970).

When TMV-RNA (U1 strain) is encapsulated within the protein

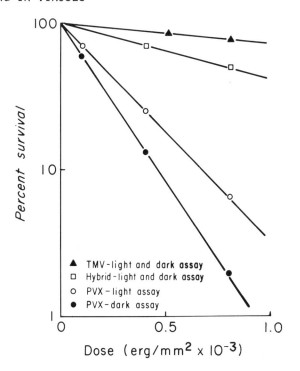

Fig. 7.   Inactivation of PVX, TMV, and TMV protein: PVX-RNA
hybrid.   The photoreactivation sector (f_p), equal to 1 - dose reduction factor, is 0.3 for PVX and 0.0 for TMV and the mixed virus.
The protection of PVX-RNA and the lack of photoreactivation of the
hybrid particle are similar to the properties of native TMV (From
Breck and Gordon, 1970).

of cowpea chlorotic mottle virus to form a spherical virus, the
RNA does not appear to be afforded any protection (Fig. 8).   The
hybrid particle also shows photoreactivation (Grouse et $al.$, 1970).

One should not generalize that viral proteins always protect
viral nucleic acids.   In the case of polio virus, the mature virion
is inactivated by 254 nm radiation more rapidly than infectious
single- or double-stranded polio RNAs (Norman, 1960; Bishop et $al.$,
1967) (Fig. 9).   There are no further experimental facts upon which
to propose an explanation for this phenomenon; however, this is an

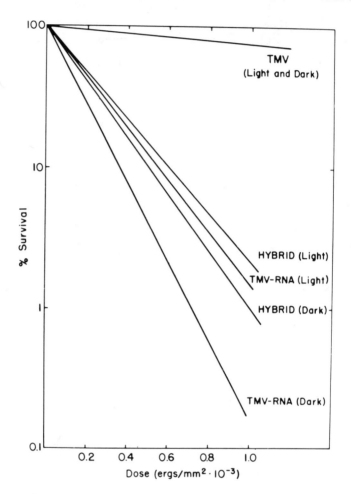

Fig. 8.   Inactivation of TMV, TMV-RNA, and Cowpea Chlorotic
Mottle Virus protein: TMV-RNA hybrid.   The curves for TMV and TMV-
RNA are a composite of curves obtained over several years in this
laboratory and are for material irradiated in distilled water.
TMV-RNA in the spherical hybrid is not protected from UV radiation
and undergoes photoreactivation (From Grouse *et al.*, 1970).

interesting, important, and easily accessible system for further
investigation.

Lettuce necrotic yellow virus is a complex lipid-containing
plant virus. It has been reported to be about eight times more
sensitive to 254 nm radiation than the U2 strain of TMV (Mclean

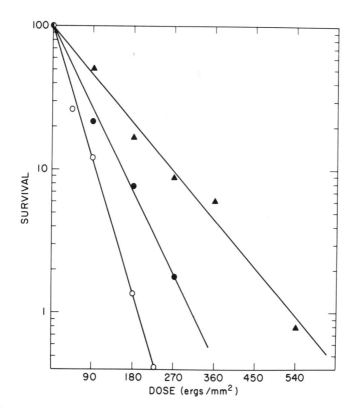

Fig. 9. UV sensitivity of polio virus and its single- and double-stranded RNAs. Virus and RNA preparations were diluted in phosphate-buffered saline, pH 7.2, and 1 ml portions irradiated in 60 mm Petri dishes, which were rocked gently during irradiation. (o---o) polio virus; (o---o) single-stranded RNA; (Δ---Δ) double-stranded RNA. The unusually high sensitivity of the intact virion should be noted (From Bishop *et al.*, 1967).

and Crowley, 1969). The photochemistry and photobiology of this virus may serve as models for the behavior of complex mammalian viruses and should be studied in greater detail.

A new and intriguing observation has been made in the case of insect nuclear polyhedrosis viruses. These viruses are of considerable interest as a means of biological control of insect pests, such as those that attack cotton and other important corps. UV light in the region below 307 nm inactivated suspensions of polyhedra of *Heliothis* nuclear polyhedrosis virus (Bullock *et al.*, 1970). Studies have shown that sunlight is the principal inactivating agency responsible for the lack of persistence of the virus. On the other hand, a recent report by Ramoska *et al.* (1975) indicated that short exposure with UV light of 320 nm produces an activation of *Autographa Californica* nuclear polyhedrosis virus *in vitro*. The techniques for the large-scale production of insect viruses and their assay are now easily available. In view of the ecological and economic importance of insect viruses, this area deserves the attention of more investigators.

An interesting new concept has been raised by the observation of the photosensitized splitting of pyrimidine cyclobutane dimers by tryptophan, 5-hydroxytryptophan, and other indole derivatives (Hélène and Charlier, 1971). In more recent work, these authors have reported that pyrimidine dimers in DNA can be split by irradiation at 313 nm in the presence of the tripeptide, Lys-Trp-Lys (Charlier and Hélène, 1975). Uracil cyclobutane dimers either free or in RNA can be photomonomerized by proteins which contain fully exposed tryptophan residues (Fig. 10). These findings suggest that fully exposed tryptophan residues when strategically positioned on the interior of capsomer proteins of virus particles could carry out *in situ* repair of UV-damaged nucleic acids. At present, no example of this type of phenomenon is known to this reviewer; however, one would predict that this type of interaction would be a positive survival trait in viruses exposed to solar radiation.

5. SUMMARY

In most of the examples discussed in this short review, the presence of the viral capsomer served to protect the encapsulated nucleic acid from inactivation by UV light. The magnitude of the protective effect of the capsomer is usually much greater than can be attributed to simple screening. In some cases, the presence of the capsomer protein led to a definite alteration in the course of the photochemical events that occurred when a high energy photon was absorbed by the virion. The mechanism whereby the energy of the absorbed photon is dissipated in an apparently harmless pathway is not known in any instance. The mechanism of the converse of this phonomenon, the sensitization of viral nucleic acids by the capsomer protein, as in the case of polio virus, is also unknown. The elucidation of the molecular nature of these processes promises to be more interesting and may serve ultimately to guide attempts to control the interaction of actinic radiation with genetic material.

Acknowledgments. The research of the author was supported by funds from the United States Atomic Energy commission [contract No. AT(45-1)2225] and the National Science Foundation (grant No. GB 24024).

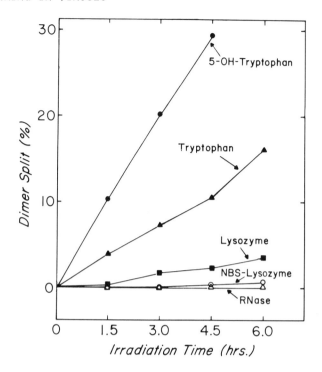

Fig. 10.   Percentage of dimers split as a function of irradiation time.   The reaction mixture containing [^{14}C] labeled uracil
dimer (2 × 10^{-4} M) and sensitizer was irradiated at 303 nm at room
temperature at an incident intensity of 2.33 × 10^4 erg/cm^2/sec.
The sensitizer concentrations were: tryptophan, lysozyme, C^{862}-
oxindolyl-lysozyme (NBS lysozyme), and ribonuclease, 3 × 10^{-3} M;
5-hydroxytryptophan, 2 × 10^{-3} M (J. Chen, C.W. Huang, L. Hinman,
M.P. Gordon, and D.A. Deranleau, unpublished observations).

References

Bishop, J.M., Quintrell, N., and Koch, G., 1967, Polio virus
     double-stranded RNA: Inactivation by ultraviolet light, *J.
     Mol. Biol.* 24:125-128.
Bohne, L., Coquerelle, T., and Hagen, U., 1970, Radiation sensi-
     tivity of bacteriophage DNA.   II.   Breaks and cross-links
     after irradiation *in vivo*, *Int. J. Radiat. Biol.* 17:205-215.

Bonhoffer, F., and Schachman, H.K., 1960, Studies on the organiza-
    tion of nucleic acids within nucleoproteins, *Biochem. Biophys.
    Res. Commun.* 2:366-371.
Breck, L.O., and Gordon, M.P., 1970, Formation, characterization,
    and some photochemical properties of a hybrid plant virus,
    Virology 40:397-402.
Bullock, H.R., Hollingsworth, J.P., and Hartstack, A.W., Jr.,
    1970, Virulence of *Heliothis* nuclear polyhedrosis virus
    exposed to monochromatic ultraviolet irradiation, *J. Invert.
    Path.* 16:419-422.
Carpenter, J.M., and Kleczkowski, A., 1969, The absence of photo-
    reversible pyrimidine dimers in the RNA of ultraviolet-
    irradiated tobacco mosaic virus, *Virology* 39:542-547.
Caspar, D.L.D., 1963, Assembly and stability of the tobacco mosaic
    virus particle, *Adv. Protein Chem.* 18:37-121.
Charlier, M., and Hélène, C., 1975, Photosensitized splitting of
    pyrimidine dimers in DNA by indole derivatives and tryptophan-
    containing peptides, *Photochem. Photobiol.* 21:31-37.
Francke, B., and Ray, D.S., 1972, Ultraviolet induced cross-links
    in the deoxyribonucleic acid of single-stranded deoxyribonu-
    cleic acid viruses as a probe of deoxyribonucleic acid pack-
    aging, *J. Virol.* 9:1027-1032.
Goddard, J., Streeter, D., Weber, C., and Gordon, M.P., 1966, Studies
    on the inactivation of tobacco masaic virus by ultraviolet light
    Photochem. Photobiol. 5:213-222.
Grouse, L., Murphy, T.M., Gordon, M.P., and Smuckler, E.A., 1970,
    The photobiology of a spherical phenotypic hybrid of tobacco
    mosaic virus, *Virology* 41:385-388.
Hawkins, R.D., 1975, Ionizing radiation induced covalent protein to
    DNA cross-links in coliphage T7. Abstr. Int. Symp. "Protein
    and Other Adducts to DNA: Their Significance to Aging, Carcino-
    genesis and Radiation Biology," Williamsburg, Virginia, May 2-
    6, 1975.
Hawkins, R.D., and Ginsberg, D.M., 1971, The physical measurement of
    radiation damage to coliphage T7 DNA, *Biophys. J.* 11:398-413.
Hayashi, T., Machida, H., Abe, T., and Kiho, Y., 1969, *In vivo*
    uncoating of tobacco mosaic virus irradiated with ultraviolet
    light, *Japan J. Microbiol.* 13:386-387.
Hélène, C., and Charlier, M., 1971, Photosensitized splitting of
    pyrimidine dimers by indole derivatives, *Biochem. Biophys.
    Res. Commun.* 43:252-257.
Huang, C.W., and Gordon, M.P., 1974, The formation of photorevers-
    ible cyclobutane-type pyrimidine dimers in ultraviolet-
    irradiated potato virus X, *Photochem. Photobiol.* 19:269-272.
Janion, C., and Shugar, D., 1967, Reaction of amines with dihydro-
    cytosine analogues and formation of amino acid and peptidyl
    derivatives of dihydropyrimidines, *Acta Biochim. Polon.* 14:
    293-302.

Katagiri, S., Hinuma, Y., and Ishida, N., 1967, Biophysical properties of polio virus particles irradiated with ultraviolet light, *Virology* 32:337-343.

Kleczkowski, A., 1971, Photobiology of plant viruses, *Photophysiology* 6:179-208.

Kleczkowski, A., and McLaren, A.D., 1967, Inactivation of infectivity of tobacco mosaic virus during ultraviolet-irradiation of the whole virus at two wavelengths, *J. Gen. Virol.* 1:441-448.

Mayo, M.A., Harrison, B.D., Murant, A.F., and Barker, H., 1973, Cross-linking of RNA induced by ultraviolet irradiation of particles of raspberry ringspot virus, *J. Gen. Virol.* 19:155-159.

McCleary, L.O., and Gordon, M.P., 1973, Ultraviolet irradiation of potato virus X, its RNA and a hybrid virus particle: Photoreactivation, kinetic isotope effects, and quantum yield of inactivation, *Photochem. Photobiol.* 18:9-15.

McLaren, A.D., and Kleczkowshi, A., 1967, Some gross changes in particles of tobacco mosaic virus caused by large doses of ultraviolet radiation, *J. Gen. Virol.* 1:391-394.

McLaren, A.D., and Moring-Claesson, I., 1961, Action spectrum for the inactivation of infectious nucleic acid from tobacco mosaic virus by ultraviolet light, *in* "Progress in Photobiology" (B. Christenson and B. Buchmann, eds.), pp. 573-575, Elsevier, Amsterdam.

McLean, G.D., and Crowley, N.C., 1969, Inactivation of lettuce necrotic yellow virus by ultraviolet irradiation, *Virology* 37:209-213.

Miller, R.L., and Plagemann, P.G.W., 1974, Effect of ultraviolet light on mengovirus: Formation of uracil dimers, instability and degradation of capsid, and covalent linkage of protein to viral RNA, *J. Virol.* 13:729-739.

Nakashima, Y., and Konigsberg, W., 1975, Photo-induced cross-linkage of gene 5 protein and Fd. Abstr. Int. Symp. "Protein and Other Adducts to DNA: Their Significance to Aging, Carcinogenesis and Radiation Biology," Williamsburg, Virginia, May 2-6, 1975.

Norman, A., 1960, Ultraviolet inactivation of polio virus ribonucleic acid, *Virology* 10:384-386.

Oster, G., and McLaren, A.D., 1950, The ultraviolet light and photosensitized inactivation of tobacco mosaic virus, *J. Gen. Physiol.* 33:215-228.

Ramoska, W.A., Stairs, G.R., and Hink, W.F., 1975, Ultraviolet light activation of insect nuclear polyhedrosis virus, *Nature* 253:628-629.

Remsen, J.F., Miller, N., and Cerutti, P.A., 1970, Photohydration of uridine in the RNA of coliphage R17. II. The relationship between ultraviolet inactivation and uridine photohydration, *Proc. Nat. Acad. Sci. USA* 65:460-466.

Rushizky, G.W., Knight, C.A., and McLaren, A.D., 1960, A comparison
    of the ultraviolet light inactivation of infectious ribonu-
    cleic acid preparations from tobacco mosaic virus with those
    of the native and reconstituted virus, *Virology* 12:32-47.
Simukova, N.A., and Budowsky, E.I., 1974, Conversion of non-
    covalent interactions in nucleoproteins into covalent bonds:
    UV-induced formation of polynucleotide-protein crosslinks in
    bacteriophage Sd virions, *FEBS Lett*. 38:299-303.
Simukova, N.A., Turchinsky, M.F., Boni, I.V., Skoblou, Y.M., and
    Budowsky, E.I., 1975, UV-induced cytosine involved polynu-
    cleotide-protein cross-linking. Abstr. Int. Symp. "Protein
    and Other Adducts to DNA: Their Significance to Aging,
    Carcinogenesis and Radiation Biology," Williamsburg, Virginia,
    May 2-6, 1975.
Small, G.D., and Gordon, M.P., 1968, Reaction of hydroxylamine and
    methoxyamine with the ultraviolet-induced hydrate of cytidine,
    J. Mol. Biol. 34:281-291.
Streeter, D.G., and Gordon, M.P., 1967, Ultraviolet photoinactiva-
    tion studies on hybrid viruses obtained by the cross-reconsti-
    tution of the protein and RNA components of U(1) and U(2)
    strains of TMV, *Photochem. Photobiol*. 6:413-421.
Streeter, D.G., and Gordon, M.P., 1968, Studies of the role of the
    coat protein in the ultraviolet photoinactivation of U(1) and
    U(2) strains of TMV, *Photochem. Photobiol*. 8:81-92.
Tao, M., Small, G.D., and Gordon, M.P., 1969, Photochemical altera-
    tions in ribonucleic acid isolated from ultraviolet-irradiated
    tobacco mosaic virus, *Virology* 39:534-541.
Turchinsky, M.F., Boni, I.V., and Budowsky, E.I., 1975, Bisulfite
    induced cytosine involved polynucleotide-protein cross-linking.
    Abstr. Int. Symp. "Protein and Other Adducts to DNA: Their
    Significance to Aging, Carcinogenesis and Radiation Biology,"
    Williamsburg, Virginia, May 2-6, 1975.
Turchinsky, M.F., Jusova, K.S., and Budowsky, E.I., 1974, Conver-
    sion of non-covalent interaction sin nucleoproteins in to
    covalent bonds: Bisulfide induced formation of polynucleo-
    tide-protein crosslinks in MS2 bacteriophage virions, *FEBS
    Lett*. 38:304-307.
Yamada, Y. Shigeta, A., and Nogu, K., 1973, Ultraviolet effects on
    biological functions of RNA phage MS2, *Biochim. Biophys. Acta*
    299:121-135.
Zech, H., 1961, Cytochemische untersuchungen zur reproduktion des
    tabakmosaikvirus, *Z. Naturforsch*. 16b:520-538.

IN VITRO STUDIES OF PHOTOCHEMICALLY CROSS-LINKED PROTEIN-NUCLEIC

ACID COMPLEXES. DETERMINATION OF CROSS-LINKED REGIONS AND

STRUCTURAL RELATIONSHIPS IN SPECIFIC COMPLEXES

Paul R. Schimmel, Gerald P. Budzik, Stella S.M. Lam, and

Hubert J.P. Schoemaker

Departments of Biology and Chemistry, Massachusetts

Institute of Technology, Cambridge, Massachusetts 02139

1. INTRODUCTION

It is well known that many enzymatic and cellular processes involve specific protein-nucleic acid associations. Examples include the interaction of a repressor with its operator DNA (see Beckwith and Zipser, 1970; Müller-Hill, 1971), of DNA polymerase with DNA (see Kornberg, 1975), of ribosomal proteins with ribosomal RNA (see Nomura *et al.*, 1974), of aminoacyl tRNA synthetases with tRNAs (see Kisselev and Favorova, 1974; Söll and Schimmel, 1974), as well as many other systems. A prime goal is to determine the mechanism by which these interactions occur; *viz*., it is desirable to understand how specificity is achieved and to determine what factors are responsible for the strength of specific protein-nucleic acid associations.

Recently it has become clear that in this context the UV radiation induced attachment of protein to nucleic acid (see Smith, 1975) is of considerable value. It appears that in proteins there is a broad spectrum of photoreactive groups available as indicated, for example, by Smith's (1969) observation that ten different amino acids react with uracil under the action of UV radiation. This broad spectrum of possibilities makes photochemical cross-linking an attractive way to join covalently sections of nucleic acid and protein that strongly interact in a specific complex. After linkage is achieved, careful analysis of the photochemically cross-linked protein-nucleic acid complex provides much insight into the molecular details of association.

This article focuses on the *in vitro* coupling of specific proteins to nucleic acids. A variety of photoinduced covalent complexes are considered. For the determination of structure-function relationships in specific complexes it is imperative that irradiations are done under conditions such that *only* specific sites are covalently joined; in this context non-specific attachment is viewed as a contamination. Once the specific complex has been covalently joined, the cross-linked regions on the nucleic acid and on the protein may then be determined. This analysis thus identifies the general location of specific receptor sites on each particle. As illustrated below, if X-ray structural information is available on one or both of the reacting partners, a molecular picture of the complex may also be constructed from the photochemical cross-linking data.

2. PHOTOCHEMICALLY CROSS-LINKED PROTEIN-NUCLEIC ACID COMPLEXES

Under the action of UV light a number of proteins have been stably attached *in vitro* to nucleic acids. These include bovine serum albumin (BSA) to DNA (Smith, 1964; Braun and Merrick, 1974), DNA polymerase to DNA and to synthetic polynucleotide duplexes (Markovitz, 1972), RNA polymerase to bromouracil (BrUra) substituted DNA and to poly(dA-dT):poly(dA-dT) (Weintraub, 1973; Strniste and Smith, 1974), the *lac* repressor to BrUra substituted DNA containing the *lac* operon (Lin and Riggs, 1974), gene 5 protein to fd DNA (Anderson *et al*., 1975), and aminoacyl tRNA synthetases to tRNAs (Schoemaker and Schimmel, 1974; Budzik *et al*., 1975; Schoemaker *et al*., 1975). In each of these cases irradiations were primarily at 254 nm, where nucleic acids have a high absorbance.

2.1. Protein-DNA Complexes

2.1.1. *BSA-DNA*. Smith (1964) reported an early observation
of protein-DNA cross-linking; BSA was stably attached to *E. coli*
DNA under the action of UV light. Of course, this is clearly an
example of a non-specific complex. The photoreaction has the
unusual property that DNA and protein are linked when they are
mixed together before irradiation or when irradiated separately
and then combined. The cross-linking has been studied in more
depth by Braun and Merrick (1975) who, using DNA from a bacteriophage, have shown that the reaction is mediated *via* an activated
protein intermediate; the activated intermediate has a half-life
of about 18 min at 37°C. Preliminary data suggest that sulfhydryl
groups on the protein somehow may be involved.

2.1.2. *DNA Polymerase-DNA*. An example where specific complex
formation is expected to occur is the association between *E. coli*
DNA polymerase and DNA. The enzyme and DNA form a stable, non-
covalent complex in low but not in high ionic strength buffers.
Complex formation may be detected with the nitrocellulose filter
assay (Jones and Berg, 1966). Free DNA passes through the filter,
but when complexed to enzyme in a low ionic strength buffer it is
retained; when the filter is washed with a high ionic strength
solvent, the bound DNA is released. However, DNA that is covalently linked to polymerase is not released from the filter by high
salt concentration, a feature that is useful for demonstrating the
formation of covalent complexes (Markovitz, 1972).

Figure 1 is a plot of the effect of UV radiation on the amount
of DNA stably attached to DNA polymerase as a function of the polymerase concentration (Markovitz, 1972). The various curves correspond to different times of radiation where the fluence rate was
2.7×10^3 erg mm^{-2} min^{-1}. The solid lines correspond to cases in
which the complexes were diluted into a high ionic strength buffer
before filtration. It is clear that in the absence of irradiation
no DNA is held by the filter. The dashed line corresponds to a
case in which the high ionic strength buffer was not added prior
to filtration. At high enzyme concentrations this curve is above
its solid line counterpart; this means that some of the polymerase
is non-covalently bound to the DNA after irradiation. Finally,
when enzyme and DNA are irradiated under dissociating conditions,
a stable complex is not formed.

The UV-induced stable complex does not dissociate upon exposure to 0.1 N NaOH or to heat. Moreover, although proteins and
nucleic acids are generally separated by phenol extraction, when
this complex is extracted DNA migrates into the phenol layer with
protein. Therefore, the data clearly suggest a covalent linkage.

Other aspects of the photoinduced reaction have also been

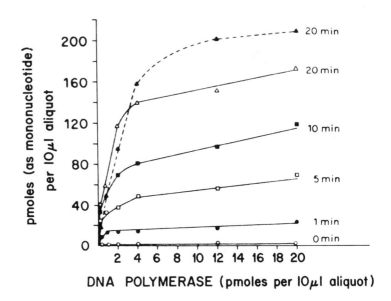

Fig. 1. The effect of the fluence of UV radiation and DNA polymerase concentration on the coupling of DNA to DNA polymerase. The fluence rate was 2.7×10^3 ergs mm^{-2} min^{-1}. The curves correspond to different times of irradiation. The solid lines correspond to samples that were diluted after irradiation into buffer containing 0.5 M NaCl, while the dashed line corresponds to a case in which the dilution buffer did not contain 0.5 M NaCl. Other methods are described in the text (From Markovitz, 1972).

studied. Under appropriate conditions the polymerase can bind to the alternating double-stranded copolymer poly(dA-dT):poly(dA-dT) and to a homopolymer duplex such as poly dA:poly dT. In experiments with poly dA:poly dT it was shown that covalent attachment of polymerase is not base specific; that is, attachment appears to occur to A and to T residues (Markovitz, 1972).

The UV-induced attachment of polymerase to DNA is in certain respects unlike that of the BSA-DNA reaction cited above. When the polymerase and DNA are separately irradiated and mixed, no covalent complex formation occurs, in contrast to the results found in the BSA reaction. Moreover, DNA polymerase is designed to bind to DNA in the course of performing its biological function; there is no evidence to suggest that a specific receptor site exists on DNA for

BSA and, in particular, on the non-eukaryotic DNAs used in studies above. On the other hand, it is not certain that the polymerase has been cross-linked to specific sites as opposed to random locations on the DNA. Irradiations were done under conditions where the enzyme binds only to nicks or ends of the DNA, and the number of linked polymerase molecules was roughly equal to or less than the number of ends plus nicks (Markovitz, 1972). These data suggest, but do not conclusively establish, that attachment occurs at specific sites--i.e., at nicks or ends.

2.1.3. *RNA Polymerase-DNA*. Similar studies to those done with DNA polymerase have been carried out by Weintraub (1973) and by Strniste and Smith (1974) with *E. coli* RNA polymerase. An example of data obtained by the filter assay described above is given in Fig. 2. This shows the amount of stable complex formed between RNA polymerase and poly(dA-dT):poly(dA-dT) as a function of UV fluence. Irradiations were performed in a low ionic strength buffer; the dashed lines in Fig. 2 show the amount of polymer retained on the filter when a low salt washing buffer is used; the solid curves show the results obtained with a high salt washing buffer. The different curves correspond to different enzyme-polymer ratios. It is clear that with a low salt wash the amount of polymer trapped is independent of UV fluence between 0 and 12.5×10^4 ergs mm^{-2}. On the other hand, high salt stable complexes do not form in the absence of UV irradiation; moreover, the yield of such complexes is directly dependent upon the fluence of radiation.

Other studies showed that the stable complex is resistant to alkali or heat treatment. Furthermore, when the protein and nucleic acid are irradiated separately and subsequently mixed, no significant amounts of stable complex are formed.

With BrUra DNA instead of the synthetic copolymer, Weintraub (1973) photoreacted *E. coli* RNA polymerase as well as other nucleic acid binding polypeptides. It was also shown that non-specific proteins such as ribonuclease A and trypsin do not significantly attach to the DNA under the irradiation conditions used. This suggests that the photoinduced complexes obtained have proteins attached at specific loci.

2.1.4. *lac Repressor-DNA*. The mechanism of gene regulation has been extensively explored in the case of the *lac* operon (see Beckwith and Zipser, 1970; Müller-Hill, 1971; Gilbert *et al.*, 1974). The expression of this operon is controllable in part by the binding of the *lac* repressor to the operator region. The association between operator and repressor is strong; it is of the order of 10^{13} M^{-1} under certain conditions (Riggs *et al.*, 1970b).

The study of the operator is conveniently done with DNA from the transducing phage λh80d*lac*; this DNA carries the *lac* operator

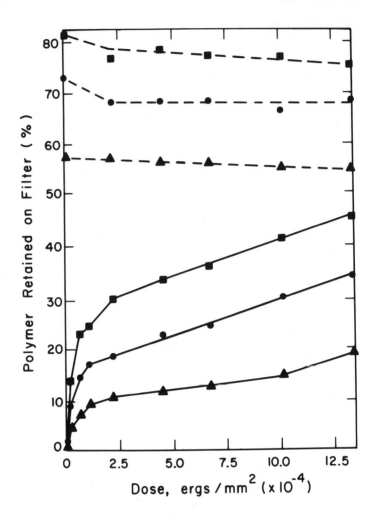

Fig. 2. The coupling of *E. coli* RNA polymerase to poly(dA-dT)· poly(dA-dT) as a function of the fluence of UV radiation. After irradiation, the complex was diluted into a high salt (solid lines) or low salt (dashed lines) buffer prior to being applied to Millipore filters. The symbols represent different enzyme-polymer molar ratios: (▲) 3:1, (●) 6:1, and (■) 12:1 (From Strniste and Smith, 1974).

while the wild-type λh80 does not. The purpose of inserting the *lac* operator into the transducing phage DNA is to heighten the proportion of the operator segment relative to its natural occurrence in the *E. coli* chromosome.

Irradiation of the *lac* repressor in the presence of λh80d*lac* DNA results in no significant stable attachment of the repressor to the DNA (Lin and Riggs, 1974). On the other hand, positive results are obtained with bromodeoxyuridine (BrdUrd) substituted DNA--BrdUrd-λh80d*lac* DNA (Lin and Riggs, 1974). This is not surprising since it is well known that BrdUrd substituted DNA is more photosensitive than normal DNA (see Setlow and Setlow, 1972; Smith, 1975); moreover, the *lac* repressor binds strongly and specifically to the derivatized DNA.

Results of photochemical cross-linking studies with BrdUrd-λh80d*lac* DNA are summarized in Fig. 3A-C. The curves show the percent of DNA retained on nitrocellulose filters *versus* the time of irradiation. The filter assay was done in the presence of IPTG (isopropyl-β-D-thiogalactoside), an inducer of the *lac* operon.* This galactoside binds to the repressor which in turn changes its conformation so that it no longer binds strongly to the *lac* operon (Riggs *et al.*, 1970a). Therefore, unless the repressor is stably attached to the DNA the nucleic acid is not retained on the filter in the presence of IPTG.

The filled circles refer to irradiations done with BrdUrd-λh80d*lac* DNA; the open circles refer to those done with BrdUrd-λh80 DNA. In Fig. 3A it is apparent that with BrdUrd-λh80d*lac* DNA, in the presence of 0.18 M KCl, stable complexes are formed in an amount that is dependent upon the time of irradiation. Under these conditions no stable complexes are formed with BrdUrd-λh80 DNA. Moreover, if irradiations with BrdUrd-λh80d*lac* DNA and repressor are done in the presence of IPTG no protein-DNA joining occurs (open triangles). If glucose--an anti-inducer that does not inhibit complex formation (Riggs *et al.*, 1970a)--is present in the irradiation mixture there is little effect on stable complex formation as detected by the filter assay. These experiments leave scarcely any doubt that in the presence of 0.18 M KCl the *lac* operator is the specific attachment site for the photo-cross-linked complexes of *lac* repressor and BrdUrd-λh80d*lac* DNA.

At lower ionic strengths the data of Fig. 3B-C show that attachment also occurs at non-specific sites. The amount of such attachment is not great in 0.13 M KCl but is substantial in 0.01 M KCl. These findings are not surprising in view of the known increased affinity of *lac* repressor for non-specific DNA at low

---

*Abbreviations used: IleRS, isoleucyl tRNA synthetase; ValRS, valyl tRNA synthetase; PheRS, phenylalanyl tRNA synthetase; TyrRS, tyrosyl tRNA synthetase; BSA, bovine serum albumin; IPTG, isopropyl-β-D-thiogalactoside; tRNA^x, the tRNA specific for amino acid x, where the standard three letter abbreviation is used for amino acids.

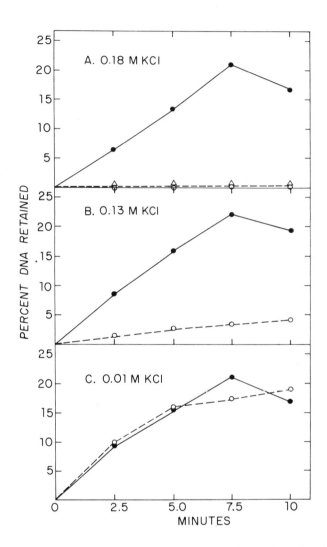

Fig. 3. Formation of IPTG-stable complex of BrdUrd-DNA and *lac* repressor as a function of the time of exposure to UV radiation. The fluence rate was 10^3 ergs mm^{-2} min^{-1}. The repressor-DNA complex was irradiated for the indicated times after which IPTG was added, followed by Millipore filtration. Each panel corresponds to a different salt concentration (as indicated) present during the irradiation. The various symbols are: •, BrdUrd-λh80d*lac* DNA; o, BrdUrd-λh80 DNA; Δ, BrdUrd-λh80d*lac* DNA with 1 mM IPTG present during irradiation (From Lin and Riggs, 1974).

ionic strengths (Lin and Riggs, 1972).

2.1.5. *Bacteriophage fd Gene 5 Protein-DNA*. The male specific filamentous coliphage fd contains single-stranded DNA (see Marvin and Hohn, 1969). The product of gene 5 (gene 5 protein) of this DNA plays an important part in the synthesis of viral single strands during phage morphogenesis. The protein appears to perform its function by binding strongly to the viral DNA, with the stoichiometry of about 1 gene 5 protein per pentanucleotide unit (cf. Pratt *et al.*, 1974). In the intact virion, however, the gene 5 protein is displaced by coat protein so that *in vivo* the gene 5 protein-DNA complex presumably has only a transient existence (Marvin and Hohn, 1969; Pratt *et al.*, 1974). But the complex may be studied in a stable form *in vitro* by simply mixing the protein with single-stranded fd DNA.

Anderson *et al.* (1975) have attempted with UV radiation to introduce covalent bonds into the complex formed *in vitro*. Some of their results are summarized in Table 1, where stable cross-linking is measured by the phenol extraction assay. The percent of DNA recovered in the aqueous phase is measured as a function of time and under different conditions. It is clear that in the presence of gene 5 protein and under non-dissociating conditions, almost all of the DNA is recovered in the phenol phase after a short time of irradiation. On the other hand, under dissociating conditions (high salt) substantially less DNA is extracted into phenol; that which is extracted into phenol, as a result of the irradiation, presumably is due to some complex formation that occurs in high salt. When fd DNA alone, or in the presence of BSA, is irradiated for 5 min, the amount of DNA that enters the phenol is not significant, especially compared with that found with gene 5 protein present under non-dissociating conditions. Interestingly enough, when the intact virion is irradiated for 5 min, there is little DNA-protein attachment. This indicates that geometric as well as photochemical constraints may operate to prevent stable photoinduced linkage formation in the virion.

The data of Table 1 suggest that the stable complex formed in low salt is not due to random, non-specific DNA-protein association. Other data more firmly establish that irradiation induces a covalent linkage between gene 5 protein and fd DNA. Recently, Nakashima and Konigsberg (1975) have reported that the photochemical attachment of the gene 5 protein to fd DNA is via cysteine 33 and probably a thymine residue.

2.2. Protein-RNA Complexes. Coupling of tRNAs to Aminoacyl tRNA
                    Synthetases

The best examples of photochemically cross-linked protein-RNA

Table 1.   DNA Recovery After Phenol Extraction
(Anderson *et al.*, 1975)*

Sample		(NaCl), M	Irradia-tion time (min)	Percent DNA recovered in aqueous phase
fd DNA (μg/ml)	Gene 5 protein (μg/ml)			
0.05	0.2	0.05	0	65
0.05	0.2	0.05	5	1
0.2	0.7	0.05	0	70
0.2	0.7	0.05	2	3
0.2	0.7	0.05	5	0
0.05	0.2	1.0	0	63
0.05	0.2	1.0	5	38
0.2	0.7	1.0	5	23
fd virion	---			
		0.05	0	67
		0.05	5	57
fd DNA	---			
2.0		0.05	0	80
2.0		0.05	5	65
2.0		1.0	5	60
2.0	70 (BSA)	0.05	5	85

*Irradiation mixtures containing gene 5 protein or the fd virion also contained 70 μg/ml of bovine serum albumin (BSA).

complexes are those of the aminoacyl tRNA synthetases with tRNAs (Schoemaker and Schimmel, 1974; Budzik *et al.*, 1975; Schoemaker *et al.*, 1975).   The synthetases are enzymes involved in the first step of protein synthesis; they specifically attach amino acids to the 3'-termini of their cognate tRNA chains (Kisselev and Favorova, 1974; Söll and Schimmel, 1974).   For each amino acid there is at least one specific synthetase and tRNA. The enzymes must match perfectly each amino acid to its cognate tRNA in order to prevent altered proteins from occurring; once an amino acid is stably attached to a tRNA its position in a growing polypeptide chain is determined by the anticodon base triplet and not by the nature of the amino acid (Chapeville *et al.*, 1962).

The tRNAs are single-stranded polynucleotide chains generally comprised of about 75-85 bases (see Zachau, 1969). Each can be folded into the same basic cloverleaf hydrogen-bonding pattern of secondary structure. An example of this structure is shown in Fig. 4 for yeast tRNA[Phe]. As indicated in the figure, the basic structure can be divided into five parts: the amino acid acceptor terminus, dihydrouridine loop, anticodon loop, extra loop, and TψC loop. Although the base sequences and chain lengths vary from one specific tRNA to another, all have the five characteristic regions of the cloverleaf. In addition, certain short sequences, such as the T-ψ-C and the C-C-A at the 3'-terminus, are common to virtually all tRNA species.

A key question is the molecular basis for specificity in synthetase-tRNA interactions. A variety of approaches have been used to pinpoint the base or bases critical for specificity. These approaches include experiments with tRNA fragments, analysis of effects of chemical modifications of specific bases, the study of consequences of single base changes (in mutant tRNAs), and others (see Kisselev and Favorova, 1974; Söll and Schimmel, 1974). In spite of these efforts, the problem remains unsolved.

Instead of focusing on specific bases or sequences, the problem can be approached in another way. One can attempt to determine those regions on a tRNA that are, and those that are not, in close proximity to the surface of the enzyme. From this information, and with the now available three dimensional structure of a specific tRNA (Kim *et al.*, 1974; Robertus *et al.*, 1974), a model can be constructed of the synthetase-tRNA complex. From this, possible sites for specificity are narrowed down to a few loci; future experiments may then be directed at these sites in order to determine precisely the mechanism of specificity.

Two approaches that have been somewhat useful are oligonucleotide hybridization and nuclease susceptibility. The oligonucleotide hybridization approach makes use of the observation that single-stranded, unshielded regions of a tRNA can hybridize to complementary tri- and tetranucleotides (Uhlenbeck *et al.*, 1970). By determining the hybridization pattern in the presence and absence of the binding protein, regions on the tRNA covered by protein may be determined (Schimmel *et al.*, 1972). The nuclease susceptibility approach has a similar rationale. A specific nuclease is used to introduce a few nicks into a tRNA in the

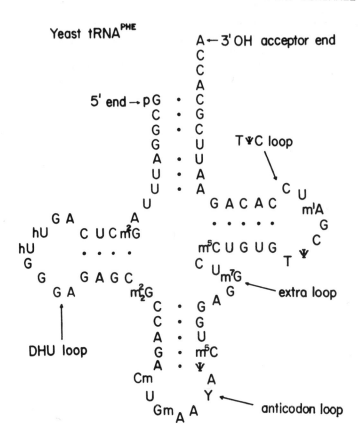

Fig. 4. Sequence and cloverleaf structure of yeast tRNA^Phe.
Familiar landmarks on the tRNA are indicated (From RajBhandary and
Chang, 1968).

presence and absence of synthetase, and the cleavage patterns for
both cases are then compared (Hörz and Zachau, 1973; Dickson and
Schimmel, 1975).

These approaches have the significant limitation that only a
few specific parts of the tRNA can be probed. For example, oligo-
nucleotides can only hybridize to single-stranded, unshielded
regions on the tRNA (Uhlenbeck *et al.*, 1970), while in the case of
nucleases one is limited by their particular base specificities
and the markedly different rates of attack on exposed *versus* buried
sites. An additional drawback to the nuclease susceptibility
approach is that the tRNA structure may be seriously altered after

the first nick is introduced into the molecule; this makes interpretation of subsequent cleavages ambiguous.

Cross-linking of enzyme and tRNA provides an alternative way
to obtain structural information. Chemical reagents that accomplish this, such as glutaraldehyde, for example, are of limited
use because they react with only a few functional groups; also,
the reaction conditions required for cross-linking with some chemicals may be too severe for delicate protein-nucleic acid complexes.
Direct photochemical cross-linking, without the aid of photoaffinity
labels or other reagents, provides an attractive alternative, since
mild solution conditions can be employed and extraneous chemicals
avoided. Also, as mentioned earlier, there appears to be a broad
spectrum of photoreactive groups available in proteins. To obtain
structural information from this approach, however, it must be
shown that cross-linking is specific and that radiation does little
damage to the tRNA or enzyme structure. If these conditions are
fulfilled, then the cross-linked regions represent close proximity
or actual contact points between the enzyme and tRNA in the native
complex.

2.2.1. *Specificity of Cross-Linking*. Figure 5 gives results
of photochemical cross-linking between a small excess of *E. coli*
tyrosyl tRNA synthetase and two purified isoaccepters of $tRNA^{Tyr}$--
$tRNA_1^{Tyr}$ and $tRNA_2^{Tyr}$. These tRNAs differ by only two bases in the
extra loop (Goodman *et al.*, 1968). The curve gives the percent
of tRNA that is joined *versus* the time of irradiation. The precent
of tRNA joined was determined by a phenol extraction assay; only
tRNA coupled to protein is extracted into phenol. The amount of
tRNA coupled to protein increases with the time of irradiation until
a plateau is reached after about 10 min; this plateau is significantly higher with $tRNA_1^{Tyr}$ than with $tRNA_2^{Tyr}$ [see Schoemaker and
Schimmel (1974) for further discussion].

The crucial question is whether the cross-linking observed is
a specific reaction. To check on this point, Table 2 gives the
results of control experiments in which different *E. coli* protein-
tRNA combinations were tested for photochemical cross-linking. It
is seen, for example, that IleRS joins to $tRNA^{Ile}$ but not to
$tRNA_1^{Tyr}$ or $tRNA^{Phe}$. BSA, a non-specific protein, cross-links
neither to $tRNA^{Ile}$ nor to $tRNA_1^{Tyr}$. On the other hand, a good
cross-linking yield is achieved between TyrRS and $tRNA_1^{Tyr}$. Also,
a small amount of joining occurs between TyrRS and $tRNA^{Ile}$; this
low yield is probably significant since other data have shown that
these two species can form a relatively stable complex. Therefore,
the data of Table 2 clearly indicate that the photochemically cross-
linked enzyme-tRNA complexes are specific.

The data of Fig. 5 show that a plateau in cross-linking is
reached before all of the tRNA is joined to enzyme. This suggests

Table 2.   Photoinduced Cross-Linking of *E. coli*-tRNAs and Enzymes
(Budzik *et al.*, 1975)*

Enzyme	tRNA	% Joining
IleRS	tRNA^{Ile}	40[a]
BSA	tRNA^{Ile}	0[b]
IleRS	tRNA^{Tyr}	0[c]
IleRS	tRNA^{Phe}	0[d]
TyrRS	tRNA^{Tyr}	50[e]
BSA	tRNA^{Tyr}	0[f]
TyrRS	tRNA^{Ile}	7[g]

*All irradiations were done for a minimum of 20 min in 10 mM
MgCl$_2$, 50 mM Na cacodylate, pH 5.2 or 5.5 (see below).
[a] 2 μM IleRS and 1.4 μM tRNA^{Ile}, pH 5.5.
[b] 3 μM BSA and 1.7 μM tRNA^{Ile}, pH 5.5.
[c] 2 μM IleRS and 1 μM tRNA^{Tyr}, pH 5.2.
[d] 4 μM IleRS and 1.8 μM tRNA^{Phe}, pH 5.5.
[e] 2 μM TyrRS and 1 μM tRNA^{Tyr}, pH 5.2.
[f] 3 μM BSA and 1 μM tRNA^{Tyr}, pH 5.2.
[g] 2 μM TyrRS and 1.4 μM tRNA^{Ile}, pH 5.5.

some photoinactivation has occurred before all molecules cross-link.
An experiment was carried out with *E. coli* IleRS and tRNA^{Ile} to
check further on this question. Enzyme and tRNA were irradiated
until the plateau was reached. At this point either fresh enzyme
or fresh tRNA was added, the irradiation was then continued, and
the amount of additional cross-linking determined. It was found
that when fresh tRNA is added no additional cross-linking is
achieved, but when fresh enzyme is added there is an additional
increment of tRNA joined. This increment roughly corresponds to
40% of the tRNA remaining after the first irradiation. Therefore,
it is clear that the plateau is due to photoinactivation of groups
on the enzyme.

Although IleRS is photoinactivated with respect to cross-
linking ability, other controls establish that it retains its tRNA
binding ability after an irradiation time of 20 min or so. The
irradiation does cause the enzyme to lose its catalytic ability;
this is possibly due to photoinactivation of an active site
sulfhydryl group known to be critical for enzymatic activity but

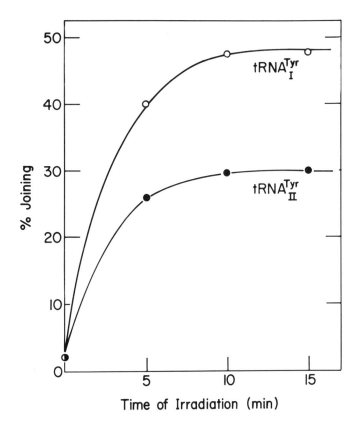

Fig. 5.   The percentage of *E. coli* tRNA$_I^{Tyr}$ and of tRNA$_{II}^{Tyr}$ that are joined to *E. coli* TyrRS as a function of the time of irradiation.   The fluence rate was ~2-3 × 10^4 ergs mm^{-2} min^{-1} (From Schoemaker and Schimmel, 1974).

not for tRNA binding (Iaccarino and Berg, 1969).   When tRNA^{Ile} alone is irradiated for 30 min or so, very little damage occurs. For example, chain breakage is about 5% or less; the amino acid acceptance activity is within experimental error of an unirradiated control; and chromatographic analyses indicate that the production of photomodified bases and intramolecular cross-links is minimal (Budzik *et al.*, 1975).   Similar results have been obtained in control experiments with other aminoacyl tRNA synthetases and tRNAs (Schoemaker and Schimmel, 1974; Schoemaker *et al.*, 1975).

2.2.2.   *Analysis for Cross-Linked Regions on tRNA.*   Having reasonable assurance that the cross-linked complex is a true representation of the native one, experiments were carried out to

identify the parts of the nucleic acid that are photojoined to the
enzyme. The most obvious approach is to use a nuclease that will
cut away all parts of the nucleic acid that are not joined to the
protein. However, care must be exercised in the choice of a
nuclease. If, for example, a non-specific endonuclease is used,
such as T2 ribonuclease, the results obtained will be of little
value. This is because the nucleic acid is made of only four basic
mononucleotide units that are each represented many times in the
sequence. Thus, if a covalent enzyme-nucleic acid complex is
degraded to the enzyme-mononucleotide level, the identity of the
attached mononucleotide units does not establish the parts of
the structure from which they arose. An alternative approach is
to use a highly specific nuclease, such as T1 ribonuclease, which
cleaves only after G's. This enzyme cuts a given tRNA into 15
or so oligonucleotide pieces; most of these have a unique size
and/or sequence and, therefore, can be assigned to a unique part
of the structure. Having established the oligonucleotide segments
to which the enzyme is attached, a T2 ribonuclease digestion of the
attached T1 fragments may be performed to determine the linked
base within each segment.

The procedure used employed T1 ribonuclease and also permitted
a statistical evaluation to be made of the frequency of cross-linking
of each T1 oligonucleotide to the enzyme (see Schoemaker and Schimmel, 1974; Budzik *et al.*, 1975). The statistical analysis is
desirable because the cross-linked complexes tend to be heterogeneous. For example, although three regions on a tRNA may join to
an enzyme, within the population of cross-linked complexes individual species may have only one or two cross-links, with different
combinations of the three possibilities existing for each species.
Data given below are reported in terms of the percent joining of
each T1 segment of a cross-linked tRNA; thus, a percent joining
of 50% for a given fragment implies that half of the cross-linked
complexes are linked at that fragment. At this point, the precise
base that is linked within each fragment has not been determined.

The results of the analysis of the cross-linked IleRS-tRNA[Ile]
complex are shown in Fig. 6. This graph plots in bar graph form
the percent joining of the various T1 fragments *versus* the fragment
number. The fragments are numbered in accordance with their positions on a two dimensional chromatogram. A percent joining of less
than 10% is considered insignificant; negative deviations in the
figure merely reflect experimental error. The figure shows that
significant cross-linking occurs to only three fragments in the
tRNA--7, 10, and 11. All the rest show no significant joining.
These data are further evidence that cross-linking occurs at
specific sites. Moreover, since the three fragments are cross-
linked 40-50%, there are on the average 1.2-1.5 cross-links in
the photojoined complexes.

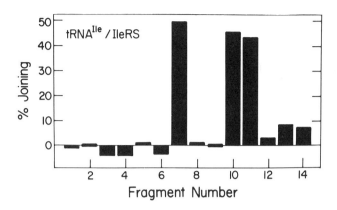

Fig. 6. Plot of the percent joining of the various T1 fragments of *E. coli* tRNA[Ile] to IleRS *versus* the fragment number (From
Budzik *et al.*, 1975).

Figure 7 gives the sequence and cloverleaf structure of *E. coli*
tRNA[Ile]. The numbered T1 fragments are enclosed by dotted outlines.
The three darkly shaded fragments correspond to the ones found cross-
linked to the isoleucyl tRNA synthetase. Two of these are in the
dihydrouridine region while the third is at the 3'-terminus of the
molecule. A discussion of the possible significance of these sites
is given elsewhere (Budzik *et al.*, 1975).

In Fig. 8 a rough sketch of the three dimensional structure of
a tRNA molecule is given. Familiar landmarks on the tRNA are indicated (compare with Fig. 4). The molecule is made up of two helical
branches that join at approximately right angles to give a L-shaped
structure. The region in which the two helical branches fuse contains a number of tertiary interactions.

Cross-linked regions are indicated by dark shading. Two of
them occur in or near the region where the two helical branches
fuse. Other data suggest that the anticodon loop is also in close
proximity to the surface of the enzyme. This fact and the cross-
linking data give the picture that the enzyme binds along and
around the "inside" of the L-shaped structure.

2.2.3. *A Non-Cognate, Heterologous Complex.* In some cases a

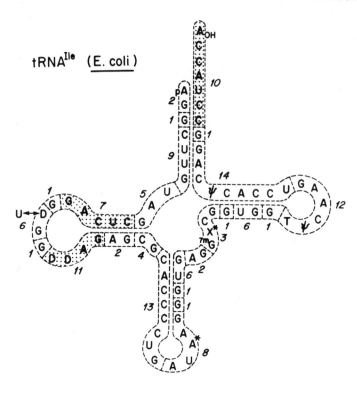

tRNA^Ile (E. coli)

tRNA^Ile / IleRS

Fig. 7. Sequence and cloverleaf structure of *E. coli* tRNA^Ile. The sequence is that determined by Yarus and Barrell (1971). T1 fragments are enclosed by dotted outlines and the darkly shaded fragments correspond to ones found cross-linked to IleRS (From Budzik *et al.*, 1975).

given aminoacyl tRNA synthetase will attach its amino acid to the "wrong" tRNA species (see Kisselev and Favorova, 1974; Söll and Schimmel, 1974). This can even occur without special reaction conditions. An example is yeast valine tRNA synthetase (ValRS) which can attach valine to *E. coli* tRNA^Ile (Kern *et al.*, 1972). The question is whether this non-cognate yeast enzyme binds to the *E. coli* tRNA by a similar or by a different topological pattern, compared to the cognate enzyme. If the pattern is similar, it suggests there is a common geometric orientation of the various synthetases on their respective tRNAs.

Photochemical cross-linking provides an ideal way to approach

tRNA^Ile / IleRS

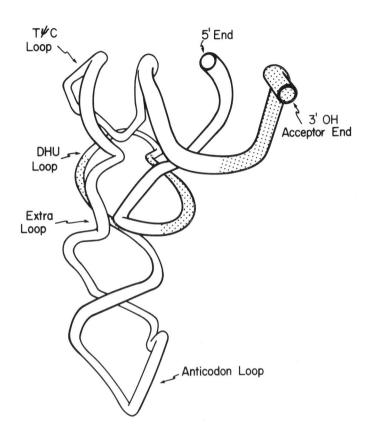

Fig. 8.   Sketch of the three dimensional structure of a tRNA molecule (see Kim *et al.*, 1973).   Regions of *E. coli* tRNA^Ile found cross-linked to *E. coli* IleRS are indicated by shading (From Budzik *et al.*, 1975).

this question. It was found that the enzyme and tRNA in the hetero-logous, non-cognate complex can be coupled together under the action of UV light. Like the cognate complex, the non-cognate one has three cross-linked regions; two of these are identical in both complexes and occur in the dihydrouridine region. The new fragment unique to the non-cognate complex is in the anticodon loop.

The regions joined to the enzyme in this special complex are indicated by shading on the three dimensional model of the tRNA structure in Fig. 9. In addition to these regions, the enzyme

tRNA^{Ile} / ValRS

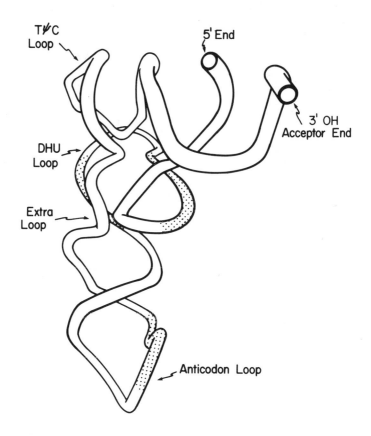

Fig. 9.   Sketch of three dimensional structure of a tRNA molecule (see Kim *et al.*, 1973) with regions on *E. coli* tRNA^{Ile} joined to yeast ValRS indicated by dark shading (From Budzik *et al.*, 1975).

must also make contact with the 3'-terminus since amino acid is attached at this site. Therefore, the data indicate that the non-cognate enzyme binds along and around the "inside" of the L, much like the cognate enzyme.

2.2.4. *Other Complexes.* The preceding data imply that two different enzymes bind to the same tRNA in a similar fashion. But there is another aspect to the above results which is also of interest to consider. Since two of the fragments that react are the same for both enzymes, each must have photochemically reactive

amino acids in similar positions. This gives rise to the speculation that the various tRNA synthetases have a similar set of amino
acids lining their tRNA binding sites; specificity could be achieved
by amino acid differences in a few key positions.

Additional data bearing on these speculations has been obtained
from three photochemically cross-linked complexes of yeast tRNA^{Phe}
(Schoemaker *et al.*, 1975). Two *E. coli* enzymes--IleRS and ValRS--
bind to this yeast tRNA in addition to the cognate yeast PheRS.
Each enzyme cross-links to three distinct parts of the tRNA^{Phe}
structure, but two of these regions are common to all three complexes. This is shown by the comparative bar graph given in Fig.
10. Here again, therefore, the enzymes appear not only to have
common features in the way they bind to yeast tRNA^{Phe}, but in
addition all three have photoactive amino acids in closely corresponding positions.

3. DISCUSSION

Since the original observations on photochemically cross-
linked BSA-DNA complexes, a number of other protein-nucleic acid
systems have been examined. Successful photochemical attachment
to an appropriate nucleic acid has been achieved with DNA polymerase, RNA polymerase, the *lac* repressor, a special DNA binding
protein, and aminoacyl tRNA synthetases. This variety of systems
in which successful cross-linking has been accomplished suggests
that nucleic acid binding proteins, under proper conditions, may
typically be capable of photojoining to their appropriate nucleic
acids.

It is now clear that the approach has considerable value for
structure-function studies. This is due to the possibility of
adjusting solution conditions so that only specific complexes are
photochemically cross-linked. Specificity is nicely illustrated
by the results of Lin and Riggs (1974) on the joining of the *lac*
repressor to BrdUrd-λh80d*lac* DNA, and the studies of complexes of
tRNAs with aminoacyl tRNA synthetases. Moreover, the results on
synthetase-tRNA complexes clearly show that the determination of
the spatial locations of cross-linking sites gives sharp insights
into topological features of protein-nucleic acid complexes.

An interesting question arises when data on the *lac* repressor
and the synthetases are compared. In the former case good cross-
linking was only achieved with BrdUrd-substituted DNA; in the case
of the synthetases no such substitution was necessary. If the *lac*
operator (the *lac* repressor binding site) is a strictly double-
stranded segment of DNA, then it might be argued that the greater
reactivity of the unsubstituted tRNAs is due to the occurrence of
single-stranded cloverleaf sections. [It is known, for example,

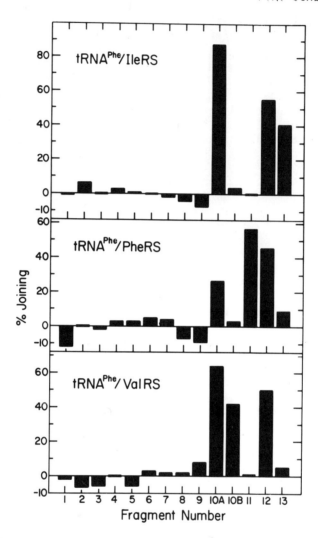

Fig. 10. Percent joining *versus* the T1 fragment number for
cross-linked complexes of yeast tRNA^Phe with yeast PheRS, *E. coli*
IleRS, and *E. coli* ValRS. Fragments are numbered in accordance
with the position of their occurrence on a two dimensional chromatogram (From Schoemaker *et al.*, 1975).

that in some photoreactions single-stranded sections are more
reactive than double-stranded ones (Smith and Meun, 1968)]. This
argument implies that in each T1 fragment of the tRNA the actual
base that is cross-linked is in a single-stranded piece. The
argument is weakened by the observation that, in one of the tRNA

complexes studied, a cross-linked fragment appears to arise entirely from a cloverleaf helical section (Schoemaker *et al.*, 1975). It should be mentioned, however, that one of the base pairs in this helical section is a G-U interaction; this might be a less stable site in the helix where cross-linking could occur.

Very little is known about the nature of the amino acid-base adducts formed under the action of UV radiation. Some of the literature on this subject has been reviewed recently by Smith (1975) and Varghese (This Volume), and only a few highlights are touched on here. It has been shown that irradiation of mixtures of cysteine and uracil gives 5-S-cysteine-6-hydrouracil as a product (Smith and Aplin, 1966); an analogous compound is formed when thymine replaces uracil [Smith, 1970; see also Varghese (1973) who discusses other photoproducts as well]. Jellinek and Johns (1970) have discussed the mechanism of this kind of reaction. The photocoupling of 1-propylamine to 1,3 dimethyluracil has been studied by Yang and coworkers (Gorelic *et al.*, 1972). In addition to the 6-position, they find, like Smith, the 5-position is a reactive site. In the case of purine nucleosides, the C-8 position is a prominent reactive site (cf. Steinmaus *et al.*, 1969).

Hopefully, sufficient quantities of the adducts formed in the cross-linked protein-nucleic acid complexes discussed above may be obtained for mass spectral or other kinds of detailed analyses. This should give a molecular picture of the covalent species that are generated. In addition, it is always of interest to sequence the amino acids in the protein, and bases in the nucleic acid, that flank the cross-linking sites. Together with other structural information on the individual reacting macromolecules, the cross-linking and sequence information may be sufficient to build a well-defined molecular model of the complex of interest. The results obtained with the tRNAs and aminoacyl tRNA synthetases are a first step in this direction and, hopefully, progress in this and other systems will soon advance to the stage where accurate models may be fashioned.

References

Anderson, E., Nakashima, Y., and Konigsberg, W., 1975, Photo-induced cross-linkage of gene-5 protein and bacteriophage fd DNA[+], *Nucleic Acid Res.* 2:361-371.
Beckwith, J.R., and Zipser, D. (eds.), 1970, "The Lactose Operon," Cold Spring Harbor Laboratory.
Braun, A., and Merrick, B., 1975, Properties of the ultraviolet light mediated binding reaction of bovine serum albumin with DNA, *Photochem. Photobiol.* 21:243-248.

Budzik, G.P., Lam, S.M., Schoemaker, H.J.P., and Schimmel, P.R., 1975, Two photo-crosslinked complexes of isoleucine specific transfer RNA with aminoacyl transfer RNA synthetases, *J. Biol. Chem.* 250:4433-4439.

Chapeville, F., Lipmann, F., von Ehrenstein, G., Weisblum, B., Ray, W.J., Jr., and Benzer, S., 1962, On the role of soluble ribonucleic acid in coding for amino acids, *Proc. Nat. Acad. Sci. USA* 48:1086-1092.

Dickson, L.A., and Schimmel, P.R., 1975, Structure of transfer RNA-aminoacyl transfer RNA synthetase complexes investigated by nuclease digestion, *Arch. Biochem. Biophys.* 167:638-645.

Gilbert, W., Maizels, N., and Maxam, A., 1974, Sequences of controlling regions of the lactose operon, *Cold Spring Harbor Symp. Quant. Biol.* 38:845-855.

Goodman, H.M., Abelson, J., Landy, A., Brenner, S., and Smith, J.D., 1968, Amber suppression: a nucleotide change in the anticodon of a tyrosine transfer RNA, *Nature* 217:1019-1024.

Gorelic, L.S., Lisagor, P., and Yang, N.C., 1972, The photochemical reactions of 1,3-dimethyluracil with 1-aminopropane and poly-L-lysine, *Photochem. Photobiol.* 16:465-480.

Hörz, W., and Zachau, H.G., 1973, Complexes of aminoacyl-tRNA synthetases with tRNAs as studied by partial nuclease digestion, *Eur. J. Biochem.* 32:1-14.

Iaccarino, M., and Berg, P., 1969, Requirement of sulfhydryl groups for the catalytic and tRNA recognition functions of isoleucyl-tRNA synthetase, *J. Mol. Biol.* 42:151-169.

Jellinek, T., and Johns, R.B., 1970, The mechanism of photochemical addition of cysteine to uracil and formation of dihydrouracil, *Photochem. Photobiol.* 11:349-359.

Jones, O.W., and Berg, P., 1966, Studies on the binding of RNA polymerase to polynucleotides, *J. Mol. Biol.* 22:199-209.

Kern, D., Giegé, R., and Ebel, J.P., 1972, Incorrect aminoacylations catalysed by the phenylalanyl- and valyl-tRNA synthetases from yeast, *Eur. J. Biochem.* 31:148-155.

Kim, S.H., Quigley, G.J., Suddath, F.L., McPherson, A., Sneden, D., Kim, J., Weinzierl, J., and Rich, A., 1973, Three-dimensional structure of yeast phenylalanine transfer RNA. Folding of the polynucleotide chain, *Science* 179:285-288.

Kim, S.H., Suddath, F.L., Quigley, G.J., McPherson, A., Sussman, J.L., Wang, A.H.J., Seeman, N.C., and Rich, A., 1974, Three-dimensional tertiary structure of yeast phenylalanine transfer RNA, *Science* 185:435-440.

Kisselev, L.L., and Favorova, O.O., 1974, Aminoacyl-tRNA synthetases: some recent results and achievements, *Adv. Enzymol. Relat. Areas Mol. Biol.* 40:141-238.

Kornberg, A., 1975, "DNA Synthesis," W.H. Freeman, San Francisco.

Lin, S.-Y., and Riggs, A.D., 1972, *lac* repressor binding to non-operator DNA: detailed studies and a comparison of equilibrium and rate competition methods, *J. Mol. Biol.* 72:671-690.

Lin, S.-Y., and Riggs, A.D., 1974, Photochemical attachment of *lac* repressor to bromodeoxyuridine-substituted *lac* operator by ultraviolet radiation, *Proc. Nat. Acad. Sci. USA* 71:947-951.

Markovitz, A., 1972, Ultraviolet light-induced stable complexes of DNA and DNA polymerase, *Biochim. Biophys. Acta* 281:522-534.

Marvin, D.A., and Hohn, B., 1969, Filamentous bacterial viruses, *Bacteriol. Rev.* 33:172-209.

Müller-Hill, B., 1971, *Lac* repressor, *Angew. Chem. Int. Ed. Engl.* 10:160-172.

Nakashima, Y., and Konigsberg, W., 1975, Photo-induced cross-linkage of gene 5 protein and Fd DNA. Abstr. Int. Symp. "Protein and Other Adducts to DNA: Their Significance to Aging, Carcinogenesis and Radiation Biology," Williamsburg, Virginia, May 2-6, 1975.

Nomura, M., Tissières, A., and Lengyel, P. (eds.), 1974, "Ribosomes," Cold Spring Harbor Laboratory.

Pratt, D., Laws, P., and Griffith, J., 1974, Complex of bacteriophage M13 single-stranded DNA and gene 5 protein, *J. Mol. Biol.* 82:425-439.

RajBhandary, U.L., and Chang, S.H., 1968, Studies on polynucleotides. LXXXII. Yeast phenylalanine transfer ribonucleic acid: partial digestion with ribonuclease T1 and derivation of the total primary structure, *J. Biol. Chem.* 243:598-608.

Riggs, A.D., Newby, R.F., and Bourgeois, S., 1970a, *lac* repressor-operator interaction. II. Effect of galactosides and other ligands, *J. Mol. Biol.* 51:303-314.

Riggs, A.D., Suzuki, H., and Bourgeois, S., 1970b, *lac* repressor-operator interaction. I. Equilibrium studies, *J. Mol. Biol.* 48:67-83.

Robertus, J.D., Ladner, J.E., Finch, J.T., Rhodes, D., Brown, R.S., Clark, B.F.C., and Klug, A., 1974, Structure of yeast phenylalanine tRNA at 3 Å resolution, *Nature* 250:546-551.

Schimmel, P.R., Uhlenbeck, O.C., Lewis, J.B., Dickson, L.A., Eldred, E.W., and Schreier, A.A., 1972, Binding of complementary oligonucleotides to free and aminoacyl transfer ribonucleic acid synthetase bound transfer ribonucleic acid, *Biochemistry* 11:642-646.

Schoemaker, H.J.P., Budzik, G.P., Giegé, R.C., and Schimmel, P.R., 1975, Three photo-crosslinked complexes of yeast phenylalanine specific transfer RNA with aminoacyl transfer RNA synthetases, *J. Biol. Chem.* 250:4440-4444.

Schoemaker, H.J.P., and Schimmel, P.R., 1974, Photo-induced joining of a transfer RNA with its cognate aminoacyl-transfer RNA synthetase, *J. Mol. Biol.* 84:503-513.

Setlow, R.B., and Setlow, J.K., 1972, Effects of radiation on polynucleotides, *Annu. Rev. Biophys. Bioeng.* 1:293-346.

Smith, K.C., 1964, The photochemical inactivation of deoxyribonucleic acid and protein *in vivo* and its biological importance, *Photochem. Photobiol.* 3:415-427.

Smith, K.C., 1969, Photochemical addition of amino acids to ^{14}C-uracil, *Biochem. Biophys. Res. Commun.* 34:354-357.

Smith, K.C., 1970, A mixed photoproduct of thymine and cysteine: 5-S-cysteine, 6-hydrothymine, *Biochem. Biophys. Res. Commun.* 39:1011-1016.

Smith, K.C., 1975, The radiation-induced addition of proteins and other molecules to nucleic acids, *in* "Photochemistry and Photobiology of Nucleic Acids" (S.Y. Wang, ed.), Academic Press, New York (in press).

Smith, K.C., and Aplin, R.T., 1966, A mixed photoproduct of uracil and cysteine (5-S-cysteine-6-hydrouracil). A possible model for the *in vivo* cross-linking of DNA and protein by UV light, *Biochemistry* 5:2125-2130.

Smith, K.C., and Meun, D.H.C., 1968, Kinetics of the photochemical addition of [^{35}S] cysteine to polynucleotides and nucleic acids, *Biochemistry* 7:1033-1037.

Söll, D., and Schimmel, P.R., 1974, Aminoacyl-tRNA synthetases, *Enzymes* 10:489-538.

Steinmaus, H., Rosenthal, I., and Elad, D., 1969, Photochemical and γ-ray-induced reactions of purines and purine nucleosides with 2-propanol, *J. Am. Chem. Soc.* 91:4921-4923.

Strniste, G.F., and Smith, D.A., 1974, Induction of stable linkage between the deoxyribonucleic acid dependent ribonucleic acid polymerase and $d(A-T)_n \cdot d(A-T)_n$ by ultraviolet light, *Biochemistry* 13:485-493.

Uhlenbeck, O.C., Baller, J., and Doty, P., 1970, Complementary oligonucleotide binding to the anticodon loop of fMet-transfer RNA, *Nature (London)* 225:508-510.

Varghese, A.J., 1973, Properties of photoaddition products of thymine and cysteine, *Biochemistry* 12:2725-2730.

Weintraub, H., 1973, The assembly of newly replicated DNA into chromatin, *Cold Spring Harbor Symp. Quant. Biol.* 38:247-256.

Yarus, M., and Barrell, B.G., 1971, The sequence of nucleotides in tRNA[Ile] from *E. coli* B, *Biochem. Biophys. Res. Commun.* 43:729-734.

Zachau, H.G., 1969, Transfer ribonucleic acids, *Angew, Chem. Int. Ed. Engl.* 8:711-727.

PHOTOSENSITIZED CROSS-LINKING OF PROTEINS TO NUCLEIC ACIDS

Claude Hélène

Centre de Biophysique Moléculaire, 45045 Orléans

Cedex, France

1. INTRODUCTION

Cross-linking of nucleic acids and proteins represents one of the many reactions that can take place when bacteria or mammalian cells are irradiated with UV light. Every cell contains a lot of potential photosensitizer molecules whose excitation in a wave-length region where neither proteins nor nucleic acids absorb light might lead to the formation of cross-links between these two macro-molecules. One might contemplate applying methods similar to those developed for the selective modification of nucleic acids, e.g., acetophenone photosensitization produces practically only cyclo-butane-type thymine dimers in DNA (Lamola, 1972). If it appeared possible to create a well-defined chemical link between a particu-lar amino acid side chain and a nucleic acid base, then the method might become an important and specific tool in the investigation

149

of protein-nucleic acid complexes. The applicability of the method
to provide evidence for the close proximity of protein and nucleic
acid species in multimacromolecular systems such as ribosomes, chromatin, etc..., might also help in understanding the architecture
of these systems. The potentialities of the photosensitization
method are therefore very diverse. In the present report photosensitized reactions leading to nucleic acid-protein cross-linking
are reviewed. Different situations may be distinguished:

i)   The photosensitizer can be a small organic molecule which
     has been added to the system under investigation and which
     absorbs light at wavelengths longer than the two macro-
     molecules.

ii) The photosensitizer may be incorporated in one of the two
     macromolecules in a covalent way. This incorporation
     could be obtained by chemical modification of the isolated
     macromolecules or by a biochemical *in vivo* pathway.

iii) The photosensitizer may be a chromophore normally present
     in one of the macromolecules or may result from a photo-
     chemical transformation of one of these chromophores.

In every case, the role of the photosensitizer molecule, once
it has been excited, will be to produce directly or indirectly
(e.g., via singlet oxygen) a reactive transient species (excited
state, radical, ion, epoxide, peroxide,...) in either the protein
or the nucleic acid. This intermediate will then react with some
chemical group of the other macromolecule. In the following review,
the term "photosensitization" will be given a broad definition,
i.e., the photosensitizer may be recovered at the end of the reaction as a separate species which has been or has not been chemically
transformed but it may also remain bound to the macromolecules and
act as a bridge between them.

2. PHOTOSENSITIZATION OF NUCLEIC ACID-PROTEIN CROSS-LINKING BY AROMATIC MOLECULES

2.1. Photodynamic Effect

It is known that irradiation of DNA with visible light in the
presence of dyes such as methylene blue or acridine orange produces damage in the DNA molecule (Simon and Van Vunakis, 1962).
Guanine bases are destroyed by a sensitized photooxidation reaction
resulting from the reaction of singlet oxygen produced by the
excited dye. Single-strand breaks are also produced in the DNA
molecule (Freifelder *et al.*, 1961).

The dye-sensitized photooxidation of proteins has been extensively investigated (see Spikes, 1968; Grossweiner, 1969; Chandra,
1970; Nilsson *et al.*, 1972). Certain amino acid side chains
(cystine, histidine, methionine, tryptophan, tyrosine) are much
more sensitive towards photooxidation than other amino acids.
Depending on the chemical nature of the sensitizer and of the
substrate and on the experimental conditions, different mechanisms
have been proposed to account for the photosensitized reactions.
The primary photochemical steps involve either singlet oxygen
production or radical formation by electron or hydrogen abstraction
reactions.

Exposure to visible light of bacterial cells which have been
pretreated with acridine orange or methylene blue results in rapid
killing of the cells and cross-linking of DNA with proteins and
membrane material (Smith, This Volume; Petrusek, 1971). The dye
which is the more efficient in inducing these cross-links is also
the more efficient in killing the bacterial cells. When λ bacteriophage are irradiated in the presence of methylated proflavine,
double-strand breaks are produced in the DNA and electron microscopy shows that the DNA pieces are strongly attached to the phage
coat protein as a result of a cross-linking reaction (Jaffe-Brachet
et al., 1971). In the absence of information on the damage created
in individual molecules (DNA, proteins, lipids...) in the cells
irradiated with visible light in the presence of dyes, it is difficult to deduce a correlation between cross-linking and killing.
Nevertheless, these investigations demonstrate that cross-linking
reactions can be photosensitized *in vivo* by dyes.

Dye-photosensitized cross-linking of DNA with proteins can also
be produced *in vitro*. For example, DNA can be cross-linked to bovine
serum albumin by the action of visible light in the presence of
acridine orange. No reaction occurs when the macromolecules are
separately irradiated in the presence of acridine orange and then
mixed (Smith, 1975). Irradiation of *B. subtilis* transforming DNA
with visible light in the presence of acridine orange results in
the inactivation of the transforming ability. However, this inactivation is much more rapid if ribonuclease, histone or spermine are
added before irradiation (Petrusek, 1971) and cross-linking between
DNA and the protein was shown to take place under these conditions.
Treatment of the DNA-RNase complex with pronase, however, led to a
dramatic increase in marker activity.

2.2. Triplet-State Energy Transfer

Photosensitized cross-linking reactions between nucleic acids
and proteins in which the photosensitizer transfers its excitation
energy either to the nucleic acid or to the protein have not been
reported yet. Acetone in its triplet state is able to transfer

its excitation energy to nucleic acid bases and probably to accessible tryptophan or tyrosine residues of proteins. Acetophenone
should be more selective in transferring its triplet state energy
only to thymine and tryptophan (Hélène, 1975). These ketones should
be able to photosensitize the cross-linking of proteins and nucleic
acids since it is known, e.g., that tyrosine and uracil form covalent bonds when UV-irradiated in aqueous solution (Smith, 1969;
Schott and Shetlar, 1974). Also reactions which are not observed
under direct excitation because, e.g., the triplet state is not
populated, may become predominant in photosensitized reactions.

Acetone and acetophenone are able to photosensitize the formation of thymine-cysteine adducts. The products formed by photosensitization are the same as those obtained by direct irradiation
and their relative yields are also the same (Fisher *et al.*, 1974).
It has been concluded that the triplet state of thymine is an
intermediate species in the formation of these adducts. When uracil
is irradiated in the presence of cysteine at least four addition
products are formed. Only two of them (5-S-cysteine-5,6-dihydro-
uracil and 5-S,S-cysteine-5,6-dihydrouracil) are obtained when
irradiation is carried out at long wavelengths ($\lambda > 290$ nm) in the
presence of acetone, suggesting that the triplet state of uracil is
involved in the formation of these two adducts (Varghese, 1974b).
The other two adducts seem to arise from the reaction of thiyl
radicals with ground-state uracil molecules.

The photoaddition of uracil and thymine to glutathione has
also been described. The main adducts (5-S-glutathione-5,6-dihyro-
pyrimidine and 5-S,S-glutathione-5,6-dihydropyrimidine) are obtained
in better yields when the irradiation is carried out in the presence
of triplet-state sensitizers such as acetophenone in the case of
thymine and acetone in the case of uracil (Varghese, 1974a).

These results show that it might prove useful to utilize
triplet-state sensitizers to initiate the selective formation of
some photoadducts involved in protein-nucleic acid cross-linking.
However, the structure of the protein-nucleic acid complex might
be such that the potentially reactive groups are not accessible to
the photosensitizer. Energy transfer processes in one of the macromolecules might possibly help overcome this difficulty. Such
processes have been reviewed recently by Longworth (1971) in the
case of proteins and polypeptides, by Eisinger and Lamola (1971)
and Hélène (1973b) in the case of nucleic acids and polynucleotides.
Energy transfer processes are responsible for the sensitized phos-
phorescence of tryptophan observed in poly(A)-oligopeptide complexes
(Hélène, 1973a). The energy absorbed by adenine bases migrates at
the triplet level until it is transferred to and trapped by the
stacked indole ring. In poly(A)-cystamine complexes, the disulfide
group also acts as a trap for the energy migrating at the triplet
level in poly(A) (Hélène, 1975; Montenay-Garestier *et al.*, to be

published). Whether this is the result of electron transfer or of
energy transfer from the adenine ring to the disulfide group remains
to be elucidated. Subsequent photochemical reactions also have to
be investigated.

2.3. Sensitizer-Mediated Cross-Linking of DNA and Proteins

In the two preceeding cases, the photosensitizer was absorbing
the exciting light but was not involved in the chemical linkage
between the nucleic acid and the protein, although it could be modified at the end of the reaction.

It may also happen that the cross-link is mediated through the
sensitizer. For example, Lesko *et al.* (1971) have reported that
irradiation of 3,4-benzpyrene-nucleohistone physical complexes at
wavelengths longer than 300 nm results in the formation of DNA-
histone cross-links. The benzpyrene molecule is chemically bound
to these complexes suggesting that the cross-linking is mediated
in some manner through benzpyrene.

Although it would be difficult in most cases to demonstrate
that the sensitizer molecule acts as a bridge between the two
macromolecules, this possibility could represent an important
reaction especially with multifunctional sensitizers. In the case
of *in vivo* studies it should also be kept in mind that the sensitizer molecule can be metabolized and that some of the metabolites
might possess several reactive groups. One might also contemplate
the possibility of forming a bridge between nucleic acids and
proteins by combining a chemical reaction in the dark on one side
and a photochemical reaction on the other side.

3. DNA-PROTEIN CROSS-LINKING INDUCED BY INCORPORATED PHOTOSENSITIZERS

In the preceeding section, the sensitizer was an organic molecule added to the DNA-protein mixture or to the cell system. This
section deals with reactions photochemically induced by a sensitizer
molecule which is incorporated in a covalent way in one of the two
macromolecules. One possibility is to chemically modify a reactive
group on the protein or the nucleic acid so that the modified molecule absorbs light at wavelengths longer than the chromophores of
the original molecule. A second possibility, which has been widely
used, is to introduce the chemical modification by a biochemical
pathway. The most common example is the incorporation of 5-bromo-
uracil (BrUra) in place of thymine in DNA.

3.1. Bromouracil Substitution

When thymine is replaced by BrUra, the sensitivity of bacterial cells to killing by UV radiation is markedly increased. At the same time, DNA-protein cross-links are produced at an enhanced rate (Smith, 1975).

In a study of the association of newly made histone with newly made DNA in chick erythroblast cultures, Weintraub (1973) has demonstrated that BrUra-DNA could be very efficiently cross-linked to proteins (mainly histones). When protein synthesis was inhibited by cycloheximide the amount of protein that could be cross-linked to newly synthesized BrUra-DNA was decreased (Fig. 1). This result supports a non-dispersive model for histone recycling in chromosome replication.

In vitro experiments clearly demonstrate the applicability of BrUra substitution to induce cross-links between DNA and proteins. As shown in Fig. 1, histone, polylysine, polyarginine, and *E. coli* RNA polymerase are efficiently cross-linked to DNA. More recently the covalent attachment of the *lac* repressor to BrUra-substituted operator has been demonstrated by Lin and Riggs (1974). Bromouracil substitution does not prevent the specific binding of the *lac* repressor to the *lac* operator. The binding constant is even increased about one order of magnitude. The repressor-operator complex is dissociated when the inducer IPTG (isopropyl-β-D-thiogalactoside) is added to the system. UV irradiation leads to the formation of IPTG-resistant complexes (see Fig. 3 in Schimmel *et al.*, This Volume). The presence during irradiation of IPTG or of other ligands known to inhibit repressor binding to operator eliminates the formation of stable complexes. Under low ionic strength conditions, the *lac* repressor binds to non-operator DNA and this binding is not sensitive to IPTG. Using BrUra-substituted DNA, it was shown that repressor can be covalently bound to non-operator DNA after UV irradiation in low salt (0.01 M KCl). At high salt (0.18 M KCl) the photochemical attachment is specific for operator DNA.

Using ^{32}P-labeled BrUra-DNA containing the *lac* operator, Ogata (1975) has prepared a *lac* repressor labeled at its operator binding site. UV irradiation was used to cross-link operator and repressor. The cross-linked complex was then subjected to DNase treatment or depurination. The labeled repressor has been isolated by gel electrophoresis and the determination of the specific locations of amino acid-nucleotide covalent bonds is now under way.

Covalent binding of catabolite gene activator protein (CAP) to BrUra-DNA has also been shown to take place after UV irradiation (Lin and Riggs, 1974). This CAP-DNA cross-linked complex is stable to high salt and cGMP (which dissociate the complex under physiological conditions).

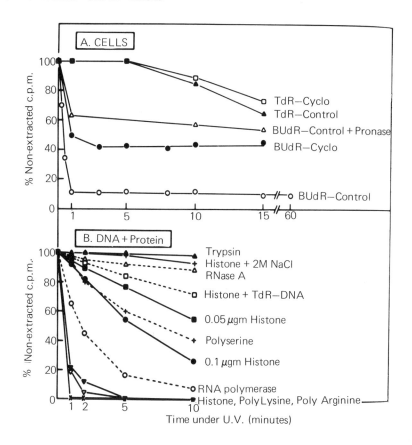

Fig. 1. Ultraviolet-induced cross-linking of protein and DNA:
(A) represents experiments involving the cross-linking of cells,
and (B) represents reconstruction experiments in which isolated
DNA is cross-linked to protein. The ordinate is the amount of
radioactivity that remains in the water phase after extraction as
a percentage of an unirradiated, control aliquot treated similarly.
The curves in (A) correspond to experiments involving control
(▲——▲) and cycloheximide cells (□——□) incubated for 30 min with
[^{3}H]thymidine (TdR); control (o——o) and cycloheximide cells
(●——●) incubated for 30 min with 5-bromodeoxyuridine (BUdR) and
[^{3}H]deoxyadenosine. Recovery of unirradiated DNA was 70% for both
control and cycloheximide cultures. The 30% of the unirradiated
DNA going to the interphase represented segments still attached to
the replication complex. Control BUdR cells digested with pronase
(Δ——Δ) had less DNA that could be extracted. All counts are
alkali stable, TCA precipitable, and DNase sensitive. In (B) DNA
was at 0.5 µg/ml and protein at 1 µg/ml, unless otherwise specified. BUdR-DNA was of hybrid density and about 90% substituted
for TdR, unless otherwise specified. All DNAs had a molecular

(Fig. 1, cont.) weight of about 10^7 daltons. The "effective dose"
of UV light received by isolated nuclei cannot at present be compared to that received by DNA in solution. (▼——▼) represents
histone and BUdR-DNA that is 50% substituted and (▽——▽) represents
protamine and fully substituted DNA (From Weintraub, 1973).

DNA and RNA polymerase can also be covalently attached to
BrUra-substituted DNA by UV irradiation, but is not known yet
whether these complexes are specific. It should be noted that
although specific covalent attachment has been shown to take place
in a few cases under direct UV irradiation (tRNA-synthetases, gene
5 protein-fd DNA; see Schimmel *et al.*, This Volume) the *lac* repressor does not appear to be photochemically bound to the *lac* operator
in the absence of BrUra-substitution.

The sensitizing activity of BrUra rests upon the photochemical
cleavage of the C-Br bond and the reactivity of the uracilyl radical
thus produced.

3.2. Chemical Modification

One of the constituents (protein or nucleic acid) of the system
under investigation can be chemically modified to introduce a chromophoric group absorbing light at wavelengths longer than the unmodified molecule. For example, in order to obtain information on the
tRNA binding sites on ribosomes, Schwartz and Ofengand (1974) have
prepared a derivative of tRNA^{Val} which can be covalently attached
to ribosomes. The 4-thiouridine of *E. coli* tRNA^{Val} was substituted
by a p-azidophenyl group (Fig. 2). The derivatized tRNA was active
in all usual reactions involving tRNA^{Val}, including amino-acylation,
non-enzymatic binding to the ribosomal P site and transfer of valine
into polypeptide. Irradiation of p-azidophenacyl-[^{3}H]valyl-tRNA
bound noncovalently to the ribosomal P site resulted in its covalent
attachment to the ribosomes. The covalent linking occurred exclusively to the 16 S RNA of the 30 S ribosomal subunit. Since the
azido group extends to about 9 Å from the sulfur atom in 4-thio-
uridine (s^{4}Urd), the above result suggests that only the 16 S RNA
molecule is within 9 Å of the s^{4}Urd residue of the tRNA.

Synthetic polynucleotides containing a modified base such as
poly-4-thiouridylic acid can be used to obtain information on the
organization of multimacromolecular systems. Poly-4-thiouridylic
acid can be used as messenger RNA for the synthesis of poly-
phenylalanine in an *in vitro* protein synthesizing system. Irradiation of the complex formed by poly-4-thiouridylic acid, ribosomes,
and phenylalanyl-tRNA at wavelengths between 300 and 400 nm where
only s^{4}Urd absorbs results in covalent attachment of the

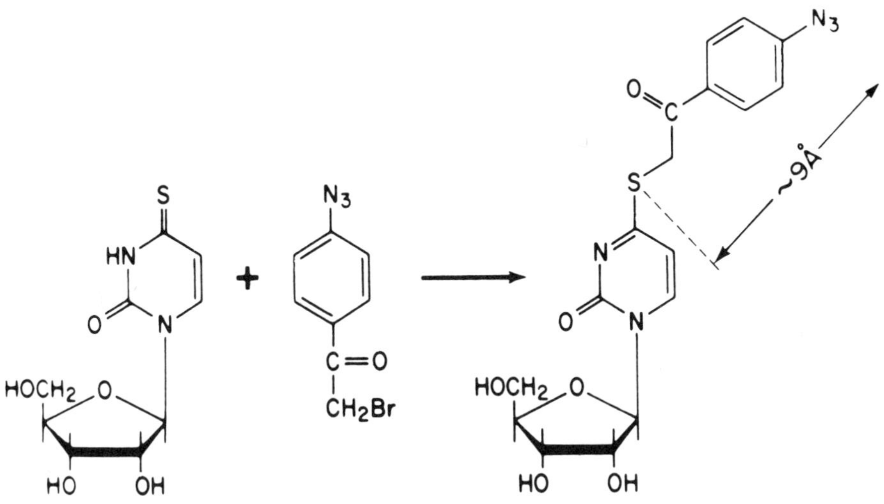

Fig. 2. Scheme for the reaction of *p*-azido phenacyl bromide with 4-thiouridine. In the maximally extended form the distance from the sulfur atom to the azido group is 9 Å and in the direction indicated (From Schwartz and Ofengand, 1974).

polynucleotide to the ribosomes (Fiser *et al.*, 1974). Using radioactive [^{3}H]poly (s^{4}Urd) it was found that the radioactive label was attached mainly to protein S1 of the 30 S ribosomal subunit suggesting that the poly (s^{4}Urd), acting as a messenger RNA, is in immediate contact with protein S1 on the ribosome.

The behavior of a complex protein system such as DNA-dependent *E. coli* RNA polymerase can also be investigated by using photoaffinity labeling. 4-Thiouridine triphosphate acts as substrate for *E. coli* RNA polymerase. Irradiation of the complexes formed by RNA polymerase and this substrate analogue in the wavelength range 300-360 nm results in covalent attachment of the sulfur derivative to the enzyme and causes irreversible inactivation (Fig. 3). The stoichiometry of the chemical modification is about 0.9. Using (^{32}P)s^{4}UTP it was found that the radioactive label was bound to β and (preferentially) β' subunits (Frischauf and Scheit, 1973).

Modified substrates which are photochemically sensitive can be used to label the active sites of enzymes involved in nucleic acid or nucleotide metabolism or of enzymes which require nucleotide coenzymes. For example, 5-iodo-2'-deoxyuridine is a substrate of thymidine kinase. This compound undergoes a dehalogenation

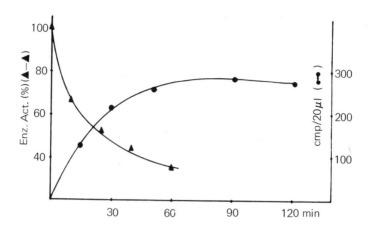

Fig. 3.   Photochemical labeling of RNA polymerase by s⁴UTP.
The reaction mixture containing 0.105 μmoles (^{32}P) s⁴UTP and 300 μg
holoenzyme in 0.2 ml was irradiated with a krypton ion laser. ▲——▲,
enzymatic activity as a function of irradiation time.   Twenty μl
aliquots of the reaction mixture were added to 1 ml of 25 mM sodium
pyrophosphate pH 8 and protein was precipitated by the addition of
2 ml of 10% trichloroacetic acid at 0°C.   The precipitate was
collected on a nitrocellulose filter, washed with 30 ml of cold 10%
trichloroacetic acid and radioactivity measured (●——●).   From the
extent of inactivation, and assuming a molecular weight for RNA
polymerase of 430,000 (30% σ-subunit), a stoichiometry s⁴UTP/enzyme =
0.9 was found (From Frischauf and Scheit, 1973).

reaction upon exposure to UV light with the formation of highly
reactive free radicals which can react with the amino acid residues
of the active site (Cysyk and Prusoff, 1972).   This method can
therefore be used to label and identify these amino acid residues.
Also, photochemically reactive derivatives of cAMP have been used
to label the active site of rabbit muscle phosphofructokinase
(Brunswick and Cooperman, 1971).   The incorporation of the label
is reversible and specific for the active site since cAMP inhibits
the photochemical binding.   Using radioactive derivatives of cAMP
this method can be used to isolate large quantities of cAMP-receptor
molecules even if only a small fraction is labeled since radioactivity can be used to follow the receptor molecules by chromatography or electrophoresis inasmuch as the label does not modify the
chromatographic or electrophoretic properties.   N⁶-(ethyl 2-diazo-
malonyl)cAMP has also been used to identify the cAMP receptor site
in human erythrocyte ghost membranes (Guthrow *et al.*, 1973).

4. SELF-PHOTOSENSITIZED REACTIONS

Direct excitation of protein and nucleic acid constituents by UV light at wavelengths shorter than 300 nm may lead to photochemical cross-linking reactions of the excited chromophores. A typical example is given by the reaction of excited thymine or uracil with cysteine (Smith, 1975; Varghese, 1974a, b). However, one must also consider the possibility that the cross-linking reaction occurs at a site far removed from the site of light absorption. This may result from different processes such as energy transfer or electron transfer. The absorbing chromophore may also undergo an internal photochemical transformation leading to the production of a molecule which can then act as a sensitizer.

Aromatic amino acids especially tryptophan form electron donor-acceptor complexes with nucleic acid bases (Montenay-Garestier and Hélène, 1971, 1973). These complexes, which involve a stacking of the two aromatic rings, have also been shown to form in oligopeptide-nucleic acid complexes (Dimicoli and Hélène, 1974). They are favored in single stranded regions of the nucleic acid (Toulmé et al., 1974). Excitation of these complexes may lead to electron transfer and subsequent reactions with other neighboring amino acid side chains may then take place. Tryptophan stacked with bases is also an energy trap for the excitation energy absorbed by nucleic acid bases (Hélène, 1973a). It has not been demonstrated yet that cross-linking between proteins and nucleic acids could occur as a result of such electron or energy transfer processes. However, recent results from our laboratory have shown that tryptophan residues of oligopeptides are able to photosensitize the splitting of thymine dimers in DNA (Charlier and Hélène, 1975; Toulmé et al., 1974). This splitting reaction is thought to involve electron transfer from the excited indole ring to thymine dimers leading to splitting and regeneration of the original thymine bases (Hélène and Charlier, 1971).

It is also tempting to speculate about the role that could be played by the photoproducts obtained by direct irradiation of the chromophores of proteins and nucleic acids. For example, it is known that tryptophan can be photooxidized under UV irradiation, and one of these photooxidation products, namely N-formylkynurenin, is a very efficient photodynamic sensitizer with respect to other amino acid residues and also to nucleotides (Walrant and Santus, 1974a). It is thus possible to convert tryptophan to formylkynurenin by irradiation at wavelengths shorter than 300 nm and then use light of wavelengths longer than 300 nm to excite selectively formylkynurenin and to photosensitize cross-linking reactions. If the photooxidation of tryptophan residues does not alter the binding of a particular protein to nucleic acid then it should be possible to use the photooxidation products as internal photosensitizers as already described for proteins (Walrant and Santus, 1974b).

Biologically-active proteins or nucleic acids may contain modified constituents which absorb light at wavelengths longer than the usual constituents. This is the case, for example, in many *E. coli* tRNAs which have sulfur-containing bases such as 4-thiouracil. Selective excitation of these modified constituents might prove useful in inducing specific cross-links with proteins interacting with tRNAs.

5. CONCLUSION

The above discussion of photosensitized cross-linking reactions between proteins and nucleic acids shows that the method can be applied to a very broad field of investigations. The possibility of introducing specific cross-links will certainly be an important tool in the study of the selectivity of protein-nucleic acid interactions (mapping of the recognition site) as well as in probing the spatial organization of multimacromolecular systems. This field is clearly at its beginning and more systematic studies have to be carried out before the many possibilities of photosensitized cross-linking reactions may be conveniently utilized.

The usefulness of triplet-state sensitizers has to be explored although in many cases the interacting chemical groups which could give rise to the cross-linking reaction might not be accessible to the sensitizer. Energy transfer processes in one of the macromolecules might possibly overcome this difficulty.

If the photosensitizer molecule can be introduced in one of the interacting macromolecules without modifying the interaction and its specificity, this could make it possible to produce cross-linking reactions which would not be observed under direct excitation. Dyes intercalated in nucleic acids may possibly play such a role.

A new field of investigation is clearly opened to photochemists who are not afraid of the complexity of biological systems.

References

Brunswick, D.J., and Cooperman, B.S., 1971, Photo-affinity labels for adenosine 3':5'-cyclic monophosphate, *Proc. Nat. Acad. Sci. USA* 68:1801-1804.

Chandra, P., 1970, Photodynamic action: a valuable tool in molecular biology, *in* "Research Progress in Organic, Biological and Medicinal Chemistry," Vol. 3, Part I, pp. 232-258, North-Holland Publishing Co., Amsterdam.

Charlier, M., and Hélène, C., 1975, Photosensitized splitting of pyrimidine dimers in DNA by indole derivatives and tryptophan-containing peptides, *Photochem. Photobiol.* 21:31-37.

Cysyk, R., and Prusoff, W.H., 1972, Alteration of ultraviolet sensitivity of thymidine kinase by allosteric regulators, normal substrates, and a photo-affinity label, 5-iodo-2'-deoxyuridine, a metabolic analog of thymidine, *J. Biol. Chem.* 247:2522-2532.

Dimicoli, J.L., and Hélène, C., 1974, Interactions of aromatic residues of proteins with nucleic acids. I. Proton magnetic resonance studies of the binding of tryptophan-containing peptides ot poly(adenylic acid) and deoxyribonucleic acid, *Biochemistry* 13:714-730.

Eisinger, J., and Lamola, A., 1971, The excited states of nucleic acids, *in* "Excited States of Proteins and Nucleic Acids" (I. Weinryb and R.F. Steiner, eds.), pp. 107-198, MacMillan, New York.

Fiser, I., Scheit, K.H., Stöffler, G., and Kuechler, E., 1974, Identification of protein S1 at the messenger RNA binding site of the *Escherichia coli* ribosome, *Biochem. Biophys. Res. Commun.* 60:1112-1118.

Fisher, G.J., Varghese, A.J., and Johns, H.E., 1974, Ultraviolet-induced reactions of thymine and uracil in the presence of cysteine, *Photochem. Photobiol.* 20:109-120.

Freifelder, D., Davison, P.F., and Geiduschek, E.P., 1961, Damage by visible light to the acridine orange-DNA complex, *Biophys. J.* 1:389-400.

Frischauf, A.M., and Scheit, K.H., 1973, Affinity labeling of *E. coli* RNA polymerase with substrate and template analogues, *Biochem. Biophys. Res. Commun.* 53:1227-1233.

Grossweiner, L.I., 1969, Molecular mechanisms in photodynamic action, *Photochem. Photobiol.* 10:183-191.

Guthrow, C.E., Rassmussen, H., Brunswick, D.J., and Cooperman, B.S., 1973, Specific photoaffinity labeling of the adenosine 3':5'-cyclic monophosphate receptor in intact ghosts from human erythrocytes, *Proc. Nat. Acad. Sci. USA* 70:3344-3346.

Hélène, C., 1973a, Energy transfer between nucleic acid bases and tryptophan in aggregates and in oligopeptide-nucleic acid complexes, *Photochem. Photobiol.* 18:255-262.

Hélène, C., 1973b, A comparison of excited states and energy transfer in polynucleotides and aggregates of nucleic acid components, *in* "Physico-Chemical Aspects of Nucleic Acids" (J. Duchesne, ed.), Vol. 1, pp. 120-142, Academic Press, New York.

Hélène, C., 1975, Excited state interactions and energy transfer processes in the photochemistry of protein-nucleic acid complexes, *in* "Excited States of Biological Molecules" (J.B. Birks, ed.), Wiley (in press).

Hélène, C., and Charlier, M., 1971, Photosensitized splitting of pyrimidine dimers by indole derivatives, *Biochem. Biophys. Res. Commun.* 43:252-257.

Jaffe-Brachet, A., Henry, N., and Errera, M., 1971, The photodynamic inactivation of λ bacteriophage particles in the presence of methylated proflavine, *Mutat. Res.* 12:9-14.

Lamola, A.A., 1972, Photosensitization in biological systems and the mechanism of photoreactivation, *Mol. Photochem.* 4:107-133.

Lesko, S.A., Hoffmann, H.D., Ts'o, P.O.P., and Maher, V.M., 1971, Interaction and linkage of polycyclic hydrocarbons to nucleic acids, *in* "Progress in Molecular and Subcellular Biology Series" (D.E. Hahn, ed.), Springer Verlag, Berlin, p. 356.

Lin, S.Y., and Riggs, A.D., 1974, Photochemical attachment of *lac* repressor to bromodeoxyuridine-substituted *lac* operator by ultraviolet radiation, *Proc. Nat. Acad. Sci. USA* 71:947-951.

Longworth, J.W., 1971, Luminescence of polypeptides and proteins, *in* "Excited States of Proteins and Nucleic Acids" (I. Weinryb and R.F. Steiner, ed.), pp. 319-484, MacMillan, New York.

Montenay-Garestier, T., and Hélène, C., 1971, Reflectance and luminescence studies of molecular complex formation between tryptophan and nucleic acid components in frozen aqueous solution, *Biochemistry* 10:300-306.

Montenay-Garestier, T., and Hélène, C., 1973, Interactions dans les agrégats de constituants des acides nucléiques et des acides aminés aromatiques, *J. Chim. Phys.* 70:1385-1390.

Nilsson, R., Merkel, P.B., and Kearns, D.R., 1972, Unambiguous evidence for the participation of singlet oxygen in photodynamic oxidation of amino acids, *Photochem. Photobiol.* 16:117-124.

Ogata, R., 1975, Affinity labeling of the operator binding site on the *lac* repressor. Abstr. Int. Symp. "Protein and Other Adducts to DNA: Their Significance to Aging, Carcinogenesis and Radiation Biology," Williamsburg, Virginia, May 2-6, 1975.

Petrusek, R.L., 1971, Ph.D. Thesis n° 7 22500, University of Chicago.

Schott, H.N., and Shetlar, M.D., 1974, Photochemical addition of amino acids to thymine, *Biochem. Biophys. Res. Commun.* 59: 1112-1116.

Schwartz, I., and Ofengand, J., 1974, Photo-affinity labeling of tRNA binding sites in macromolecules. I. Linking of the phenacyl-p-azide of 4-thiouridine in (*Escherichia coli*) valyl-tRNA to 16S RNA at the ribosomal P site, *Proc. Nat. Acad. Sci. USA* 71:3951-3955.

Simon, M.I., and Van Vunakis, H., 1962, The photodynamic reaction of methylene blue with deoxyribonucleic acid, *J. Mol. Biol.* 4:488-499.

Smith, K.C., 1969, Photochemical addition of amino acids to ^{14}C-uracil, *Biochem. Biophys. Res. Commun.* 34:354-357.

Smith, K.C., 1975, The radiation-induced addition of proteins and other molecules to nucleic acids, *in* "Photochemistry and Photobiology of Nucleic Acids" (S.Y. Wang, ed.), Academic Press, New York (in press).

Spikes, J.D., 1968, Photodynamic action, *Photophysiology* 3:33-64.

Toulmé, J.J., Charlier, M., and Hélène, C., 1974, Specific recognition of single-stranded regions in ultraviolet-irradiated and heat-denatured DNA by tryptophan-containing peptides, *Proc. Nat. Acad. Sci. USA* 71:3185-3188.

Varghese, A.J., 1974a, Photochemical addition of glutathione to uracil and thymine, *Photochem. Photobiol.* 20:339-343.

Varghese, A.J., 1974b, Photoaddition products of uracil and cysteine, *Biochim. Biophys. Acta* 374:109-114.

Walrant, P., and Santus, R., 1974a, N-formyl-kynurenine, A tryptophan photooxidation product, as a photodynamic sensitizer, *Photochem. Photobiol.* 19:411-417.

Walrant, P., and Santus, R., 1974b, Ultraviolet and N-formyl-kynurenine-sensitized photoinactivation of bovine carbonic anhydrase: an internal photodynamic effect, *Photochem. Photobiol.* 20:455-460.

Weintraub, H., 1973, The assembly of newly replicated DNA into chromatin, *Cold Spring Harbor Symp. Quant. Biol.* 37:247-256.

IONIZING RADIATION-INDUCED DNA-PROTEIN CROSS-LINKING

Osamu Yamamoto

Research Institute for Nuclear Medicine and Biology

Hiroshima University, Kasumi 1-2-3, Hiroshima, Japan

1. INTRODUCTION

Ionizing radiation-induced damage in DNA includes deamination and ring scission of the purine and pyrimidine bases, base elimination by scission of the glycoside bond, and strand breaks produced by scission of the ester bond between sugar and phosphate groups or by scission of the sugar moiety. In addition, cross-linking between DNA and other substances and also intra- or inter-molecular cross-linking of DNA are produced by ionizing radiation.

The binding or cross-linking of DNA with DNA or with the other substances may be important to the inhibition of cell multiplication and to the production of mutation or cancer in irradiated cells. Interactions have been found between DNA and protein after *in vivo* irradiation, but a covalent cross-link is still only suggestive at

the present time. The covalent binding of amino acids with DNA
and of nucleic acid bases with protein have been observed *in vitro*,
however, and the covalent binding of RNA with protein has been
observed *in vivo*.

This review is confined to the interaction or cross-linking
in biochemical aqueous systems (*in vitro*) and biological cell
systems (*in vivo*) exposed to ionizing radiation. However, some
data from experiments with UV radiation will be referred to for
comparison.

2. EVIDENCE OF INTERACTION OR CROSS-LINKS BETWEEN DNA AND PROTEIN
IN VIVO

2.1. Unextractability of DNA

Butler (1959) described in his review that it was difficult
to extract DNA completely from the nucleoprotein after irradiation
with appreciable doses, although the data were not presented.
Alexander and Stacey (1959) found that a substantial fraction of
DNA was unextractable when sperm heads of fish were irradiated
with 1 MeV electrons. Smith (1962) observed an increase in
unextractability of *E. coli* DNA following irradiation with
increasing fluences of UV radiation, and with visible light plus
dye. However, after X-irradiation, a 5% loss in extractable of
DNA was observed after a dose of 1 kR but this value was not altered
even after a dose of 40 kR. It was discussed that the question of
whether or not the cross-linking of DNA and protein by X-rays occurs
in bacteria should be reevaluated by analytical procedures less
dependent upon the molecular weight of DNA and protein, because
the chain breaks produced in macromolecules by X-rays could interfere with the selective precipitation procedure (Smith, 1975).

Similar studies have been made by Russian workers since 1967.
Sklobovskaya and Ryabchenko (1970a) observed an increase in unextractability of DNA from calf thymus deoxyribonucleoprotein (DNP)
with increasing doses of UV- and γ-radiation (Fig. 1). However,
no unextractability of DNA was observed when treated with trypsin.
They also compared unextractability under different conditions for
DNP and artificial DNA-protein complexes (Table 1). Unextractability
was found in 0.4 mM Na$^+$ for DNP and in 0.01 M phosphate buffer
(p.b.), pH 4.8 for DNA + BSA, but not in 1 M NaCl and in 0.4 mM Na$^+$
+ 0.2% SDS for DNP and in 0.01 M p.b., pH 6.8 for DNA + BSA.
Alexander and Stacey (1959) found a loss in extractable DNA with
increasing radiation dose in 2 M NaCl but observed no loss of
DNA when the solution was centrifuged at 20,000 g for 2 h.

Sklobovskaya and Ryabchenko (1970b) studied the unextractability

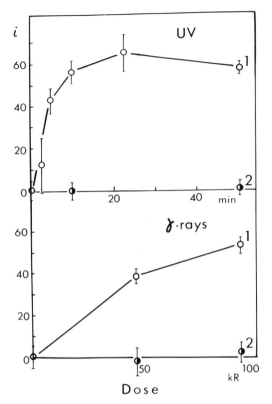

Fig. 1.   Dependence of the percent unextractability of DNA (i) on the dose of UV- and γ-radiation. 1: Calf thymus deoxyribonucleoprotein in 0.4 mM $NaHCO_3$ solution; 2: the same conditions plus treatment with trypsin after irradiation (Sklobovskaya and Ryabchenko, 1970a).

of DNA after UV- and γ-irradiation using DNA and artificial DNA-histone complexes prepared from calf thymus. They observed the dependence of unextractability on the amount of protein in the artificial complex (Fig. 2). The DNA-histone complexes were analyzed by gel filtration after irradiation. Most of the protein was separated from the DNA, while only a few percent of protein [non-irradiated: 3%, UV-irradiated (2.5×10^5 ergs/mm^2): 5% and γ-irradiated (100 kR): 7%] remained in the DNA fraction. This DNA fraction, bound with the small amount of protein, showed an unextractability of DNA (about 50%) as much as the initial complex did. No difference in unextractability between the initial complex and the separated fraction of DNA in which a small amount of protein remained indicates that the small amount of protein associated with DNA should participate in the unextractability.

Table 1. Percent Unextractability of DNA After Deproteinization of
Nucleoproteins Irradiated Under Various Conditions (Sklobovskaya
and Ryabchenko, 1970a)

Preparations*	UV irradiation (min)			γ-irradiation (kR)		
	5	10	50	50	100	200
DNP, solution in 0.4 mM Na+	43±6	56±6	57±3	38±4	53±5	-
DNP, solution in 1 M NaCl	23±9	40±6	43±4	0±2	1±1	-
DNP, dry preparation	-	-	-	-	-	-
DNP, solution in 0.4 mM Na+ + 0.2% SDS	-	-3±2	-	-1±2	-3±2	-
DNA + BSA, solution in 0.01 M p.b., pH 4.8	-	60±10	-	-	27±5	-
DNA + BSA, solution in 0.01 M p.b., pH 6.8	-	39±9	-	-	-4±2	-

*DNP, calf thymus deoxyribonucleoprotein; SDS, sodium dodecyl
sulfate; p.b., phosphate buffer; BSA, bovine serum albumin.

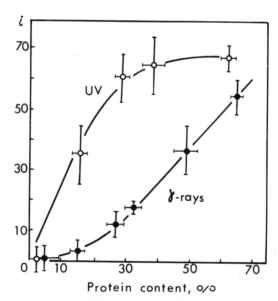

Fig. 2. Dependence of the percent unextractability of DNA (i)
in the deproteinization of irradiated DNA-histone complexes on the
protein content in the complex. UV: 2.5×10^5 ergs/mm^2; γ-rays:
100 kR (Sklobovskaya and Ryabchenko, 1970b).

In addition, each component of the DNA-histone complex was separately irradiated or one of the two components was irradiated prior to the formation of the DNA-histone complex. The results (Table 2) show that the unextractability of DNA was mostly DNA-irradiation dependent.

Table 2. Percent Unextractability of DNA After Deproteinization of Irradiated (irr) Complexes and Complexes Formed After Irradiating the Components Separately (Sklobovskaya and Ryabchenko, 1970b)

Type of complex	UV 2.5×10^5 ergs/mm^2	γ-rays 100 kR
(DNA + histone)$_{irr}$	65 ± 8	35 ± 6
DNA$_{irr}$ + histone$_{irr}$	47 ± 7	43 ± 4
DNA$_{irr}$ + histone	21 ± 4	28 ± 6
DNA + histone$_{irr}$	5 ± 2	2 ± 1

Strazhevskaya *et al.* (1969) observed an increase in unextractable DNA after [137]Cs γ-ray irradiation not only for *in vitro* experiments with calf thymus but also for *in vivo* experiments with rat thymus. A dose of 100 R *in vitro* produced a distinct increase (62%) in the amount of DNA firmly bound to protein as judged by deproteinization in alkaline phenol (pH 8.5) in 1 M NaCl. Higher doses progressively increased this amount (e.g., 470% after 10 kR). A dose of 1 kR *in vivo* produced a 41% increase in the amount of DNA firmly bound to protein. In the deproteinization of various artificial complexes of DNP, Strazhevskaya *et al.* (1971) turned their attention to the "interphase" (an intermediate layer at the phenol-water interface). In order to evaluate the role of radiation damage to each of the components of DNP, the effect was judged according to the amount of DNA transferred during deproteinization to "interphase". Radiation damage in the structure of DNA was the basic prerequisite for the appearance of a strengthened bond between DNA and protein. From an amino acid analysis of the proteins associated with the DNA in the "interphase", it was found that the proteins were not histones but were acidic proteins, because the ratio of bound acidic to basic amino acids was 1.5-1.7 versus a ratio of 0.5-0.7 that is characteristic for histones.

The data permit the conclusion that irradiation increases the amount of DNA-bound protein and that acidic proteins take part in the binding. They also suppose that the DNA-acid protein bond is not covalent, but is accomplished according to the type of hydrophobic interaction, since treatment with SDS led to removal of the radiation effect though raising the pH and ionic strength did not remove the effect (Strazhevskaya and Troyanovskaya, 1970) in contradiction to the data of Sklobovskaya and Ryabchenko (1970a).

The unextractability of DNA after ionizing irradiation has been studied *in vivo* by many workers but the conclusion appears to be that the unextractability of DNA may be caused by some structural change in DNA which induces some close association with protein that is not covalent.

2.2. Residual Protein in Isolated DNA

As evidence of an ionizing radiation-induced interaction between DNA and protein other than the unextractability of DNA, an increase in the residual protein content of DNA isolated after exposure to ionizing radiation has been presented. The hindered removal of a small portion of protein from DNA isolated from γ-irradiated nucleoprotein was reported by Tseĭtlin *et al.* (1967) and from γ-irradiated rats by Skalka and Matyasova (1967). An increased amount of protein in the bone marrow DNA of a locally irradiated rabbit was noted in the work of Kritskiĭ (1967). Also, Ivannik and Ryabchenko (1969) reported an increase in the protein content of DNA isolated immediately after ^{60}Co γ-irradiation of the liver and thymus gland of rats, though the latter was not statistically significant.

Strazhevskaya *et al.* (1971), compared the amino acid compositions of the protein associated with DNA in the "supernatant" and "interphase" and noted that the residual protein in DNA of both the "supernatant" and "interphase" were acidic proteins. Strazhevskaya *et al.* (1972) also showed that the residual protein associated with DNA was also acidic in the case of *in vivo* irradiation. They observed, however, that treatment with SDS stripped off the increased residual protein produced by irradiation.

Hawkins (1975) observed that protein distributed as if it had an affinity for the aqueous phase and the DNA distributed as if it had an affinity for the phenolic phase in a two phase phenol-water system, after phage T7 was irradiated in 0.01 M phosphate buffer (pH 7.5) media. But when irradiated in 1% tryptone broth + 0.5% NaCl, such results could not be obtained.

Zimmerman *et al.* (1965) reported that RNA polymerase, an acidic protein, binds with irradiated DNA. The mechanism of the binding of RNA polymerase with irradiated DNA may be similar to that of the DNA-protein interaction which resulted in the unextractability of DNA and the increase of residual protein of DNA, and the hydrophobic or hydrophilic nature of the bound structure may be subordinate. Hagen *et al.* (1970), through the binding of RNA polymerase with irradiated DNA, found that the length of the RNA chains synthesized decreased markedly, whereas the number of RNA

chains synthesized was much less affected and concluded that the
formation of binding sites ineffective for RNA synthesis contri-
butes less than 10% to the inactivation of the priming ability of
DNA and that the loss of priming activity is mainly due to formation of critical lesions along the DNA strand. Strazhevskaya *et
al*. (1971, 1972) concluded that the radiation effect on nuclear
structure is complicated and the interaction may damage the regulating system for replication and transcription of DNA because
acidic proteins are specific regulators of gene activity of the
template and may lead to early aging of the organism (see Cutler,
This Volume).

From the published work on the unextractability and residual
protein of DNA after ionizing irradiation, there is still no clear
evidence for covalent cross-links between DNA and protein. A
decrease of histidine (25%) and phenylalanine (37%) in the residual
protein or DNA of "supernatant" (Strazhevskaya *et al*., 1972) and a
decrease of phenylalanine (34%) in the residual protein of DNA
from rat thymus and of histidine (76%) in that from rat liver
(Strazhevskaya *et al*., 1972) after irradiation might suggest
undetectable amounts of covalent bonding cross-links between DNA
and protein because these aromatic amino acid residues have a
specific radiation-induced binding activity, as will be discussed
in Section 4.1.

Rhase (1968) has identified adenine-7-N-oxide as one of oxidized
products from oligo- and mono-deoxyadenylic acids reacted with OH·
radicals. One possible interaction appears to be a hydrogen bonding between an oxygen atom in the NO group produced in the base
and a hydrogen atom in the carboxyl group of an acidic protein.

$$
\begin{array}{c}
\text{NH}_2 \\
\end{array}
\quad \text{N} \rightarrow \text{O} \cdots\cdots \text{H} - \text{O} - \overset{\overset{\displaystyle \cdot\cdot}{\|}}{\underset{\displaystyle O}{C}} - \text{R}
$$

Carboxyl groups newly produced in protein by irradiation might
also participate in this kind of interaction. The formation of
adenine-7-N-oxide was found not to be a mutagenic base analogue
for point mutations in T4 phage (Rhase, 1968).

2.3. Sedimentation Analysis

Using sedimentation analysis, Bohne *et al*. (1970) studied the
radiation sensitivity of T1 phage. In Table 3, G-values for the
inactivation of plaque-forming ability, the formation of strand
breaks, and cross-links in phage DNA are shown in comparison with
those for T7 phage studied by Freifelder (1965, 1968). G-values
for DNA cross-links with other molecules were higher than those

Table 3, G-values for the Inactivation of Plaque-Forming Ability,
and the Formation of DNA Strand Breaks, and Cross-Links in Phage
(Modified from Bohne *et al.*, 1970)

Radiation-induced lesion	T1 phage*	T7 phage†
Inactivation of plaque-forming ability	0.33	0.27
Single-strand breaks	1.15	1.00
Double-strand breaks	0.058	0.088‡
DNA-DNA cross-links	0.009	0.014‡
DNA cross-links with other molecules	0.023	0.035‡

*Bohne *et al.*, 1970.
†Freifelder, 1965, 1968.
‡A total value for T7 phage of 0.137, was distributed pro-
portionally to the values of these three categories for T1 phage.

of DNA-DNA cross-links but less than those of DNA double-strand
breaks.

Recently Yamamoto (1975) exposed L5178Y mammalian cells to
γ-rays in the presence of amino acids and nucleic acid bases and
the cells were lysed with SDS. The covalent binding of low molecular weight compounds with nucleic acid constituents in cells
was observed (dotted lines in Fig. 3). Also, the radiation-induced
binding yields of cysteine with each macromolecular substance in
cells were obtained (Table 4). Among them the binding yield of
cysteine with DNA was the lowest. Sedimentation analysis was
also made with a sucrose gradient (Fig. 4). Degradation of DNA
to smaller molecules was observed upon irradiation, while the
cysteine peak increased with increasing dose. The increase of the
cysteine peak with increasing dose indicates an increased binding
with macromolecular substances. However, the main substance bound
with cysteine was not DNA. Radioactive counts due to RNA were
very low without irradiation, probably due to hydrolysis by the
alkali used for cell lysis. Interestingly, the RNA radioactivity
on the gradient increased with increasing dose. This indicates
that nucleotide or nucleoside portions of RNA become bound to
macromolecular substances by irradiation. The proximity of the RNA
radioactivity peaks to the protein peaks strongly suggests a covalent cross-linkage between RNA and protein. It appears that DNA
may also bind with protein or RNA to a small extent.

Also in studies on the binding of hydrocarbon carcinogens to
macromolecular compounds of exponentially growing cells, it was
found that the carcinogens bound readily to RNA and protein, but
only to a small extent to DNA (Kuroki *et al.*, 1971/72).

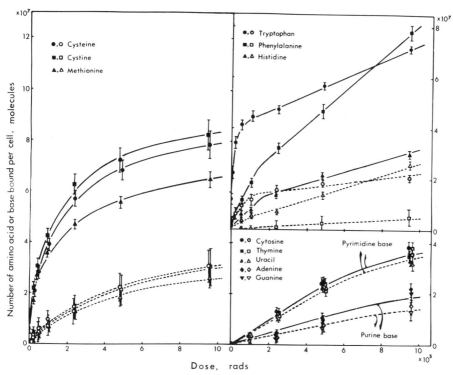

Fig. 3. Binding yield of amino acids and bases with macromolecular substances in intact cells of L5178Y vs radiation dose.
Amino acid concentration: 0.84×10^{-4} M (5×10^{16} molecules/ml);
cell concentration: 5×10^7 cells/ml. ——: After heating in the
presence of TCA; ---: difference [(before heating with TCA)—(after
heating with TCA)] (Yamamoto, 1975).

     Such a small yield of covalent DNA-protein cross-links in
biological systems may be caused by the highly folded form or the
condensed volume of DNA which makes reaction difficult, i.e., there
is a low binding efficiency except possibly for some stages of the
cell cycle. However, the covalent binding of DNA with some substance can be very biologically important, and a study of cell
cycle dependency for the covalent cross-link between DNA and DNA,
DNA and protein, or DNA and other molecules should be made.

     In addition, it is necessary to study whether the covalent
links between DNA and DNA, or DNA and other substances are easily
repairable. Smith (1975) has suggested that DNA-protein cross-
links appear to be at least partially repairable. The repair of
carcinogen bound DNA (Kuroki, 1973) would seem to support this
view.

Table 4. Radiation-Induced Binding Yields of Cysteine with
Macromolecular Substances in Intact Cells of L5178Y (Percent of
the Added Total Cysteine, 5×10^{16} molecules/ml) (Yamamoto, 1975)*

Cell component Dose	Protein†	DNA†	RNA†	Lipid†	Total†
0 rad	0.22	0.02	0.04	0.36	0.64
2.41×10^5 rads	5.75	0.92	2.35	7.69	16.71
	(34.4)	(5.5)	(14.1)	(46.0)	(100)
4.83×10^5 rads	8.39	1.21	3.47	9.38	22.55
	(37.2)	(5.8)	(15.4)	(41.6)	(100)

*^{35}S-cysteine concentration: 2.5 μCi/ml (32 mCi/mmol);
cell concentration: 6×10^7 cells/ml. Standard deviation <±0.5.
†Values in parentheses: Percentage of total binding yield.

3.   COVALENT LINKS BETWEEN NUCLEIC ACID AND PROTEIN AND THEIR CONSTITUENTS *IN VITRO*

Yamamoto (1967) reported the radiation-induced binding of
amino acids with protein and nucleic acid. In an enzymatic reaction, phenylalanine + tRNA → phenylalanyl-tRNA, it was found that
the ^{14}C-activity of phenylalanine in the TCA-precipitate after
γ-irradiation was much more than that for unirradiated solutions
and increased with dose.

A competitive reaction of 20 amino acids with ^{14}C-phenylalanine
suggested high binding activities of aromatic amino acids and sulfur-
containing amino acids (Fig. 5).

Byfield *et al.* (1970) reported the binding of amino acids to
DNA. They irradiated ^{3}H-leucine and several concentrations of DNA
in aqueous solution with increasing doses of 6 MeV electrons. The
conversion of acid soluble radioactivity to acid insolubility was
proportional to radiation dose. They also irradiated ^{14}C-labeled
amino acids and DNA, and chromatographed after the hydrolysis of
DNA. The label was found to be distributed over the entire chromatogram suggesting that many different amino acids may have become
bound to the DNA.

Yamamoto (1973a) studied the binding of tryptophan to DNA,
RNA, and serum albumin and the effect of the presence of salt on

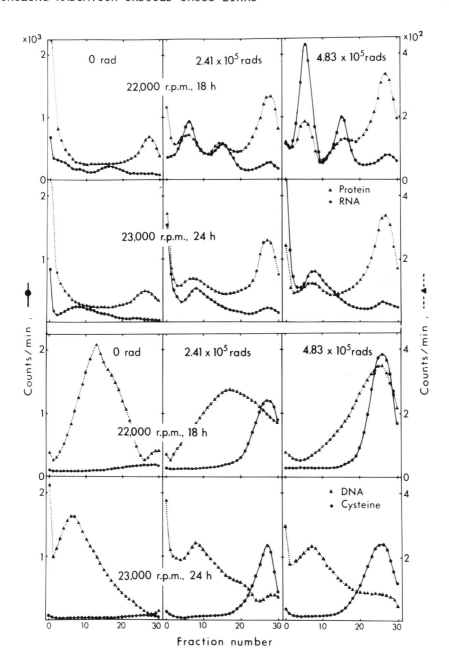

Fig. 4.   Sedimentation profiles in alkaline sucrose gradients.

(Fig. 4, cont.) Protein: tryptophan-^{14}C radioactivity incorporated into protein before irradiation; RNA: uridine-^{14}C radioactivity incorporated into RNA before irradiation; DNA: thymidine-^{3}H radioactivity incorporated into DNA before irradiation; cysteine: cysteine-^{35}S radioactivity bound to macromolecular substances by γ-irradiation (Yamamoto, 1975).

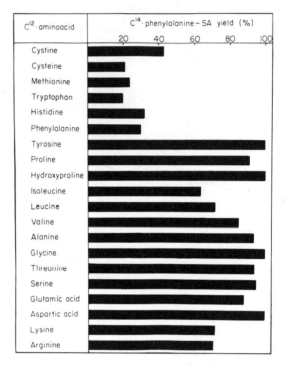

Fig. 5. Comparison of competing effects of twenty ^{12}C-amino acids (10^{-4} M) on γ-radiation-induced binding of ^{14}C-phenylalanine (0.5 μCi/ml, 50 mCi/mmol) with serum albumin (1 mg/ml) in aqueous solution. Radiation dose: 5×10^5 R (Yamamoto, 1967).

the binding yield. As seen in Fig. 6, the binding yields of tryptophan with DNA or RNA increased up to 1.93×10^5 rads and then decreased with higher doses of radiation. The decrease in yield may indicate strand breakage of DNA and RNA. At higher concentrations of nucleic acid, the peak moved to a higher dose, and the presence of sodium citrate (0.015 M) produced no peak but an increasing binding yield up to 10^6 rads (Yamamoto, unpublished). In Fig. 6, the binding yield of tryptophan with DNA was much greater than with RNA in 0.25 M NaCl solution. This could be due

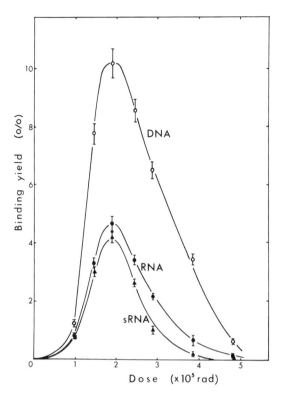

Fig. 6. The radiation-induced binding yields of tryptophan (10^{-4} M, 0.5 μCi-^{14}C/ml) with DNA, RNA, or sRNA (0.25 mg/ml) in NaCl (0.25 M) solution as a function of the gamma-radiation dose in air (Yamamoto, 1973a).

to the increase of the tryptophan-DNA binding yield and no increase of the tryptophan-RNA binding yield with increasing concentration of NaCl, i.e., both yields should be similar to each other in the absence of NaCl as shown in Fig. 7.

Yamamoto (1973a) showed a clear indication for the chemical specificity of the binding of amino acids with serum albumin and RNA (Table 5). Compared to the binding yields of aromatic amino acids and sulfur-containing amino acids, those of aliphatic amino acids ere very low. Nucleic acid bases and the specific amino acids bound comparably with protein, but the former bound less with nucleic acid than did the latter. As for the binding of the specific amino acids, the highest reactivity was of cysteine, tryrosine, and phenylalanine in the addition of amino acids to uracil (Smith, 1969) and the binding of tyrosine, phenylalanine and methionine with ribonuclease (Kuntz *et al.*, 1975) by UV light,

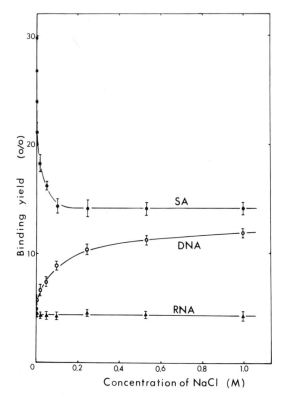

Fig. 7. The effect of concentration of NaCl on the radiation-induced binding of yield of tryptophan (10^{-4} M, 0.5 μCi-^{14}C/ml) with DNA, RNA, or serum albumin (SA) (0.25 mg/ml) in aqueous solution in air. Radiation dose: 1.93×10^5 rads (Yamamoto, 1973a).

and the binding yield of cystine much higher than that of aspartic acid (Friedberg, 1972) and methionine and tyrosine were the most effective in the attachment of amino acids to ribonuclease (Kuntz *et al.*, 1975) by ionizing radiation.

Links between specific amino acids and nucleic acid bases were studied with paper chromatography after γ-irradiation in aqueous solution (Yamamoto, 1973a). In the presence of amino acids, one peak was observed at the origin of the chromatogram which was not seen when only nucleic acid bases were used. These results indicate that the bases bind less with other bases than they do with specific amino acids. Concurrently, the binding of bases with albumin or amino acids suggests that the binding site of nucleic acid with protein or amino acids is the base portion in the nucleic acid molecule. This was proved by the comparison

Table 5.   Comparison of the γ-Radiation-Induced Binding of Amino
    Acids and Nucleic Acid Bases with Serum Albumin (SA) and RNA.
    Gamma-Ray Dose: 4.83×10^5 rads in Air (Yamamoto, 1973a)

Amino acids and bases (10^{-4} M)	Binding yield (%)	
	SA (1 mg/ml)	RNA (1 mg/ml)
Alanine	3.9 ± 0.2	<1
Leucine	2.9 ± 0.1	<1
Methionine	32.2 ± 0.2	4.5 ± 0.2
Cysteine	43.1 ± 1.0	4.5 ± 0.2
Cystine	42.3 ± 2.4	4.4 ± 0.5
Histidine	40.3 ± 3.0	4.3 ± 0.7
Phenylalanine	54.6 ± 1.8	4.6 ± 1.0
Tryptophan	59.0 ± 2.3	5.4 ± 1.0
Cytosine	43.7 ± 2.8	1
Uracil	46.6 ± 1.2	<1
Thymine	45.2 ± 2.2	<1
Adenine	28.5 ± 1.1	<1
Guanine	25.2 ± 2.0	<1

of binding yields of various nucleic acid constituents with albumin.

Binding yields of five bases with albumin as a function of
radiation dose are shown in Fig. 8.   There were observed no great
difference of the yield among three pyrimidine bases and between
two purine bases, and higher yields of pyrimidine bases than those
of purine bases.   When the binding yields of bases were compared
with those of the corresponding nucleosides and nucleotides the
yields of nucleosides and nucleotides were slightly less than
those of the bases.   Ribose and ribose phosphate bound very little
with albumin.   Therefore, the base portion of DNA should mainly
participate in the binding (Yamamoto, 1973a).

Lynn (1974) worked on the γ-radiolysis of a DNA complex with
trypsin, chymotrypsin and chymotrypsinogen but did not report their
cross-linking.   Kasche (1974), however, reported a binding of α-
chymotrypsin with DNA.

As to the mutual binding of DNA, a report of the radiation-
induced cross-linking in DNA gels was presented by Lett and Alexander
(1961) who observed the magnitude of the cross-linking process
depended on the water content.   For a dose of 10^6 rads there was a
progressive increase in cross-linking when the water content was
increased from 0-175% and thereafter a progressive decrease to zero
at a water content of about 300%.   The presence of oxygen prevented

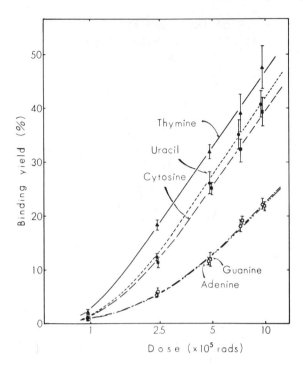

Fig. 8. The radiation-induced binding yields of bases (5 × 10⁻⁴
M, 0.5 μCi-¹⁴C/ml) with serum albumin (1 mg/ml) in phosphate buffer
solution (5 × 10⁻³ M, pH 7.6) as a function of the gamma-radiation
dose in air (Yamamoto, 1973a).

the DNA-DNA cross-linking. These authors suggested that the direct
action of the radiation leads to the rupture of polynucleotide chain
to give reactive ends that can combine intermolecularly to give a
cross-link if there is no oxygen present.

    Relevant to the above work on DNA-DNA cross-links, the poly-
merization of nucleotides was observed after ¹³⁷Cs γ-irradiation
and the presence of oxygen prevented this polymerization (Aguilera
et al., 1965, 1968).

    The inhibition by oxygen is a common characteristic in the
radiation-induced cross-linking reactions of macromolecules in
aqueous systems. Typical binding patterns in the presence of N_2,
air, or O_2 are compared in Fig. 9 (Yamamoto and Okuda, 1975).
Here it should be noted that in the binding of macromolecular substances in the intact cells or the cell lysates with amino acids
and nucleic acid bases under air, the dose-yield curve becomes
similar to Curve II but not to Curve I. Cells consist of a great

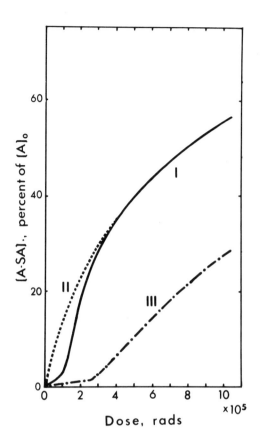

Fig. 9. Typical curves of radiation dose vs binding yield of
various compounds with serum albumin or nucleic acid. Example:
Phenylalanine (5×10^{-4} M) plus serum albumin (1 mg/ml) in aqueous
solution. I: Under air; II: N_2-saturated; III: O_2-saturated.
$[A_0]$: Original concentration of amino acid; [A-SA]: binding yield
of amino acid with serum albumin (Yamamoto and Okuda, 1975).

number of components. Some of them are high oxygen receptors or
reactants, e.g., unsaturated fatty acid molecules. Such substances
may be the efficient oxygen consumers.

4. MECHANISM OF COVALENT BINDING REACTION

4.1. Formation of Amino Acid Radicals in Proteins

In order to elucidate the mechanism of radical formation and
binding, the binding yields of aromatic amino acids with serum
albumin (Yamamoto, 1973b; Yamamoto and Okuda, 1975) and with DNA
(Yamamoto, unpublished) were compared under different conditions.
For non-OH-substituted aromatic amino acids, the yield decreased
in the presence of OH· scavengers (e.g., methanol or potassium
thiocyanate) and the yield increased in the presence of e_{aq}^-
scavengers (e.g., nitrous oxide; $N_2O + e_{aq}^- \rightarrow N_2 + OH· + OH^-$).
There should be a participation of OH· radicals in the formation
of these amino acid radicals. Two possible types of radicals, the
phenyl-type radical and cyclohexadienyl-type radical, will be discussed. Hatano and Tanei (1971) have observed the formation of both
types of radicals in aromatic compounds utilizing ESR spectroscopy
after γ-irradiation. However, Yamamoto (1973b) concluded that only
phenyl-type radicals are active in cross-linking reactions. In the
formation of phenyl-type radicals, there should be an abstraction
of one hydrogen atom on the ring by a OH· radical. For OH-substi-

tuted aromatic amino acids, OH· and e_{aq}^- scavenger effects were
decreased with increasing numbers of OH-groups. Therefore, phenyl-
type radicals formed by OH· radicals and phenoxyl-type radicals
formed by unknown mechanisms may participate in cross-linking
reactions and the phenoxyl-type radical may be formed in larger
yields than the phenyl-type with an increasing number of OH-groups
on the aromatic ring.

Scavenger effects on the binding yields of sulfur-containing
amino acids with albumin (Yamamoto, 1972a, b) and with DNA (Yamamoto,
unpublished) were also studied. Various mechanisms for the formation of thiyl radicals from cysteine and cystine have been presented
by many workers (Littman *et al.*, 1957; Markakis and Tappel, 1960;
Grant *et al.*, 1961; Packer, 1963; Brdička *et al.*, 1963; Armstrong

and Wilkening, 1964; El Samahy *et al.*, 1964; Purdie, 1967; Wilkening *et al.*, 1967, 1968; Al-Thannon *et al.*, 1968, 1974; Owen *et al.*, 1968; Packer and Winchester, 1968). On the binding of cysteine and cystine to albumin and DNA, no scavenger effect of nitrous oxide, methanol, and potassium thiocyanate was observed. The lack of OH⋅ radical scavenging effect and e_{aq}^- scavenging effect in the binding of cysteine and cystine as observed in the binding of OH-substituted aromatic amino acids suggests that the mechanism of radical formation for the S atom is similar to that for the O atom, and that there should be a mechanism of thiyl or oxyl radical formation without the participation of OH⋅ radical and e_{aq}^-.

$$\left.\begin{array}{l} R\text{-}S\text{-}H \\ R\text{-}S\text{-}S\text{-}R \end{array}\right\rangle \longrightarrow R\text{-}S\cdot$$

The binding yield of methionine, however, was affected by the scavengers. There may be the participation of OH⋅ radicals fo methionine radical formation as follows.

$$H_3C\text{-}\ddot{S}\text{-}R \xrightarrow{\ +OH\cdot\ } H_2\dot{C}\text{-}\ddot{S}\text{-}R \quad + \quad (H_2O)$$
$$\updownarrow$$
$$H_2C\text{=}\dot{S}\text{-}R$$
$$\updownarrow$$
$$\underset{R}{H_2C\text{---}\ddot{S}:} \rightleftharpoons \underset{R}{H_2C\text{-}S\cdot}$$

Oxidized derivatives of sulfur-containing amino acids, such as cysteic acid, cystine disulfoxide, methionine sulfoxide, and methylsulfonic acid, do not bind with protein (Yamamoto, 1972a, b). Therefore, oxidized thiyl radicals such as R-OS⋅ or ⋅SOH, R-O$_2$S⋅ or ⋅SO$_2$H, and ⋅SO$_3$H may have no binding activity toward protein and nucleic acid. This could be due to a decrease of electronegativity of the S atom affected by O atom(s). This suggests that the specific amino acid radical may act as an electrophilic reagent. If there are passive reaction sites in proteins, these sites should be the rings of the aromatic amino acids.

Aliphatic amino acids show very little reactivity as mentioned in Section 3. In those cases, the larger chain length of the aliphatic amino acid, the greater the binding yield as shown in Fig. 10 (Yamamoto, unpublished). Their binding yields with DNA was almost equal to those with albumin, and an OH⋅ radical scavenging effect was observed on their yield. The binding of aliphatic amino acids to DNA or albumin might be due to a radical-radical reaction.

In addition, after irradiation little reactivity of the peptide bonds in protein molecules was suggested (Yamamoto, 1973b).

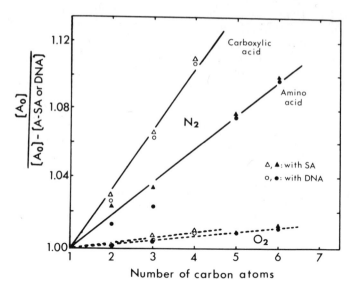

Fig. 10. Radiation-induced binding of aliphatic amino acids and carboxylic acids with serum albumin or DNA. Concentration of amino acid and carboxylic acid: 5×10^{-4} M, 0.5 μCi-^{14}C/ml; concentration of albumin and DNA: 1 mg/ml. [A_0]: Original concentration of amino acid or carboxylic acid; [A-SA or DNA]: binding yield of acid with serum albumin or DNA (Yamamoto, unpublished).

4.2. Passive Reactions of the Nucleic Acids

The 5- or 6-OH substituted pyrimidine bases (Khattak and Green, 1966a-c; Pleticha-Lánský, 1968; Smith and Hays, 1968; Shragge et al. 1974) and 8-OH substituted adenine (Conlay, 1963; Ponnamperuma et al., 1963; van Hemmen, 1971; van Hemmen and Bleichrodt, 1971) have been reported as the radiolytic products from pyrimidine bases and adenine, respectively. Their formation schemes were presented as follows.

Cytosine (Khattak and Green, 1966a):

Adenine (van Hemmen and Bleichrodt, 1971):

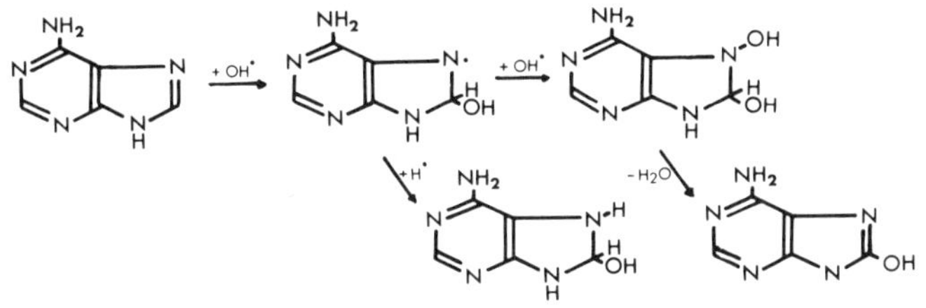

Quantum biochemical data support the above schemes because such positions are nucleophilic to which the electrophilic reagents act (Pullman and Pullman, 1963). The nucleophilic nature of the 6-position in the pyrimidine bases and the 8-position in the purine bases does not change even when the hydrogen bond is formed. Indeed, no difference was found between the binding yields of tryptophan with single-stranded DNA and double-stranded DNA (Yamamoto, unpublished). In addition, other data showed that about 80% of 6-H in thymine and 8-H in adenine was eliminated through binding with albumin (Yamamoto, 1973a).

Also, Bjorksten and Andrews (1964) have had an idea that nucleophilic centers of nucleic acids and proteins are available for the cross-linkage due to the free radicals generated by ionizing radiation. Electrophilic amino acid radicals may first attack mainly the 6-position in pyrimidine bases and the 8-position in purine bases, exactly similar to the attack of OH· radicals. There are two possible ways for the binding. For example, the reaction scheme of uracil is given below. One way is the formation of a partially

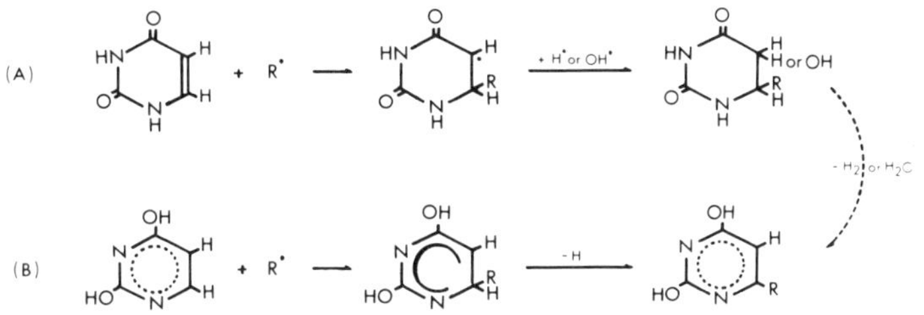

saturated compound through the addition of the specific active radical and the further addition of H· or OH· (Reaction A) as well as the formation of 5-hydro-6-hydroxypyrimidine bases, 5,6-dihydroxy-pyrimidine bases, 8-hydroxy-9-hydropurine bases, and 8,9-dihydroxy-purine bases (Ekert, 1962; Latarjet et al., 1963; Conlay, 1963; Kamal and Garrison, 1965; Khattak and Green, 1966a-c; Castro and Jiménez, 1968; Pleticha-Lánský, 1968; Smith and Hays, 1968; Drásil et al., 1968; van Hemmen, 1971; van Hemmen and Bleichrodt, 1971; Shragge et al., 1974). The other way is the substitutional reaction (B) as postulated for the binding mechanism of aromatic amino acids

(Yamamoto, 1973b; Yamamoto and Okuda, 1975). There is the possibility of dehydrogenation or dehydration of the partially saturated
compounds. The formation of partially saturated compounds, as mentioned above, suggests that the main pathway would be via Reaction A.

Recently, Shragge *et al.* (1974) reported an addition reaction
between two molecules of uracil. They isolated by irradiation at
pH 8.5 in N_2 a small amount of two kinds of product (I and II) from
a fraction eluted by column chromatography and suggested that
others probably are 2-pyrimidone derivatives similar to II. In

I   II

these structures, one of two uracil rings in the product is linked
at the 6-position with the other uracil. This result may support
the preceding binding scheme, although an easy 4'-OH elimination
in these postulated structures is still questionable because its
OH-band is larger than that of cyclobutyl type dimer in IR spectrum
(Khattak and Wang, 1969). At any rate, these kinds of addition
reactions of the bases may be related to DNA-DNA cross-links.

The participation of the 5- and 6-positions in the pyrimidine
ring in the binding reaction have been observed from UV radiation
experiments (Smith and Aplin, 1966; Smith, 1970; Varghese, 1970).

5.   CONCLUSIONS

The unextractability of DNA and the increase of residual protein of isolated DNA which have been observed after ionizing irradiation are prevented under different medium conditions. The interaction between DNA and protein was DNA-irradiation dependent and
protein-irradiation independent, which was supported by the fact
that RNA polymerase interacts with irradiated DNA. Thus, it is
suggested that the DNA-protein interaction observed in biological
systems may not be covalent. In addition, the participation of
acidic protein was suggested in the interaction.

Calculations from the sedimentation distributions showed the
number of covalent DNA-protein cross-links to be less than the
number of DNA double-strand breaks produced per nucleotide (Bohne
et al., 1970). In the patterns of alkaline sucrose gradient
observed by other workers, the DNA-protein cross-link was only

suggestive, though the RNA-protein cross-link was clearly observed (Yamamoto, 1975).

In aqueous biochemical systems, clear evidence of the covalent binding of the constituents of protein and nucleic acid mutually and with each other has been reported (Yamamoto, 1973a). Aromatic amino acids and sulfur-containing amino acids are particularly reactive and aliphatic amino acids show very little reactivity. In the latter case, the longer the chain length of the aliphatic amino acid the greater their binding yield. It is also concluded that the base portion of nucleic acid participates in the binding. These radiation-induced covalent bindings are inhibited by the presence of oxygen.

For the mechanism of the covalent cross-links between DNA and protein, it can be concluded that the thiyl radicals from sulfur-containing amino acid residues and the phenyl-type radicals and phenoxyl-type radicals from aromatic amino acid residues in protein may mainly attack the 6-position in pyrimidine base rings and the 8-position in purine base rings in nucleic acid.

References

Aguilera, A., Colombara, E., and Tohá, J., 1965, Synthesis of poly-uridylic acid by γ-radiation, *Biochim. Biophys. Acta* 95:569-577.

Aguilera, A., Gampel, Z., Pieber, M., and Tohá, J., 1968, Polymeri-zation of nucleotides by gamma radiation, *Photochem. Photobiol.* 7:711-720.

Alexander, P., and Stacey, K.A., Cross-linking of deoxyribonucleic acid in sperm heads by ionizing radiations, 1959, *Nature* 184:958-960.

Al-Thannon, A.A., Barton, J.P., Packer, J.E., Sims, R.J., Trumbore, C.N., and Winchester, R.V., 1974, The radiolysis of aqueous solutions of cysteine in the presence of oxygen, *Int. J. Radiat. Phys. Chem.* 6:233-248.

Al-Thannon, A.A., Peterson, R.M., and Trumbore, C.N., 1968, Studies in the aqueous radiation chemistry of cysteine. I. Deaerated acidic solutions, *J. Phys. Chem.* 72:2395-2399.

Armstrong, D.A., and Wilkening, V.G., 1964, Effects of pH in the γ-radiolysis of aqueous solutions of cysteine and methyl mercaptan, *Can. J. Chem.* 42:2631-2635.

Bjorksten, J., and Andrews, F., 1964, Chemical mechanisms under-lying the biological mechanisms of the aging process, *J. Am. Genet. Soc.* 12:627-631.

Bohne, L., Coquerelle, Th., and Hagen, U., 1970, Radiation sensi-tivity of bacteriophage DNA. II. Breaks and cross-links after irradiation *in vivo*, *Int. J. Radiat. Biol.* 17:205-215.

Brdička, R., Spurný, Z., and Fojtík, A., 1963, Effect of the dose intensity on the rate of radio-oxidation of cystine in aqueous solutions, *Colln Czech. Chem. Commun.* 28:1491-1498.

Butler, J.A.V., 1959, Changes induced in nucleic acids by ionizing radiation and chemicals, *Radiat. Res. Suppl.* 1:403-416.

Byfield, J.E., Lee, Y.C., and Bennett, L.R., 1970, Binding of small molecules to DNA following ionizing radiation, *Nature* 225:859-860.

Castro, E., and Jiménez, R., 1968, The effects of gamma radiation on aqueous solutions of 2'-3' uridylic acid, *Photochem. Photobiol.* 7:721-726.

Conlay, J.J., 1963, Effect of ionizing radiation on adenine in aerated and de-aerated aqueous solutions, *Nature* 197:555-557.

Drášil, V., Rýznar, L., and Jurašková, V., 1968, Incorporation of hydrogen into products of thymine radiolysis, *Biochim. Biophys. Acta* 166:600-602.

Ekert, B., 1962, Effect of γ-rays on thymine in de-aerated aqueous solutions, *Nature* 194:278-279.

El Samahy, A., White, H.L., and Trumbore, C.N., 1964, Scavenging action in γ-irradiated aqueous cysteine solutions, *J. Am. Chem. Soc.* 86:3177-3178.

Freifelder, D., 1965, Mechanism of inactivation of coliphage T7 by X rays, *Proc. Nat. Acad. Sci. USA* 54:128-134.

Freifelder, D., 1968, Physicochemical studies on X-ray inactivation of bacteriophage, *Virology* 36:613-619.

Friedberg, F., 1972, Covalent binding of amino acids to proteins due to gamma irradiation, *Z. Naturforsch.* 27b:85.

Grant, D.W., Mason, S.N., and Link, M.A., 1961, Products of the γ-radiolysis of aqueous cystine solutions, *Nature* 192:352-353.

Hagen, U., Ullrich, M., Petersen, E.E., Werner, E., and Kröger, H., 1970, Enzymatic RNA synthesis on irradiated DNA, *Biochim. Biophys. Acta* 199:115-125.

Hatano, H., and Tanei, T., 1971, A comparative aspect of radical species produced from several benzene derivatives by photo and ionizing radiations, *Bull. Inst. Chem. Res. (Kyoto Univ.)* 49:38-42.

Hawkins, R.B., 1975, Ionizing radiation induced covalent protein to DNA cross-links in coliphage T7. Abstr. Int. Symp. "Protein and Other Adducts to DNA: Their Significance to Aging, Carcinogenesis, and Radiation Biology," Williamsburg, Virginia, May 2-6, 1975.

Ivannik, B.P., and Ryabchenko, N.I., 1969, Some physicochemical changes in DNA isolated from the organs of irradiated rats (In Russian), *Radiobiologiya* 9:7-14.

Kamal, A., and Garrison, W.M., 1965, Radiolytic degradation of aqueous cytosine: Enhancement by a second organic solute, *Nature* 206:1315-1317.

Kasche, V., 1974, Radiation-induced cross-linking of α-chymotrypsin to DNA and agarose gel, *Int. J. Radiat. Biol.* 26:455-465.

Khattak, M.N., and Green, J.H., 1966a, Gamma-irradiation of nucleic-acid constituents in de-aerated aqueous solutions. I. Cytosine, *Int. J. Radiat. Biol.* 11:131-136.

Khattak, M.N., and Green, J.H., 1966b, Gamma-irradiation of nucleic-acid constituents in de-aerated aqueous solutions. II. 5-Methyl cytosine, *Int. J. Radiat. Biol.* 11:137-143.

Khattak, M.N., and Green, J.H., 1966c, Gamma-irradiation of nucleic-acid constituents in de-aerated aqueous solutions. III. Thymine and uracil, *Int. J. Radiat. Biol.* 11:577-582.

Khattak, M.N., and Wang, S.Y., 1969, Uracil photoproducts from uracil irradiated in ice, *Science* 163:1341-1342.

Kritskiĭ, G.A., 1967, Marrow nucleic acid fractions, normal and after irradiation *in vivo* (In Russian), *Radiobiologiya* 7:193-198.

Kunts, E., and Olson, P., 1975, Attachment of amino acids to ribonuclease by electron beam, UV light or photosensitization. Abstr. Int. Symp. "Protein and Other Adducts to DNA: Their Significance to Aging, Carcinogenesis, and Radiation Biology," Williamsburg, Virginia, May 2-6, 1975.

Kuroki, T., 1973, Chemical carcinogenesis *in vitro, J. Radiat. Res. (Japan)* 14:51.

Kuroki, T., Huberman, E., Marquardt, H., Selkirk, J.K., Heidelberger, C., Grover, P.L., and Sims, P., 1971/72, Binding of K-region epoxides and other derivatives of benzanthracene and dibenzanthracene to DNA, RNA, and proteins of transformable cells, *Chem.-Biol. Interactions* 4:389-397.

Latarjet, R., Ekert, B., and Demersman, P., 1963, Peroxidation of nucleic acids by radiation: Biological implications, *Radiat. Res. Suppl.* 3:247-256.

Lett, J.T., and Alexander, P., 1961, Crosslinking and degradation of deoxyribonucleic acid gels with varying water contents when irradiated with electrons, *Radiat. Res.* 15:159-173.

Littman, F.E., Carr, E.M., and Brady, A.P., 1957, The action of atomic hydrogen on aqueous solutions, *Radiat. Res.* 7:107-119.

Lynn, K.R., 1974, γ-Radiolysis of trypsin, chymotrypsin, and chymotrypsinogen when associated with DNA, *Radiat. Res.* 57:395-402.

Markakis, P., and Tappel, A.L., 1959, Products of γ-irradiation of cysteine and cystine, *J. Am. Chem. Soc.* 82:1613-1617.

Owen, T.C., Rodriguez, M., Johnson, B.G., and Roach, J.A.G., 1968, The radiation chemistry of biochemical disulfides. I. The low-dose X-radiolysis of cystine, *J. Am. Chem. Soc.* 90:196-200.

Packer, J.E., 1963, The action of ^{60}Co-gamma-rays on aqueous solutions of hydrogen sulphide and of cysteine hydrochloride, *J. Chem. Soc.* 2320-2325.

Packer, J.E., and Winchester, R.V., 1968, Radiolysis of neutral aqueous solutions of cysteine in the presence of oxygen, *Chem. Commun.* 826-827.

Pleticha-Lánský, R., 1968, Oscillo-polarographic studies of the effects of γ-radiation on adenine in aqueous solution, *Int. J. Radiat. Biol.* 14:331-339.

Ponnamperuma, C., Lemmon, R.M., and Calvin, M., 1963, The radiation decomposition of adenine, *Radiat. Res.* 18:540-551.

Pullman, B., and Pullman, A., 1963, "Quantum Biochemistry," pp. 683-835, Interscience Publishers, New York.

Purdie, J.W., 1967, γ-Radiolysis of cystine in aqueous solution. Dose-rate effects and a proposed mechanism, *J. Am. Chem. Soc.*

Rhase, H.-J., 1968, Chemical analysis of DNA alterations. III. Isolation and characterization of adenine oxidation products obtained from oligo- and mono-deoxyadenilic acids treated with hydroxyl radicals, *Biochim. Biophys. Acta* 166:311-326.

Shragge, P.C., Varghese, A.J., Hunt, J.W., and Greenstock, C.L., 1974, Radiolysis of uracil in the absence of oxygen, *Radiat. Res.* 60:250-267.

Skalka, M., and Matyášová, J., 1967, The effect of radiation on deoxyribonucleoproteins in animal tissue. III. The character of the polydeoxyribonucleotides released from irradiated tissues, *Folia Biologica (Cze.)* 13:457-464.

Sklobovskaya, M.V., and Ryabchenko, N.I., 1970a, Reduction of the yield of DNA in the deproteinization of UV or gamma-irradiated solutions of deoxyribonucleoprotein. I. Dependence of the magnitude of the effect on the completeness of the complexation of DNA with protein (In Russian), *Radiobiologiya* 10:14-18.

Sklobovskaya, M.V., and Ryabchenko, N.I., 1970b, Reduction of the yield of DNA in the deproteinization of UV or gamma-irradiated solutions of deoxyribonucleoprotein. II. Some problems of the formation of damage (In Russian), *Radiobiologiya* 10:332-337.

Smith, K.C., 1962, Dose dependent decrease in extractability of DNA from bacteria following irradiation with ultraviolet light or with visible light plus dye, *Biochem. Biophys. Res. Commun.* 8:157-163.

Smith, K.C., 1968, The biological importance of UV induced DNA-protein cross-linking *in vivo* and its probable chemical mechanism, *Photochem. Photobiol.* 7:651-660.

Smith, K.C., 1969, Photochemical addition of amino acids to ^{14}C-uracil, *Biochem. Biophys. Res. Commun.* 34:354-357.

Smith, K.C., 1970, A mixed photoproduct of thymine and cysteine: 5-S-Cysteine, 6-hydrothymine, *Biochem. Biophys. Res. Commun.* 39:1011-1016.

Smith, K.C., 1975, The radiation-induced addition of proteins and other molecules to nucleic acids, *in* "Photochemistry and Photobiology of Nucleic Acids" (S.Y. Wang, ed.), Academic Press, New York (in press).

Smith, K.C., and Aplin, R.T., 1966, A mixed photoproduct of uracil and cysteine (5-S-Cysteine-6-hydrouracil). A possible model for the *in vivo* cross-linking of deoxyribonucleic acid and protein by ultraviolet light, *Biochemistry* 5:2125-2130.

Smith, K.C., and Hays, J.E., 1968, The response of uracil-2-^{14}C to X-irradiation under nitrogen and oxygen and to treatment with ascorbic acid, *Radiat. Res.* 33:129-141.

Strazhevskaya, N.B., Krivtsov, G.G., Krasichlova, Z.I., and Struchkov, V.A., 1972, Change in the complex of supermolecular DNA. Residual protein in the thymus and liver of γ-irradiated rats (In Russian), *Radiobiologiya* 12:19-25.

Strazhevskaya, N.B., and Troyanovskaya, M.L., 1970, Method of investigating the radiation effect on chromatin deoxyribonucleoprotein (In Russian), *Radiobiologiya* 10:808-814.

Strazhevskaya, N.B., Troyanovskaya, M.L., and Krivtsov, G.G., 1971, Mechanism of the radiation damage to the deoxyribonucleoprotein in animal cell chromatin (In Russian), *Radiobiologiya* 11:329-334.

Strazhevskaya, N.B., Troyanovskaya, M.L., Struchkov, V.A., and Krasichlova, Z.I., 1969, Disturbance of the state of the DNA-protein complex of chromatin in the cell nucleus under the influence of ionizing radiation (In Russian), *Radiobiologiya*

Tseĭtlin, P.I., Ryabchenko, N.I., Gorin, A.I., Tronov, V.A., Sklobovskaya, M.V., and Ivannik, B.P., 1967, The influence of ionizing radiation on the macromolecular organization of DNA and DNP (In Russian), *Radiobiologiya* 7:658-669.

van Hemmen, J.J., 1971, 6-Amino-8-hydroxy-7,8-dihydropurine: Radiation product of adenine, *Nature N. Biol.* 231:79-80.

van Hemmen, J.J., and Bleichrodt, J.F., 1971, The decomposition of adenine by ionizing radiation, *Radiat. Res.* 46:444-456.

Varghese, A.J., 1970, 5-Thyminyl-5,6-dihydrothymine from DNA irradiated with ultraviolet light, *Biochem. Biophys. Res. Commun.* 38:484-490.

Wilkening, V.G., Lal, M., Arends, M., and Armstrong, D.A., 1967, The γ-radiolysis of cysteine in deaerated 1 N HClO$_4$ solutions, *Can. J. Chem.* 45:1209-1214.

Wilkening, V.G., Lal, M., Arends, M., and Armstrong, D.C., 1968, The cobalt-60 γ radiolysis of cysteine in deaerated aqueous solutions at pH values between 5 and 6, *J. Phys. Chem.* 72:185-190.

Yamamoto, O., 1967, Biochemical studies of radiation damage. I. Inactivation of the pH 5 fraction in amino acyl sRNA synthesis *in vitro* and the binding of amino acids with protein and nucleic acid by gamma-ray irradiation, *Int. J. Radiat. Biol.* 12:467-476.

Yamamoto, O., 1972a, Radiation-induced binding of cysteine and cystine with aromatic amino acids or serum albumin in aqueous solution, *Int. J. Radiat. Phys. Chem.* 4:227-236.

Yamamoto, O., 1972b, Radiation-induced binding of methionine with serum albumin, tryptophan or phenylalanine in aqueous solution, *Int. J. Radiat. Phys. Chem.* 4:335-345.

Yamamoto, O., 1973a, Radiation-induced binding of nucleic acid constituents with protein constituents and with each other, *Int. J. Radiat. Phys. Chem.* 5:213-229.

Yamamoto, O., 1973b, Radiation-induced binding of phenylalanine,
     tryptophan and histidine mutually and with albumin, *Radiat.
     Res.* 54:398-410.
Yamamoto, O., 1975, Radiation-induced binding of some protein and
     nucleic acid constituents with macromolecular components in
     cell systems, *Radiat. Res.* 61:261-273.
Yamamoto, O., and Okuda, A., 1975, Radiation-induced binding of OH-
     substituted aromatic amino acids, tyrosine and dopa, mutually
     and with albumin in aqueous solution, *Radiat. Res.* 61:251-260.
Zimmerman, F.K., Kröger, H., and Lücking, T., 1965, Interaction of
     RNA polymerase with irradiated DNA, *Biochemische Zeitschrift*
     342:115-119.

CHEMICALLY-INDUCED DNA-PROTEIN CROSS-LINKS

John O. Thomas

Department of Biochemistry, Stanford University Medical

School, Stanford, California 94305[*]

1. INTRODUCTION

Naturally occurring nucleic acids are found in intimate association with proteins. Viral DNA or RNA is folded within a protein
capsid; the bacterial chromosome is associated with polyamines,
proteins, and membrane components (Worcel and Burgi, 1975); and the
DNA of eukaryotes is associated with histones and non-histone proteins. Cross-links between nucleic acids and the surrounding proteins have been generated by UV radiation both *in vitro* and *in vivo*
(Smith, This Volume). They have been employed in studies of nucleic
acid-protein interactions (Schimmel *et al.*, This Volume), and may
lead to viral inactivation (Gordon, This Volume), cell death (Smith,
This Volume; Todd and Han, This Volume), and perhaps carcinogenesis.

In principle, many chemicals should also be capable of inducing

---

*Present address: Department of Biochemistry, New York
University Medical School, New York, New York 10016.

DNA-protein cross-links, but in practice, only a few have been investigated. DNA-protein cross-links may be induced by chemicals
through any of several possible modes of action. These include:
     a) activation of the proteins allowing them to react directly
with DNA.
     b) activation of DNA allowing it to react directly with pro-
teins,
     c) cross-linking by a bifunctional reagent,
     d) an indirect effect of the chemicals inducing a cellular
cross-linking mechanism.
Reagents which cross-link through one of the first two mechanisms
have been used extensively in studies of nucleic acid-protein interactions. Reagents which induce DNA-protein cross-links through the
second two mechanisms however, have been investigated with a primary
emphasis on their cytotoxic effects.

2.   CROSS-LINKING VIA AN ACTIVATED INTERMEDIATE

2.1.   Aldehydes

     Formaldehyde has long been used as a cross-linking reagent.
It reacts readily with both nucleic acids and protein, and is
capable of polymerizing so that cross-links of various sizes can
be produced (Walker, 1964). It is employed for the inactivation
of viruses and for vaccine production, and has found wide use as a
fixative for microscopy and for physical studies of macromolecular
complexes.

     With proteins, formaldehyde reacts with a large variety of side
chains, forming methylol derivatives (Means and Feeney, 1971). Methylol derivatives are also formed by the reaction of formaldehyde
with the amino and imino groups of nucleic acids (Feldman, 1973;
McGhee and Von Hipple; 1975a, b). These methylol derivatives, which
are unstable, are capable of reacting further with other proteins or
nucleic acids to form a stable product cross-linked by a methylene
bridge.

$$RNH_2 + CH_2O \rightleftharpoons RNH-CH_2OH$$
$$R'NH_2 + RNH-CH_2OH \rightarrow RNH-CH_2-NHR' + H_2O$$

The rate of reaction of formaldehyde with amino acids is much faster
than the rate of reaction with nucleic acids (Semin *et al.*, 1974).
One might expect, therefore, that in inducing nucleic acid-protein
cross-links, formaldehyde first reacts with an amino acid side
chain, forming a methylol derivative. This methylol derivative
then reacts with one of the bases of the nucleic acid, forming a
product cross-linked by a methylene bridge. This scheme is supported by the results reported by Siomin *et al.* (1973) and Semin

et al. (1974). The reaction of nucleic acids with formaldehyde in the presence of amino acids (glycine and lysine) was shown to differ substantially from the reaction of nucleic acids with formaldehyde in the absence of amino acids. The rate of formation of the DNA-formaldehyde-amino acid adduct was about 100 times faster than the rate of reaction of DNA with formaldehyde alone, and the spectra of the products of the nucleotide-formaldehyde-amino acid reaction were substantially different from those of the nucleotide-formaldehyde adduct (Semin *et al.*, 1974). McGhee and von Hippel (1975a) have also observed an acceleration in the rate of reaction between formaldehyde and nucleotides in the presence of morpholine. The product of the reaction between DNA, [^{14}C]lysine, and formaldehyde is stable to dialysis. After dialysis for 24 h against 0.5 M NaCl, measurement of the remaining [^{14}C] indicated that lysine was bound in the ratio of one residue per six bases. In control experiments lacking either DNA or formaldehyde, the lysine was completely dialyzable. Experiments in which [^{14}C]glycine was incubated with DNA and formaldehyde failed to produce a stable complex. It was also observed in the experiments with glycine that the DNA was markedly more susceptible to degradation. The possibility that the [^{14}C] glycine was dialyzable due to a degradation of the DNA was not excluded.

Jackson and Chalkley (1974) have observed that the fixation of histones to DNA by formaldehyde (1% formaldehyde for 30 min) can be "reversed" by dialysis at 37° or 60°C for 48 h. Fixation was determined by the ability to extract the histones with 0.4 N H_2SO_4. The possibility that the observed "reversability" of the fixation was due to degradation of the DNA was not discounted.

Formaldehyde has been used to cross-link ribosomes for electron microscopy (Huxley and Zubay, 1960; Bayley, 1964), and for physical studies (Cox, 1969; Tal, 1970; Spirin *et al.*, 1965; Roberts and Walker, 1970). These studies demonstrated that following treatment with formaldehyde, ribosomes are resistant to unfolding by CsCl (Spirin *et al.*, 1965), urea (Robert and Walker, 1970), or sodium dodecyl sulfate (Cox, 1969). Amos and Moller (1972) have presented data which they claim demonstrate that this resistance to denaturation is not a consequence of rRNA-protein cross-links, but results exclusively from protein-protein cross-links. Following treatment of ribosomes with formaldehyde, the rRNA was digested with ribonuclease, and the proteins separated from the digested rRNA using slab gel electrophoresis. At most, one or two 30-nucleotide lengths of rRNA migrated with the ribosomal proteins. The possibility that 30 mono or dinucleotides could have remained after ribonuclease digestion rather than one or two 30 nucleotide fragments was not excluded. Other evidence presented by these authors tends to support the existence of rRNA-protein cross-links. No protein can be extracted from rRNA by urea-LiCl, acetic acid, or phenol treatment of formaldehyde treated ribosomes. Also, the ribosomal proteins

of formaldehyde treated ribosomes will not enter an SDS gel during
electrophoresis unless they are first treated with ribonuclease.
The ribosomal proteins from untreated ribosomes readily enter the
gel.

Formaldehyde has also found extensive use as a cross-linking
agent in studies of chromatin structure (Doenecke and McCarthy,
1975; Jackson and Chalkley, 1974; Varshavskii and Ilyin, 1974a,
1974b; Clark and Felsenfeld, 1971; Brutlag *et al.*, 1969; Ilyin and
Georgiev, 1969), and has been employed in studies on the packaging
of DNA in phage (Tikchonenko *et al.*, 1974; Chatteraj and Inman,
1974).

Formaldehyde has been reported to induce mutations in viruses,
bacteria, Neurospra and Drosophila (Feldman, 1973; Nishioka, 1973).
There is also a report that formaldehyde is a possible carcinogen
(Rosenkranz, 1972). The nature of the direct mutagen is not known,
but three possibilities have been suggested. Mutation of Drosophila
larvae by introduction of formaldehyde into the media appears to
involve methelene-bis adenylic acid formed by the action of formaldehyde on adenylic acid or RNA in the culture media (Alderson,
1973). Whether this product actually becomes incorporated into the
DNA (or RNA) or whether it blocks the action of an enzyme system
is not clear. The possibility that formaldehyde reacts with hydrogen peroxide to form dihydrodimethyl peroxide has been suggested
(Sobels, 1963), but little evidence has been presented to support
this hypothesis. Poverenny *et al.* (1974) have suggested that formaldehyde forms monomethyl derivatives of amino acids which then
form cross-links with the DNA as described above. In support of
this, they have shown that *E. coli* is inactivated by monomethylol
glycine and formaldehyde at the same rate. This result is not
surprising since there is a rapid equilibrium between formaldehyde
and the methylol compounds. *E. coli polA1* (deficient in DNA polymerase I) is also inactivated by monomethylol glycine and formaldehyde at the same rate although more rapidly than is *E. coli pol*[+].
The inactivation of *E. coli polA1* is accompanied by an accumulation
of DNA single-strand breaks.

Glutaraldehyde is another widely employed cross-linking reagent
and fixative, which was used by Delius *et al.* (1972) to cross-link
bacteriophage T4 gene-32 protein to DNA. The mechanism by which
glutaraldehyde cross-links is, however, poorly understood.

Malonaldehyde (malondialdehyde) is generated as a product of
the peroxidation of unsaturated lipids. It has been shown to induce
tumors when applied to the shaved backs of mice, and skin treated
with 7, 12-dimethylbenz[a]-anthracene, benzo[a]pyrene, or 3-methyl-
cholanthrene shows an increased level of malonaldehyde (Shamberger
et al., 1974). An increased level of malonaldehyde also accompanies
irradiation (Wills, 1970). Although malonaldehyde reacts with both

proteins (Chio and Tappel, 1969) and DNA (Reiss *et al.*, 1972; Brooks and Klamerth, 1968), its ability to induce DNA-protein cross-links has not been investigated.

Formaldehyde and glutaraldehyde are very effective cross-linking agents, and their small size minimizes problems of steric hinderance. As a tool for the molecular biologist however, they suffer from the disadvantage that they are capable of polymerizing, thus forming cross-links of variable size. They are also rather indiscriminate in their reactions, producing not only nucleic acid-protein cross-links, but also protein-protein and nucleic acid-nucleic acid cross-links. These problems can be reduced by using reagents such as those discussed in the following section which activate the nucleic acid rather than the protein.

2.2. Nucleophilic Activating Agents

Hydroxylamine, O-methyl hydroxylamine and bisulfite induce DNA-protein cross-links by activating cytosine, allowing it to undergo a transamination with a neighboring protein. An interesting feature of the reaction is its "reversibility." Under conditions of acid pH, the cross-linked protein can be displaced by water, hydroxylamine, or O-methyl hydroxylamine. These reactions are discussed in detail by Shapiro (This Volume).

2.3. Other Activating Agents

The water soluble carbodiimide, N-cyclohexyl-N'-β-(4-methyl-morpholinium) ethyl carbodiimide *p*-toluene sulfonate, has been used as a DNA-protein cross-linking agent in studies of the organization of DNA inside of the bacteriophage lambda (Thomas, 1974). The mechanism of cross-linking has not been elucidated, but probably involves the activation or a protein carboxyl or nucleic acid phosphoester which then reacts to form an amide, ester, phosphodiester, phosphoramidate or mixed anhydride (Kurzer and Douraghi-Zadeh, 1967).

DNA-protein cross-links have been demonstrated as a product of nitrous acid inactivation of the coliphage T7, but these cross-links only account for a small fraction of the inactivation (Dussault *et al.*, 1970). The chemical identity of the cross-links and the mechanism by which they are generated is unknown.

A variety of activated analogues of t-RNA have been prepared for structural studies of ribosomes, t-RNA synthetase and amino-acyl-t-RNAs by affinity labeling. These studies are discussed in the chapters by Cooperman and Schimmel *et al.* in this volume.

3. CROSS-LINKING BY CYTOTOXIC CHEMICALS

3.1. Bifunctional Alkylating Agents

In general, bifunctional alkylating agents are much more cytotoxic, and are far better carcinogens than their monofunctional
analogs.[*] These observations prompted Elmore *et al.* (1948) and
Goldacre and Ross (1949) to propose that the cytological effects
of these reagents are due, to a large extent, to a cross-linkage
between cellular components. A considerable amount of evidence has
been presented showing that bifunctional alkylating agents, particularly nitrogen mustard [methyl bis(2-chloroethyl) amine] and sulfur
mustard [bis(2-chloroethyl) sulfide], are capable of inducing both
intrastrand and interstrand DNA-DNA cross-links (Jolley, 1973; Yin
et al., 1973; Ball and Roberts, 1971; Walker, 1971; Chun *et al.*,
1969; Lawley *et al.*, 1969; Brookes, 1966). There is much less evidence to support the suggestion that DNA-protein cross-links can
be generated by bifunctional alkylating agents, even though DNA
and proteins are both readily alkylated.

Several workers have observed that the treatment of animal
cells with bifunctional alkylating agents produces an increase in
the amount of protein which remains associated with DNA after various extraction procedures. Rutman *et al.* (1961) noticed that DNA
recovery from phenol extracted Ehrlich ascites cells decreased as
the extent of alkylation increased. Steele (1962) demonstrated
that upon incubation of Ehrlich ascites cells with nitrogen,
chloroquine, L-phenylalanine, or sulfur mustard, protein bound to
DNA as measured by salt-phenol extraction increased almost linearly
with the concentration of mustard. Monofunctional alkylating agents
however, did not produce an increased binding of proteins to DNA.
Golder *et al.* (1963) demonstrated that a nitrogen mustard treatment
of Swiss mice bearing 6 - 7 day ascites increased the amount of
protein bound to DNA by about six-fold (from 1.2% protein to 7.7%
protein). The DNA bound protein was isolated by repeated extraction
with phenol-p-aminosalicylate. The DNA was alkylated to the extent
of one alkylation/10^4 nucleotides. Klatt *et al.* (1969) studied the
effect of nitrogen mustard on the bouyant density of DNA extracted
from resistant and sensitive Ehrlich cells. Cells were disrupted
for 10 min in 2% SDS at 60°C, then banded in CsCl. The amount of
material banding at the position of DNA decreased as the concentration of nitrogen mustard in the medium was increased. This effect
was far greater for sensitive cells than for resistant cells. The
material displaced from the band could be found at the top of the

---

[*]The bifunctional alkylating agents are, however, less cytotoxic and poorer carcinogens than the carcinogenic nitroso compounds,
which are monofunctional alkylating agents.

gradient, and if treated with trypsin, banded at the position characteristic of DNA.

Since mustard induced DNA-protein cross-links have not been shown to contain bis-ethylamine bridges, they may have been generated by another mechanism. Lett (This Volume) and Balis (This Volume) have presented evidence suggesting that DNA-protein cross-links are produced in normal cells, and that the extent of cross-linking depends on the metabolic state of the cell. Nothing is known about the mechanisms by which these cross-links are produced and perhaps excised. It is possible, therefore, that mustard-induced cross-links may result indirectly from an alteration in the metabolism of the cell, the altered cell containing a greater number of such cross-links.

Many of the ambiguities associated with experiments using animal cells are eliminated in studies employing *in vitro* systems. Results from this laboratory indicate that chlorambucil [4-*p*-(bis (2-chloroethyl)amino)phenyl butyric acid] and nitrogen mustard are capable of cross-linking the DNA of the bacteriophage lambda to the coat proteins (J.O. Thomas, in preparation).

3.2. Other Cytotoxic Agents

Bifunctional alkylating agents are not unique in their ability to induce DNA-protein cross-links in animal cells. Grunicke *et al.* (1973) showed that an increased binding of protein to DNA could be obtained by treating cells with the monofunctional alkylating agent methyl methanesulfonate (MMS) at sufficiently high concentrations to inhibit cell multiplication (Ehrlich ascites cells). Increasing the concentration of MMS resulted in a decrease in the extractability of DNA by phenol (the unextracted DNA could be found in the interphase) which paralleled the decrease in cell multiplication. Other metabolic inhibitors were investigated with the result that arsenate, arsenite, N-ethylmaleimide, iodoacetate, and *p*-chloromercuribenzoate (all of which react with sulfhydryl groups) decreased the phenol extractability of DNA from the Ehrlich cells. Deoxyglucose, dinitrophenol, fluoroacetate, KCN, and oligomycin had little effect on the extractability of DNA at the concentrations used. The alkylating agents trenimon (2,3,5-triethyleneiminobenzoquinone-1,4), cyclophosphamide [N,N-bis(2-chloroethyl)-N',O-propylene phosphodiamide], TEM (2,4,6-triethylenimino-1,3,5-triazine, triethylenemelamine), and nitrogen mustard were also shown to decrease the extractability of the DNA.

Actinomycin D has also been found to influence the DNA extractability (Helgeland and Reistad, 1967). Chick embryo cells were treated with actinomycin D, lysed with SDS, then extracted with chloroform-butanol or phenol. With either solvent, the DNA

partitioned between the aqueous phase and the interphase. The migration of the DNA from the aqueous phase to the interphase was related
to both the concentration of actinomycin D (0-50 μg/ml) and the
length of treatment.

Salzer and Balis (1970) investigated the effect of actinomycin
D, mitomycin C, proflavin, and nitrogen mustard on the DNA-associated
amino acids isolated from various organs of rats. They found that
both the relative and absolute amounts of the amino acids bound to
DNA changed markedly after treatment. There were both increases
and decreases in the amounts bound, depending on the drug, tissue,
and amino acid. It was also observed that tumors differ from normal
cells in the composition of the DNA-associated amino acids (Salzer
and Balis, 1968; Salzer *et al.*, 1969). The amino acid compositions
reported probably reflect the amino acid compositions of DNA-bound
proteins.

These data show that DNA-protein cross-links can be induced
by many (but not all) cytotoxic chemicals. As mentioned in the
last section, DNA-protein cross-links might be generated by a
normal cellular mechanism operating in response to an alteration
of the cell. It is also possible that the DNA-protein cross-links
may have been generated through the action of naturally occurring
cross-linking agents such as malonaldehyde and free radicals. The
non-alkylating compounds which induce DNA-protein cross-links
(Grunicke, 1973) all react with sulfhydryls, one of the cells main
defenses against free radicals.

In vitro studies have shown that at least two potent carcinogens are capable of inducing DNA-protein cross-links. Neitert *et
al.* (1974) have presented evidence which suggests that the carcinogenic, monofunctional alkylating agent, β-propiolactone, induces
DNA-protein cross-links *in vitro* when DNA is mixed with bovine serum
albumin in the presence of β-propiolactone. The chemical identity
of the product is unknown, as is the mechanism of production.
Another carcinogen, benz[a]pyrene has been shown to cross-link DNA
and histones *in vitro* when irradiated with UV light (Lesko *et al.*,
1971).

4.   CONCLUSIONS

Evidence has been presented which demonstrates that DNA-protein
cross-links may be induced by the following compounds.

formaldehyde	hydroxylamine	chlorambucil
glutaraldehyde	O-methyl hydroxylamine	β-propiolactone
carbodiimide	bisulfite	benz[a]pyrene
nitrous acid	nitrogen mustard	

Two notable omissions from the above list are the nitroso compounds and free radicals. Free radicals have been implicated (Smith, This Volume) as being important intermediates in the photochemically induced cross-linking of DNA and proteins. Chemically generated free radicals (such as from microsomal oxidation of carcinogens) might also lead to DNA-protein cross-links.

To date, many of the studies have been conducted using animal cells, and clear cut results were not obtained due to the complexity of the system. Bacteriophage (in conjunction with microsomal activating systems where required) provide a much simpler system for investigating the chemistry of DNA-protein cross-links; a DNA (or RNA) molecule in intimate contact with protein without the complexities of cellular systems. Another advantage of the bacteriophage system is the sensitivity with which DNA-protein cross-links can be detected. A reaction product involving several nucleotides per chromosome may be quite important biologically, but unimportant chemically, involving only $10^{-6}\%$ of the nucleotides in the chromosome. This sensitivity is, therefore, a desirable feature.

The importance of chemically induced DNA-protein cross-links to carcinogenesis and aging can only be assessed after a larger number of chemicals have been studied. Of particular interest in this respect are free radicals, malonaldehyde, the nitrosamines, and polycyclic hydrocarbons. Although the nitrosamines and polycyclic hydrocarbons may not be cross-linking agents themselves, their oxidation products may be very effective. Another important consideration is the excision of DNA-protein cross-links by cellular repair processes. Unfortunately, very little is known about the repair of DNA-protein cross-links, but four questions are of prime importance. 1) How does a repair enzyme distinguish between a noncovalent DNA-protein association and a covalently bound protein? 2) What is the efficiency of repair? 3) What is the fidelity of repair? And 4) what are the consequences of an unrepaired crosslink for transcription and replication?

It is obvious that investigations of DNA-protein cross-linking in general, and chemically induced DNA-protein cross-links in particular are in their infancy. Future investigations will undoubtedly yield important new tools for the molecular biologist, and important new knowledge for the clinician.

Acknowledgment. This review was written during the tenure of a Senior Fellowship from the California Division of the American Cancer Society.

References

Alderson, T., 1973, Chemotherapy for a selective effect on mammalian tumour cells, *Nature New Biol.* 244:3-6.

Amos, R., and Moller, W., 1972, On the mode of reaction of formaldehyde with ribosomes, *Biochim. Biophys. Acta* 272:95-107.

Ball, C.R., and Roberts, J.J., 1971, Estimation of interstrand DNA cross-linking resulting from mustard gas alkylation of He La cells, *Chem-Biol. Interactions* 4:297-303.

Bayley, S.T., 1964, Physical studies on ribosomes from pea seedlings, *J. Mol. Biol.* 8:231-238.

Brookes, P., 1966, Quantitative aspects of the reaction of some carcinogens with nucleic acids and the possible significance of such reactions in the process of carcinogenesis, *Cancer Res.* 26:1994-2003.

Brooks, B.R., and Klamerth, O.L., 1968, Interaction of DNA with bifunctional aldehydes, *Eur. J. Biochem.* 5:178-182.

Brutlag, D., Schlehuber, C., and Bonner, J., 1969, Properties of formaldehyde-treated nucleohistone, *Biochemistry* 8:3214-3218.

Chattoraj, D.K., and Inman, R.B., 1974, Location of DNA ends in P2, 186, P4 and lambda bacteriophage heads, *J. Mol. Biol.* 87:11-22.

Chio, K.S., and Tappel, A.L., 1969, Inactivation of ribonuclease and other enzymes by peroxidizing lipids and by malonaldehyde, *Biochemistry* 8:2877-2832.

Chun, E.H.L., Gonzales, L., Lewis, F.S., Jones, J., and Rutman, R.J., 1969, Differences in *in vivo* alkylation and cross-linking of nitrogen mustard sensitive and resistant lines of Lettre-Ehrlich ascites tumours, *Cancer Res.* 29:1184-1194.

Clark, R.J., and Felsenfeld, G., 1971, Structure of chromatin, *Nature New Biol.* 229:101-106.

Cox, R.A., 1969, A study of the effects of reaction with formaldehyde on some optical and physical properties of reticulocyte ribosome *Biochem. J.* 114:743-751.

Delius, H., Mantell, N.J., and Alberts, B., 1972, Characterization by electron microscopy of the complex formed between T4 bacterio phage gene 32-protein and DNA, *J. Mol. Biol.* 67:341-350.

Doenecke, D.,and McCarthy, B.J., 1975, The nature of protein association with chromatin, *Biochemistry* 14:1373-1378.

Dussault, D., Bourgault, J.M., and Verly, W.G., 1970, T7 coliphage inactivation by nitrous acid, *Biochim. Biophys. Acta* 213:312-319.

Elmore, D.T., Gulland, J.M., Jordan, D.O., and Taylor, H.F.W., 1948, Reaction of nucleic acids with mustard gas, *Biochem. J.* 42:308-316.

Feldman, H.Yu., 1973, Reactions of nucleic acids and nucleoproteins with formaldehyde, *in* "Progress in Nucleic Acid Research and Molecular Biology" (J.N. Davidson and W.E. Cohn, eds.), Vol. 13, pp. 1-49, Academic Press, New York.

Goldacre, R.J., and Ross, W.C.J., 1949, Mode of production of chromosome abnormalities by nitrogen mustard, *Nature* 163:667-669.

Golder, R.H., Martin-Guzman, G., Jones, J., Goldstein, N.O., Roten-
    berg, S., and Rutman, R.J., 1964, Experimental chemotherapy
    studies. III. Properties of DNA from Ascites cells treated
    in vivo with nitrogen mustard, *Cancer Res.* 24:964-968.
Grunicke, H., Bock, K.W., Becher, H., Gang, V., Schnierda, J., and
    Pushendorf, B., 1973, Effect of alkylating antitumor agents on
    the binding of DNA to protein, *Cancer Res.* 33:1048-1053.
Helgeland, K., and Reistand, K., 1967, Effect of actinomycin D on
    tissue culture cells: An altered DNA distribution after
    extraction with phenol or chloroform-butanol, *Biochim. Biophys.
    Acta* 145:214-217.
Huxley, H.E., and Zubay, G., 1960, Electron microscope observations
    on the structure of microsomal particles from *Escherichia coli*,
    J. Mol. Biol. 2:10-18.
Ilyin, Yu.V., and Gerorgiev, G.P., 1969, Heterogeneity of deoxynu-
    cleoprotein particles as evidenced by ultracentrifugation in
    cesium chloride density gradient, *J. Mol. Biol.* 41:299-303.
Jackson, V., and Chalkley, R., 1974, Separation of newly synthesized
    nucleohistone by equilibrium centrifugation in cesium chloride,
    Biochemistry 13:3953-3956.
Jolley, G.N., and Omerod, M.G., 1973, An improved method for measur-
    ing cross-links in the DNA of mammalian cells: The effect of
    nitrogen mustard, *Biochim. Biophys. Acta* 308:242-251.
Klatt, O., Stehlin, J.S., Jr., McBridge, C., and Griffin, A.C.,
    1969, The effect of nitrogen mustard treatment on the deoxyri-
    bonucleic acid of sensitive and resistant Ehrlich tumor cells,
    Cancer Res. 29:286-290.
Kurzer, F., and Douraghi-Zadeh, K., 1967, Advances in the chemistry
    of carbodiimides, *Chemical Rev.* 67:107-152.
Lawley, P.D., Lethbridge, J.H., Edwards, P.A., and Shooter, K.V.,
    1969, Inactivation of bacteriophage T7 by mono-and difunc-
    tional sulfur mustards in relation to cross-linking and depuri-
    nation of bacteriophage DNA, *J. Mol. Biol.* 39:181-189.
Lesko, S.A., Hoffmann, H.O., Ts'o, P.O.P., and Maher, W.H., 1971,
    in Progress in Molecular and Subcellular Biology Series (F.E.
    Hahn, ed.), Springer-Verlag, Berlin 2 356.
McGhee, J.D., and von Hippel, P.H., 1975a, Formaldehyde as a probe
    of DNA structure. I. Reaction with exocyclic amino groups
    of DNA bases, *Biochemistry* 14:1281-1296.
McGhee, J.D., and von Hippel, P.H., 1975b, Formaldehyde as a probe
    of DNA structure. II. Reaction with endocyclic imino groups
    of DNA bases, *Biochemistry* 14:1297-1303.
Means, G.E., and Feeney, R.E., 1971, "Chemical Modification of
    Proteins," pp. 125-128, Holden-Day Inc., San Francisco.
Nietert, W.C., Kellicutt, L.M., and Kubinski, H., 1974, DNA-protein
    complexes produced by a carcinogen, β-propiolactone, *Cancer
    Res.* 34:859-864.
Nishioka, H., 1973, Lethal and mutagenic action of formaldehyde in
    Hcr[+] and Hcr[−] strains of *Escherichia coli*, *Mutat. Res.* 17:261-
    265.

Poverenny, A.M., Siomin, Yu.A., Saenko, A.S., and Sinzinis, B.I.,
    1975, Possible mechanisms of lethal and mutagenic action of
    formaldehyde, *Mutat. Res.* 27:123-126.
Reiss, V., Tappel, A.L., and Chio, K.S., 1972, DNA-malonaldehyde
    reaction; formation of fluorescent products, *Biochem. Biophys.
    Res. Commun.* 48:921-926.
Roberts, M.E., and Walker, I.O., 1970, Structural studies on
    Escherichia coli ribosomes III. Denaturation and sedimen-
    tation of ribosomal subunits unfolded in urea, *Biochim.
    Biophys. Acta* 199:184-193.
Rosenkranz, H.S., 1972, Formaldehyde as a possible carcinogen,
    Environ. Contam. Toxicol. 8:242-244.
Rutman, R.J., Steele, W.J., and Price, C.C., 1961, Experimental
    chemotherapy studies. I. Chemical and metabolic investiga-
    tions of chloroquine mustard, *Cancer Res.* 21:1134-1140.
Salser, J.S., and Balis, M.E., 1968, Amino acids associated with
    DNA of tumors, *Cancer Res.* 28:595-600.
Salser, J.S., and Balis, M.E., 1970, Alterations in deoxyribonucleic
    acid-bound amino acids after the administration of deoxyribo-
    nucleic acid-binding drugs, *Biochem. Pharmacol.* 19:2375-2387.
Salser, J.S., Teller, M.N., and Balis, M.E., 1969, Changes in DNA-
    bound amino acids in experimental tumor transplants, *Cancer
    Res.* 29:1002-1007.
Semin, Yu.A., Kolomyitsera, E.N., and Poverenny, A.M., 1974, Effects
    of formaldehyde and amino acids on nucleotides and DNA, *Mol.
    Biol.* (Eng. Ed.) 8:220-227.
Shramberger, R.J., Andreone, T.L., and Willis, C.E., 1974, Atioxi-
    dants and cancer. IV. Initiating activity of malonaldehyde
    as a carcinogen, *J. Natl. Cancer Inst.* 53:1771-1773.
Siomin, Yu.A., Simonov, V.V., and Poverenny, A.M., 1973, The reaction
    of formaldehyde with deoxynucleotides and DNA in the presence
    of amino acids and lysine-rich histone, *Biochim. Biophys. Acta*
    331:27-32.
Sobels, F.H., 1963, Peroxides and the induction of mutations by X-
    rays, ultraviolet, and formaldehyde, *Radiat. Res. Suppl.* 3:171-
    183.
Spirin, A.S., Celitsina, N.V., and Lerman, M.I., 1965, Use of for-
    maldehyde fixation for studies of ribonucleoprotein particles
    by cesium chloride density-gradient centrifugation, *J. Mol.
    Biol.* 14:611-615.
Steele, W., 1962, Cross-linking of DNA to nuclear proteins by di-
    functional alkylating agents, *Proc. Am. Assoc. Cancer Res.*
    3:364.
Tal, M., 1970, Formaldehyde and ribosomal conformation, *Biochim.
    Biophys. Acta* 224:470-476.
Thomas, J.O., 1974, Chemical linkage of the tail to the right-hand
    end of bacteriophage lambda DNA, *J. Mol. Biol.* 87:1-9.
Tikohonenko, T.I., Kislina, O.S., and Dobrov, E.N., 1974, Peculiari-
    ties of the secondary structure of bacteriophage DNA *in situ*.
    V. Change in DNA conformation inside the phages under the

influence of formaldehyde, *Arch. Biochem. Biophys.* 160:1-13.

Varsharskii, A.Ya., and Ilin, Yu. V., 1974a, Salt treatment of chromatin induces redistribution of histones, *Biochim. Biophys. Acta* 340:207-217.

Varshavskii, A.Ya., and Ilin, Yu. V., 1974b, Structure of the chromosomal deoxyribonucleoproteins. VI. Redistribution of histones during salt treatment of the chromatin, *Mol. Biol.* (Eng. Ed.) 8:334-340.

Walker, I.G., 1971, Intrastrand bifunctional alkylation of DNA in mammalian cells treated with mustard gas, *Can. J. Biochem.* 49:332-336.

Walker, J.F., 1964, "Formaldehyde," 3rd Edition, Reinhold, New York.

Wills, E., 1970, Effects of irradiation on subcellular components I. Lipid peroxide formation in the endoplasmic reticulum, *Int. J. Radiat. Biol.* 17:217-228.

Worcel, A., and Burgi, E., 1974, Properties of a membrane-attached form of the folded chromosome of *Escherichia coli*, *J. Mol. Biol.* 82:91-105.

Yin, L., Chun, E.H.L., and Rutman, R.J., 1973, A comparison of the effects of alkylation on the DNA of sensitive and resistant Lettre-Ehrlich cells following *in vivo* exposure to nitrogen mustard, *Biochim. Biophys. Acta* 324:472-481.

PHOTOCHEMICAL ADDITION OF AMINO ACIDS AND RELATED COMPOUNDS TO

NUCLEIC ACID CONSTITUENTS

Alummutil J. Varghese

Physics Division, Ontario Cancer Institute

500 Sherbourne Street, Toronto, Ontario, Canada

1. INTRODUCTION

The most vital cell constituents of all living systems are the nucleic acids. Consequently, alterations in nucleic acid molecules are of utmost biological significance. These alterations can be either addition of molecules to nucleic acids or degradation of purine, pyrimidine, or sugar phosphate residues. From a biological point of view, the former type of alteration is of greater significance and it is the subject of this symposium. As shown by Smith (1975) in his review, a wide variety of compounds add to nucleic acids and their constituents under the influence of radiation (UV, visible, and ionizing).

The aim of the present discussion is to describe the chemical nature of addition products of nucleic acid constituents with other molecules. The discussion will be limited to addition products derived from pyrimidine bases. Very few addition reactions of

207

purine residues are known and these are discussed by Elad (This Volume). Addition products of sugar phosphate residues are not known.

2. ACTIVATED OLEFINS

The formation of cyclobutane derivatives is a general photo-reaction (Chapman, 1967) of "activated olefins" (e.g., small ring olefins, rigid multiring olefins, α, β-unsaturated carbonyl compounds). The C_5-C_6 double bond in the pyrimidine base has the characteristics of an activated double bond. Consequently the pyrimidine base can form cyclobutane addition products with other "activated olefins". Thus, uracil (I) adds on to another uracil molecule, II, to form III, generally referred to as a cyclobutane

dimer (for a recent review of this class of products see Fisher and Johns, 1975); to acrylonitrile (IV) forming an adduct of type V (Helene and Brun, 1970); and to furocoumarins (VI) forming products of the type VII (Musajo and Rodighiero, 1972). Polynuclear hydrocarbons also form these types of products (Rice, 1964). Since the addition of an excited molecule to a ground-state molecule leads to a cyclobutane derivative, excitation of either molecule could lead to this type of product. For example, III is formed when the irradiation is carried out at 254 nm, while VII is formed at 365 nm. Consequently the absorption characteristics of the 'activated olefins' will determine the excitation wavelengths. Many isomers are possible for these addition products. The predominance of a particular isomer depends on the experimental conditions (Varghese, 1972).

Among these adducts, only the pyrimidine dimers have been extensively studied. A number of chemical mutagens (e.g., afla-toxins, maleic hydrazide; Fishbein *et al.*, 1970) have the charac-teristics of activated olefins and absorb light in the visible region. It is highly probable that they form addition products readily with nucleic acid constituents. This appears to be a fertile field for further study.

3. KETONES AND SIMILAR COMPOUNDS

The simplest example for this type of product is the uracil-acetone adduct (IX) (where $X = 0$; $R_1 = R_2 = CH_3$) (Varghese, 1975a).

$X = 0, S, NH$

Generally, photocycloaddition products of this type are very unstable. The uracil-acetone adduct undergoes degradation in acid, alkali, and when heated in aqueous solution. It is converted to uracil and acetone when exposed in aqueous solution to shortwave UV radiation.

Other ketones that are known to add to pyrimidine bases include acetophenone (Charlier and Helene, 1972) and benzophenone (von Wilucki *et al.*, 1967). Under certain conditions, thymine and uracil exhibits photochemical properties of ketones and form oxetanes (X, XI, XII). For example, when irradiated ($\lambda = 254$ nm) in frozen aqueous solution, thymine and thymidine form adducts derived from oxetanes (Varghese and Wang, 1968; Varghese, 1970). Uracil and uridine also form similar adducts (Varghese, 1971a). Thioketones add to pyrimidine bases in an analogous manner. The photochemical addition of 4-thiouracil to cytosine and uracil (Bergstrom and Leonard, 1972) probably involves a thietane inter-mediate ($X = S$). The formation of cytosine-cytosine adduct (Varghese, 1971b) and cytosine-thymine adduct (Varghese and Patrick, 1969) in UV-irradiated calf thymus DNA is best explained through an azetidine ($X = NH$) intermediate.

X = O,S,NH

4. HYDROXY COMPOUNDS

When pyrimdine bases are irradiated in aqueous solution with
UV light, addition of water across the C_5-C_6 double bond is the
major reaction and the corresponding 5,6-dihydro-6-hydroxy derivative is the major product. According to earlier reports alcohols
add to pyrimidine bases photochemically giving rise to the corresponding 6-alkoxy-5,6-dihydro pyrimidine (Moore and Thompson, 1956).
However, results of recent studies show that the type of addition
product depends on the irradiation conditions. According to Shetlar
(1975a) XVI is a major product when 1,3-dimethyluracil (XIII; R =
CH_3) is irradiated (λ >260 nm) in ethanol (10^{-3} M), and XVII is
the major addition product when the irradiation (λ >290 nm) was
carried out in methanol in the presence of di-t-butylperoxide.
Another interesting photoreaction of XIII is the addition to
tetrahydrofuran to form adducts of the type XV (R = CH_3) (Shetlar,
personal communication). Leonov et al. (1973) have reported the
identification of a 2-propanol adduct corresponding to XVI from
1,3-dimethyluracil and 2-propanol. Concerning the mechanism of
formation of these adducts, most of the evidence suggests that free
radicals are the primary reactive species. It should be mentioned
that the formation of alcohol addition products similar to that of
XVI from thymine exposed to ionizing radiation has been reported
(Brown et al., 1968; Zarebska and Shugar, 1972).

The structures of radiolysis products of uracil (Smith and
Hays, 1968; Shragge et al., 1974) shown in Fig. 1 provide a model
for the possible types of free radical-initiated pyrimidine products.

The addition of hydroxy compounds to pyrimidine bases are of
particular significance for two reasons. First, Smith (1969) and
more recently Schott and Shetlar (1974) have shown that UV light

causes the addition of the hydroxy amino acids serine and tyrosine to uracil. Secondly, radiation induced addition of tyrosine to nucleic acids has been demonstrated (Yamamoto, 1973, 1975).

5. AMINO COMPOUNDS

In spite of its possible importance in the cross-linking of nucleic acids to protein, very few studies have been reported on the addition of amino acids to nucleic acid constituents. As mentioned in Section 3, one possible reaction is the formation of azetidine-type products. Another system where considerable effort has been made to characterize the products is that of propylamine and 1,3-dimethyluracil, XVII (Gorelic et al., 1972). A large number of products have been identified. Of particular interest are adducts XIX and XX, where the addition occurs at the C_5 carbon atom and both C-C and C-N addition occur. According to Gorelic et al. (1972), XX is also formed under conditions where the pyrimidine does not absorb (λ >297 nm). This suggests that photolysis of the amine is the primary reaction under these conditions, and addition of these radicals to the pyrimidine leads to the different products.

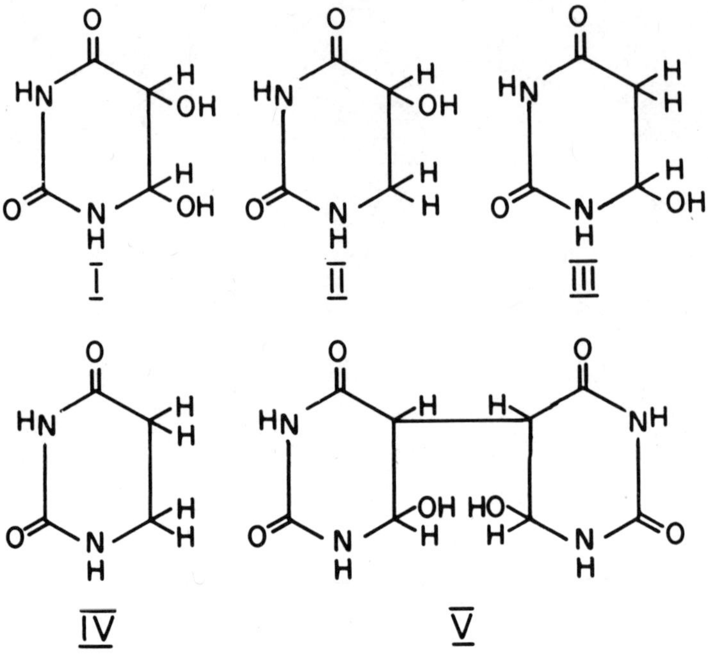

Fig. 1.   Radiolysis products of uracil.

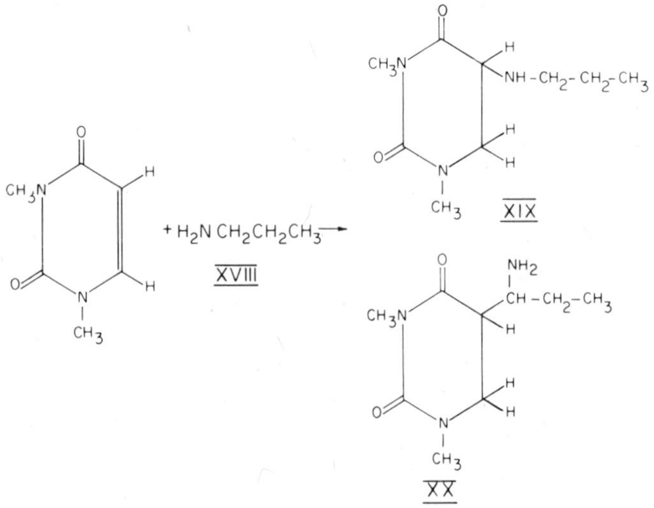

6.   SULFHYDRYL COMPOUNDS

In 1965, Rupp and Prusoff showed that cysteamine adds to iodouracil photochemically. Subsequently, Smith and Aplin (1966) demonstrated the addition of cysteine to uracil and isolated 5-S-cysteine-5,6-dihydrouracil (I in Fig. 2) as the major photoaddition product. Since then, the number of nucleic acid derivatives that add to sulfhydryl compounds have increased considerably (Table 1). Exposure to shortwave UV, longwave UV and to ionizing radiation lead to the addition of sulfhydryl compounds to nucleic acid constituents.

When uracil is irradiated in deaerated aqueous solution in the presence of cysteine, the yields of cyclobutane-type dimers and uracil photohydrates are considerably reduced (Jellinek and Johns, 1970). As shown by Smith and Aplin (1966), the addition of cysteine to uracil is the major reaction. About six products (Fig. 2) are present in the irradiated solution and the relative amounts of the individual products can be altered by changing the irradiation conditions (Varghese, 1974a).

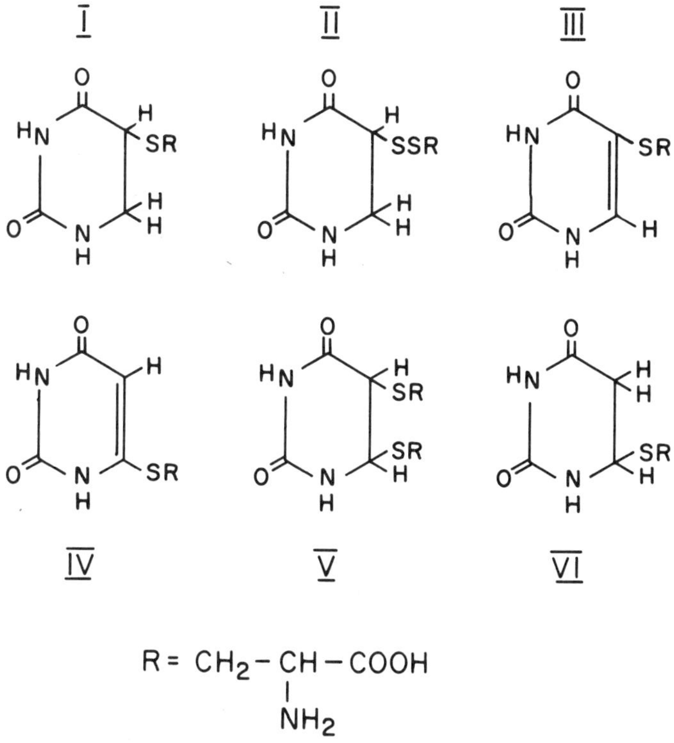

$$R = CH_2 - CH - COOH$$
$$|$$
$$NH_2$$

Fig. 2. Uracil-Cysteine Adducts.

Table 1.   Radiation-Induced Addition of Sulfhydryl Compounds to
           Nucleic Acid Derivatives.

Sulfhydryl Compound	Nucleic Acid Derivative	Sensitizer	Reference
A. Shortwave UV Radiation			
cysteamine	5-iodouracil		Rupp and Prusoff, 1965
cysteine	uracil		Smith and Aplin, 1966
			Jellinek and Johns, 1970
			Varghese, 1974a
			Fisher *et al.*, 1974
	thymine		Smith, 1970
			Varghese, 1973
			Fisher *et al.*, 1974
	polynucleotides		Smith and Meun, 1968
	RNA		
	DNA		
	cytosine		
	5-bromouracil		Varghese, 1974
	TpBrU		Haug, 1964
glutathione	uracil		Varghese, 1974b
	thymine		
	5-bromouracil		Varghese, 1974c
B. Longwave UV Radiation in the Presence of Sensitizers			
cysteine	uracil	acetone	Jellinek and Johns, 1970
		riboflavin	
	thymine	acetophenone	Varghese, 1973
glutathione	uracil	acetone	Varghese, 1974c
	thymine	acetophenone	
C. Gamma and X-Rays			
cysteine	RNA		Yamamoto, 1974, 1975
	uracil		Varghese, 1975b
	5-bromouracil		
	thymine		

The amounts of the various adducts under different irradiation
conditions (Table 2) provide valuable information on the mechanism.
The adducts I and II (Fig. 2) are formed in high yields when the
irradiation was carried out with light of wavelength >290 nm in
the presence of acetophenone (Varghese, 1974a). This suggests
that the uracil triplet-state is involved in the formation of I
and II. Adduct III is a major product when the irradiation
(λ = 254 nm) was carried out in aerated solution or in the presence

Table 2. Relative Distribution of Uracil-Cysteine Adducts Under
Different Irradiation Conditions.

Irradiation Conditions	Percentage Distribution*					% Ura Reacted	% Ura-Cys Adducts Formed
	I	II	III	IV	V		
In nitrogen λ >240 nm	25	45	10	4	16	32	75
In nitrogen; acetone added λ >290 nm	20	65	6	2	7	80	55
In air λ >240 nm	5	-	40	15	40	10	70

*See Fig. 2 for the structure of the products. (From Varghese 1974a)

of riboflavin with long wavelength (λ >290 nm) light. This suggests the involvement of free radical intermediates. One possibility
is that III is derived from V which is the primary product. This
mechanism is further supported by the fact that III is formed when
uracil is irradiated with X-rays in aqueous solution in the presence
of cysteine (Varghese, unpublished data).

    Adducts I and II (Fig. 2) are fairly stable to heat and acid,
and unstable in alkali. They are photoreversible; III and IV are
stable under these conditions, V and VI are the least stable.
These differences in properties indicate that no single test or
procedure is suitable for their detection in biological systems.

    The photoreactions of thymine in the presence of cysteine
have also been extensively studied (Smith, 1970; Varghese, 1973;
Fisher *et al.*, 1974); and in general, are found to be similar to
those of uracil. One big difference was in the formation of addition products in which the methyl group was involved in the addition (see Section 7).

7. ADDITION PRODUCTS SPECIFIC FOR INDIVIDUAL BASES

    In addition to the general reactions discussed above, which
involve addition at the C_5 or C_6 positions, individual pyrimidine
bases may undergo specific additions. For example, addition to
the methyl carbon of thymine is an important reaction. Addition

of another thymine molecule to thymine to form XXI occurs under
certain conditions (Varghese, 1970). Cysteine forms addition products of the type XXII and XXIII (Varghese, 1973). It is to be

emphasized that the γ-irradiation of thymine in the presence of
cysteine in aqueous solution produces XXIII (Varghese, 1975b).
Structure analysis of XXIII by X-ray crystalography indicate that
the formation of XXIII could cause considerable distortion in the
DNA by newly formed hydrogen bonds between the amino acid residue
and the adjacent base (Berman *et al.*, 1975).

5-Hydroxymethyl-cytosine is another base which undergoes
specific alteration. Recently we have isolated an addition product
analogous to XXIII from 5-hydroxymethylcytosine and cysteine.

Irradiation of 5-bromouracil (XXIV) with γ-rays (Varghese,
1975b) or UV light (Varghese, 1974c) results in the formation of
addition products of the type XXV and XXVI. These products may
contribute to the enhanced extent of nucleic acid-protein cross-
links in cells substituted with 5-bromouracil (Smith, 1975).

8.   OTHER TYPES OF ADDITION PRODUCTS

This discussion was limited to systems where precise knowledge of the products was available. A large variety of compounds
are presently known to form radiation-induced addition products.
They are listed in Table 3. As can be seen, UV, visible and

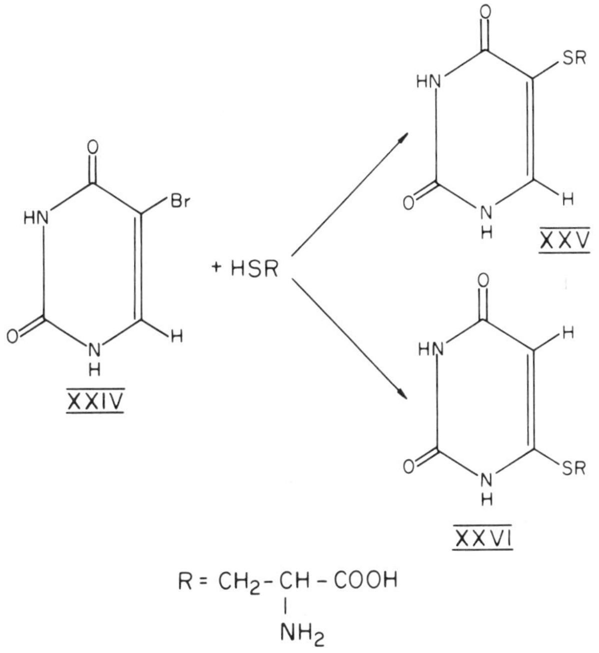

$R = CH_2-CH-COOH$
$|$
NH_2

ionizing radiations are effective in causing addition reactions.

9.   ADDITION PRODUCTS OF DNA

It has been questioned whether addition reactions of pyrimidine bases observed under *in vitro* conditions are of any relevance to nucleic acids in a cell since most of the *in vitro* reactions have been observed after very high doses of radiation. The answer is definitely in the affirmative. For example, about five thymine derived products have been isolated from DNA and bacterial cells irradiated with biological fluences of UV light (for a review, see Varghese, 1972). All these products have been isolated as well from thymidine under appropriate radiation conditions. Similarly, the identification of a cytosine-cytosine adduct from cytidine irradiated in frozen solution has led to its detection in UV-irradiated calf thymus DNA (Varghese, 1971). Another example is the identification of thymine-cysteine adducts from mammalian cells exposed to biological fluences of UV light (Varghese and Rauth, 1974).

As shown in Table 3, a large number of compounds add to nucleic acids. However, very little is known about the chemical nature of these adducts. Information from model systems could be of immense value in this respect. Finally, both nucleic and protein are made up of a large number of constituents and a clear knowledge of the

Table 3. Miscellaneous Addition Reactions

Compound	Nucleic Acid Derivative	Reference
A. Shortwave UV Radiation		
glycine	uracil	Smith, 1969
serine		
phenylalanine		
cystine		
histidine		
tryptophan		
methionine		
arginine		
lysine		
tyrosine		
lysine	thymine	Schott and Shetlar, 1974
arginine		
cystine		
tyrosine	DNA, RNA	Smith and Meun, 1968
threonine		
serine		
methionine	RNA	
poly-L-lysine	1,3-dimethyluracil	Gorelic *et al.*, 1972
protein	phage T1 DNA	Bohne *et al.*, 1970
CH_3NH_2	uracil	Summers *et al.*, 1973
N_2H_4		
ethylene	uracil	Krajewska and Shugar, 197
	uridine	
50S ribosomal	rRNA	Gorelic, 1975
proteins		
DNA polymerase	DNA	Markovitz, 1972
	poly (dA-dT)	
RNA polymerase	$d(A-T)_n \cdot d(A-T)_n$	Strinste and Smith, 1974
albumin	DNA	Braun and Merrick, 1975
gene-5 protein	fd DNA	Anderson *et al.*, 1975
lac repressor	bromodeoxyuridine	
protein	substituted *lac* operator	Lin and Riggs, 1974
DNA-polymerase	BrdU-DNA	
RNA-polymerase		
poly lysine		
poly arginine		Weintraub, 1973
B. Longwave UV Radiation		
benzo(a)pyrene	DNA	Rapaport and Ts'o, 1966
	cytosine	Rice, 1964
	1-methylcytosine	Cavalieri and Calvin, 197

Table 3. (cont.)

benzophenone	1,3-dimethyluracil thymine	von Wilucki *et al.*, 1967
acetophenone		Charlier and Helene, 1972
acetone	cytosine, uracil	Varghese, 1975
furocoumarin	DNA	Musajo and Rodighiero, 1970
	pyrimidine bases	Musajo *et al.*, 1967
acrylonitrile		Helene and Brun, 1970

C. <u>Gamma and X-Rays</u>

phenylalanine	DNA	Byfield *et al.*, 1970
	RNA	Yamamato, 1973
tryptophan	RNA, DNA	
histidine	RNA	
albumin	pyrimidine bases	
N-ethylmaleimide	DNA	Johansen *et al.*, 1968
	thymine	Ward *et al.*, 1969
nitrofurans	DNA	Chapman *et al.*, 1973
nitroimidizoles	DNA	Willson *et al.*, 1975
triacetoneamine-N-oxyl	DNA	Brustad *et al.*, 1973
fluorescein	DNA	Andersson, 1969

types of possible products provides a handle to look into the chemical basis of nucleic acid-protein cross-links.

10. CONCLUSION

Pyrimidine bases are very reactive compounds and they form addition products with a variety of compounds under a wide variety of conditions. Our knowledge on the chemical nature of the products as well as on the mechanisms of formation is very limited. In those instances, where the identity of the products are known, very little is known about their properties. These aspects need special emphasis in future studies in this field. Another important aspect is the development of new mild procedures for the detection of these adducts in biological systems. Results of studies of model compounds suggest that these adducts are unstable to the acid hydrolysis procedures generally employed for the isolation of photoproducts of nucleic acid constituents from biological systems. Chemical identification of radiation-induced adducts could give valuable information on the arrangement of cell constituents inside a cell.

<u>Acknowledgements</u>. The author is indebted to H. E. Johns for his continued interest in this work. This work was supported by the National Cancer Institute and the Medical Research Council of Canada.

References

Anderson, E., Nakashima, Y., and Konigsberg, W., 1975, Photoinduced cross-linkage of gene-5 protein and bacteriophage fd DNA, *Nucleic Acid Res.* 2:361-371.

Andersson, L.O., 1969, Coupling of dyes to various macromolecules by gamma-irradiation, *Nature* 222:374-375.

Bergstrom, D.E., and Leonard, N.J., 1972, Photoreaction of 4-thio-uracil with cytosine. Relation to photoreactions in *Escherichia coli* transfer ribonucleic acids, *Biochemistry* 11:1-9.

Berman, H.M., Zacharias, D.E., Carrel, H.L., and Varghese, A.J., 1975, αS-cysteinyl-thymine: A model for radiation-induced cross-linking of deoxyribonucleic acid to protein, *Biochemistry* (submitted).

Bohne, L., Coquerelle, T., and Hagen, U., 1970, Radiation sensitivity of bacteriophage DNA. II. Breaks and cross-links after irradiation *in vivo*, *Int. J. Radiat. Biol.* 17:205-215.

Braun, A., and Merrick, B., 1975, Properties of the ultraviolet light-mediated binding of bovin serum albumin to DNA, *Photochem. Photobiol.* 21:243-247.

Brown, P.E., Calvin, M., and Newmark, J.F., 1968, Thymine addition to ethanol; Induction by gamma-irradiation, *Science* 151:68-70.

Brustad, T., Jones, W.B.G., and Wold, E., 1973, Reactions between nitroxyls and radiation-induced long lived DNA-transients, *Int. J. Radiat. Biol.* 24:33-43.

Byfield, J.E., Lee, Y.C., and Bennet, L.R., 1970, Bonding of small molecules to DNA following ionizing radiation, *Nature* 225:859-86

Cavalieri, E., and Calvin, M., 1971, Photochemical coupling of benzo-(a)pyrene with 1-methylcytosine; Photoenhancement of carcinogenicity, *Photochem. Photobiol.* 14:641-653.

Chapman, O.L., 1967, "Organic Photochemistry", Vol. 1, Marcel Dekker, New York.

Chapman, J.D., Greenstock, C.L., Reuvers, A.P., McDonald, E., and Dunlop, I., 1973, Radiation chemical studies with nitrofurazone as related to its mechanism of radiosensitization, *Radiat. Res.* 53:190-203.

Charlier, M., and Helene, C., 1972, Photochemical reactions of aromatic ketones with nucleic acids and their components. 1. Purine and pyrimidine bases and nucleosides, *Photochem. Photobiol.* 15:71-87.

Cysyk, R., and Prusoff, W.A., 1972, Alteration of U.V. sensitivity of thymidine kinase by allosteric regulators, normal substrates and IUdR, a metabolic analogue of TdR, *J. Biol. Chem.* 247:2522.

Fishbein, L., Flamm, W.G., and Falk, H.L., 1970, Chemical Mutagens, 98-141, Academic Press, New York.

Fisher, G.J., Varghese, A.J., and Johns, H.E., 1974, Ultraviolet-induced reactions of thymine and uracil in the presence of cysteine, *Photochem. Photobiol.* 20:109-120.

Fisher, G.J., and Johns, H.E., 1975, Pyrimidine dimers, *in* Photo-chemistry and Photobiology of Nucleic Acids" (S.Y. Wang, ed.), Academic Press, New York.

Gorelic, L., 1975, Photoinduced covalent linkage *in situ* of *Escherichia coli* 50s ribosomal proteins to rRNA, *Biochim. Biophys. Acta* 390:209-225.

Gorelic, L., Lisagor, P., and Yang, N. C., 1972, The photochemical reactions of 1,3-dimethyluracil with 1-aminopropane and poly-L-lysine, *Photochem. Photobiol.* 16:465-480.

Haug, A., 1964, Influence of cysteine on the photochemical decom-position of thymidyl-(5'-3')-bromodeoxyuridine, *Biochim. Biophys. Acta* 173:435-437.

Helene, C. and Brun, F., 1970, Photochemical reactions of pyrimidine derivatives with acrylonitrile in aqueous solutions, *Photochem. Photobiol.* 11:77-84.

Jellinek, T. and Johns, R. B., 1970, The mechanism of photochemical addition of cysteine to uracil and formation of dihydrouracil, *Photochem. Photobiol.* 11:349-359.

Johansen, I., Ward, J. F., Siegel, K., and Sletten, A., 1968, X-ray induced binding of N-ethylmaleimide to DNA in aqueous solution, *Biochem. Biophys. Res. Commun.* 33:949-953.

Krajewska, E., and Shugar, D., 1971, Photochemical transformation of 5-alkyl-uracils and their nucleosides, *Science* 173:435-437.

Leonov, D., Salomon, J., Sasson, S., and Elad, D., 1973, Ultra-violet- and α-ray-induced reactions of nucleic acid constituents with alcohols on the selectivity of these reactions for purines, *Photochem. Photobiol.* 17:465-468.

Lin, S. Y., and Riggs, A. D., 1974, Photochemical attachment of *lac* repressor to bromodeoxyuridine-substituted *lac* operator by ultraviolet radiation, *Proc. Nat. Acad. Sci.*, USA, 71:947-951

Markovitz, A., 1972, Ultraviolet light-induced stable complexes of DNA and DNA polymerase, *Biochim. Biophys. Acta* 281:522-528.

Moore, A. M. and Thomson, C. H., 1957, Ultraviolet irradiation of pyrimidine derivatives. I. 1,3-dimethyluracil, *Can. J. Chem.* 35:163-169.

Musajo, L., Bordin, F., Caporale, G., Marciani, S., and Rigatti, G., 1967, Photoreactions of 3655 Å between pyrimidine bases and skin-photosensitizing furocoumarins, *Photochem. Photobiol.* 6:711-719.

Musajo, L. and Rodighiero, G., 1970, Studies on the photo-cyclo-addition reactions between skin photosensitizing furocoumarins and nucleic acids, *Photochem. Photobiol.* 11:27-35.

Musajo, L. and Rodighiero, G., 1972, Mode of photosensitizing action of furocoumarins, *Photophysiology* 7:115-147.

Rapaport, S. A. and Ts'o, P.O.P., 1966, Interaction of nucleic acids. III. Chemical linkage of the carcinogen 3,4-benzpyrene to DNA induced by X-ray irradiation, *Proc. Nat. Acad. Sci.* USA 55: 381-387.

Rice, J. M., 1964, Photochemical addition of benzo(a)pyrene to py-rimidine derivatives, *J. Amer. Chem. Soc.* 86:1444-1446.

Rupp, W.D., and Prusoff, W.H., 1965, Photochemistry of iodouracil. Effects of sulfur compounds, ethanol and oxygen, *Biochem. Biophys. Res. Commun.* 18:158-164.

Schott, N., and Shetlar, M. D., 1974, Photochemical addition of amino acids to thymine, *Biochem. Biophys. Res. Commun.* 59: 1112-1116.

Shetlar, M. D., 1975, Photoreactions and free radical induced reactions of 1,3-dimethyluracil in methanol and other alcohols, *Photochem. Photobiol.* (submitted).

Shetlar, M. D., Schott, H. N., Martinson, H. G., and Lin, E. T., 1975, Formation of thymine-lysine adducts in irradiated DNA-lysine systems, *Biochem. Biophys. Res. Commun.* (submitted).

Shragge, P. C., Varghese, A. J., Hunt, J. W., and Greenstock, C. L., Radiolysis of uracil in the absence of oxygen, *Radiat. Res.* 60:250-267.

Smith, K. C., 1969, Photochemical addition of amino acids to ^{14}C-uracil, *Biochem. Biophys. Res. Commun.* 34:354-357.

Smith, K. C., 1970, A mixed photoproduct of thymine and cysteine; 5-S-cysteine, 6-hydrothymine, *Biochem. Biophys. Res. Commun.* 39:1011-1016.

Smith, K. C., 1975, Radiation-induced addition of proteins and other molecules to nucleic acids *in* Photochemistry and Photobiology of Nucleic Acids (S.Y. Wang, ed.) Academic Press, New York.

Smith, K. C. and Aplin, R. T., 1966, A mixed photoproduct of uracil and cysteine (5-S-cysteine-6-hydrouracil). A possible model for the *in vivo* cross-linking of deoxyribonucleic acid and protein by ultraviolet light, *Biochemistry* 5:2125-2130.

Smith, K. C. and Meun, D.H.C., 1968, Kinetics of the photochemical addition of [^{35}S]cysteine to polynucleotides and nucleic acids, *Biochemistry* 7:1033-1037.

Stein, M. T., Berman, H. M. and Varghese, A. J., 1975, The crystal structure of a uracil-acetone photoaddition product, *Biochim. Biophys. Acta* (in press).

Strniste, G. F., and Smith, D. A. 1974, Induction of stable linkage between the deoxyribonucleic acid dependent ribonucleic acid polymerase and d(A-T)$_n$. d(A-T)$_n$ by ultraviolet light, *Biochemistry* 13:485-493.

Summers, Jr., W. A., Enwall, C., Burr, J. G., and Letsinger, R. L., 1973, The photoaddition of nucleophiles to uracil, *Photochem. Photobiol.* 17:295-301.

Varghese, A. J., 1970, 5-Thyminyl-5,6-dihydrothymine from DNA irradiated with ultraviolet light, *Biochem. Biophys. Res. Comm.* 38:484-490.

Varghese, A. J., 1971a, Photochemistry of uracil and uridine, *Biochemistry* 10:4283-4290.

Varghese, A. J., 1971b, Photochemistry of cytosine nucleosides in frozen aqueous solution and in DNA, *Biochemistry* 10:2194-2199.

Varghese, A. J., 1972, Photochemistry of nucleic acid and its components, *Photophysiology* 7:207-274.

Varghese, A. J., 1973, Properties of photoaddition products of
    thymine and cysteine, *Biochemistry* 14:2725-2730.
Varghese, A. J., 1974a, Photoaddition products of uracil and
    cysteine, *Biochim. Biophys. Acta* 374:109-114.
Varghese, A. J., 1974b, Photochemical addition of glutathione to
    uracil and thymine, *Photochem. Photobiol.* 20:339-343.
Varghese, A. J., 1974c, Photoreactions of 5-bromouracil in the pre-
    sence of cysteine and glutathione, *Photochem. Photobiol.* 20:
    461-464.
Varghese, A. J., 1975a, Photocycloaddition of acetone to uracil and
    cytosine, *Photochem. Photobiol.* 21:147-151.
Varghese, A. J., 1975b, Ionizing radiation induced addition of cy-
    steine to thymine, uracil and 5-bromouracil, *Biochem. Biophys.
    Res. Commun.* (submitted).
Varghese, A. J., and Patrick, M. H., 1969, Cytosine derived hetero-
    adduct formation in ultraviolet-irradiated DNA, *Nature* 223:
    299-300.
Varghese, A. J., and Rauth, A. M., 1974, Evidence for the addition
    of sulfhydryl compounds to thymine in UV-irradiated mammalian
    cells, American Society for Photobiology Abstr., p. 65.
Varghese, A. J., and Wang, S. Y., 1968, Thymine-thymine adduct as
    a photoproduct of thymine, *Science* 160:186-187.
Ward, J. F., Johansen, I., and Aasen, J., 1969, Radiosensitization
    by N-ethylmaleimide - a model chemical system, *Int. J. Radiat.
    Biol.* 15:163-170.
Weintraub, H., 1973, The assembly of newly replicated DNA into
    chromatin, Cold Spring Harbor Symp. Quant. Biol. 38:247-256.
Willson, R. L., Cramp, W. A., and Ings, R.M.J., 1974, Metronidazole
    ('Flagyl') Mechanisms of radiosensitization, *Int. J. Radiat.
    Biol.* 26:557-569.
von Wilucki, I., Mätthaus, H., and Krauch, C. H., 1967, Photosensi-
    bilisiente cyclodimerisation von thymin in Lösung, *Photochem.
    Photobiol.* 6:497-500.
Yamamoto, O., 1973, Radiation-induced binding of nucleic acid con-
    stituents with protein constituents and each other, *Int. J.
    Radiat. Phys. Chem.* 5:213-229.
Yamamoto, O., 1975, Radiation-induced binding of some protein and
    nucleic acid constituents with macromolecular components in
    cell systems, *Radiat. Res.* 61:261-273.
Zarebska, Z., and Shugar, D., 1972, Radio-products of thymine in
    the presence of ethanol, *Int. J. Radiat. Biol.* 21:101-114.

Addendum

X-ray crystallographic studies of uracil-acetone adduct (Stein
et al., 1975) show that the formation of oxetane-type products
could cause more distortion in the DNA helix than that produced by
the formation of cyclobutane-type pyrimidine dimers.

ADDITION OF AMINO ACIDS AND RELATED SUBSTANCES TO NUCLEIC ACIDS BY

NUCLEOPHILIC CATALYSIS

Robert Shapiro

Department of Chemistry, New York University

New York, New York 10003

1. INTRODUCTION

Little attention has been paid to nucleophilic reactants when considering the biologically important transformations of nucleic acids. The role of free radical processes in the radiation chemistry and photochemistry of nucleic acids is well appreciated (Smith, 1975). In the case of chemical carcinogenesis, it has been suggested that the ultimate carcinogens are often, or perhaps

225

always, strong electrophilic reagents (Miller, 1970; Heidelberger, This Volume). Nucleic acids, do, however, contain a number of sites susceptible to nucleophilic attack, and there is no obvious reason why alterations at these positions should be of less significance then changes produced at other locations by other mechanisms. In fact, nucleophilic reactions on nucleic acid are involved in a number of biologically important processes.

This review will cover the most significant type of nucleophilic nucleic acid alteration: saturation of the 5-6 double bond of cytosine, followed by displacement of its amino group. This process has been shown to cause cross-linking of proteins and nucleic acids, and to be involved in mutagenesis. Reagents of this type have been valuable in studying the structure and function of nucleic acids. Nucleophilic reagents have not yet been implicated as carcinogens. However, in model studies at the oligonucleotide level, they have been shown to induce conformational transitions similar to those produced by the electrophilic carcinogen, N-acetoxy-acetylaminofluorene (Nelson *et al.*, 1971).

2. CHEMISTRY OF THE REACTIONS

2.1. General Scheme

In its most general form, the reaction involves nucleophilic attack at two distinct sites on the cytosine ring: C-4 and C-6. A single reagent, or two different nucleophilic species, may be involved. The transformations are summarized in Fig. 1. The initial step involves attack at C-6 of cytosine (I) by the *addition reagent*, HX, to give a dihydrocytosine (II). This intermediate is in equilibrium with the starting material. This reaction is fastest in acidic solution, and primarily involves cytosine cation, rather than the free base. The next step is displacement of the cytosine amino group by a *substitution reagent*. If this reagent is an amine, hydroxylamine, or hydrazine, transamination to III takes place. In the absence of such a reagent, deamination of II by water occurs, giving the dihydrouracil, V. The last step involves the reversible loss of the addition reagent from III, to give the substituted cytosine, VI, or from V, to give the uracil, IV.

2.2. Dihydrocytosine Transformations

In the simplest form of the reaction, the starting material is a dihydrocytosine. It was observed by Janion and Shugar (1967) that dihydrocytosine, dihydrocytidine, and reduced oligocytidylic acid reacted with glycine to give a product of type III, Fig. 1 (X=R=H, R=CH$_2$CO$_2$H). Similar reactions were observed with dihydrocytosine

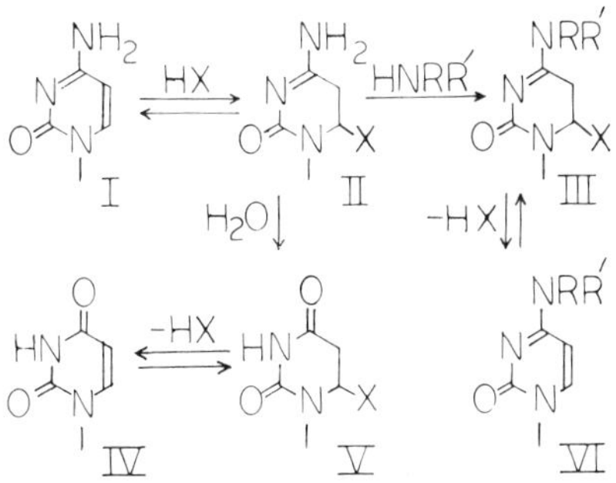

Fig. 1. General scheme for deamination and transamination of cytosine derivatives by nucleophilic catalysis. HX represents the addition reagent. The substitution reagent HNRR' may be an amine, hydroxylamine, or hydrazine.

and several other amino acids and dipeptides, methylamine, and semicarbazide. In the absence of a suitable amine, dihydrocytosine derivatives are hydrolyzed by water to give dihydrouracil V (Brown and Hewlins, 1968; Shapiro *et al.*, 1974).

The photohydrate of cytidine, 5,6-dihydro-6-hydroxycytidine (II, X=OH) exhibits similar reactivity. With hydroxylamine and its O-methyl derivative, cytidine photohydrate gives III (X=OH, R=H, R'=OH or OCH3) (Small and Gordon, 1968; Simukova *et al.*, 1975). The ready deamination of cytidine photohydrate to 5,6-dihydro-6-hydroxyuridine has also been studied (Johns *et al.*, 1965).

2.3. Catalysis by Addition Reagents

In the more general form of the reaction, the starting material is a derivative of cytosine, and the various steps in Fig. 1 take place concurrently. Although a number of nucleophiles can function as the addition reagent, sodium bisulfite and hydroxylamine (and its O-methyl derivative) are especially effective and have come into wide use.

2.3.1. *Sodium Bisulfite*. The reaction scheme involved in bisulfite-catalyzed deamination and transamination is given in Fig. 2 (Shapiro *et al.*, 1970; Hayatsu *et al.*, 1970a, b). The initial step involves addition of sulfite to protonated cytosine to give 2. Deamination proceeds most rapidly between pH 5 and 6, and the actual deamination step 2→3 (Fig. 2) is catalyzed by

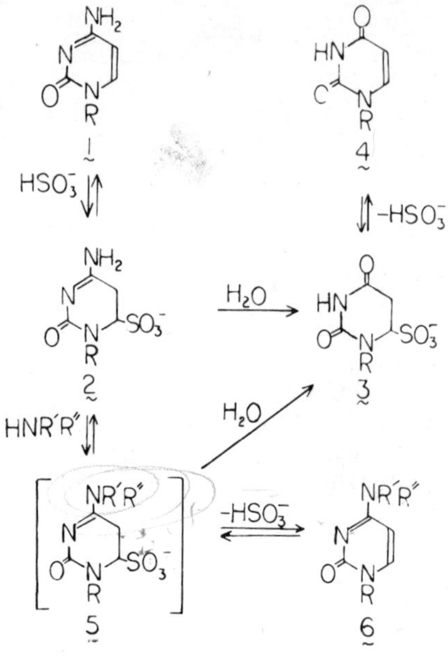

Fig. 2. Reactions of bisulfite with cytosine derivatives
(From Shapiro and Weisgras, 1970).

bisulfite (Sono *et al.*, 1973; Shapiro *et al.*, 1974). This reaction
has found use as a synthetic tool with nucleoside analogs and oligo-
nucleotides (Hayatsu, 1975).

At neutral pH, in the presence of a suitable amine, transamination predominates over deamination; the product is an N^4-substituted
cytosine (Shapiro and Weisgras, 1970). Products of structure 6
(Fig. 2) have been obtained from cytosine or cytidine and the
following amines: methylamine, dimethylamine, pyrrolidine, glycine,
aniline, *o*-aminophenol, β-naphthylamine (Shapiro and Weisgras,
1970), and glycylglycine (Boni and Budowsky, 1973). As bisulfite
catalyzes the deamination step, the extent of deamination under
these conditions can be limited by restricting the bisulfite concentration to 0.2 M (Boni and Budowsky, 1973).

When O-methylhydroxylamine is used as the substitution reagent,
in combination with bisulfite as the addition reagent, the final
product is 5, which is unusually stable to elimination of bisulfite
(Budowsky *et al.*, 1972a; Verdlov *et al.*, 1974). The application
of this reaction to the determination of the base composition and
sequence of oligodeoxynucleotides has been proposed (Sverdlov *et
al.*, 1972a, b).

2.3.2. *Hydroxylamine Derivatives*. Sodium bisulfite is active
as an addition reagent, but not as a substitution reagent, which
allows its use in transamination reactions with other amines.
Hydroxylamine and its O-methyl derivative are active in both addition and substitution. Their reactions with cytosine are illustrated in Fig. 3. The only case in which another nucleophile
competes with hydroxylamine for substitution at C-4 is the protein-
nucleic acid cross-linking reaction (see Section 3.1.2).

The mechanisms of the reactions in Fig. 3 have been the subject
of intensive investigation. For a complete account of these studies,
consult the following works and the references cited therein:
Phillips and Brown (1967), Lawley (1967), Brown and Hewlins (1968),
Budowsky *et al.* (1971), Budowsky *et al.* (1972b). The principal
features of the reaction are the following: The optimal pH is
about 6 for hydroxylamine and 5 for O-methylhydroxylamine. The
initial product of addition (II, Fig. 3) is unstable and the final
products of the reaction are the N^4-substituted cytosine (IV, Fig.
3) and the bis-adduct (III, Fig. 3). The proportion of the two
products depends on the reaction conditions. The N^4-substituted
cytosine is formed primarily through the addition-elimination route,
but also directly from cytosine (I→IV, Fig. 3), in a slower reaction. In the case of 5-substituted cytosines, addition products
are not observed, and the direct formation of the N^4-substituted
cytosine from cytosine is believed to be the principal pathway.

In the reaction of N-methylhydroxylamine with cytosine derivatives, no addition products are observed, and the principal product

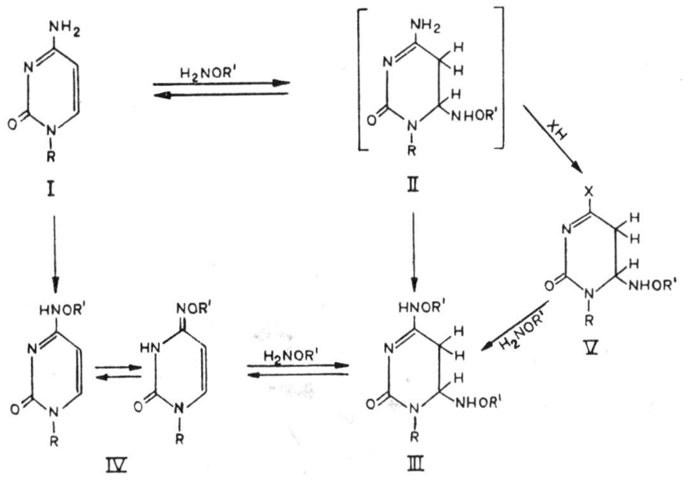

Fig. 3. Reactions of hydroxylamine and O-methylhydroxylamine
with cytosine derivatives (From Budowsky *et al.*, 1972b).

is the N^4-hydroxy-N^4-methylcytosine. No reaction is observed between N-methylhydroxylamine and a 5-substituted cytosine derivative (Janion and Shugar, 1971).

2.3.3. *Hydrazine Derivatives*. N-methylhydrazine, hydrazine, N,N'-dimethylhydrazine (Lingens and Schneider-Bernlöhr, 1966), semicarbazide (Hayatsu and Ukita, 1964; Hayatsu, Takeishi, and Ukita, 1966), Girard-P reagent ("acetohydrazide pyridinium chloride," $NH_2NHCOCH_2C_5H_5N^+Cl^-$) (Kikugawa *et al.*, 1967), acetylhydrazide, and other acylhydrazines (Gal-Or *et al.*, 1967) have been shown to react with cytosine derivatives to give the product of direct substitution at C-4. For example, the reaction of cytosine derivatives with semicarbazide proceeds as illustrated in Fig. 4. Although intermediate addition products have not been observed in these reactions, no evidence has been reported to exclude the formation of these intermediates in low concentration. Such a reaction course is probable, by analogy of these reactions with the hydroxylamine reaction. In fact, under more vigorous conditions, the reaction of hydrazine with cytosine proceeds with ring cleavage to give 3-aminopyrazole (Baron and Brown, 1955; Temperli *et al.*, 1964; Lingens and Schneider-Bernlöhr, 1966; Hayes and Baron, 1967). A plausible pathway for this cleavage is attack by hydrazine at C-6 of cytosine, followed by intramolecular substitution by the other amino group of the hydrazine molecule at C-4. Hydrazinolysis of DNA to give apyrimidinic acid tracts has been considered as a possible aid to the sequencing of DNA (Cashmore and Petersen, 1969; Havelaar and de Waard, 1973).

2.3.4. *Other Nucleophiles*. In principal, almost any nucleophile can act as the addition reagent in the scheme in Fig. 1. In most cases, the equilibrium for addition is poor. Intermediates corresponding to II, III, and IV, Fig. 1, are seldom detected, but their existence can be inferred by kinetic studies. Thus, Shapiro and Klein (1966) demonstrated that deamination of cytosine derivatives was catalyzed at pH 4 by carboxylate buffers such as acetate,

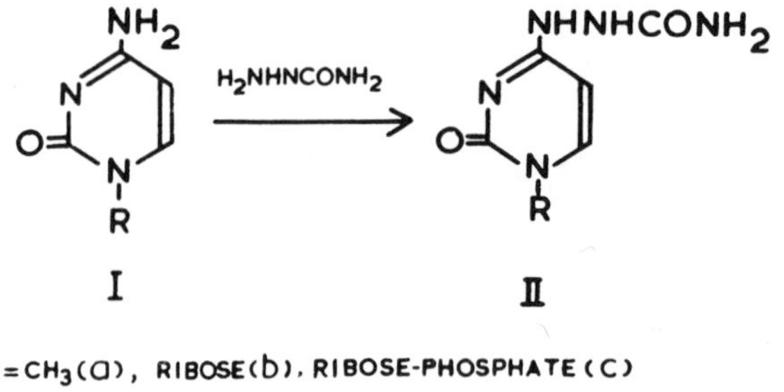

R=CH₃(a), RIBOSE(b), RIBOSE-PHOSPHATE (c)

Fig. 4. Reaction of semicarbazide with cytosine derivatives (From Hayatsu and Ukita, 1964).

formate, oxalate, lactate, citrate and mercaptoacetate, and by
pyridine. When aromatic amine buffers, such as aniline, o-hydroxy-
aniline, or β-naphthylamine were used at pH 4, transamination as
well as deamination took place (Shapiro and Klein, 1967). Further
studies on the mechanism of the deamination reaction confirmed the
addition-elimination route, and demonstrated the effectiveness of
additional buffers such as phosphate and carbonate (Notari, 1967;
Notari *et al.*, 1970; Wechter and Kelly, 1970; Garrett and Tsau,
1972).

3. APPLICATIONS

3.1. Cross-Linking of Proteins and Nucleic Acids

3.1.1. *Bisulfite Catalysis.* The prediction that bisulfite
could catalyze the cross-linking of proteins and nucleic acids was
made at the time of the discovery of the bisulfite-catalyzed transamination of glycine and cytosine (Shapiro and Weisgras, 1970).
Subsequently, Boni and Budowsky (1973) prepared the transamination
products of glycylylycine with cytidine and cytidine-5'-phosphate.
They demonstrated that concentrated bisulfite, pH 7.4, was capable
of causing the covalent binding of cytidine to poly-L-lysine. The
bound cytidine was released on treatment by 0-methylhydroxylamine.

In further studies, MS2 phage was treated with 1 M bisulfite
at pH 7 (Turchinsky *et al.*, 1974). Following the modification,
the phage protein was treated with N-[^{14}C]acetoxysuccinimide to
introduce a radioactive label, and the phage RNA was separated
from protein either by phenol treatment or gel filtration. Between
1 and 2% of the protein remained with the RNA fraction during this
treatment. After pancreatic ribonuclease treatment of the RNA, the
presence of both coat and maturation proteins in the RNA fraction
was demonstrated by gel electrophoresis. When the bisulfite treatment was conducted at a more acidic pH, the amount of protein bound
to RNA reached a peak within an hour, and then declined. This
result was attributed to deamination of the initially formed transamination products (6 →5 →3, Fig. 2). The loss of the cross-links
was not observed at pH 7.4, as deamination is slow at that pH. In
more recent work (Turchinsky *et al.*, 1975), the isolation of ε-N-
(2-ketopyrimidyl-4)-lysine, after severe hydrolysis of the modified
phage, has been reported. This substance is the expected product
of transamination of cytosine in RNA with the amino group of a
lysine side chain of a phage protein.

3.1.2. *0-Methylhydroxylamine Catalysis.* An extensive series
of experiments have demonstrated the cross-linking of DNA and
protein in Sd phage treated with 0-methylhydroxylamine (Andronikova
et al., 1974; Tikchonenko *et al.*, 1971, 1973). Upon treatment of

this phage with 1 M O-methylhydroxylamine, pH 5.1, three reversible decreases in the viscosity of the phage DNA were observed successively, after approximately 5 min, 1 h, and 3 h. Phage DNA, isolated after a 3 h modification period, differed from unmodified DNA in its bouyant density (cesium sulfate gradient). When phage with ^{35}S-labeled protein was used, this label was found in the DNA fraction. Electron microscopy indicated that globular material was attached to the DNA. A minimum in the infectivity of the phage and in the extent of injection of the phage DNA into bacteria, was also found after 3 h of modification. After longer modification periods, the physical properties described above returned to normal, and a portion of the infectivity was restored. More limited experiments were also performed on other bacteriophage. Waves of reversible inactivation were observed on modification of phage T7 with O-methylhydroxylamine, but the extent of inactivation was less than that observed with Sd phage (Andronikova et al., 1974).

The above transformations have been interpreted in terms of the chemistry illustrated in Fig. 3. Although double helical DNA is inert to O-methylhydroxylamine (see Section 3.2), 20% of the cytosines of Sd phage DNA reacted readily. It was suggested that these bases were in an unusual conformation, complexed intimately with phage protein. In this complex, C-6 of cytosine was readily available for reaction, but C-4 was shielded by protein. After reaction at C-6, transamination of the intermediate (II, Fig. 3) with a nearby protein amino group afforded a transient cross-link (V, Fig. 3). Upon longer treatment with O-methylhydroxylamine, this bond was broken. The bis-adduct (III, Fig. 3) was produced as the sole final product of the reaction.

3.1.3. *UV Catalysis.* UV light was also found to cross-link Sd phage, as measured by changes in DNA viscosity and bouyant density, and the persistent attachment of ^{35}S-labeled protein to DNA. In this case the amount of DNA-bound protein increased with the extent of irradiation, with no reversibility (Simukova and Budowsky, 1974). Cross-linking was also observed on UV irradiation of RNA phage MS2. A number of photochemical causes can lead to protein-nucleic acid cross-linking, but recent degradate studies have implicated a nucleophilic process in the case of MS2. Strong acidic hydrolysis of this irradiated phage led to the isolation of the same transamination product of cytosine with lysine that was encountered in the bisulfite-induced cross-linking of this phage (Simukova et al., 1975).

3.1.4. *Summary.* A unified scheme which relates the three cross-linking processes described above is illustrated in Fig. 5. A cytosine, within a phage nucleic acid, is shown in close association with a free protein nucleophile, presumably a lysine amino group. Saturation of the 5-6 double bond by addition of bisulfite or O-methylhydroxylamine, or by photohydration, leads to the

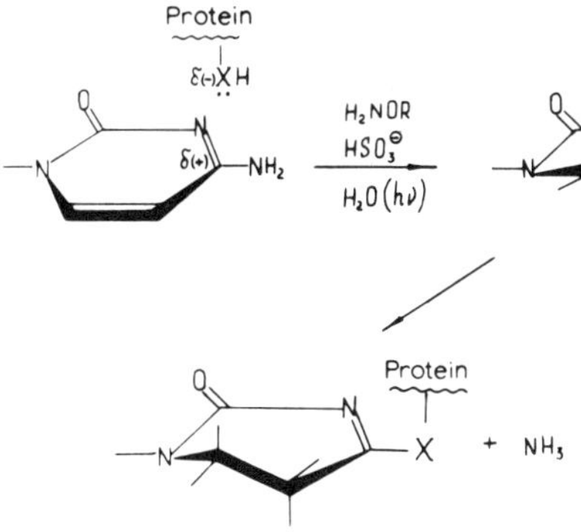

Fig. 5. Cross-linking of proteins and nucleic acids by nucleophilic displacement of the cytosine amino group (From Simukova and
Budowsky, 1974).

formation of a reactive dihydrocytosine (the 6-substituent is not
shown in Fig. 5). This intermediate reacts with the nearby amine
to give the cross-linked dihydrocytosine intermediate. In the
case of bisulfite modification (at pH 7.4) or UV irradiation, the
cross-link is stabilized by elimination of bisulfite or water. In
the O-methylhydroxyl case, the cross-link is eventually opened up
under the influence of excess reagent.

3.2. Study of the Structure and Function of Nucleic Acids

Both the deamination and transamination reactions of bisulfite,
and the addition of O-methylhydroxylamine, show a strong conformational preference (Shapiro *et al.*, 1972; Shapiro *et al.*, 1973;
Cashmore *et al.*, 1971; Tikchonenko *et al.*, 1971). Cytosines in
single-stranded nucleic acids react hundreds of times faster than
those in double helical areas. For this reason, bisulfite and O-
methylhydroxylamine have been widely employed in studies on the
secondary structure of various tRNA species. As bisulfite deamination converts cytosine to another normal RNA component, uracil,
this reagent has been a valuable aid to studies of the function of
tRNA. For a summary of the applications of bisulfite to tRNA, see
Hayatsu (1975), Schulman and Her (1973), and Schulman (1974). A
typical secondary structure study, using transamination with
$^{14}CH_3NH_2$, is illustrated in Fig. 6 (Schulman *et al.*, 1974). For
applications of O-methylhydroxylamine to tRNA, see Chang and Ish-
Horowitz (1974), Robertus *et al.* (1974), and the earlier references
cited in these articles. The conformations of phage f2 RNA
(Filipowicz *et al.*, 1972) and of the DNA within intact Sd phage,
have also been explored with the aid of O-methylhydroxylamine
(Tikchenenko *et al.*, 1971).

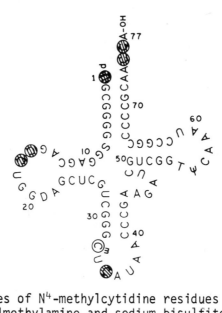

Fig. 6. Sites of N⁴-methylcytidine residues in tRNAfMet treated with [¹⁴C]methylamine and sodium bisulfite. ⊗ indicates heavily modified residues, ⊘ indicates residues modified to an intermediate extent, and Ⓒ indicates residues which have only undergone limited reaction (From Schulman *et al.*, 1974).

3.3. Mutagenesis

The very nature of the change involved in the deamination of cytosine to uracil by bisulfite made this reagent an obvious candidate for mutagenic studies. It was predicted, in advance of any genetic data, that bisulfite would be a mutagen (Shapiro *et al.*, 1970). This prediction has been confirmed in five systems: the phages λ (Hayatsu and Miura, 1970) T2 (Summers and Drake, 1971), and φX174 (Linney *et al.*, 1972), *E. coli* (Mukai *et al.*, 1970), and yeast (Dorange and Dupuy, 1972). The specificity of mutagenesis was tested in *E. coli* and phage T4, and the observed GC→AT transitions were exactly in accord with chemical expectations. The mutagenic effects of bisulfite are attributed to uracil formation; the intermediate uracil adduct (3 in Fig. 2) appears to be inactive in biochemical systems (Shapiro and Braverman, 1972; Kai *et al.*, 1974). The biological properties of the dihydrocytosine intermediate (2 in Fig. 2) are uncertain; it may be too unstable to be of biological significance.

It has been suggested that the same general route, but with carboxylate catalysis instead of bisulfite catalysis, is responsible for transition mutations observed on heating phage T4 in acidic buffers (Shapiro and Klein, 1966).

The mutagenic properties of hydroxylamine and its O-methyl derivative have been recognized for considerably longer than those of bisulfite. A large amount of literature on the subject has accumulated. The reader interested in the full details should consult Freese (1971), Fishbein *et al.* (1970), Drake (1970), Phillips and Brown (1967), and the additional references cited in the following summary: In studies with transforming DNA, T-even phages, and certain other viruses, hydroxylamine and its O-methyl derivative exhibit GC→AT specificity. The N^4-hydroxy (or methoxy) cytosine product is a cause of mutagenesis (Flavell *et al.*, 1974; Budowsky *et al.*, 1972; Banks *et al.*, 1971). This product can exist in two tautomeric forms, as shown in IV, Fig. 3. The rightmost (oxime) tautomer is predominant (Brown *et al.*, 1968; Sverdlov *et al.*, 1971). In this form, the product has the hydrogen-bonding properties of thymine, and pairs with adenine, leading to a mutation. There is fairly general agreement that formation of the bis-adduct (III, Fig. 3) is inactivating. Opinion is divided upon the properties of the dihydrocytosine intermediate (II, Fig. 3), with some workers feeling that its existence is too transient to be of great significance (Budowsky *et al.*, 1972; Fraenkel-Conrat and Singer, 1972) and others supporting an important role in mutagenesis for this intermediate (Banks *et al.*, 1971; Phillips and Brown, 1967).

At any event, the mutagenic specificity of hydroxylamine is not observed in phage φ80, bacteria, and in a number of other unicellular and higher organisms. These effects have been ascribed to free radical reactions (Freese, 1971) rather than the nucleophilic transformations described in this article.

3.4. Carcinogenesis

The critical target attacked by chemicals in the initiation of the carcinogenic process has not yet been conclusively identified. Electrophilic substitution has, however, been advocated as the unifying mechanism of attack by the ultimate carcinogens (Miller, 1970; Heidelberger, This Volume). One of the best developed models of chemical carcinogenesis has been the "base displacement model" of Weinstein, Grunberger, and their co-workers (Levine *et al.*, 1974). It is proposed that an acetylaminofluorene residue, after attachment by electrophilic substitution to the 8-position of guanine, stacks with the neighboring bases in a DNA or RNA chain. In doing so, it displaces the guanine from its normal position in the helix. One of the more compelling studies that support this mechanism has been circular dichroism measurements on oligonucleotides modified by N-2-acetylaminofluorene (Nelson *et al.*, 1971).

In our laboratory, we have shown that an analogous effect can be produced as the result of a nucleophilic substitution mechanism. β-Naphthylamine is a potent bladder carcinogen whose ultimate reactive metabolite has not been established. The product of transamination of cytosine with β-naphthylamine (N^4-β-naphthylcytidine, abbreviated CNap below) is shown in Fig. 7. We have prepared, using bisulfite catalysis, a number of diribonucleoside monophosphates modified with β-naphthylamine (Shapiro and Brown, unpublished). The modified compounds GpCNap and ApCNap exhibited dramatic alterations in their circular dichroism spectra, when compared to the unmodified compounds. These changes resemble those observed in the acetylaminofluorine series. A base displacement effect may be operative in these cases. No such dramatic effects were observed with the phenyl-substituted analogs of the above compounds, nor with other β-naphthyl-modified diribonucleoside monophosphates, including CNappG and CNappA. We conclude that it is the specific geometry in an altered compound that determines whether base displacement takes place. The mechanism of attachment of the aromatic residue is irrelevant. Similar conclusions may well apply to the initiation of carcinogenesis on a nucleic acid target.

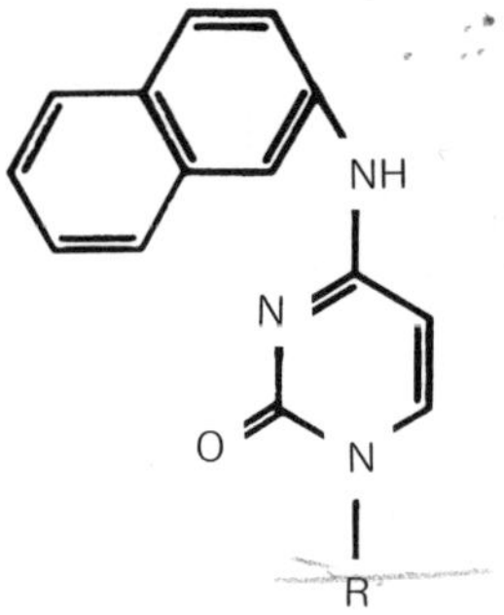

Fig. 7. The product of transamination of β-naphthylamine with a cytosine derivative (From Shapiro and Klein, 1967).

4. CONCLUSIONS AND DIRECTIONS FOR FUTURE RESEARCH

It is striking that many of the biological effects attributed to radiation, such as mutations and cross-linking of proteins and nucleic acids, can also be produced by nucleophilic reagents. In the production of energy, nucleophilic reagents and radiation may be released into the environment. Sulfur dioxide (the gaseous form of bisulfite) is an air pollutant primarily produced by burning fossil fuels in conventional power plants; radiation maybe released from nuclear power plants.

In order to make intelligent decisions as to which method of energy production is more ecologically acceptable, we will need a much better understanding of the biological effects of sulfur dioxide. Considerable data has accumulated on the long range adverse effects of this pollutant on the health of human beings, animals, and plants (U.S. Department of Health, Education, and Welfare, 1969). No biochemical mechanisms for these effects have as yet been established. Cross-linking of proteins and nucleic acids is certainly one plausible mechanism. A particularly vulnerable site would appear to be chromosomes, where DNA exists in intimate association with lysine-rich histones. A number of strongly suggestive observations have already been reported that support this idea. Cultures of human lymphocytes treated with sulfur dioxide show chromosomal abnormalities, lowered levels of DNA synthesis and reduced mitotic indices (Schneider and Calkins, 1970). Similar observations have been made in pollen tube cultures of *Tradescantia poludosa* (Ma *et al.*, 1973), the root meristem of *Vicia faba* (Brandle and Erismann, 1973), and in *Chlorella pyrenoidosa* (Das and Runeckles, 1974). Further exploration of these effects would certainly seem in order. A direct analysis for protein-DNA cross-links would be very desirable.

It seems unlikely that the list of nucleophilic reagents with potent reactivity for nucleic acids will end with those described in this article. It is possible that a search for additional reagents would lead to the discovery of as yet unsuspected new classes of mutagens, carcinogens, and other toxic agents. The prediction that carcinogens are electrophilic reagents may have been self-fulfilling, in that it discouraged the testing of nucleophilic reagents. I hope that future experiments will clarify the uncertainty in this area, and give us a clearer understanding of the importance of these processes in aging, carcinogenesis and radiation biology.

Acknowledgment. The author holds a Career Development Award from the National Institutes of General Medical Sciences, N.I.H.

References

Andronikova, M.L., Velikodvorskaya, G.A., Tkhruni, F., and Tikhonenko, T.O., 1974, Biological effects associated with the modification of intraphage DNA with O-methylhydroxylamine, *Molecular Biology* 8:3-11.

Banks, G.R., Brown, D.M., Streeter, D.G., and Grossman, L., 1971, Mutagenic analogues of cytosine: RNA polymerase template and substrate studies, *J. Mol. Biol.* 60:425-439.

Baron, F., and Brown, D.M., 1955, Nucleotides. XXXIII. The structure of cytidylic acids a and b, *J. Chem. Soc.* 1955: 2855-2860.

Boni, I.V., and Budowsky, E.I., 1973, Transformation of non-
    covalent interactions in nucleoproteins into covalent bonds
    induced by nucleophilic reagents. I. The preparation and
    properties of the products of bisulfite ion-catalyzed reac-
    tion of amino acids and peptides with cytosine derivatives,
    J. Biochem. (Tokyo) 73:821-830.
Brandle, R., and Erismann, K.M., 1973, Bee influssung der DNS-
    Synthese durch sulfit im wurzelmeristem der puffbohne
    (vicia faba), *Experienta* 29:586-587.
Brown, D.M., and Hewlins, M.J.E., 1968a, The reaction between
    hydroxylamine and cytosine derivatives, *J. Chem. Soc. (C)* 1968:
    1922-1924.
Brown, D.M., and Hewlins, M.J.E., 1968b, Dihydrocytosine and
    related compounds, *J. Chem. Soc. (C)* 1968:2050-2055.
Brown, D.M., Hewlins, M.J.E., and Schell, P., 1968, The tautomeric
    state of N(4)-hydroxy- and of N(4)-amino-cytosine derivatives,
    J. Chem. Soc. (C) 1968:1925-1929.
Budowsky, E.I., Sverdlov, E.D., Shibaeva, R.P., Monastyrskaya, G.S.,
    and Kochetkov, N.K., 1971, Mechanism of the mutagenic action
    of hydroxylamine. III. Reaction of hydroxylamine and O-
    methylhydroxylamine with the cytosine nucleus, *Biochim. Biophys.*
    Acta 246:300-319.
Budowsky, E.I., Sverdlov, E.D., and Monastyrskaya, G., 1972a, New
    method of selective and rapid modification of the cytidine
    residues, *FEBS Lett.* 25:201-204.
Budowsky, E.I., Sverdlov, E.D., and Spasokukotskaya, T.N., 1972b,
    Mechanism of the mutagenic action of hydroxylamine. VII.
    Functional activity and specificity of cytidine triphosphate
    modified with hydroxylamine and O-methylhydroxylamine,
    Biochim. Biophys. Acta 287:195-210.
Cashmore, A.R., Brown, D.M., and Smith, J.D., 1971, Selective
    reaction of methoxyamine with cytosine bases in transfer
    ribonucleic acid, *J. Mol. Biol.* 59:359-371.
Cashmore, A.R., and Petersen, G.B., 1969, The degradation of DNA
    by hydrazine: a critical study of the suitability of the
    reaction for the quantitative determination of purine nucleo-
    tide sequences, *Biochim. Biophys. Acta* 174:591-603.
Chu, B.F.C., Brown, D.M., and Burdon, M.G., 1973, Effect of nitrogen
    and of catalase on hydroxylamine and hydrazine mutagenesis,
    Mutat. Res. 20:265-270.
Das, G., and Runeckles, V.C., 1974, Effects of bisulfite on meta-
    bolic development in synchronous chlorella pyrenoidosa,
    Environ. Res. 7:473-483.
Dorange, J.-L., and Dupuy, P., 1972, Mise en evidence d'une action
    mutagene du sulfite de sodium sur la levure, *C.R. Acad. Sci.*
    Paris, Ser. D. 274:2798-2800.
Drake, J.W., 1970, "The Molecular Basis of Mutation," Holden-Day,
    San Francisco.
Filipowicz, W., Wodnar, A., Zagorska, L., and Szafranski, P., 1972,
    f2 RNA structure and peptide chain initiation: fMet-tRNA

binding directed by methoxyamine-modified unfolded or native-like f2 RNA's, *Biochim. Biophys. Res. Commun.* 49:1272-1279.

Fishbein, L., Flamm, W.G., and Falk, H.L., 1970, "Chemical Mutagens, Environmental Effects on Biological Systems," Academic Press, New York.

Flavell, R.A., Sako, D.L., Bandle, E.F., and Weissman, C., 1974, Site-directed mutagenesis: generation of an extracistronic mutation in bacteriophage Qβ RNA, *J. Mol. Biol.* 89:255-272.

Fraenkel-Conrat, H., and Singer, B., 1972, The chemical basis for the mutagenicity of hydroxylamine and methoxyamine, *Biochim. Biophys. Acta* 262:264-268.

Freese, A., 1971, Molecular mechanisms of mutations, *in* "Chemical Mutagens, Principles and Methods for Their Detection," (A. Hollaender, ed.), Vol. 1, pp. 1-56, Plenum Press, New York.

Gal-Or, L., Mellema, J.E., Moudrianakis, N., and Beer, M., 1967, Electron microscopy study of base sequence in nucleic acids. VII. Cytosine-specific addition of acyl hydrazides, *Biochemistry* 6:1909-1915.

Garrett, E.R., and Tsau, J., 1972, Solvolyses of cytosine and cytidine, *J. Pharm. Sci.* 61:1052-1060.

Havelaar, K.J., and de Waard, A., 1973, Isolation of purine oligo-nucleotides after hydrazinolysis of deoxyribonucleic acid, *Rec. Trav. Chim. Pays-Bas* 92:132-144.

Hayatsu, H., 1975, Bisulfite modification of nucleic acids and their constituents, *Progr. Nucleic Acid Res. Mol. Biol.* 16 (in press).

Hayatsu, H., and Miura, M., 1970, The mutagenic action of sodium bisulfite, *Biochem. Biophys. Res. Commun.* 39:156-160.

Hayatsu, H., Takeisha, K.-I., and Ukita, T., 1966, The modification of nucleosides and nucleotides. III. A selective modification of cytidine with semicarbazide, *Biochim. Biophys. Acta* 123:445-457.

Hayatsu, H., and Ukita, T., 1964, Selective modification of cytidine residue in ribonucleic acid by semicarbazide, *Biochem. Biophys. Res. Commun.* 14:198-203.

Hayatsu, H., Wataya, Y., and Kai, K., 1970a, The addition of sodium bisulfite to uracil and to cytosine, *J. Amer. Chem. Soc.* 92:724-726.

Hayatsu, H., Wataya, Y., Kai, K., and Iida, S., 1970b, Reaction of sodium bisulfite with uracil, cytosine, and their derivatives, *Biochemistry* 9:2858-2865.

Hayes, D.H., and Baron, F.H., 1967, Hydrazinolysis of some purines and pyrimidines and their related nucleosides and nucleotides, *J. Chem. Soc. (C)* 1967:1528-1533.

Janion, C., and Shugar, D., 1967, Reaction of amines with dihydro-cytosine analogs and formation of amino acid and peptidyl derivatives of dihydropyrimidines, *Acta Biochim. Polon.* 14:293-302.

Janion, C., and Shugar, D., 1971, Chemical mutagenesis: reaction of N-methylhydroxylamine with cytosine analogues, *Acta*

Biochim. Polon. 18:403-418.

Johns, H.E., LeBlanc, J.C., and Freeman, K.B., 1965, Reversal and deamination rates of the main ultraviolet photoproduct of cytidylic acid, *J. Mol. Biol.* 13:849-861.

Kai, K., Tsuruo, T., and Hayatsu, H., 1974, The effect of bisulfite modification on the template activity of DNA for DNA polymerase I, *Nucleic Acids Res.* 1:889-899.

Kikugawa, K., Hayatsu, H., and Utika, T., 1967, Modification of nucleosides and nucleotides. V. A selective modification of cytidylic acids with Girard-P reagent, *Biochim. Biophys. Acta* 134:221-231.

Lawley, P.D., 1967, Reaction of hydroxylamine at high concentration with deoxycytidine or with polycytidylic acid: evidence that substitution of amino groups in cytosine residues by hydroxylamine is a primary reaction, and the possible relevance to hydroxylamine mutagenesis, *J. Mol. Biol.* 24:75-81.

Levine, A.F., Fink, L.M., Weinstein, I.B., and Grunberger, D., 1974, Effect of N-2-acetylaminofluorene modification on the conformation of nucleic acids, *Cancer Res.* 34:319-327.

Lingens, F., and Schneider-Bernlöhr, H., 1966, Uber die unsetzung naturlich vorkommender pyrimidinbasen mith hydrazin und methylsubstituierten hydrazinen, *Justus Liebigs Ann. Chem.* 686:134-144.

Linney, E.A., Hayashi, M.N., and Hayashi, M., 1972, Gene A of ϕX174. I. Isolation and identification of its products, *Virology* 50:381-387.

Ma, T.-H., Isbandi, D., Khan, S.H., and Tseng, Y.-S., 1973, Low level of SO_2 enhanced and chromatid aberrations in tradescantia pollen tubes and seasonal variation of the aberration rates, *Mutat. Res.* 21:93-100.

Miller, J.A., 1970, Carcinogenesis by chemicals: an overview, *Cancer Res.* 30:559-575.

Mukai, F., Hawryluk, I., and Shapiro, R., 1970, The mutagenic specificity of sodium bisulfite, *Biochem. Biophys. Res. Commun.* 39:983-988.

Nelson, J.H., Grunberger, D., Cantor, C.R., and Weinstein, I.B., 1971, Modification of ribonucleic acid by chemical carcinogens. IV. Circular dichroism and proton magnetic resonance studies of oligonucleotides modified with N-2-acetylaminofluorene, *J. Mol. Biol.* 62:331-346.

Notari, R.E., 1967, A mechanism for the hydrolytic deamination of cytosine arabinoside in aqueous buffer, *J. Pharm. Sci.* 56:804-809.

Notari, R.E., Chin, M.L., and Cardoni, A., 1970, Intermolecular and intramolecular catalysis in deamination of cytosine nucleosides, *J. Pharm. Sci.* 59:28-32.

Phillips, J.H., and Brown, D.M., 1967, The mutagenic action of hydroxylamine, *Progr. Nucleic Acid Res. Mol. Biol.* 7:349-367.

Robertus, J.D., Ladner, J.E., Finch, J.T., Rhodes, D., Brown, R.S., Clark, B.F.C., and Klug, A., 1974, Correlation between three-dimensional structure and chemical reactivity of transfer RNA, *Nucleic Acids Res.* 1:927-932.

Schneider, L.K., and Calkins, C.A., 1970, Sulfur-dioxide-induced lymphocyte defects in human peripheral blood cultures, *Environ. Res.* 3:473-483.

Schulman, L.H., and Her, M.O., 1973, Reaction of altered *E. coli* formylmethionine transfer RNA by bacterial T factor, *Biochem. Biophys. Res. Commun.* 51:275-283.

Schulman, L.H., Shapiro, R., Law, D.C.F., and Louis, J.B., 1974, A simplified method for study of RNA conformation-reaction of formylmethionine transfer RNA with [^{14}C]methylamine-bisulfite, *Nucleic Acids Res.* 1:1305-1316.

Shapiro, R., and Braverman, B., 1972, Modification of polyuridylic acid by bisulfite: effect on double helix formation and coding properties, *Biochem. Biophys. Res. Commun.* 47:554-550.

Shapiro, R., Braverman, B., Louis, J.B., and Servis, R.E., 1973, Nucleic acid reactivity and conformation. II. Reaction of cytosine and uracil with sodium bisulfite, *J. Biol. Chem.* 248:4060-4064.

Shapiro, R., DiFate, V., and Welcher, M., 1974, Deamination of cytosine derivatives by bisulfite. Mechanism of the reaction, *J. Amer. Chem. Soc.* 96:906-912.

Shapiro, R., and Klein, R.S., 1966, The deamination of cytidine and cytosine by acidic buffer solutions. Mutagenic implications, *Biochemistry* 6:2358-2362.

Shapiro, R., and Klein, R.S., 1967, Reactions of cytosine derivatives with acidic buffer solutions. II. Studies on trans-amination, deamination, and deuterium exchange, *Biochemistry* 7:3576-3582.

Shapiro, R., Law, D.C.F., and Weisgras, J.M., 1972, A new chemical probe for single-stranded RNA, *Biochem. Biophys. Res. Commun.* 49:358-366.

Shapiro, R., Servis, R.E., and Welcher, M., 1970, Reactions of uracil and cytosine derivatives with sodium bisulfite. A specific deamination method, *J. Amer. Chem. Soc.* 92:422-424.

Shapiro, R., and Weisgras, J.M., 1970, Bisulfite-catalyzed trans-amination of cytosine and cytidine, *Biochem. Biophys. Res. Commun.* 40:839-843.

Simukova, N.A., and Budowsky, E.I., 1974, Conversion of non-covalent interactions in nucleoproteins into covalent bonds: UV-induced formation of polynucleotide-protein crosslinks in bacteriophage Sd virions, *FEBS Lett.* 38:299-303.

Simukova, N.A., Turchinsky, M.F., Boni, I.V., Skoblov, Yu. M., and Budowsky, E.I., 1975, UV-induced cytosine involved poly-nucleotide-protein cross-linking. Abstr. Int. Symp. "Protein and Other Adducts to DNA: Their Significance to Aging, Carcinogenesis and Radiation Biology," Williamsburg, Virginia, May 2-6, 1975.

Smith, K.C., 1975, The radiation-induced addition of protein and other molecules to nucleic acids, *in* "Photochemistry and

Photobiology of Nucleic Acids" (S.Y. Wang, ed.), Academic Press, New York (in press).

Small, G.D., and Gordon, M.P., 1968, Reaction of hydroxylamine and methoxyamine with the ultraviolet-induced hydrate of cytidine, *J. Mol. Biol.* 34:281-291.

Sono, M., Wataya, W., and Hayatsu, H., 1973, Role of bisulfite in the deamination and the hydrogen isotype exchange of cytidylic acid, *J. Amer. Chem. Soc.* 95:4745-4749.

Summers, G., and Drake, J.W., 1971, Bisulfite mutagenesis in bacteriophage T4, *Genetics* 68:603-607.

Sverdlov, E.D., Krapivko, A.P., and Budowsky, E.I., 1971, Tautomeric equilibrium of 1-β-D-ribofuranosyl-2-keto-4-(N-methoxyamino) pyrimidine, *Khim. Geterotsikl. Soedin* 9:1264-1267.

Sverdlov, E.D., Monastyrskaya, G.S., and Budowsky, E.I., 1972a, Determination of the number of cytidine residues in oligo-nucleotides, *FEBS Lett.* 28:236-238.

Sverdlov, E.D., Monastryrskaya, G.S., Budowsky, E.I., and Grachev, M.A., 1972b, A novel approach to structural analysis of oligo-nucleotides, *FEBS Lett.* 28:231-235.

Temperli, A., Turler, H., Rust, P., Danon, A., and Chargaff, E., 1964, Studies in the nucleotide arrangement in deoxyribonucleic acid. IX. Selective degradation of pyrimidine deoxyribonu-cleotides, *Biochim. Biophys. Acta* 91:462-476.

Tikchonenko, T.I., Budowsky, E.I., Sklyadneva, V.B., and Khromov, I.S., 1971, The secondary structure of bacteriophage DNA in situ. III. Reaction of S_d phage with O-methylhydroxylamine *J. Mol. Biol.* 55:535-547.

Tikchonenko, T.I., Kisseleva, N.P., Zintshenko, A.I., Ulanov, B.P., and Budowsky, E.I., 1973, Peculiarities of the secondary structure of bacteriophage DNA in situ. IV. Covalent cross-links between DNA and protein that arise in the reaction of S_d phage with O-methylhydroxylamine, *J. Mol. Biol.* 73:109-119.

Turchinsky, M.F., Boni, I.V., and Budowsky, E.I., 1975, Bisulfite-induced cytosine involved polynucleotide-protein crosslinking. Abstr. Int. Symp. "Protein and Other Adducts to DNA: Their Significance to Aging, Carcinogenesis and Radiation Biology," Williamsburg, Virginia, May 2-6, 1975.

Turchinsky, M.F., Kusova, K.S., and Budowsky, E.I., 1974, Conver-sion of non-covalent interactions in nucleoproteins into covalent bonds: bisulfite-induced formation of polynucleo-tide-protein crosslinks in MS2 bacteriophage virions, *FEBS Lett.* 38:304-307.

Verdlov, E.D., Monastyrskaya, G.S., Guskova, L.I., Levitan, T.L., Sheichenko, V.I., and Budowsky, E.I., 1974, Modification of cytidine residues with a bisulfite-O-methylhydroxylamine mixture, *Biochim. Biophys. Acta* 340:153-165.

U.S. Department of Health, Education, and Welfare, 1969, "Air Quality Criteria for Sulfur Oxides," National Air Pollution Control Administration Publication No. AP-50, Washington, D.C.

Wechter, W.J., and Kelly, R.C., 1970, The mechanism of the deamina-tion of cytidine, *Collect Czech. Chem. Commun.* 35:1991-2002.

PHOTOCHEMICALLY-INDUCED ADDUCTS OF DNA

Dov Elad

Department of Organic Chemistry

The Weizmann Institute of Science, Rehovot, Israel

1. INTRODUCTION

Amongst the most important detrimental effects of light on living systems are mutations, aging, and carcinogenesis. In order to study these effects of light on man it is necessary to focus attention upon the effect of UV light on the genetic material, namely, DNA. It is of particularly great importance to identify the chemical make up of the photoinduced lesions in the genetic material and elucidate their origin and mechanism of formation.

Until recently photobiology has been primarily concerned with the photochemistry of pure DNA. The DNA in a cell, however, is surrounded by proteins, lipids, carbohydrates, and low molecular weight precursors. It is not unlikely that the cellular environment of the nucleic acid plays a most important role in the determination

of the types and relative yields of photoproducts formed in nucleic
acids. Indeed, many compounds have been shown to readily combine
covalently with DNA or its constituents when irradiated *in vitro*
or *in vivo* (Smith, 1975). In these photoinduced reactions we can
distinguish between two real possibilities: (a) the excited species
are primarily produced in DNA and proceed to interact with substrates in the surrounding environment; or (b) the reactive species
are generated in the environment with DNA moieties serving as substrates or scavengers. Indeed, both these possibilities do occur.
In fact, the heterocyclic bases in DNA at times serve as the light
absorbing system, while under other conditions these moieties play
the role of scavengers for the reactive species. In both these
roles, however, pyrimidines and purines undergo hetero-adduct formation. This involves in the pyrimidine case the addition of the
reactant across the 5,6-double bond in uracil or thymine, as well
as substitution at the C-5 methyl group of thymine. With purines
from nucleic acids, hetero-addition involves mainly reactions at
the C-8 position of the purine nucleus, resulting in the substitution of the appropriate entity for the hydrogen atom at this position

The multiplicity of products formed in irradiated DNA com-
plicates the chemical identification of products, and further inter-
fers with the correlation between a given photoproduct and the accompanying biological effect. The induction of selective photochemical modification in one of the constituents of the nucleic
acid can serve as a most powerful tool for the study of this correlation. Photosensitization, mainly with ketonic compounds, has
been used for the selective production of pyrimidine dimers in DNA.
Ketonic sensitizers, such as acetone and acetophenone, are known to
participate in energy transfer processes; thus, the use of these
reagents should lead eventually to excited purines and pyrimidines
as the active species. On the other hand, peroxidic photoinitiation,
which is also employed for the production of selective modifications
in nucleic acids, produces free radicals as the active agents.
Consequently, different photoproducts might be expected to be formed
in reactions initiated by these differing modes. Thus, photosensitization and selective photoinitiation can be applicable to the
selective production of a variety of hetero-adduct to DNA, with the
proviso that the appropriate photosensitizer, chemical reagent and
wavelength of light are employed. Such an approach aids in elucidating the effect that cellular environment as a whole or its individual components in particular have upon the type and ratio of
photoproducts produced in DNA, and in discerning the contributing
chemical elements of the various biological effects.

2. PHOTOHYDRATION OF PYRIMIDINES

It has been demonstrated that UV light irradiation of uracil
or its derivatives in aqueous solution leads to the formation of

photohydrates and photodimers, the former resulting from the addition of a water molecule across the 5,6-double bond (Varghese, 1972; Sinsheimer and Hasting, 1949). Similarly, uridine photohydrates are produced in irradiated polynucleotides and in nucleic acids, e.g., TMV-RNA (Small *et al.*, 1968) where, in solvents of low ionic strength, the inactivation by UV light is assumed to be mainly due to pyrimidine hydrate formation. Lomant and Fresco (1972) have recently reviewed the aspects of UV photochemistry that can probe the polyribonucleotide conformation.

$$\text{uracil} + H_2O \xrightarrow{h\nu} \text{6-hydroxy-5,6-dihydrouracil}$$

Among the typical features of uracil photohydrates is the spontaneous loss of water and the reversion to the parent compound. This reversal proceeds rapidly on heating, and its rate is faster in acidic solution. These properties of heat and acid reversibility are generally used to follow the rate of formation, as well as the reversal, of pyrimidine photohydrate. Another interesting property of pyrimidine hydrates is the easy exchangeability of the C-5 hydrogen for deuterium or tritium (Chambers, 1968; Grossman and Rogers, 1968; Wechter and Smith, 1968).

The photohydration reaction of uracil and its derivatives must involve an excited singlet state precursor, since it is not quenched by oxygen (Greenstock *et al.*, 1967) and cannot be photosensitized by triplet sensitizers (Brown and Johns, 1968). Burr *et al.*, (1968) suggested that the precursor is a protonated singlet; however, it has been shown recently (Burr *et al.*, 1972) that the neutral excited species reacts faster with water than anionic or cationic species. It follows, therefore, that some energetic species other than the conventional singlet is the precursor to the pyrimidine hydrate.

Cytosine and its derivatives form photohydrates similar to those of uracil. This addition of water across the 5,6-double bond proceeds in high yields (De Boer *et al.*, 1970; Grossman and Rogers, 1968; Setlow and Carrier, 1963; Shugar and Wierzchowski, 1957). In addition, these photohydrates, like those of uracil, reversibly lose the elements of water and undergo C-5 hydrogen exchange.

Cadet and Teoule (1971) have shown that both *cis* and *trans* isomers of thymine hydrate (6-hydroxy-5,6-dihydrothymine) are produced when thymine in aqueous solution is exposed to γ-radiation, while Fisher and Johns (1973) have demonstrated the formation of the *cis* thymine hydrate upon UV irradiation. The yield of the

thymine hydrate is three orders of magnitude smaller than for uracil.
There is no direct evidence which indicates that hydrates are formed
on UV irradiation in aqueous solution of other thymine-containing
systems. However, the detection of deoxyribosylurea as a photo-
reduction product of thymine with NaBH$_4$ (Kondo and Witkop, 1968)
suggests the formation of 6-hydroxy-5,6dihydrothymine as a product
of thymidine irradiated in aqueous solution. Though there is no
conclusive evidence for the formation of thymine photohydrates in
DNA, there is, however, indications that they are formed and undergo
dehydration (Varghese, 1972).

3.   PHOTOCHEMICAL REACTIONS OF PYRIMIDINES WITH ALCOHOLS

As compared to the photohydration reactions, considerably
less research has been carried out on the photochemical reactions
of uracil and its derivatives with alcohols. Two types of photoadducts have been reported. Wang (1961) showed that irradiation
of a methanolic solution of uracil led to the addition of the alcohol across the 5,6-double bond of uracil resulting in an ether
type adduct: an ether type adduct was also obtained upon photolysis of an ethanolic solution of uracil.

In addition to the ether type photoadducts, alcohol type products have also been discovered (Leonov et al., 1973). In particular, uracil, uridine, and uridine-3'-phosphate react with 2-propanol
across their 5,6-double bond to give the corresponding 5,6-dihydro-
6-iso-propanol adduct.

These photoaddition reactions of alcohols to uracil can be
induced directly with UV light of λ>260 nm, photosensitized with
ketonic sensitizers, or photoinitiated with peroxides and light
of λ>290 nm. Only in the latter case is a single photoproduct,

i.e., the uracil-alcohol of the alcohol type, produced; otherwise, photodimers of uracil and dihydrouracil are also formed in considerable amounts (Leonov *et al.*, 1973). The ether type adducts are generally produced only in reactions which are induced directly by UV light. Shetlar (1975) has shown, however, that the formation of an ether type or an alcohol type photoadduct in the photolysis of 1,3-dimethyluracil (DMU)-ethanol mixtures depends on the concentration of DMU in the irradiated mixture.

The two types of photoadducts result from different chemically reactive species produced during irradiation. The ether type photoadducts result from the interaction of the alcohol molecule with an excited uracil molecule and proceeds via polar intermediates. The formation of the alcohol type adducts, on the other hand, involves the attack of the alcohol free radical $\dot{C}(R_1R_2)OH$ on uracil (Jellinek and Johns, 1970). The alcohol radical is generated through the interaction of the alcohol with either excited uracil, excited photosensitizer or oxy radicals, the latter resulting from the photofragmentation of the peroxide. Further study is still required to determine the optimal conditions for the production of one or the other of these two precursors and thereby of the resulting photoadducts.

In contrast to the uracil system, the photochemical reactions of thymine and thymine derivatives with alcohols has been less explored. In the reactions studied so far, substitution of an alcohol moiety for a hydrogen atom at the C-5 methyl group of thymine occurred (Leonov *et al.*, 1973). However, the generality of this reaction at the various molecular levels of thymine derivatives and

under the various reaction conditions has still to be proved. Indeed, γ-ray radiolysis of an ethanolic solution of thymine led to the addition of ethanol across the 5,6-double bond of thymine to produce an alcohol type adduct (Brown *et al.*, 1966). It is also noteworthy, that the acetone photosensitized or peroxide photoinitiated reactions of denatured DNA with 2-propanol resulted in the formation of a thymine-alcohol adduct with the alcohol moiety substituting for a hydrogen atom at the C-5 methyl group of the thymine moiety (Ben-Ishai *et al.*, 1973).

4. PHOTOCHEMICAL REACTIONS OF PURINES WITH ALCOHOLS

4.1. Photoadduct Formation

There is a dearth of information concerning the effect of radiation on purines and purine moieties in nucleic acids. A few UV light- and γ-ray-induced reactions of purines and purine moieties in nucleic acids have been described recently, and include reactions with alcohols, amines, and acetals (Leonov and Elad, 1974a; Salomon and Elad, 1973, 1974a; Stankunas *et al.*, 1971; Yang *et al.*, 1971; Evans and Wolfenden, 1970; Jerumanis and Martel, 1970; Connolly and Linschitz, 1968). These may be of importance in evaluating the effect of the environment on the type of photoproduct in DNA. However, due to the lack of sufficient chemical data, it is still too early to evaluate the biological importance of purine photochemical modification. A systematic study of the photochemical reactions of purines will supply the chemical data required for such an evaluation.

With the exception of purine itself, the photoreactions of purines and purine nucleosides with alcohols resulted in the substitution of the appropriate alcohol moiety for the hydrogen atom at the C-8 position of the purine system (Salomon and Elad, 1973; Steinmaus *et al.*, 1971).

The parent compound (i.e., purine itself), on the other hand is attacked at the C-6 position (Connolly and Linschitz, 1968; Yang *et al.*, 1971). This is consistent with order of reactivities of the various sites of purines towards alcohol free radicals, which has been shown to be C-6 > C-8 > C-2 (Steinmaus *et al.*, 1971).

These reactions can be induced directly with UV light ($\lambda > 260$ nm), which is absorbed by the purine, or indirectly, with light of longer wavelength ($\lambda > 290$ nm) through the use of ketonic photosensitizers or peroxidic photoinitiators. In the "direct" reaction the excited purine molecule abstracts a hydrogen atom from the alcohol to yield the alcohol free radical $\overset{\bullet}{C}(R_1R_2)OH$. The subsequent step involves the attack of an alcohol free radical on the carbon end of the C=N group of a ground state purine molecule, which eventually leads to product. In the sensitized reactions, the ketone absorbs most of the incident light. Two routes for the generation of alcohol free radicals may now operate. On one hand, the excitation energy may in turn be transferred to the purine, which initiates the reaction as described above. On the other hand, excited ketone may also abstract a hydrogen atom from the alcohol generating the alcohol free radical. In the peroxide-induced reaction most of the incident light ($\lambda>290$ nm) is absorbed by the peroxide. It is, therefore, suggested that the initiation occurs as a result of the splitting of the peroxide into oxy radicals, which in turn abstract a hydrogen atom from the alcohol, generating alcohol free radicals (Salomon and Elad, 1973).

Ben-Ishai *et al.*, (1973) have shown that similar reactions take place in the purine moieties of DNA when irradiated with UV light of $\lambda>260$ nm in the presence of 2-propanol or longer wavelengths ($\lambda>290$ nm), using acetone as a photosensitizer. The data indicate that irradiation of native DNA at 313 nm leads to a very limited production of purine photoproducts. Photoproducts could, however, be induced if, prior to exposure to UV light of 313 nm (a) DNA was heat or alkali denatured, (b) single-strand breaks were introduced into DNA by limited treatment with deoxyribonuclease or by irradiation at $\lambda>300$ nm, or (c) DNA exposed to direct UV irradiation. It is evident that denaturation as well as induction of single-strand breakage occurring in the photosensitized reactions may in fact be partially responsible for the greater production of purine photoproducts in the nucleic acid by sensitization than by direct UV irradiation.

It is noteworthy that adenine and guanine in DNA are photoalkylated to a similar extent; in this respect the photoalkylation reaction differs from alkylation by chemical agents, since the latter react preferentially with guanine at the N-7 position. The difference in site of attack is most probably due to the different mechanisms operating. In the photochemical reaction, alkylation proceeds through free radical intermediates, whereas the chemical alkylation proceeds through polar intermediates (Lawly, 1966).

In contrast to the purine moieties in DNA, the pyrimidine constituents, upon direct or indirect irradiation in alcoholic media, gave primarily the corresponding dimers. In the photosensitized reaction, the amount of pyrimidine dimers formed in the presence of 2-propanol is smaller significantly as compared to that produced in the absence of the alcohol (Steinmaus *et al.*, 1970; Ben-Ishai *et al.*, 1973). This gives some indication as to the effect environment of DNA has on the type and yields of the various photoproducts produced in the nucleic acid during irradiation. To account for the quenching of thymine dimer formation in the presence of 2-propanol, it is assumed that there is a competition for the excited acetone by the alcohol and the hetero-cyclic bases in DNA. Since the alcohol is present in excess as compared to DNA, a large amount of excited acetone might be converted to ketyl radicals $(CH_3)_2COH$, thus facilitating the hydroxyalkylation reaction of purines at the expense of thymine dimer formation. In denatured DNA a thymine-2-propanol adduct is produced in addition to the purine photoadducts and pyrim-

idine dimers. The former results from the interaction of a ketyl
radical and thymine radical (Ben-Ishai *et al.*, 1973).

The selective production of 8-α-hydroxy-*iso*-propyl-adenine and
-guanine in native DNA, without any formation of pyrimidine dimers,
has been reported recently (Salomon and Elad, 1974b). This was
achieved by irradiating the nucleic acid in the presence of 2-propano
with di-*tert.*-butyl peroxide [(t-BuO)$_2$] as a photoinitiator. The
presence of (t-BuO)$_2$ during irradiation enhanced the production of
chain breaks in DNA and it is assumed that these strand breaks
allowed for easier access of the alcohol free radicals to the purine
moieties.

4.2. Reversibility

The photoalkylation of purines with alcohols is a reversible
reaction and it has been shown (Salomon and Elad, 1974c) that irradiation of C-8-α-hydroxyalkyl purines and purine nucleosides in
the presence of photosensitizers, such as hydroquinone or N,N-
dimethylaniline, results in the dealkylation of the side-chain at
the 8-position, leading to the regeneration of the original purine.

These photosensitized reactions are induced by UV light of
λ>290 nm, which is absorbed by the photosensitizer. It has been
found that photosensitizers possessing high triplet energies, such
as acetophenone, fail to initiate the reactions, and that the reactions are quenched only partially by triplet quenchers. In
addition, photosensitizers possessing low triplet energies are extremely effective in these photoreversions. It was concluded,
therefore, that this restoration of the original purine does not
involve a transfer of triplet energy. It is likely that a negative
charge is transferred from the excited sensitizer to the 8-hydroxy-
alkylpurine and evidence for this charge-transfer step has recently
been presented (Salomon and Elad, 1974c).

This process can also be viewed as a photochemical repair of
lesions in the purine moieties of nucleic acids. It is noteworthy
that the photosensitized monomerization of pyrimidine photodimers,
which imitates the light-requiring step of the enzymic photoreactivation, also involves the transfer of an electron, however, in the
opposite direction (Sasson and Elad, 1972).

The observation that the mechanism of the regeneration of the original purine and that of the photosensitized monomerization of pyrimidine dimers both involve an electron transfer process, leads us to propose that there may exist a general photochemical mechanism for the repair of radiation-induced lesions of different chemical nature in the nucleic acid. This mechanism may involve a redox turnover in the chromophore responsible for the light absorption.

4.3. Selectivity

Since it has been found that purines and purine moieties in nucleic acids participate in photochemical reactions, the development of irradiation conditions under which one group of the nucleic acid bases would react selectively is of major importance. Leonov and Elad (1974b) have examined the selectivity in reactions of mixtures of pyrimidines and purines or their nucleosides with 2-propanol, employing light of $\lambda > 290$ nm and $(t\text{-}BuO)_2$ as a photoinitiator. In these reactions uracil and its derivatives yield 6-α-hydroxyalkyl-5,6-dihydrouracil, thymine undergoes substitution at the C-5 methyl group, while purines give the appropriate 8-α-hyroxyalkyl derivatives. Irradiation of mixtures of purines and pyrimidines led to the predominant formation of purine photoproducts. It has further been found that the qunatum yields for the formation of the pyrimidine-alcohol photoadducts were usually higher than those of the purine-alcohol photoproducts when each base is irradiated separately. This indicates that the selectivity of the photochemical reactions of 2-propanol for the purines results primarily from the suppression of the pyrimidine reactivity in the presence of the purines. It is assumed that this effect results from the association (stacking) of the heterocyclic bases.

5. PHOTOCHEMICAL REACTIONS OF PYRIMIDINES AND PURINES WITH AMINES

Nucleic acids in cells are frequently associated with basic proteins (histones) or amines (e.g. cadaverine and spermine). A study of the photochemistry of nucleic acid constituents in the presence of amines or basic amino acids might provide a clearer picture of the interaction of these substances under irradiation, the cross-links formed, and the molecular basis of the resultant biological effects. Gorelic *et al.*, (1972) have shown that irradiation of DMU and 1-aminopropane with UV light resulted in the formation of reduced DMU, DMU dimers, and adducts between DMU and 1-aminopropane. The latter results from the addition of 1-aminopropane across the 5,6-double bond of DMU. The formation of these photoproducts may be rationalized by assuming the excitation of either DMU or 1-aminopropane. These excited species would be responsible for the generation of the chemically reactive species, which seem to be mainly free radicals.

Similarly, irradiation with UV light of DMU with poly-L-lysine in water resulted in the extensive binding of DMU to poly-L-lysine. In these photoadducts the pyrimidine is probably attached in its 6-position to the ε-carbon of the polypeptide chain (Gorelic et al., 1972).

Purines and purine nucleosides have also been shown to undergo photoreactions when irradiated with UV light in the presence of amines (Salomon and Elad, 1974a; Stankunas et al., 1971; Yang et al., 1971). In purines or purine moieties of nucleic acids the reactions resulted in the substitution of the appropriate group for the 8-hydrogen atom in the purine system. The side chain obtained at the C-8 position in the photoadduct depended both on the purine and the amine employed. Thus, alicyclic amines afforded only one photo-product (the α-amino alkyl derivative), while the side-chain of the photoproducts derived from the aliphatic amines depended on substitution of the carbon α to the NH$_2$ groups of the free amine. [For example, amines possessing a secondary α-carbon atom (e.g. n-butyl amine) afforded mostly the appropriate alkyl derivative, while α-amino alkyl derivatives were formed preferentially with amines possessing a tertiary α-carbon atom (e.g. *iso*-propyl amine) (Salomon and Elad, 1974a)].

These reactions can be induced by light of $\lambda > 260$ nm or $\lambda > 290$ nm in the presence of ketonic sensitizers or peroxidic photoinitiators. In the former case, light is undoubtedly absorbed exclusively by the purine, since amines absorb at shorter wavelengths. The reaction further proceeds through formation of amine free radicals of the type $R_1R_2CNH_2$, via hydrogen atom abstraction from the amine by an excited purine molecule, and this radical is subsequently scavenged by a neighbor ground-state purine molecule, to yield the observed photoproducts, through a pathway similar to that of the reactions of the alcohols. In the peroxide-induced photoreactions, the peroxide absorbs most of the incident light ($\lambda > 290$ nm), and then fragments into oxy radicals which abstract a hydrogen atom from the amine, leading to an amine free radical which in turn reacts further. In the reactions initiated by acetone, the latter absorbs the incident light ($\lambda > 290$ nm) and in its excited state abstracts a hydrogen atom from an amine molecule. The formation of 8-α-aminoalkyl purines in the acetone-sensitized reaction of purines and amines is best explained in terms of this pathway (Stankunas *et al.*, 1971).

6. MISCELLANEOUS PHOTOCHEMICAL REACTIONS

6.1. Pyrimidines

Photoadduct formation between pyrimidine bases and furocoumarins is among the best known reaction of pyrimidines. These reactions, which result in the formation of a cyclobutane ring between the reactants, have been thoroughly reviewed recently. (Musajo and Rodighiero, 1972; Musajo *et al.*, 1974). When irradiated at 365 nm furocoumarins react with nucleic acids to give a C_4-cyclo-addition to the 5,6-double bond of the pyrimidine bases through either their 3,4 or 4',5'-double bond (Krauch *et al.*, 1967; Musajo and Rodighiero, 1970, 1972; Dall'acqua *et al.*, 1974). Consequently, two types of 1:1 pyrimidine-furocoumarin photoadducts might be expected. It has been shown (Dall'acqua *et al.*, 1970, 1972) that photoadducts derived from one molecule of furocoumarin and two pyrimidine bases are also formed when DNA is irradiated in the presence of psoralen. Here the furocoumarin acts as a bifunctional reagent for cross-linking. Differences exist in the photochemical behavior of the various

furocoumarins, thus, dimethylpsoralen reacts to a greater extent
with native DNA as compared to monomethylpsoralen and psoralen itself. These photoreactions are not accompanied by breaks in the
polynucleotide chain or by conformational modifications of the
macromolecule. In the case of native DNA, a dark-occurring intercalation of furocoumarins between two adjacent base pairs of the
double helix is suggested as the first step of the reaction.
Harter *et al.*, (1974) have found that benzo(1,2-b; 4,5-b')dipyran-
2,7-dione (*trans*-benzodipyrone) is significantly more reactive towards pyrimidine bases in solution than the other coumaryl derivatives. It has further been shown that the excited triplet states
of the benzodipyrones resemble those of other coumaryl derivatives
in their spectroscopic assignments and characteristics.

Another reaction of pyrimidines which involves an addition of
an olefin to form a cyclobutane ring at one of its stages is the
photofragmentation of 5-alkyl uracils to uracil. Krajewska and
Shugar (1971) have shown that the reaction proceeds via the following route,

Pyrimidine bases react with ketones photochemically to yield
oxetanes (Charlier and Helene, 1972). Wilucki *et al.*, (1967) have
isolated oxetanes from the photoreaction of thymine and benzophenone.
Similarly, oxetanes are formed in irradiated mixtures of uracil or
cytosine with acetone (Varghese, 1972). The oxetanes of cytosine
undergo deamination readily to yield the corresponding uracil

derivative.

Summers *et al.*, (1973) have shown that hydrazine, HCN, HSO_3^-, methyl amine, and BH_4^- add to uracil when irradiated with UV light of λ 254 nm. Sulfide, nitrite, and thiocyanante failed to add under

$$X = CN, HNNH_2, CH_2NH_2, SO_3^-, BH_3^-$$

these conditions. Since triplet sensitizers do not sensitize nucleophile addition reactions, it is concluded that the precursor of these photoadducts is an excited singlet state. A possible candidate for this state might be a hidden n,π* singlet, which would appear to be planar and polarized as is the ground state.

The photochemical reaction of 3,4-benzopyrene with either cytosine or thymine resulted in the attachment of benzopyrene to the C-5 or 6-position of the pyrimidine ring through a single covalent bond (Ts'o and Lu, 1964; Cavalieri and Calvin, 1971; Blackburn *et al.*, 1972; Moore *et al.*, 1973).

UV irradiation of pyrimidine derivatives in aqueous solutions containing acrylonitrile lead to polymerization of acrylonitrile and the pyrimidine (Helene and Brun, 1970). By using ^{14}C-labelled orotic acid it has been shown that the polymer contained the pyrimidine entity. These processes involve free radicals derived from excited orotic acid molecules, and it has been further shown that photoaddition proceeds entirely by way of the triplet state of orotic acid.

The photoaddition of enol acetates of 6-azauracils has been described (Swenton and Balchunis, 1974). These reactions yield labile
bicyclic azetidines which decompose in turn to yield 5-substituted-
5,6-dihydro-6-azauracils.

6.2. Purines

Purines undergo photochemical reactions with a variety of hydrogen donors besides alcohols and amines. Thus, irradiation with
UV light or γ-rays of caffeine, adenine, or guanosine with ethers,
hydroxyethers or acetals led to the substitution of the appropriate
moiety for the hydrogen atom at the 8-position of the purine
(Jerumanis and Martel, 1970; Leonov and Elad, 1974a). The site of
binding to the purine in the ether moiety is at the carbon atom
alpha to the ether oxygen, whereas in dioxolane it is at the acet-
alic carbon.

$$R = CH_2; O; CH_2O; (CH_2)_2$$

These reactions could be induced directly by UV light of $\lambda > 260$
nm or the presence of photosensitizers with light of $\lambda > 290$ nm. They
involve free radical intermediates and proceed in a fashion similar
to that of the reactions of alcohols or amines with purines. These
reactions can serve as models for the study of the interaction of
purines and sugars in photochemical reactions.

Blackburn *et al.*, (1974) have shown that diethylstilbestrol
binds to DNA as a result of the action of long-wavelength UV irradiation. A level of binding of one molecule of diethylstilbestrol
per thousand bases can be achieved by photochemical means; while
iodine-mediated binding of diethylstilbestrol to DNA was approximately three times as effective in overall linkage. Analysis of
the adduct indicates a 2:1 selectivity for binding to purine rather
than to pyrimidine bases.

7. SUMMARY

It has been found recently that purine moieties in nucleic acids are sensitive sites for photochemical reactions, e.g., photo-alkylation, and under certain reaction conditions are even more reactive than the pyrimidines. Thus, it is feasible that the purines can serve as binding-sites for cross-linking and covalent bond formation between nucleic acids and proteins under radiation. This presents an additional aspect for the cross-linking reactions. It is noteworthy, that the photochemical reactions of the purines are mostly with reagents present in the surrounding environment of the nucleic acids. Thus, the study of the photochemical reactions of the purines can serve as a tool for understanding the effect of the environment of the nucleic acid on the types and relative yields of the photoproducts formed.

The multiplicity of products formed in irradiated DNA compli-cates the chemical identification of products, and further inter-feres with the correlation between a given photoproduct and the accompanying biological effect. The induction of selective photo-chemical modification in one of the constituents of the nucleic acid can serve as a most powerful tool for the study of this cor-relation. Thus, the development of such photochemical reactions is of major importance and should, perhaps, be a line to be followed. Photosensitization in its broad aspects can be applicable to the selective production of a variety of hetero-adducts to DNA. Such an approach aids in elucidating the effects that the cellular en-vironment as a whole, or its individual components in particular, has upon the type and ratio of photoproducts formed in DNA, and in discerning the contributing chemical elements of the various bio-logical effects.

References

Ben-Ishai, R., Green, M., Graff, E., Elad, D., Steinmaus, H., and Salomon, J., 1973, Photoalkylation of purines in DNA, *Photo-chem. Photobiol.* 17:155-167.

Blackburn, G.M., Fenwick, R.G., and Thomson, M.H., 1972, The struc-ture of the thymine:3,4-benzopyrene photoproduct, *Tetrahedron Lett.* 589-592.

Blackburn, G.M., Flavel, A.J., and Thompson, M.H., 1974, Oxidative and photochemical linkage of diethylstilbestrol to DNA *in vitro*, *Cancer Res.* 34:2015-2019.

Brown, P.E., Calvin, M., and Newmark, J.F., 1966, Thymine addition to ethanol:induction by γ-irradiation, *Science* 151:68-70.

Brown, I.H., and Johns, H.E., 1968, Photochemistry of uracil. In-tersystem-crossing and dimethylation in aqueous solution, *Photochem. Photobiol.* 8:273-286.

Burr, J.G., Gordon, B.R., and Park, E.H., 1968, The mechanism of photohydration of uracil and N-substituted uracils, *Photochem. Photobiol.* 8:73-78.

Burr, J.G., Park, E.H., and Cahn, A., 1972, Nature of the reactive species in the photohydration of uracil and cytosine derivatives, *J. Amer. Chem. Soc.* 94:5866-5872.

Cadet, J., and Teoule, R., 1971, γ-Irradiation of thymine in de-aerated media. *Cis*- and *trans*-6-hydroxy-5,6-dihydrothymine isomers, *Int. J. Appl. Radiat. Isotop.* 22:273-280.

Cavalieri, E., and Calvin, M., 1971, Photochemical coupling of benzo[a]pyrene with 1-methylcytosine:photoenhancement of carcinogenicity, *Photochem. Photobiol.* 14:641-653.

Chambers, R.W., 1968, Synthesis of trithiouridine 5'-phosphate via the photohydrate of uridylic acid, *J. Amer. Chem. Soc.* 90 2191-2193.

Charlier, M., and Helene, C., 1972, Photochemical reactions of aromatic ketones with nucleic acids and their components. 1. Purine and pyrimidine bases and nucleosides, *Photochem. Photobiol.* 15:71-87.

Dall'acqua, F., Marciani, S., Vedaldi, D., and Rodighiero, G., 1972, Formation of inter-strand cross-linking on DNA of Guinea pig skin after application of psoralen and irradiation at 365 nm, *Febs Lett.* 27 (2):192-194.

Dall'acqua, F., Marciani, S., Vedaldi, D., and Rodighiero, G., 1974, Studies of the photoreactions (365 nm) between DNA and some methylpsoralens, *Biochim. Biophys. Acta* 353:267-273.

De Boer, G., and Johns, H.E., 1970, Hydrogen exchange in photohydrates of cytosine derivatives, *Biochim. Biophys. Acta* 204: 18-30.

De Boer, G., Klinghoffer, O., and Johns, H.E., 1970, Reversal mechanisms for the photohydrates of cytosine and its derivatives, *Biochim. Biophys. Acta* 213:253-268.

Evans, B., and Wolfenden, R., 1970, Potential transition state analog for adenosine deaminase, *J. Amer. Chem. Soc.* 92:4751-4752.

Fisher, G.J., and Johns, H.E., 1973, Thymine hydrate formed by ultraviolet and γ-irradiation of aqueous solutions, *Photochem. Photobiol.* 18:23-27.

Gorelic, L.C., Lisagor, P., and Yang, N.C., 1972, The photochemical reactions of 1,3-dimethyluracil with 1-aminopropane and poly-L-lysine, *Photochem. Photobiol.* 16:465-480.

Greenstock, C.L., Brown, I.H., Hunt, J.W., and Johns, H.E., 1967 Photodimerization of pyrimidine nucleic acid derivatives in aqueous solution and effect of oxygen, *Biochem. Biophys. Res. Commun.* 27:431-436.

Grossman, L., and Rogers, E., 1968, Evidence for the presence of cytosine photohydrates in UV irradiated nucleic acids, *Biochem. Biophys. Res. Commun.* 33:975-983.

Harter, M.L., Felkner, I.C., Mantulin, W.W., McInturff, D.L., Marx, J.N., and Song, P.S., 1974, Excited states and photobiological properties of potential DNA cross-linking agents, the benzodipyrones, *Photochem. Photobiol.* 20:407-413.

Helene, C., and Brun, F., 1970, Photochemical reactions of pyrimidine derivatives with acrylonitrile in aqueous solutions, *Photochem. Photobiol.* 11:77-84.

Jellinek, T., and Johns, R.B., 1970, The mechanism of photochemical addition of cysteine to uracil and formation of dihydrouracil, *Photochem. Photobiol.* 11:349-359.

Jerumanis, S., and Martel, A., 1970, Photochemical reactions of caffeine with ethers, *Can. J. Chem.* 48:1716-1721.

Kondo, Y., and Witkop, B., 1968, The stereochemistry of the catalytic and light-induced reduction of thymidine to dihydrothymidine and ureido alcohols, *J. Amer. Chem. Soc.* 90:764-770.

Krauch, C.H., Kraemer, D.M., and Wacker, A., 1967, Photoreactions of psoralen-(4-^{14}C) with DNA. RNA, homopolynucleotides and nucleotides, *Photochem. Photobiol.* 6:341-354.

Krojewska, E., and Shugar, D., 1971, Photochemical transformation of 5-alkyluracils and their nucleosides, *Science* 173:435-437.

Lawly, P.D., 1966, Effects of some chemical mutagens and carcinogens on nucleic acids, *Prog. Nucl. Acid Res. Mol. Biol.* 5:89-131.

Leonov, D., and Elad, D., 1974a, Ultraviolet and γ-ray-induced reactions of nucleic acid constituents. Reactions of purines with ethers and dioxolane, *J. Org. Chem.* 39:1470-1473.

Leonov, D., and Elad, D., 1974b, Photochemical and γ-ray-induced reactions of nucleic acid constituents. Suppression of the reactivity of pyrimidines in the presence of purines, *J. Amer. Chem. Soc.* 96:5635-5637.

Leonov, D., Salomon, J., Sasson, S., and Elad, D., 1973, Ultraviolet- and γ-ray-induced reactions of nucleic acid constituents with alcohols. On the selectivity of these reactions for purines, *Photochem. Photobiol.* 17:465-468.

Lomant, A.J., and Fresco, J.R., 1972, Ultraviolet photochemistry as a probe of polyribonucleotide conformation, *Prog. Nucl. Acid Res. Mol. Biol.* 12:1-27.

Moore, T.A., Mantulin, W.W., and Song, P.S., 1973, Excited states and reactivity of carcinogenic benzpyrene; a comparison with skin-sensitizing coumarins, *Photochem. Photobiol.* 18:185-194.

Musajo, L., and Rodighiero, G., 1970, Studies on the photo-C_4-cycloaddition reactions between skin photosensitizing furocoumarins and nucleic acids, *Photochem. Photobiol.* 11:27-35.

Musajo, L., and Rodighiero, G., 1972, Mode of photosensitizing action of furocoumarins, *Photophysiology* 7:115-147.

Musajo, L., Rodighiero, G., Caporale, G., Dall'acqua, F., Marciani, S., Bordin,F., Bacuchetti, F., and Bevilacqua, R., 1974, Photoreactions between skin photosensitizing furocoumarins and nucleic acids, *in* "Sunlight and Man" (Fitzpatrick, T.B., ed), University of Tokyo Press, pp. 369-387.

Salomon, J., and Elad, D., 1973, Photochemical reactions of nucleic acid constituents. Peroxide-initiated reactions of purines with alcohols, *J. Org. Chem.* 38:3420-3421.

Salomon, J., and Elad, D., 1974a, Ultraviolet and γ-ray-induced reactions of nucleic acid constituents. Reactions of purines with amines, *Photochem. Photobiol.* 19:21-27.

Salomon, J., and Elad, D., 1974b, Selective photochemical alkylation of purines in DNA, *Biochem. Biophys. Res. Commun.* 58:890-894.

Salomon, J., and Elad, D., 1974c, Photochemical and γ-ray-induced reactions of nucleic acid constituents. Dealkylation of 8-α-hydroxyalkyl purines, *J. Amer. Chem. Soc.* 96:3295-3299.

Sasson, S., and Elad, D., 1972, Photosensitized monomerization of 1,3-dimethyluracil photodimers, *J. Org. Chem.* 37:3164-3167.

Setlow, R.B., and Carrier, W.L., 1963, Identification of ultra-violet induced thymine dimers in DNA by absorbance measurements, *Photochem. Photobiol.* 2:49-57.

Shetlar, M.D., 1975, The photoreaction of N,N-1,3-dimethyluracil with ethanol, *Tetrahedron Lett.* 477-480.

Shugar, D., and Wierzchowski, K.L., 1957, Reversible photolysis of pyrimidine derivatives, including trials with nucleic acids, *Biochim. Biophys. Acta.* 23:657-658.

Sinsheimer, R.L., and Hasting, R., 1949, A reversible photochemical alteration of uracil and uridine, *Science* 110:525-526.

Small, G.D., Tao, M., and Gordon, M.P., 1968, Pyrimidine hydrates and dimers in ultraviolet irradiated TMV-RNA, *J. Mol., Biol.* 38:57-87.

Stankunas, A., Rosenthal, I., and Pitts, J.N., 1971, Photochemical and radiochemical alkylation of caffeine by alkyl amines, *Tetrahedron Lett.* 4779-4782.

Steinmaus, H., Elad, D., and Ben-Ishai, R., 1970, Ultraviolet light-induced purine-modified DNA, *Biochem. Biophys. Res. Commun.* 40:1021-1025.

Steinmaus, H., Rosenthal, I., and Elad, D., 1971, Light- and γ-ray-induced reactions of purines and purine nucleosides with alcohols, *J. Org. Chem.* 36:3594-3598.

Summers, W.A., Enwall, C., Burr, J.G., and Letsinger, R.L., 1973, The photoaddition of nucleophiles to uracil, *Photochem. Photobiol.* 17:295-301.

Swenton, J.S., and Blachunis, R.J., 1974, Photochemical functionalization of 6-azauracils to 5-substituted-6-azauracils, *J. Heterocycl. Chem.* 11:917-910.

Ts'o, P.O.P., and Lu, P., 1964, Interaction of nucleic acids. II. Chemical linkage of the carcinogen benzpyrene to DNA induced by photoradiation, *Proc. Natl. Acad. Sci. USA* 51:272-280.

Varghese, A.J., 1972, Photochemistry of nucleic acids and their constituents, *Photophysiology* 7:207-274.

Wang, S.Y., 1961, Photochemical reactions in frozen solutions, *Nature* 190:690-694.

Wechter, W.J., and Smith, K.C., 1968, The structure and chemistry of uridine photohydrate, *Biochemistry* 7:4064-4069.

Wilucki, V.I., Matthaus, H., and Krauch, C.H., 1967, Photosensitized cyclodimerization of thymine in solution, *Photochem. Photobiol.* 6:497-500.

Yang, N.C., Gorelic, L.S., and Kim, B., 1971, A new photochemical reaction of purine. Photochemical alkylation of purine by 1-propylamine, *Photochem. Photobiol.* 13:275-277.

IONIZING RADIATION-INDUCED ATTACHMENT REACTIONS OF NUCLEIC ACIDS

AND THEIR COMPONENTS

Lawrence S. Myers, Jr.

Laboratory of Nuclear Medicine and Radiation Biology

and the Department of Radiological Sciences, University

of California, Los Angeles, 900 Veteran Avenue, Los

Angeles, California 90024

1. INTRODUCTION

This paper is concerned with reactions which are initiated by ionizing radiations (γ-rays, X-rays, etc.) and which result in the formation of new bonds involving nucleic acids or nucleic acid constituents. These reactions may differ from those initiated by near-UV radiation because identity of the substances affected by the radiation, the nature of the primary chemical species, and their distribution in the irradiated volume all differ. With ionizing radiations the amount of energy deposition in various molecules depends on their electron fraction, not their absorption spectra, and results in formation of significant yields of electrons separated from their parent molecules, cation radicals, and excited states ranging from the lowest excitation levels to superexcited states. These primary species are distributed along the path of

261

each ionizing particle in small clusters in which the probability
of interactions within the clusters is comparable to the probability
of escape from the clusters. If escape occurs, reaction may occur
at a considerable distance (1-100 nm) from the site of energy deposition. Many of the secondary and subsequent reactions started by
the cation radicals and electrons involve free radicals similar to
those frequently observed following absorption of near-UV radiation.
There is thus a large overlap between ionizing and UV radiation
chemistry in spite of the differences noted above, and the fields
contribute to a large degree to one another.

The emphasis in this paper is on non-protein molecules. An
extensive review of protein-DNA attachment reactions is given by
Yamamoto (This Volume).

Several lines of evidence suggest that attachments of organic
molecules to DNA are likely to occur in living systems exposed to
ionizing radiations. Among these are the following:

a) Although ionizing radiation is frequently thought of as
destroying organic molecules, it is well known that it also can
cause increases in size and complexity of molecules. Among important examples are radiation induced polymerization reactions (Dole,
1973), and grafting of molecules onto cellulose (Arthur, 1970);

b) Increasing information about 1) the microenvironment in
the neighborhood of nucleic acids in cells, 2) the patterns of
energy deposition by ionizing radiations, 3) the properties of
initial chemical products of energy deposition, and 4) the subsequent reactions of these products suggests that *in vivo* conditions
are favorable for formation of covalent bonds between DNA and molecules in the vicinity of DNA (Myers, 1973a, b, 1974; Ward, 1975);

c) Preliminary experiments with isolated nuclei of *T. pyri-
formis* have demonstrated that radiation induced binding of small
molecules with DNA does indeed occur. In these experiments, [^{14}C]-
D-phenylalanine in the medium became attached to DNA during irradiation in such a way that it remained during standard DNA isolation
and purification procedures (Byfield *et al.*, 1970).

The significance of attachment reactions to radiation biology
arises from the possibilities that they may be important lesions
leading to the biological effects of ionizing radiation, and that
they may account, at least in part, for the action of substances
which modify radiation effects in living organisms. Regarding the
former, DNA inactivation, and phage and cell death are by no means
entirely accounted for by the most frequently studied molecular
lesions in irradiated DNA, single- and double-strand breaks
(Freifelder, 1974). Van der Schans and Bleichrodt (1974) report
that 85% of the inactivation of PM2 bacteriophage in frozen solution

is not associated with a chain break. Clearly other lethal lesions must be identified. One obvious candidate is base destruction. Another which, in view of the above discussion, must be considered is modification of DNA by attachment of organic molecules to base or pentose moieties. Such modifications might well include forma- tion of DNA-protein cross-links, intra or intermolecular DNA-DNA cross-links, and attachment of various non-protein compounds to DNA. With respect to sensitization, several substances (discussed below) which sensitize anoxic cells to ionizing radiation have been shown to form bonds with DNA or DNA constituents (Emmerson and Willson, 1968; Ward *et al.*, 1969; Brustad *et al.*, 1971; Chapman *et al.*, 1973a; Willson *et al.*, 1974). It has not been proven that the binding is the cause of the sensitization because other reactions, especially electron transfer also occur; but it may well be. The general subject of this paper has been reviewed briefly (Myers, 1974; Smith, 1975).

2. MECHANISMS OF IONIZING RADIATION INDUCED SUBSTITUTION AND ADDITION REACTIONS

In considering the effects of ionizing radiations on nucleic acids in cells, it is important to keep in mind that the nucleic acids are in more or less intimate contact with many other kinds of substances. These are reasonably certain to include water, proteins, especially histones or protamines, membrane components, various other organic compounds, and metal counter-ions. When such a system is exposed to ionizing radiation, a single 'hit', or act of energy deposition is very likely to involve two or more of the substances. A brief discussion of typical reactions follows.

If energy is deposited in a water molecule the initial reaction is believed to be separation of an electron with formation of the highly reactive cation radical, $H_2O^{\dot{+}}$ (the dot signifies an unpaired electron). The $H_2O^{\dot{+}}$ reacts almost immediately with H_2O to give a hydroxyl free radical ($\cdot OH$). The electron may interact with water molecules to give a hydrated electron, e_{aq}^-, or with a compound which has an appreciable electron affinity. In dilute aqueous solutions yields of $\cdot OH$ and e_{aq}^- per 1000 rad, with X- or γ-rays, are about 2.7×10^{-6} mol/liter. Small yields of hydrogen atoms, H_2, and H_2O_2 ($\sim 0.5 \times 10^{-6}$ mol/liter) also are observed. With α-radiation, yields of H_2 and H_2O_2 are larger, and of $\cdot OH$ and e_{aq}^-, smaller.

Analogous reactions occur if energy is deposited in any of the organic compounds, including DNA. These may be written formally

$$RH \xrightarrow{} RH^{\dot{+}} \quad + \quad e^- \tag{2-1}$$

$$DNA \xrightarrow{} DNA^{\dot{+}} \quad + \quad e^- \tag{2-2}$$

The cation radicals may react with other molecules, or may undergo deprotonation reactions, possibly with water, to form neutral free radicals.

$$RH^{\ddot{+}} \longrightarrow R^{\cdot} \quad + \quad H^{+} \qquad\qquad (2\text{-}3)$$

$$DNA^{\ddot{+}} \longrightarrow DNA^{\cdot} \quad + \quad H^{+} \qquad\qquad (2\text{-}4)$$

The fate of the electrons is the same as that of the electron from water.

Secondary reactions include a) capture of hydrated electrons by organic molecules, b) transfer of electrons from substances of lower electron affinity to substances with higher electron affinities (Adams *et al.*, 1968), c) reaction of hydroxyl free radicals with organic compounds to produce organic free radicals, and d) interactions involving the organic free radicals to give nucleic acid with organic substances incorporated as adducts or substituents. Items a) and b) will not be discussed further. The hydroxyl free radical (item c) reacts by addition to unsaturated bonds of organic compounds, or by abstraction of hydrogen atoms from saturated $\geq$C-H bonds. With nucleic acids, it has been shown to add to the 5,6-double bond of pyrimidine bases [illustrated for thymine (Thy)] and to the 4, 5, or possibly the 7,8-double bond of purine bases.

$$(2\text{-}5)$$

The radical shown will be referred to as the Thy-·OH adduct radical in the rest of this paper. The ·OH free radical abstracts hydrogen from the deoxyribose or ribose part of nucleic acids, but the site of attack is not certain. The reaction with ethyl alcohol is illustrative:

$$(2\text{-}6)$$

On absorption by aqueous DNA solutions of several thousand rads, it has been shown that about 80% of the ·OH reacts with base and about 20% with the deoxypentose moieties (Scholes *et al.*, 1960). Evidence is accumulating, however, which is consistent with the notion that the proportion of attack on the bases as compared with that on the pentose in native double-stranded DNA is less until after the molecule has become partially uncoiled as a result of strand breakage (Ward, 1975). The proportion of attack on the various bases is in proportion to the amount of each base in the DNA (Scholes *et al.*, 1969; Myers *et al.*, 1973b).

The rate constants for reaction of ·OH with nucleic acids and the organic compounds in the vicinity of nucleic acids are very large, of the order of 10^8 - 10^9 liter mol^{-1} s^{-1}, or close to the limit imposed by the rate of diffusion. It may be anticipated, therefore, that ·OH will react at a site close to its site of formation with almost any organic compound which is available.

Relatively little is known about structure and reactivity of cation radicals formed by deposition of energy in nucleic acids or of their deprotonated derivatives. Cation radicals are reported to have been observed by EPR spectroscopy at 77°K of irradiated thymine, cytosine, and DNA [unpaired spin localized on cytosine or guanine (Gräslund *et al.*, 1971)], and several neutral free radicals that could have been formed by deprotonation of cation radicals have been observed at higher temperatures (for a review see Myers, 1974). Among the latter is a substituted methyl radical observed in both irradiated thymine and DNA (Hartig and Dertinger, 1971).

$$(2-7)$$

Interactions involving the organic free radicals may lead to formation of covalent bonds between nucleic acids and organic compounds by several reaction paths. These include reactions between a) organic molecules and nucleic acid radicals (neutral or charged):

$$RH \quad + \quad DNA· \longrightarrow Bonding \qquad (2-8)$$

b) organic radicals (neutral or charged) and nucleic acid molecules:

$$R· \quad + \quad DNA \longrightarrow Bonding \qquad (2-9)$$

and c) organic radicals and nucleic acid radicals:

R˙   +   DNA˙————————▶ Bonding   (2-10)

In the remainder of this paper experimental results, obtained
for the most part with model systems, will be reviewed. These will
show that each of the three pathways may play a role in radiolysis
of DNA *in vivo*.

3. REACTIONS WITH WATER, FORMATE, AND ALCOHOLS (TABLE 1)

3.1. Addition of Water or Parts of Water

Reactions of nucleic acid constituents and nucleic acids with
water have been studied extensively (for reviews see Scholes, 1968;
Ward, 1975) and only sufficient information will be given here to
provide examples.

On radiolysis of oxygen-free dilute aqueous solutions of
thymine, the thymine is converted in less than stoichiometric
amounts to compounds with elements of water added to the 5,6-
double bond or substituted into the methyl group. Among the

Table 1.   Attachment Reactions of Nucleic Acids Induced by Ionizing
Radiations: Water, Formate, and Alcohols

Compound	Nucleic acid derivative	Reference
H_2O	Thymine	Teoule *et al.*, 1972
"	"	Infante *et al.*, 1973
"	Uracil	Smith and Hays, 1968
O_2	Base-˙OH adduct	Scholes *et al.*, 1960
Formate	Cytosine	Kamal and Garrison, 1965
Ethanol	"	"
"	Thymine	Brown *et al.*, 1966
"	N,N'-dimethylthymine	"
"	Thymine	Zarebska and Shugar, 1972
"	Caffeine	Elad *et al.*, 1969
2-Propanol	"	"
"	Adenine	Steinmaus *et al.*, 1969, 1971
"	Adenosine	"
"	Guanosine	"
"	2-Deoxyguanosine	"
"	6-Ethoxypurine	"
"	Thymine plus adenine	Leonov *et al.*, 1975
"	"	"

products are the hydrate, the glycol, and dihydrothymine (Teoule
et al., 1972; Teoule and Cadet, 1975; Infante *et al.*, 1973). Similar
products are obtained with uracil (Smith and Hays, 1968). The
formulas show only the atoms at positions 5 and 6 of the ring. The
rest of the molecule is shown in (2-5).

$$(3\text{-}1)$$

These substances, in turn, appear to have H_2O, H_2O_2, and H_2 added
to the base. They are probably formed by disproportionation reactions of the electron or $\cdot OH$-adduct radicals. For example,

$$(3\text{-}2)$$

Analogous reactions with inclusion of protonation steps would give
dihydrothymine and the hydrates. Formation of these products by
consecutive reactions with two $\cdot OH$, 2 e_{aq}^-, or $\cdot OH + e_{aq}^-$ can be
excluded by kinetic considerations.

Yields for thymine disappearance are well below the amounts
of $\cdot OH$ and e_{aq}^- produced by the radiolysis of water. This was
recognized many years ago (Scholes *et al.*, 1960) and it was proposed that reactions occur which regenerate the parent molecule.
The disproportionation reactions for formation of products are
among these. These reactions reduce the maximum yield to half the
initial amount of $\cdot OH$ and e_{aq}^-; yields are lower than this, and
variable, however, so that other reconstitution reactions must occur.
Recently it has been shown that the glycol can be converted to thymine by radiation (Namiki and Hayashi, 1970), and it is well known
that the hydrates reconstitute the parent molecule. Further, the
yields of the disproportionation reactions may be reduced by reactions such as

$$\text{Thy-}\cdot OH \quad + \quad (\text{Thy})^- \longrightarrow 2 \text{ Thy} \quad + \quad OH^- \qquad (3\text{-}3)$$

If oxygen is present a different set of reactions occurs.
First, the oxygen reacts with e_{aq}^- to give the anion radical of
HO_2

$$e_{aq}^- \quad + \quad O_2 \longrightarrow \cdot O_2^- \qquad (3\text{-}4)$$

The anion radical is the stable form at physiological pH. The reaction prevents e_{aq}^- from reacting with Thy (or DNA) but 'OH can still
add to give the Thy-'OH adduct radical. Oxygen adds to this radical
to give the 5-hydroxy-6-hydroperoxy radical (Scholes *et al.*, 1960).

$$(3-5)$$

This radical is reduced by electron transfer from $'O_2^-$ to give the
anion of the hydroxy hydroperoxide.

$$RO_2^{\cdot} \quad + \quad 'O_2^- \longrightarrow RO_2^- \quad + \quad O_2 \qquad (3-6)$$

This addition of oxygen blocks the restitution reactions and increases
the yield for thymine destruction to the yield of 'OH produced by
radiation. Several products, especially the glycol, are formed in
addition to the hydroxy hydroperoxide.

Radiation induced reactions of other bases, and of nucleosides
and nucleotides have not been studied as extensively as those of
thymine. The reactions appear to be similar to those of thymine
in that 'OH adds to unsaturated bonds of all the bases, restitution
reactions occur, and O_2 adds to the base-'OH adduct radicals and
with nucleosides and nucleotides, to radicals on the pentose moiety.
Some of the secondary reactions leading to final products differ,
however (Scholes, 1968; Cadet and Teoule, 1972; Ward, 1975). The
hydroxyhydroperoxides of thymine and cytosine have been observed
in DNA irradiated *in vitro* (Schweibert and Daniels, 1971) and of
thymine *in vivo* (Cerutti, 1974).

3.2. Addition of 'COO⁻ Ion Radical and Related Reactions

Formate ion in oxygen free irradiated solutions can also block
restitution reactions (Kamal and Garrison, 1965). In solutions of
cytosine (the formulas show only the 5,6-double bond of cytosine)
the following occurs.

$$'OH \quad + \quad HCOO^- \longrightarrow H_2O \quad + \quad 'COO^- \qquad (3-7)$$

This is followed by the addition reactions:

$$(3-8)$$

$$(3\text{-}9)$$

These radicals undergo disproportionation to give cytosine and

The effect is to increase the yield for cytosine destruction, just
as does oxygen. Other substances which accomplish the same result
are ethanol (Kamal and Garrison, 1965), cysteine, and ascorbic
acid (Holian and Garrison, 1969). The latter two compounds are
believed to react by transfer of an H-atom to the base anion radical, i.e., the H-atom adds. In the absence of any additive the
restitution reaction can be written

$$\dot{B}^{-} \; + \; \dot{B}OH \longrightarrow 2B \; + \; OH^{-} \qquad\qquad (3\text{-}10)$$

In the presence of cysteine, RSH, this reaction is stopped by

$$H^{+} \; + \; \dot{B}^{-} \; + \; RSH \longrightarrow BH_2 \; + \; RS^{\cdot} \qquad (3\text{-}11)$$

The yield of BH_2 is equal to the yield of e_{aq}^{-}. This reaction illustrates very well a non-protective reaction of sulfhydryl compounds.

3.3.   Reactions with Alcohols

Ethyl alcohol (EtOH) has been shown to add to thymine by reactions which involve the hydroxyethyl radical (Brown *et al.*, 1966).
In oxygen free aqueous solutions containing about 5×10^{-3} M thymine and 0.1 M EtOH nearly all ·OH produced by the radiolysis of
water react with the alcohol to give the hydroxyethyl radical
(Eq. 2-6). The product isolated is shown in Eq. (3-12). Both *cis*
and *trans* isomers are formed. These compounds are probably formed
by a disproportion reaction between the thymine anion radical
(formed by capture of the hydrated electron) and the thymine hydroxyethyl adduct radical. The yield is about one-third of the yield
of ·OH. N,N'-Dimethylthymine undergoes a similar reaction with
EtOH with a yield nearly equal to the ·OH yield. The 0,0-dimethyl-
thymine does not undergo the addition reaction.

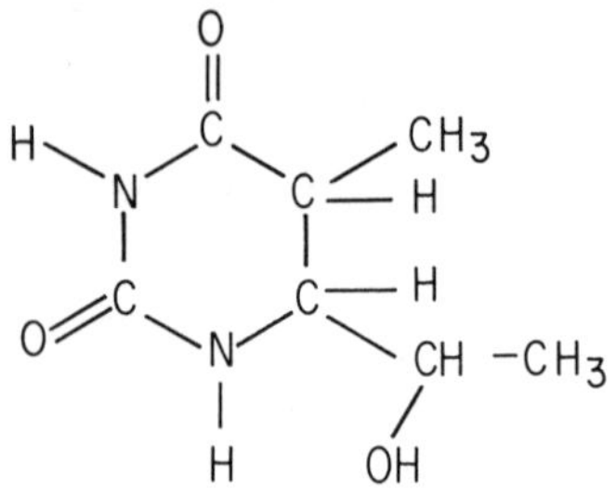

(3-12)

The thymine-alcohol adduct compound undergoes a secondary
reaction on continued irradiation of oxygen-free nitrogen-saturated
solutions which leads to formation of 6-ethylthymine, in which the
5,6-double bond has been restored (Zarebska and Shugar, 1972).

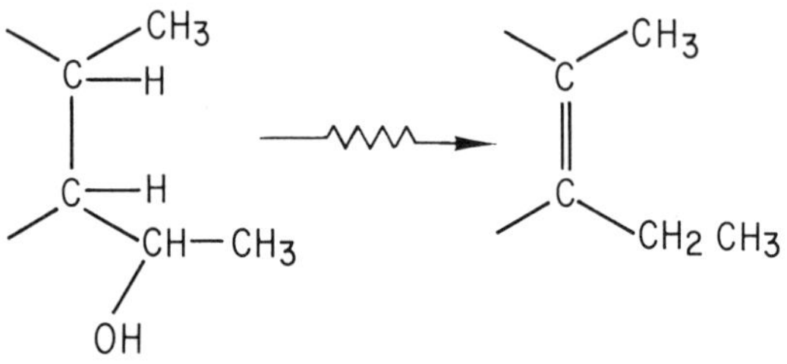

(3-13)

Both ˙OH and electrons appear to be essential for this reaction, but
the mechanism is not known. It should be noted, however that while
it appears that substitution of ethyl for hydrogen has occurred,
the mechanism is not that of a simple substitution reaction. Confirming that ethylthymine is a secondary product, the yield (amount
formed per unit radiation does) increases with increasing radiation do

Purine bases have been shown to undergo radiation-induced
reactions with alcohols which result in substitution at the C(8)
position. The reaction is shown for caffeine (Elad et $al.$, 1969).

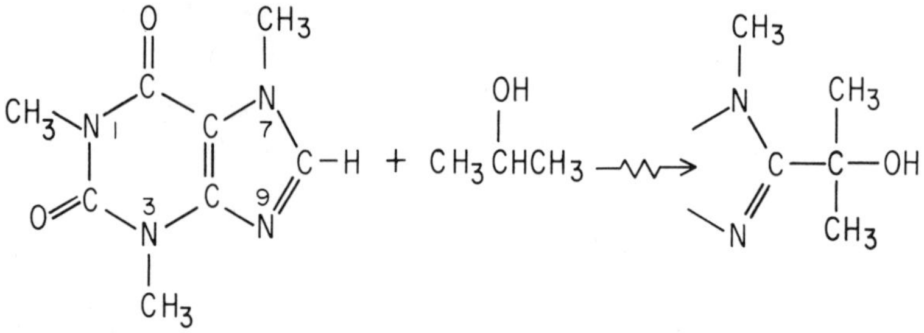

(3-14)

Ethyl alcohol forms the analogous product plus 8-ethylcaffeine in
a 1-1 ratio.

$$CH_3$$

$$(3-15)$$

Structure with N-CH$_3$, C—C$_2$H$_5$, and N groups.

Substitution of 2-propanol into adenine, adenosine, guanosine, 2-deoxyguanosine, and 6-ethoxypurine has also been observed (Steinmaus *et al.*, 1969, 1971).

These particular experiments were carried out under very different conditions from those for the pyrimidine reactions described above. Unfortunately, experiments have not been carried out under comparable conditions with both purines and pyrimidines. Steinmaus *et al.* (1969, 1971) dissolved small amounts of the purine compound in the alcohol or a solution of approximately equal amounts of the alcohol and acetone. In some experiments a little water was present, but in all cases most of the energy was absorbed by the alcohol and acetone. The apparent substitution is believed to occur by addition of alcohol free radicals and H$\cdot$ (or e$^-$ + H$^+$) generated by the radiation, to the 8,9-double bond of caffeine or the 7,8-double bond of other purines, followed by an oxidation step during isolation of the compound which gives the observed product. Yields range from 15 to 80% conversion of the initial material after radiation doses of the order of 10^7 rads, and for the reaction of 2-propanol with caffeine, are larger by a factor of about two if acetone is present in the solution.

The relative reactivity of purines and pyrimidines was investigated by Leonov *et al.* (1973). Mixtures of about equal amounts of thymine and adenine (~3 mmol each) in 2-propanol were irradiated. Although both bases react with alcohol when irradiated separately, in the mixture, all of the reaction was with the purine. A similar result was obtained with a mixture of adenosine and thymine. Leonov and Elad (1974a) suggested that the suppression of the reactivity of the pyrimidines may be related to association of the pyrimidines with purines in alcohol solutions. An alternative explanation may be that the rate constants for reactions between the alcohol radical and the two kinds of bases differ.

4. REACTIONS WITH AMINES AND OTHER SMALL MOLECULES (TABLE 2)

Many alkyl amines react with purines to give substitution of an α-aminoalkyl or an alkyl group for the hydrogen atom at C(8) of the purine. Irradiation of deoxygenated 5 M aqueous amine solutions

containing caffeine is reported to give the alkyl substituent
(Stankunas *et al.*, 1971). Thus, ethyl-, diethyl-, and triethylamine
all give 8-ethylcaffeine. Normal propylamine gives 8-n-propylcaf-
feine, and isopropylamine gives 8-isopropylcaffeine. Tertiary-
butylamine does not react with caffeine, suggesting that a hydrogen
atom on the α-carbon atom is necessary for reaction. The composition of the solutions used for these experiments is such that 25-
50% of the energy from the radiation is deposited in the amine,
and the rest in water. Thus, all of the products from both water
and amine radiolysis are available for the reaction, and it is
impossible with the available data to suggest a mechanism. It may
be suggested by analogy with the alkylation of thymine and purines
by alcohol that the reactions proceed by addition to the 8,9-double
bond, and that secondary reactions lead to formation of the substituted compound.

In similar experiments in which energy deposition was almost
entirely in the amine, i.e., the solutions contained much less
water, Elad and Salomon (1971) and Salomon and Elad (1974) obtained
α-aminoalkyl substituents of purines as well as the alkyl substituents. Thus, radiolysis of isopropylamine solutions containing
adenine gave 8-α-amino-isopropyladenine. Under similar conditions
piperidine formed 8-(2'-piperidyl)-caffeine and 8-(2'-piperidyl)-

Table 2. Attachment Reactions of Nucleic Acids Induced by Ionizing
Radiations: Amines and Other Small Molecules

Compound	Nucleic acid derivative	Reference
D-Phenylalanine	DNA *in vivo*	Byfield *et al.*, 1970
Ethylamine	Caffeine	Stankunas *et al.*, 1971
Diethylamine	"	"
Triethylamine	"	"
n-Propylamine	"	"
iso-Propylamine	"	"
t-Butylamine	" (no reaction)	"
iso-Propylamine	Adenine	Salomon and Elad, 1974
Piperidine	"	"
"	Caffeine	"
Tetrahydrofuran	"	Leonov and Elad, 1974
"	Adenine	"
Dioxane	Caffeine	"
Thyroxine	DNA *in vitro*	Byfield *et al.*, 1970
Glyceraldehyde	"	"
Leucine	"	"
Benz(a)pyrene	DNA	Chan and Ball, 1971
Pyrene	"	"
Fluorescein	"	Andersson, 1969

adenine.

Available evidence indicates that the cyclic ether, tetrahydro-furan (THF), and dioxane react with purines under the influence of ionizing radiation by reactions analogous to those of the amines and alcohols discussed above (Leonov and Elad, 1974b). THF gives the appropriate 8-substituted caffeine and adenine derivatives, and dioxane the 8-substituted derivatives of caffeine. The substituant is attached to the purine C(8) atom by a bond to the carbon *alpha* to a ring oxygen. The substitution reaction is believed to take place by means of free radical addition reactions followed by secondary reactions which give the observed product.

Several small molecules have been observed to become attached to DNA or RNA on irradiation of aqueous solutions. These include thyroxine, glyceraldehyde, leucine, and other amino acids (Byfield *et al.*, 1970). The attachment of [C^{14}]leucine, as determined by acid insolubility, is proportional to DNA concentration (0.05 to 0.2%) and to radiation dose to 10^6 rads. On hydrolysis and paper chromatographic separation of components of the irradiated DNA, the [C^{14}] was not localized, suggesting that several products may have been formed.

What appears to be an entirely different kind of reaction has been observed with polycyclic aromatic compounds such as benz(a)-pyrene (BP) and pyrene (P) (Chan and Ball, 1971). When a physical complex between either of these compounds and calf thymus DNA was irradiated in a dilute cacodylate solution, the hydrocarbon became covalently bonded to the DNA. The degree of binding was negligible to a dose of about 8000 rads, but then increased rapidly. After a dose of 17 krads, the amount of binding of BP and P, respectively, was 1 mol/100 and 1 mol/270 DNA nucleotides (initial ratios 1 to 48 and 1 to 27). The criteria for binding were unextractability by ethanol or cyclohexane, and shifts in the UV absorption spectra. The template activity of DNA containing bound BP (1 mol/370 nucleo-tides) in an *in vitro* RNA synthesizing system at short (15 min) incubation times was the same as that of control DNA (no BP) exposed to the same amount of radiation (10 krads)--about 45% of that of unirradiated DNA. After 30 min of incubation, the acti-vity was only 80% of that of the control DNA. The results suggest that the covalently bound BP does not block binding of the RNA polymerase or interfere with the initiation of transcription, but that it does result in retardation or termination of transcription when a growing RNA chain encounters a bound BP molecule.

Irradiation of a 0.1% calf thymus DNA solution containing fluorescein has been reported to result in binding of the dye to the macromolecule (Andersson, 1969).

5. NUCLEIC ACID-NUCLEIC ACID INTERACTIONS (TABLE 3)

5.1. Base-Base Attachment Reaction to Give Dimers on Radiolysis
of Uracil

In spite of many investigations of the radiolysis of pyrimidine bases in the absence of oxygen, a satisfactory understanding
of the reactions has not been obtained. It has recently been
reported (Shragge *et al.*, 1974), however, that several major
dimeric products of uracil radiolysis have been overlooked. The
products formed at pH 5 in N_2-saturated solutions have structures
such as:

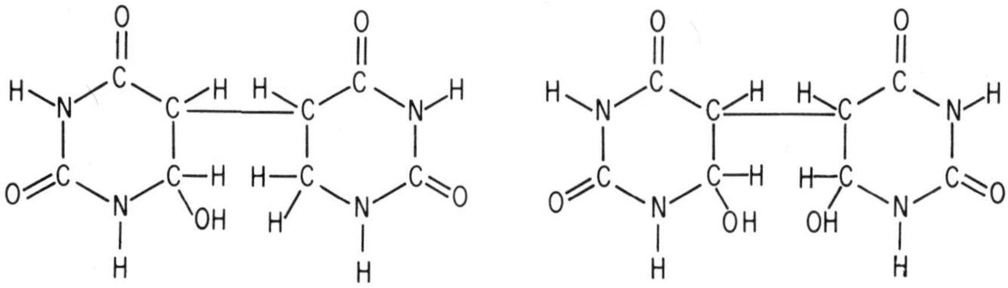

(5-1)

The corresponding 6-6 and 5-6 dimers are also possible. The dimers
are believed to be formed by the combination of Ura-'OH with a
protonated anion radical $(Ura^{\cdot})^{-}(H^{+})$ or of two Ura-'OH radicals,
respectively. At pH 8.5, also in N_2, dimers have been obtained
in which the 5,6 bonds of the rings are unsaturated, for example

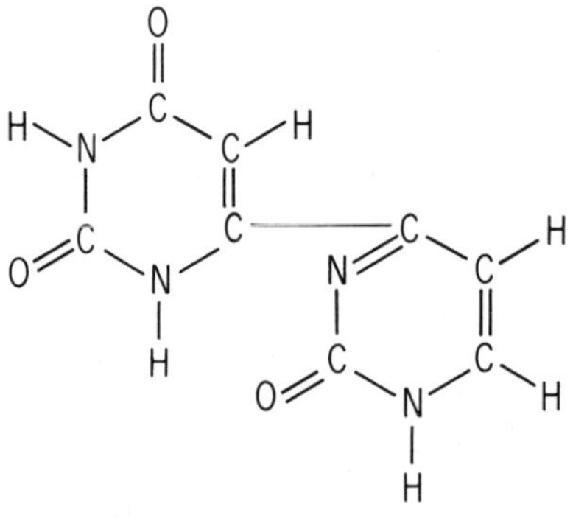

(5-2)

The 2-pyrimidone derivative is probably formed, as well.

Dimers of the cyclobutane type produced by photolysis are not
reported to be formed by ionizing radiation.

Table 3. Attachment Reactions of Nucleic Acids Induced by Ionizing
Radiations: Nucleic Acid-Nucleic Acid Interactions

Compound	Nucleic acid derivative	Reference
Uracil	Uracil	Shragge *et al.*, 1974
Adenosine mono-phosphate	(Intramolecular)	Keck *et al.*, 1966
		Raleigh and Kramers, 1975
Uracil	RNA	Yamamoto, 1973
Thymine	"	"
Cytosine	"	"
Adenine	"	"
Guanine	"	"
DNA	DNA	Lett *et al.*, 1961
"	"	Lett and Alexander, 1961
"	"	Coquerelle *et al.*, 1969
"	"	Bohne *et al.*, 1970

5.2. Intramolecular Attachment of Pentose and Base Moieties of Nucleotides

Keck *et al.* (1966) reported that irradiation of adenosine monophosphate (AMP) in deoxygenated solutions resulted in attachment of the ribose to the base at the C(8) position, giving a cyclonucleotide. Raleigh and Kramers (1975) have identified the compound as the 8,5' cyclo-compound. The yield is equal to the yield for inorganic phosphate release over a wide pH range and is doubled when N_2O is substituted for oxygen (N_2O converts e_{aq}^- to ·OH), suggesting that ·OH brings about the reaction. Oxygen inhibits formation of the cyclonucleotide. Attack on the base by the lesion on the pentose moiety may be a significant event in the radiolysis of intact DNA, in which bases appear to be at least partly shielded from attack by ·OH (Ward, 1975).

5.3. Attachment of Bases to Nucleic Acids

Nucleic acid bases become attached to RNA (Sigma Type XI from Baker's yeast) when aqueous solutions (about 1% RNA, 5×10^{-4} M bases) are exposed to γ-rays at near neutral pH (Yamamoto, 1973). The criterion for attachment was precipitation of the bases ([[14C] labeled) with RNA by 5% trichloroacetic acid. Binding yields in the presence of air were less than 1% of the starting materials for doses up to 10^6 rads, and were less than yields for binding to serum albumin (25-45%) under comparable conditions. In the absence of air, binding yields were likewise small when an ·OH scavenger such as methanol or thiocyanate was present. With a nitrogen atmosphere and no ˙OH scavenger, binding yields of about 1.5% were obtained for pyrimidine bases, and about 0.5% for purine bases. With N_2O, which converts e_{aq}^- to ˙OH, binding yields in solution were increased to about 2% (4.8×10^4 rads) for pyrimidines and 1% for purines. This results suggest that the binding reaction is initiated by ˙OH, but the reaction mechanisms and product structures are unknown.

5.4.   Cross-linking of Nucleic Acids

Cross-linking of DNA with DNA has been observed on irradiation of isolated salmon or herring sperm DNA containing 0 to 300% of its weight in water (Lett *et al.*, 1961; Lett and Alexander, 1961). The criteria used to establish occurrence of cross-linking was a combination of measurements of viscosity, radius of gyration, and determination of molecular weight by light scattering. The radiation was 1-2 MeV electrons; doses were of the order of a megarad. The cross-linkage reaction competes with chain scission. In dry DNA or DNA containing 25% of its weight in water, cross-linking predominates slightly with the result that branched molecules are formed. Oxygen decreases the yield of cross-links slightly. Increasing the water content to 200% of the weight of DNA increased the amount of cross-linking in the absence of oxygen, and resulted in the formation of a gel by a dose of 10^6 rads. Oxygen has a greater inhibitory effect in moist than in dry DNA. Further increases in water content gave a relative increase in the scission reaction; with water contents greater than 300% no gel was formed. It is hypothesized that the absorption of energy from the radiation by DNA causes a rupture of the chain with the formation of "active centers," probably free radicals. Under sterically favorable conditions, two of these combine to give a cross-link if no oxygen is present. Small amounts of water increase the probability of the active centers coming together, but larger amounts increase the efficiency of degradation processes.

Radiolysis of DNA from *E. coli* bacteriophage T1 in dilute aqueous solution (200 µg DNA/ml, 0.165 M NaCl) gave a small yield of cross-links up to doses of about 2 krads. No further cross-linkage occured as the dose was increased (Coquerelle *et al.*, 1969). When the intact phage was irradiated under conditions in which most of the products of water radiolysis are scavenged it was found that per inactivated phage, 0.03 DNA-DNA cross-links were formed. This yield is small compared with other lesions: 3.5 single-strand breaks, 0.17 double-strand breaks, and 0.06 DNA-protein cross-links (Bohne *et al.*, 1970).

Recent results indicate that the decay of tritium situated at the 2-position of adenine causes cross-linking between the strands of double-stranded DNA. Cross-linkage does not occur if the tritium is at any other position on adenine or on the other bases. The 2-position of adenine faces the second DNA strand (personal communication from S. Person reporting work done with F. Hutchinson and F. Krasin).

6. REACTIONS WITH RADIATION SENSITIZERS (TABLE 4)

The sensitizers considered here are substances which increase the sensitivity of living cells, usually relatively anoxic, to the effects of ionizing radiation. They must not be confused with the sensitizers used in photochemistry.

6.1. 5-Bromouracil (BrUra)

Under certain conditions, this substance can be made to replace some of the thymine in DNA. Cells in which such replacement has been made are generally more radiosensitive than normal cells. A chemical mechanism to explain the increased sensitivity has been proposed (Adams, 1967; Zimbrick *et al.*, 1969a, b). BrUra reacts with electrons by a rapid dissociative attachment reaction to give a uracilyl radical (Ura·).

(6-1)

The electron source may be a hydrated electron, an anion radical such as ·COO⁻, or some other substance capable of transferring an electron. Ura· is highly reactive and will add a hydrogen atom from a donor to form Ura and another organic free radical.

$$\text{Ura·} \quad + \quad \text{HR} \longrightarrow \text{Ura} \quad + \quad \text{·R} \qquad (6\text{-}2)$$

The donor may well be a neighboring pentose moiety on the DNA main chain. An alternative reaction of the uracilyl radical is addition of oxygen (Gilbert *et al.*, 1971; Gilbert and Wagner, 1972). The rate constant for oxygen addition is 24 times greater than that for H-abstraction from methanol (which should behave kinetically somewhat like the deoxyribose moiety of DNA). Which reaction occurs will depend on the local oxygen concentration. If the abstraction reaction occurs, the DNA will have a foreign base,

Table 4. Attachment Reactions of Nucleic Acids Induced by Ionizing
Radiations: Radiation Sensitizers

Compound	Nucleic acid derivative	Reference
Electrons	5-Bromouracil (BrUra)	Adams, 1967; Zimbrick *et al.*, 1969a
"	BrUra-DNA	Zimbrick *et al.*, 1969b
N-Ethylmaleimide	Thy-˙OH adduct radical	Ward *et al.*, 1969
"	DNA	Johansen *et al.*, 1968
Nitrofurazone	"	Chapman *et al.*, 1972
"	"	Chapman *et al.*, 1973
Metronidazole	"	Willson *et al.*, 1974
TAN	Thy-˙OH adduct	Willson and Emmerson, 1968; Cadet *et al.*, 1975
"	Base-˙OH adducts	Brustad *et al.*, 1972; Wold and Brustad, 1973
"	DNA *in vitro*	Brustad *et al.*, 1971
"	"	Wold and Brustad, 1974

uracil, and a lesion on a deoxyribose moiety which may lead to a
strand break or other chemical change. If oxygen adds, a peroxy-
radical will be present in the DNA where a thymine base ought to
be. Either event would be expected to cause difficulty in DNA
function.

6.2. N-Ethylmaleimide (NEM)

This compound, when present in solution during irradiation,
sensitizes anoxic cells to the lethal effects of ionizing radiation.
It undergoes several kinds of reactions, including binding to DNA,
which may contribute to its effects. The binding is dose dependent
and appears to involve a reaction between DNA radicals and NEM
molecules. Oxygen competes with NEM for binding sites, and in oxygen saturated solutions, the binding of NEM does not occur (Johansen *et al.*, 1968; Ward *et al.*, 1969).

A suggestion as to the mechanism of binding has been obtained
in model experiments with thymine and other bases. These show that
NEM binds to the Thy-˙OH adduct radical. It also is expected to
bind at a radical site formed by H˙ abstraction from the pentose
moiety of DNA. At either site, competition with oxygen would be
expected.

The relation between NEM binding and sensitization of DNA is

not certain because NEM undergoes other reactions. It reacts
rapidly with e_{aq}^- and $\cdot OH$ [$k(e_{aq}^- + NEM) = 3.2 \times 10^{10}$ M^{-1} s^{-1},
$k(\cdot OH + NEM) = 5 \times 10^9$ M^{-1} s^{-1}], with Thy-$\cdot OH$ adduct in part by
electron transfer, and with other base radicals. It is certain,
however, that in cellular systems, NEM will react with organic
radicals produced by radiation, thus altering yields and types of
radiation-induced products.

6.3. Nitrofurans

Various derivatives of nitrofuran appear to have good potential as sensitizing agents in anoxic or hypoxic cells. Many of
these compounds have the general structure:

$$\text{[structure]} = RX \qquad (6\text{-}3)$$

Nitrofurazone is R-CH=NNHCONH$_2$. Metronidazole has a somewhat
different structure:

$$\text{[structure]} \qquad (6\text{-}4)$$

Structures of related compounds are given by Chapman *et al.* (1973b).

These compounds undergo several reactions in irradiated systems.
Among them are reactions with e_{aq}^-, with $\cdot OH$, with organic free
radicals (observed with metronidazole), binding with DNA, and
binding with protein (observed with nitrofurazone) (Chapman *et al.*,
1972; Chapman *et al.*, 1973a; Willson *et al.*, 1974). The binding
reaction with DNA is decreased by oxygen, i.e., the sensitizer and
oxygen appear to compete for the same site. Conditions for binding
indicate that the sensitizer molecule reacts with a DNA free radical generated by $\cdot OH$. The binding efficiency is small, only about
4% with metronidazole, but since the amount of binding required
for cell death is unknown, it is possible that the reaction may
play an important role in sensitization.

6.4. TAN (2,2,6,6-tetramethyl-4-piperidone-N-oxyl)

Since the report by Emmerson and Howard-Flanders (1964) of the ability of nitroxides to sensitize anoxic cells to radiation, this family of compounds has been studied extensively. The compounds differ from the other sensitizing agents discussed above in that they are "stable" free radicals, i.e., they have an unpaired electron. The structure of TAN is:

$$\text{(6-5)}$$

This compound reacts with the Thy-·OH adduct with the large bimolecular rate constants k = 3.5 × 10^8 M^{-1} s^{-1} (Emmerson and Willson, 1968). Similar values have been obtained for reaction with Cyt-·OH and Gua-·OH, but the adenine adduct appears to react much more slowly (k < 10^{-7} M^{-1} s^{-1}) (Brustad et al., 1972). The adenosine-·OH adduct reacts normally (Wold and Brustad, 1973). The major products of the reaction with Thy-·OH adduct (Cadet et al., 1975) have been identified as the cis- and trans-isomers of TAN-Thy-·OH adducts in which attachment has occurred by radical-radical reactions.

$$\text{(6-6)}$$

A minor product was the product of a reaction with the methyl group, also a radical-radical reaction as shown in Eq. (6-7). Radiolysis of thymidine in the presence of TAN gives a mixture of pyrimidine and nucleoside products. The binding of TAN to sugar free radicals seems to be a minor process. The main thymidine products were identified as the (+) and (-) diastereoisomers of cis- and trans-TAN-Thy-·OH adducts with the TAN on the 6-position of the

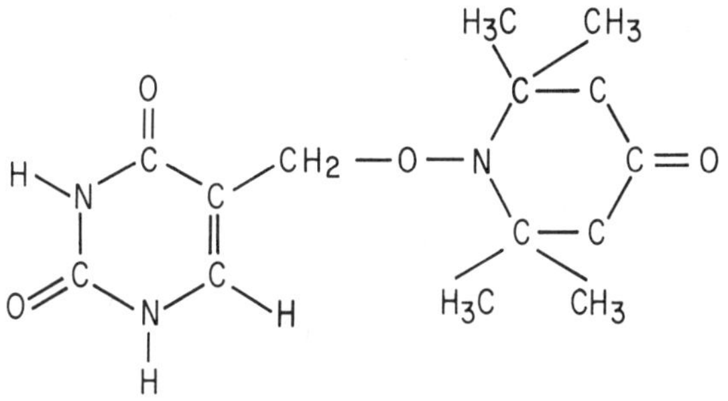

$$
\begin{array}{c}
H_3C \quad CH_3 \\
\end{array}
$$

(structure of thymine-TAN adduct)

$$(6-7)$$

pyrimidine ring.

In experiments with DNA (calf thymus) it has been found that TAN binds with DNA radicals (Brustad *et al.*, 1971) induced primarily by reactions of ·OH with the DNA. In addition to binding, TAN reacts with a transient DNA species by electron transfer, to give reduced TAN.

The binding of TAN to DNA during and immediately after the irradiation of *E. coli* K-12 has been observed and compared with the degree of sensitization (Wold and Brustad, 1974). These experiments made use of the long lifetimes of DNA radicals. It was found that binding can occur without sensitization, but radio-sensitization is always accompanied by some binding. It may be that binding is necessary, but not sufficient, for sensitization. It also was noted that sensitization is delayed compared with entrance of TAN into the bacterium, suggesting that the lethal event may be interaction of TAN with sterically hindered DNA radical sites in base pairs.

7. IMPORTANCE OF ATTACHMENT REACTIONS IN RADIATION BIOLOGY

In the foregoing material it has been shown that explanations of effects of ionizing radiations on living organisms are by no means complete, and that mechanisms for modifying radiation effects are even less well understood. It has also been pointed out on the basis of fundamental concepts that the environment within a cell is such that complex radiation-induced reactions between different substances should be expected and that these should include attachment reactions. The possibility of such reactions has been confirmed by studies with model systems which have shown that attachment and other reactions occur between nucleic acid constituents and numerous compounds related to those existing in the vicinity of nucleic acids in cells. Studies of reaction mechanisms have shown that many of the reactions take place by radical-molecule reactions, with the radical sometimes initially on the nucleic acid constituent and sometimes on the other molecule.

Other attachment reactions have been shown to occur by radical-radical reactions. Radiation modifiers have been shown to become attached to nucleic acids *in vitro* and *in vivo*, and there are indications that attachment may be necessary for the action of certain sensitizers.

This accumulated evidence suggests that further investigation of attachment and related reactions which may be reasonably expected to occur in cells will be an important and critical part of our continuing efforts to understand radiation effects and develop ways to modify them.

Acknowledgment. Preparation of this article and work done in the author's laboratory was supported by the U.S. Energy Research and Development Administration.

References

Adams, G.E., 1967, The general applications of pulse radiolysis to current problems in radiobiology, *Current Topics Radiat. Res.* 3:37-93.

Adams, G.E., Michael, B.D., and Willson, R.L., 1968, Electron studies by pulse radiolysis, *in* "Radiation Chemistry" (E.J. Hart, ed.), Advances in Chemistry, Series 81, American Chemical Society, Washington, D.C., Vol. I, pp. 289-308.

Andersson, L.O., 1969, Coupling of dyes to various macromolecules by means of gamma-irradiation, *Nature* 220:374-375.

Arthur, J.C., 1970, Graft polymerization onto polysaccharides, *in* "Advances in Macromolecular Chemistry" (W.M. Pasika, ed.), Academic Press, New York, Vol. 2, pp. 1-87.

Bohne, L., Coquerelle, Th., and Hagen, U., 1970, Radiation sensitivity of bacteriophage DNA. II. Breaks and cross-links after irradiation *in vivo*, *Int. J. Radiat. Biol.* 17:205-215.

Brown, P.E., Calvin, M., Newmark, J.F., 1966, Thymine addition to ethanol: induction by gamma irradiation, *Science* 151:68-70.

Brustad, T., 1971, Covalent binding of an organic nitroxide free radical to radiation-induced lysozyme transients under anoxic conditions, *Int. J. Radiat. Phys. Chem.* 3:63-69.

Brustad, T., Bugge, H., Jones, W.B.G., and Wold, E., 1972, Reactions between organic nitroxyl free radicals and radiation-induced transicents in the DNA bases, *Int. J. Radiat. Biol.* 22:115-129.

Brustad, T., Jones, W.B.G., and Nakken, K.F., 1971, On the binding of an organic nitroxide free radical to radiation-induced deoxyribonucleic acid (DNA) radicals under anoxic conditions, *Int. J. Radiat. Phys. Chem.* 3:55-61.

Byfield, J.E., Lee, Y.C., Bennett, L.R., 1970, Bonding of small molecules to DNA following ionizing radiation, *Nature* 225:859-860.

Cadet, J., Guttin-Lombard, M., and Teoule, R., 1975, Gamma

radiolysis of thymine and thymidine in deaerated aqueous solutions containing electron affinic radiosensitizers: formation and identification of stable adducts, Abstr. Int. Symp. "Protein and Other Adducts to DNA: Their Significance to Aging, Carcinogenesis and Radiation Biology," Williamsburg, Virginia, May 2-6, 1975.

Cadet, J., and Teoule, R., 1972, γ-irradiation of thymidine in aerated aqueous solution, *Tetrahedron Lett.* 31:3225-3228.

Cerutti, P.A., 1974, Effects of ionizing radiation on mammalian cells, *Naturwiss.* 61:51-59.

Chan, E.W., and Ball, J.K., 1971, Polycyclic aromatic hydrocarbons: covalent binding to DNA and effects on template function, *Biochim. Biophys. Acta* 238:46-59.

Chapman, J.D., Greenstock, C.L., Reuvers, A.P., McDonald, E., and Dunlop, I., 1973a, Radiation chemical studies with nitrofurazone as related to its mechanism of radiosensitization, *Radiat. Res.* 53:190-203.

Chapman, J.D., Reuvers, A.P., and Borsa, J., 1973b, Effectiveness of nitrofuran derivatives in sensitizing hypoxic mammalian cells to x-rays, *Brit. J. Radiol.* 46:623-630.

Chapman, J.D., Reuvers, A.P., Borsa, J., Petkau, A., and McCalla, D.R., 1972, Nitrofurans as radiosensitizers of hypoxic mammalian cells, *Cancer Res.* 32:2630-2632.

Coquerelle, T., Bohne, L., and Hagen, U., 1969, Radiation sensitivity of bacteriophage DNA I: breaks and crosslinks after irradiation *in vitro*, *Z. Naturforsch.* 24b:885-893.

Dole, Malcolm (ed.), 1973, "The Radiation Chemistry of Macromolecules" Vols. I and II, Academic Press, New York.

Elad, D., Rosenthal, I., and Steinmaus, H., 1969, Radiation- and ultraviolet-induced reactions of caffeine with alcohols, *Chem. Commun.* pp. 305-306.

Elad, D., and Salomon, J., 1971, Ultraviolet- and radiation-induced reactions of caffeine with amines, *Tetrahedron Lett.* 50:4783-4784.

Emmerson, P.T., and Howard-Flanders, P., 1964, Sensitization of anoxic bacteria to x-rays by di-t-butyl nitroxide and analogues, *Nature* 204:1005-1006.

Emmerson, P.T., and Willson, R.L., 1968, Pulse radiolysis of aqueous solutions of thymine and triacetoneamine n-oxyl, *J. Phys. Chem.* 72:3669-3671.

Freifelder, D., 1974, Radiobiology of simple microbiol systems, *in* "Physical Mechanisms in Radiation Biology" (R.D. Cooper and R.W. Wood, eds.), U.S. Atomic Energy Commission Report CONF-271001, pp. 207-219.

Gilbert, E., and Wagner, G., 1972, Photochemistry of 5-ioduracil in aqueous oxygenated solution in presence of primary and secondary alcohols, *Z. Naturforsch.* 27b:644-648.

Gilbert, E., Wagner, G., and Schulte-Frohlinde, D., 1971, Photochemistry of 5-iodouracil in aqueous solution in presence of oxygen and methanol, *Z. Naturforsch.* 26b:209-213.

Gräslund, A., Ehrenberg, A., Rupprecht, A., and Strom, G., 1971,
    Ionic base radicals in γ-irradiated DNA, *Biochim. Biophys.
    Acta* 254:172-186.
Hartig, G., and Dertinger, H., 1971, A computer-controlled EPR
    analysis of free radical formation in dry thymine and deriva-
    tives after electron irradiation, *Int. J. Radiat. Biol.* 20:
    577-588.
Holian, J., and Garrison, W.M., 1969, Reconstitution mechanisms in
    the radiolysis of aqueous biochemical systems: inhibitive
    effects of thiols, *Nature* 221:57.
Infante, G.A., Jirathana, P., Fendler, J.H., and Fendler, E.J.,
    1973, Radiolysis of pyrimidines in aqueous solutions. I.
    Product formation in the interaction of e^-_{aq}, ˙H, ˙OH, and
    ˙Cl^-_2 with thymine, *J. Chem. Soc. Faraday Trans. I.* 69:1586-
    1596.
Johansen, I., Ward, J.F., Siegel, K., and Sletten, A., 1968, X-ray
    induced binding of n-ethylmaleimide to DNA in aqueous solution,
    Biochem. Biophys. Res. Commun. 33:949-953.
Kamal, A., and Garrison, W.M., 1965, Radiolytic degradation of
    aqueous cytosine: enhancement by a second organic solute,
    Nature 206:1315-1317.
Keck, K., Hagen, U., and Friebolin, H., 1966, Bildung eines cyclo-
    nucleotids bei röntgenbestrahlung von adenosin-monophosphat,
    Naturwiss. 53:204-205.
Leonov, D., and Elad, D., 1974a, Photochemical and γ-ray-induced
    reactions of nucleic acid constituents. Suppression of the
    reactivity of pyrimidines in the presence of purines, *J.
    Am. Chem. Soc.* 96:5635-5637.
Leonov, D., and Elad, D., 1974b, Ultraviolet- and γ-ray-induced
    reactions of nucleic acid constituents. Reactions of purines
    with ethers and dioxane, *J. Org. Chem.* 39:1470-1473.
Leonov, D., Salomon, J., Sasson, S., and Elad, D., 1973, Ultraviolet-
    and γ-ray-induced reactions of nucleic acid constituents with
    alcohols. On the selectivity of these reactions for purines,
    Photochem. Photobiol. 17:465-468.
Lett, J.T., and Alexander, P., 1961, Crosslinking and degradation
    of deoxyribonucleic acid gels with varying water contents when
    irradiated with electrons, *Radiat. Res.* 15:159-173.
Lett, J.T., Stacey, K.A., and Alexander, P., 1961, Crosslinking of
    dry deoxyribonucleic acids by electrons, *Radiat. Res.* 14:349-
    362.
Myers, L.S., Jr., 1973a, Free radical damage of nucleic acids and
    their components by ionizing radiation, *Fed. Proc.* 32:1882-
    1894.
Myers, L.S., Jr., 1973b, Radiation chemistry of nucleic acids,
    proteins, and polysaccharides, *in* "The Radiation Chemistry
    of Macromolecules" (M. Dole, ed.), Academic Press, Inc. New
    York, Vol. II, pp. 323-374.
Myers, L.S., Jr., 1974, Radiation effects on simple biological sys-
    tems, *in* "Physical Mechanisms in Radiation Biology" (R.D.

Cooper and R.W. Wood, eds.), U.S. Atomic Energy Commission, CONF-721001 (available from Natl. Techn. Information Services, U.S. Dept. of Commerce, Springfiled, Va. 22151), pp. 185-206.

Namiki, M., and Hayashi, T., 1970, Radiation-induced thymine formation from thymine glycol, *Int. J. Radiat. Biol.* 17:197-200.

Raleigh, J.A., and Kremers, W., 1975, Intramolecular transfer of radiation damage in γ-irradiated nucleotides: 8,5'-cyclo-adenosine 5'monophosphate (8,5'-cyclo AMP), Abstract Fe-4, 23rd Annual Meeting of the Radiation Research Society, Miami, Beach, Fla., May 11-15, 1975.

Salomon, J., and Elad, D., 1974, Ultraviolet and γ-ray-induced reactions of nucleic acid constituents. Reactions of purines with amines, *Photochem. Photobiol.* 19:21-27.

Scholes, G., 1968, Radiolysis of nucleic acids and their components in aqueous solutions, *in* "Radiation Chemistry of Aqueous Systems," (G. Stein, ed.), Weizman Science Press, Jerusalem, pp. 259-285.

Scholes, G., Ward, J.F., and Weiss, J., 1960, Mechanism of the radiation induced degradation of nucleic acids, *J. Mol. Biol.* 2:379-391.

Scholes, G., Willson, R.L., and Ebert, M., 1969, Pulse radiolysis of aqueous solutions of deoxyribonucleotides and of DNA: Reactions with hydroxy-radicals, *Chem. Commun.* 17-18.

Schweibert, M.C., and Daniels, M., 1971, ^{60}Co γ-ray induced peroxidation of DNA in aqueous solution, *Int. J. Radiat. Phys. Chem.* 3:353-366.

Shragge, P.C., Varghese, A.J., Hunt, J.W., and Greenstock, C.L., 1974, Radiolysis of uracil in the absence of oxygen, *Radiat. Res.* 60:250-267.

Smith, K.C., 1975, The radiation induced addition of proteins and other molecules to nucleic acids, *in* "Photochemistry and Photobiology of Nucleic Acids" (S.Y. Wang, ed.), Academic Press, New York (in press).

Smith, K.C., and Hays, J.E., 1968, The response of uracil-2-^{14}C to x-irradiation under nitrogen and oxygen and to treatment with ascorbic acid, *Radiat. Res.* 33:129-141.

Stankunas, A., Rosenthal, I., and Pitts, J.N., Jr., 1971, Photochemical and radiochemical alkylation of caffeine by alkyl amines, *Tetrahedron Lett.* 50:4779-4782.

Steinmaus, H., Rosenthal, I., and Elad, D., 1969, Photochemical and γ-ray-induced reactions of purines and purine nucleosides with 2-propanol, *J. Am. Chem. Soc.* 91:4921-4923.

Steinmaus, H., Rosenthal, I., and Elad, D., 1971, Light- and γ-ray-induced reactions of purines and purine nucleosides with alcohols, *J. Org. Chem.* 36:3594-3598.

Teoule, R., and Cadet, J., 1975, ESR spectra and radiolysis products of thymine and thymidine, *Int. J. Radiat. Biol.* (in press).

Teoule, R., Cadet, J., and Polverelli, M., 1972, Effets des radiations sur les bases constitutives des acides nucleiques, *in* "Peaceful Uses of Atomic Energy" Int. Atomic Energy Agency,

Vienna, United Nations, New York, A/CONF/49/P/633, pp. 447-458.

Van Der Schans, G.P., and Bleichrodt, J.F., 1974, Contribution of various types of damage to inactivation of bacteriophage PM2 DNA in frozen solution by gamma radiation, *Int. J. Radiat. Biol.* 26:121-126.

Ward, J.F., 1975, Molecular mechanisms of radiation induced damage to nucleic acids, *Adv. Radiat. Biol.* 5:181-239.

Ward, J.F., Johansen, I., and Aasen, J., 1969, Radiosensitization by N-ethyl maleimide-a model chemical system, *Int. J. Radiat. Biol.* 15:163-170.

Willson, R.L., Cramp, W.A., and Ings, R.M.J., 1974, Metronidazole ('flagyl'): mechanisms of radiosensitization, *Int. J. Radiat. Biol.* 26:557-569.

Wold, E., and Brustad, T., 1973, Reactions between nitroxyl free radicals and radiation-induced transients in nucleosides, *Int. J. Radiat. Biol.* 24:153-160.

Wold, E., and Brustad, T., 1974, Binding of nitroxyls to radiation-induced DNA-transients in *E. coli* K-12 under *in vivo* conditions and its relevance for radiosensitization, *Int. J. Radiat. Biol.* 25:225-233.

Yamamoto, O., 1973, Radiation-induced binding of nucleic acid constituents with protein constituents and with each other, *Int. J. Radiat. Phys. Chem.* 5:213-229.

Zarebska, Z., and Shugar, D., 1972, Radio-products of thymine in the presence of ethanol, *Int. J. Radiat. Biol.* 21:101-114.

Zimbrick, J.D., Ward, J.F., and Myers, L.S., Jr., 1969a, Studies on the chemical basis of cellular radiosensitization by 5-bromouracil substitution in DNA. I. Pulse and steady state radiolysis of 5-bromouracil and thymine, *Int. J. Radiat. Biol.* 16:505-523.

Zimbrick, J.D., Ward, J.F., and Myers, L.S., Jr., 1969b, Studies on the chemical basis of cellular radiosensitization by 5-bromouracil substitution in DNA. II. Pulse and steady state radiolysis of bromouracil substituted and unsubstituted DNA, *Int. J. Radiat. Biol.* 16:525-534.

REPAIR OF DNA ADDUCTS PRODUCED BY ALKYLATION

Bernard S. Strauss

Department of Microbiology, The University of Chicago

Chicago, Illinois 60637

1. INTRODUCTION

Auerbach and Robson's discovery (1942) that mustard gas is mutagenic was released after the close of the second World War (Auerbach and Robson, 1946, 1947) and quickly led to the finding that many simple alkylating agents are mutagenic. Some of these compounds were found to be useful in cancer chemotherapy because of their cytotoxic effect but, at the same time, were carcinogenic themselves, the ratio of therapeutic to carcinogenic activity varying mysteriously from compound to compound (see Whitelock, 1958). It was natural that the reactivity of these alkylating agents with cellular constituents should be investigated. The reactivity with protein was especially studied during the 1950's because of the general biochemical importance of this class of compound. However, the gradual acceptance of the view that the genetic material is only DNA focused attention on alkylation of this substance. The reaction of alkylating agents with nucleic acid, particularly with DNA has therefore been extensively studied during the 1960's and 1970's for the theoretical reason that mutation must involve a change in DNA structure, rather than because of any direct demonstration that alkylation of DNA is uniquely important. Demonstration of the metabolic activation of hydrocarbon and other carcinogens to form electrophilic reagents with the reactivity characteristic of alkylating agents (Cramer *et al.*, 1960; Miller *et al.*, 1960) intensified the search for DNA adducts since this discovery made it likely that the initial reaction leading to carcinogenesis must be the formation of a covalently bound adduct, presumably to DNA.

The result of the investigation of DNA adducts was, at first, confusing. The bifunctional alkylating agents were found to introduce cross-links into DNA (Geiduschek, 1961) and this reaction is likely to be cytotoxic and to lead to chromosomal but not to gene mutations. It was first proposed that the reaction of DNA with alkylating agents resulted in the formation of phosphotriesters (Stacey *et al.*, 1958). Later it was shown that the evidence was compatible with the formation of a 7-alkylguanine which was isolated as a major reaction product (Brookes and Lawley, 1961). Ten years later, phosphotriester formation was clearly demonstrated as a minor reaction pathway (Bannon and Verly, 1972) with the amount of reaction depending on the particular reagent. In addition, a number of other reaction products resulting from the interaction of DNA with alkylating agents were described (see Section 2) and helped account for what seemed an inexplicable specificity in the action of alkylating agents (Loveless, 1969).

An additional factor was introduced as a result of work in radiation biology and particularly as a result of the isolation of radiation-sensitive mutants (Hill, 1958) which by their existence demonstrated the importance of the response of the organism to a lesion. Adducts can be either removed (Setlow and Carrier, 1964) or by-passed (Rupp and Howard-Flanders, 1968). Consideration of the biological importance of a particular adduct therefore requires some information as to the permanence of that lesion in a particular organism and tissue. The discussion of DNA adducts must therefore be extended to include more than chemistry since a judgement of the relevance of particular adduct requires knowledge of whether it remains in the DNA and what its effect on DNA replication may be.

Although the chemical studies are quite advanced, biological evaluation of the importance of individual adducts is far from complete. This paper discusses some of the adducts produced, the repair mechanisms which affect their stability and the relevance of the findings to the processes of mutagenesis and carcinogenesis.

2. ADDUCTS TO DNA

Simple compounds can be both mutagenic and carcinogenic (Table 1). The particular listing shown is not meant to be exhaustive but rather is designed to indicate the large number of compounds of relatively simple structure which possess both important biological properties of mutagenicity and carcinogenicity.

Table 1.   Some Compounds Reported to be Both Mutagenic and
Carcinogenic (From Zimmerman, 1971)

Dimethyl-nitrosoamine	Diazomethane
Diethyl-nitrosamine	Dimethylsulphate
Methyl-vinyl-nitrosamine	Methylmethanesulfonate
Methyl-butylnitrosamine	Diethylsulphate
N-methyl-N'-nitrosopiperazine	β-Propiolactone
N-methyl-N-nitrosourea	Ethylenimine
N-methyl-N-nitrosourethane	Triethylene melamine
1-Methyl-3-nitro-1-nitrosoguanidine	1,2:3,4-Diepoxybutane
N-methyl-N-nitrosoacetamide	1,2-Dimethyl-hydrazine
N-ethyl-N-nitrosourea	Nitrogen mustards
N-butyl-N-nitrosourea	Sulfur mustards
1-Nitroso-imidazolidone-2	Propanesultone

The simplicity of the compounds discourages any attempt to understand the process by a listing of substances which are carcinogenic,
particularly in view of the wide range of possible products which
occur as a result of the reaction of these compounds with cells.
This complexity can be illustrated by diagramming a section of a
DNA chain with the possible reaction sites with electrophilic reagents indicated by arrows (Fig. 1). If it is possible to write a
theoretical reaction between an alkylating, electrophilic reagent
and some reactive group in the DNA, then that reaction has already
been demonstrated or, I suppose, will be demonstrated shortly
(Table 2)! The relative proportion of reaction products is determined both by the reaction site and by the nature of the alkylating
agents which therefore show specificity even though the N-7 position of guanine is the most reactive site for most, but not all,
electrophilic reagents (Lawley, 1974a).

Unfortunately, organic chemistry tells us only little of
biological importance because of the implications of Avogadros
number.   I calculate that a relatively rare reaction product,
formed to an extent of only one per cent of the total and acting
with an efficiency of one per cent is still capable of producing
important biological effects although almost impossible to detect
radiochemically (Table 3). Notwithstanding this difficulty of
direct detection, such a product, if it is excised, will induce
sufficient repair synthesis to be easily observed (Table 4).

Chemical methodology is therefore necessary but not sufficient
for the identification of the biologically important reaction pro-
duct(s) although there is, of course, no *a priori* reason why the
major chemical reaction should not also be the major biological
reaction.   However, the evidence is clear that the major reaction
product of alkylation, the 7-alkyl derivative of guanine, is

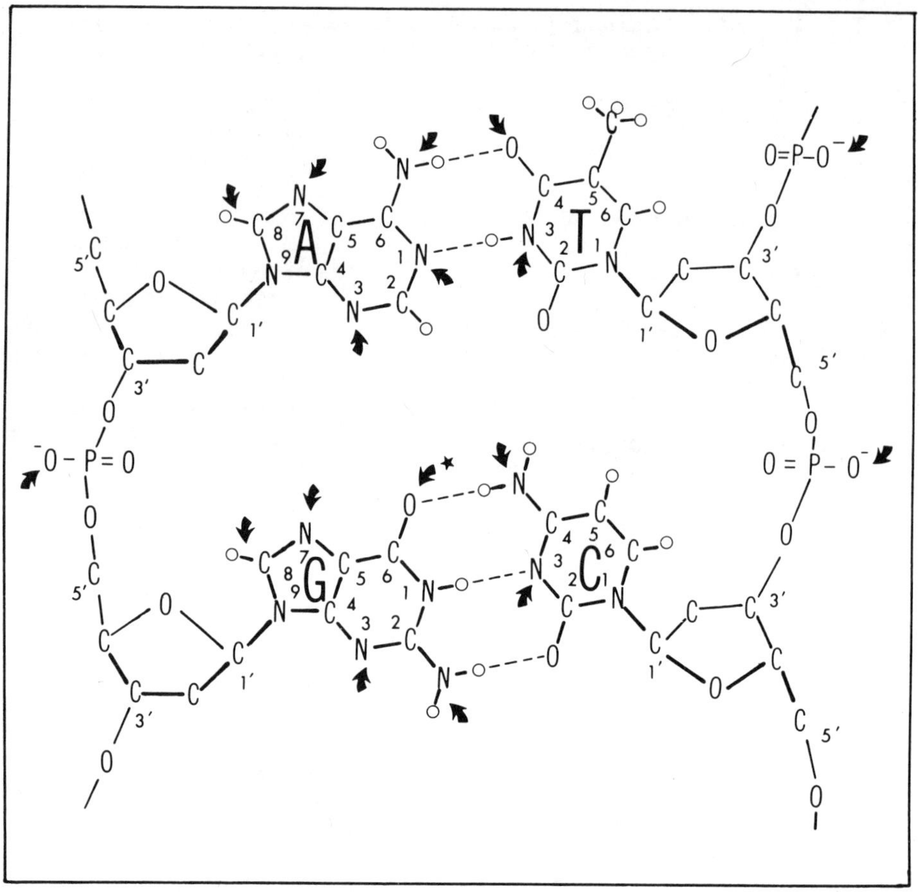

Fig. 1.   Section of DNA showing reported sites of reaction
with electrophilic reagent (see legend to Table 2 for references).

largely ignored by cells since bacteria methylated with MMS* are
able to replicate the methylated DNA without extensive excision
(Prakash and Strauss, 1970), and direct determinations by Lawley
and Orr (1970) indicate that the production of 7-methyl guanine
does not make DNA a substrate for the DNA excision repair system
and that the adduct is lost only by spontaneous (chemical)

---

*Abbreviations: AAAF, N-acetoxy-2-acetylaminofluorene; BMBA,
7-bromomethyl benz (α) anthracene; BND-cellulose, benzoylated
naphthoylated DEAE cellulose; BrdUrd, bromodeoxyuridine; MMS,
methyl methanesulfonate; MNNG, N-methyl-N'-nitro-N-nitrosoguanidine;
MNNU, methyl nitrosourea; dT, thymidine; HPBL, human peripheral
blood lymphocytes.

Table 2. Sites of Reaction in DNA of Several Alkylating Agents

Reaction site in DNA		Compounds				
		MMS[1]	MNNG[2]	MNNU[3]	BMBA[4]	AAAF[5]
Adenine	1	++	+	+		
	3	++	++	++		
	6-NH$_2$				+	+
	7			+		
	8					+
Guanine	2-NH$_2$				+++	
	3	±	+	+		
	6-0	±	++	++		
	7	+++	+++	+++		
	8					+++
Thymine	3			±		
	4-0			±		
Cytosine	3	+	+	+		
	4-NH$_2$				+	
Phosphate		+		++		

(Note: lack of entry means only that a reaction has not been reported)
[1]Lawley and Shah, 1972.
[2]Lawley and Thatcher, 1970.
[3]Lawley and Shah, 1973; Lawley, 1973.
[4]Dipple *et al.*, 1971.
[5]Miller and Miller, 1969.

depurination in both bacterial and mammalian cells.

Apurinic (and apyrimidinic) sites are the end result of alkylation reactions which result in quaternary ring nitrogens destabilizing the glycosidic bond in DNA (Lawley and Brookes, 1963). Large numbers of such sites result from alkylation. In a recent experiment (Scudiero *et al.*, 1975) we found that treatment of HEp.2 cells with 2.5 mM MMS for 1 h would add about 2.8×10^{12} methyl groups per µg to the DNA. Depurination occurs simultaneously with the methylation reaction and we estimate that a 1 h treatment with MMS followed by a 1 h post-treatment incubation would result in about 6×10^{10} apurinic sites per µg, or, since there are about 12 pg of DNA per HEp.2 cell, about 7.4×10^5 apurinic sites per cell. Since the apurinic site is a good substrate for endonuclease action (Hadi and Goldthwait, 1971; Ljungquist and Lindahl, 1974), these sites should be quickly

Table 3. The Inefficiency of Radiochemical Methods as Compared to Biological Tests for the Detection of Minor Alkylation Products.

---

1. Lawley and Thatcher (1970) show that 0.23 mM MNNG yields 2.3 μmol of methyl groups per gram of DNA.

2. Assume a minor reaction product is formed to only 1% of the total and that mutation occurs 1% of the time at this minor reaction site. There will then be 2.3×10^{-4} μmol of methyl groups per gram of DNA at which mutation occurs, corresponding to 2.3×10^{-10} mol $\times$ 6.023 $\times 10^{23}$ molec/mol = 1.38×10^{14} methyl groups at which mutation occurs per gram of DNA. Since there are 4.2×10^{-15} g DNA per *Escherichia coli* there are 0.58 mutations induced per *E. coli*. Assuming 4000 genes per *E. coli*, this corresponds to an induced mutation frequency of 0.58/4000 = 1.4×10^{-4} mutations per gene per *E. coli*. Such mutation frequencies are readily detected using no more than about 10^7 organisms.

3. Suppose that MNNG is available at 3 mCi/mmol (1.6×10^9 cpm/mmol at an actual counting efficiency), then 2.3 μmol of methyl groups per gram of DNA = 3.7×10^6 cpm/g DNA for all products and 3.7×10^4 cpm/g DNA for a minor reaction product formed to one percent of the total. Since there are 4.2×10^{-15} g DNA/*E. coli*, there will be $3.7 \times 10^4 \times 4.2 \times 10^{-15} = 1.55 \times 10^{-10}$ cpm/organism. At least 10,000 more organisms would be required to barely detect a rare product radiochemically than would be required to detect induced mutation (e.g., at least 10^{11} organisms to give 15 cpm above background).

---

converted into single-strand breaks leading to single-strand pieces of about 10^7 daltons. Lindahl and Nyberg (1972) calculate that a mammalian cell spontaneously loses about 10^4 purines in a cell cycle of 20 h or about 10^3 in a 2 h period. The alkylation-induced frequency of apurinic sites at a dose leading to about ten per cent survival (Coyle *et al.*, 1971) is therefore about 740 times the spontaneous frequency. There must be very active repair mechanisms which restore DNA damaged by spontaneous depurination and these processes might be able to cope with some of the apurinic sites resulting from the aftermath of alkylation. Although apurinic sites might well be lethal once the repair mechanisms are saturated and at a level 700 times the spontaneous, it is hard to imagine that a product formed in such large numbers as a result of spontaneous processes should produce significant amounts of mutation or be responsible for carcinogenesis. It may be that faithful repair of such lesions always occurs and that the alternative is inactivation, not post-replication repair (see Section 3).

The discovery of the minor alkylation product, O^6 alkylguanine

Table 4. The Relative Efficiency of Repair Measurements for the
Detection of Minor Reaction Sites at which Excision Occurs

---

1. Suppose that treatment with an alkylating agent results in
a variety of methylated sites in DNA. If the alkylating agent is
radioactive, the reaction will produce: $(m \cdot s_1 \cdot e \cdot C/A)$ cpm per unit
of DNA, where m is the total number of methylations of all sorts
per unit of DNA, s_1 is the specific radioactivity of the alkylating
agent in Ci/mmol, e is the efficiency of counting, C is the number
of disintegrations per Curie per minute and A is Avogadros number.

2. If repair of a fraction, f, of the alkylation products is
measured using thymidine of specific activity s_2 Ci/mmol, and if
an average of B nucleotide bases are inserted at each repaired
site, then, assuming a thymidylic acid content for eucaryotic DNA
of 30%, there will be $(s_2 \cdot C \cdot e/A)$ cpm per dT molecule and $(s_2 \cdot C \cdot e/A)$
$\cdot(0.3f \cdot m \cdot B)$ cpm per unit of DNA due to repair.

3. The relative detectability of a repair-inducing lesion
(present as any fraction, f, of the total lesions) will be:

$$\frac{(s_2 \cdot C \cdot e/A) \cdot (0.3f \cdot m \cdot B)}{(m \cdot s_1 \cdot e \cdot C/A)} = 0.3f \cdot B \ (s_2/s_1)$$

when both alkylating agent and thymidine are labeled with the same
isotope and therefore have the same counting efficiency.

4. As an example consider the repair of MNNG-induced lesions:
[^{3}H]MNNG = 3 mCi/mmol; [^{3}H]dT = 46 Ci/mmol; B = 50 for large patch
repair; f = 1% of MNNG lesions inducing large patch repair (probably a 7- to 10-fold underestimate); the ratio will be:

$$\frac{(0.3 \times 10^{-2} \times 50 \times 46 \times 10^3) \ \text{mCi/mmol}}{3 \ \text{mCi/mmol}} = 2,300$$

There will be over 2000 times more radioactivity introduced by
repair per unit of DNA than by direct alkylation assuming normally
available specific radioactivities and assuming a negligible thymidylic acid pool (Derivation by P. Karran).

---

by Loveless (1969) helped resolve many questions about the different specificity and mutagenicity of alkylating agents at equivalent
total alkylation levels. This adduct is recognized by the excision
repair system; it is not excised by the B_{s-1} *uvr*$^-$ *exr*$^-$ double mutant
of *E. coli* (Lawley and Orr, 1970). There are two general modes of
alkylation (see Lawley, 1974b). The first, S_N1 type, occurs with
unimolecular kinetics *via* an ionic intermediate. The second, S_N2
type, requires the formation of a transition complex and occurs with

bimolecular reaction kinetics. S_N1 type reagents such as MNNG are
more efficient in the formation of O^6 alkylguanine derivatives
although the separation is not absolute since S_N2 reagents do make
smaller amounts of O^6 alkylguanine and 3-alkylguanine. Consideration of the minor DNA reaction products such as O^6 methylguanine,
which interfere with H-bonding of the DNA molecule (Fig. 1), does
help to correlate the carcinogenicity of compounds with their
reaction products. The S_N1 type reagents seem to be more mutagenic
and carcinogenic, but, depending on the cell line, not necessarily
more lethal per mole of alkylation adduct than their S_N2 counterparts (Roberts *et al.*, 1971) and therefore the minor reaction products, such as the O^6 methylguanine derivative which is formed
more readily by S_N1 type reagents, are major candidates for consideration as the carcinogenic and mutagenic but not inactivating
lesions. However, I do not see how data on reactivity alone can
permit the choice of any particular minor reaction product as a
biologically significant lesion. For example, after many years of
effort, it now seems well established that the phosphotriesters
make up a significant fraction of the products formed as a result
of the reaction of S_N1 reagents with DNA both *in vitro* and *in vivo*
(Bannon and Verly, 1972; O'Connor *et al.*, 1975). Phosphotriester
formation does lead to chain breakage in RNA but not in DNA (Shooter
et al., 1974), but it is not known what biological effects might
result from the introduction of this particular adduct into DNA.

3. THE ROLE OF EXCISION REPAIR

The important biological problem, of course, is the identification of the lesions responsible for inactivation, for mutation
and for carcinogenesis. A variety of DNA adducts have been isolated
from animals fed alkylating agents or agents such as the nitrosamines
which give electrophilic intermediates as the result of metabolic
activation (Magee, 1969). The gamut of reaction products observed
in vitro can also be observed *in vivo* (as one example, see Craddock,
1973; 1975).

How are the important lesions to be identified? I propose,
as a working hypothesis, that the simplest test of the relevance
to carcinogenesis of a lesion or a compound is the induction or
inhibition of excision type repair. I think that the induction of
excision repair will turn out to be more closely correlated with
carcinogenicity than the mutagenic potential of particular compounds.
The importance of the excision repair system for carcinogenesis
and for some types of mutation can be illustrated by two correlations: a) the evidence that individuals with xeroderma pigmentosum
(XP) who are deficient in excision repair are particularly susceptible to squamous cell carcinoma (Robbins *et al.*, 1974), and the
finding that cells from XP patients are particularly susceptible
to induced mutation (Maher and McCormick, 1975); b) the observation

that there is an inverse correlation between the ability of a tissue
to excise a lesion and the development of tumors in that tissue.
Goth and Rajewsky (1974) have shown that the brain, which is relatively susceptible to tumorigenesis by N-ethyl-N-nitrosourea, is
deficient in its ability to excise 6-ethoxyguanine as compared to
liver, although 7-ethylguanine has a similar half-life in both
tissues. Nicoll *et al.* (1975) have shown that after a large dose
of dimethylnitrosamine, O^6-methylguanine is much longer lived in
the kidney than in the liver and it is in the kidney that tumors
develop. These authors (*loc. cit.*) propose that "the differing
susceptibilities of organs towards carcinogenic stimuli may be
determined by the ability to repair certain alterations produced
by the carcinogen in DNA."

I suggest that although there may be a good correlation between
carcinogenicity and mutagenicity, many mutagens may not be carcinogens. The operational identification of putative carcinogens can
therefore best be made by first measuring the ability of compounds
to elicit the reactions of excision repair or to inhibit the process
(Trosko *et al.*, 1975). Mutagens like BrdUrd, iododeoxyuridine,
and hydroxylamine which do not induce excision repair should not
be expected to be (efficient) carcinogens. This suggestion, which
clearly requires further testing against an extensive body of data,
does not require, or even suggest, that excision by itself is carcino-
genic--especially since the evidence suggests that the reverse is
true, and that *failure* of excision repair is identifiable with the
onset of carcinogenic reactions--but rather that excision repair
acts as the molecular analog of "immune surveillance" and that its
induction may signal the presence of biologically important potentially carcinogenic lesions. Those lesions which act to hold up
DNA synthesis, either by altering hydrogen bonding sites or by
sterically interfering with the polymerase reaction, but which
nonetheless can be bypassed by the special mechanisms of post-
replication repair (e.g., are not lethal) are likely to result in
DNA alterations which lead to tumorigenesis. Such adducts are
likely to be recognized by the scanning mechanism which selects
sections of the DNA for excision and replacement for the same
reason, e.g., because of the alteration of the DNA structure.

A second part of the hypothesis is that only those lesions
subject to large patch excision repair are likely to be carcinogenic.
Not all lethal lesions can be excised. For example, it seems
likely that BMBA produces lesions which block DNA synthesis but
which are not subject to excision [e.g., "inactivating lesions"
Freese (1971)]. The total number of adducts required to inhibit
DNA synthesis is the same for either AAAF or BMBA (Fig. 2a, b).
Nonetheless, AAAF adducts are excised much more rapidly than BMBA
(Fig. 3) and data in the literature (Venitt and Tarmy, 1972;
Lieberman and Dipple, 1972) suggest that only about 15% of the
BMBA lesions can be excised. It therefore seems likely that there

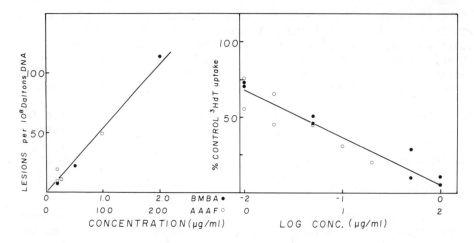

Fig. 2a. Fixation of AAAF or BMBA residues to DNA as a function of drug concentration. RAJI cells were reacted with labeled
drug and the DNA was isolated and purified by CsCl density gradient
centrifugation. The lesions fixed per 10^8 daltons DNA were determined from measurements of radioactivity and absorbancy at 260 nm
of DNA isolated at a density of 1.70. b. Inhibition of thymidine
incorporation as a function of AAAF or BMBA concentration. Cells
were incubated with drug and [^{3}H]dT (11 Ci/mmol; 1 μCi/ml) was
added for 15 min. Acid insoluble radioactivity was then determined (Unpublished data of P. Karran).

are lesions produced by BMBA addition to DNA which inhibit DNA
synthesis and are not excised and that the proportion of such
lesions is much smaller after AAAF treatment. It is those sites
susceptible to repair processes which are likely to be important
for carcinogenesis because it is at those sites that an abnormal
DNA replication may take place (see Section 4).

Excision repair can be readily detected after treatment of cells
with alkylating agents (Strauss, 1975). Different compounds produce different patterns of repair, and excision of certain adducts
might, theoretically, occur preferentially in certain parts of the
genome, such as the DNA growing point. We have recently developed
a simple methodology (Fig. 4) which permits the ready investigation of the different types of repair (Scudiero *et al.*, 1975).
This method depends upon the ability of columns of BND-cellulose
to distinguish fragments of DNA with single-stranded regions from
totally native regions. Such fragments adhere to the column and
elute with solutions of caffeine or formamide in contrast to fragments of native DNA which elute from the column with 1 M NaCl. In
the presence of an inhibitor of DNA synthesis such as hydroxyurea
or cytosine arabinoside, the progression of the DNA chain is

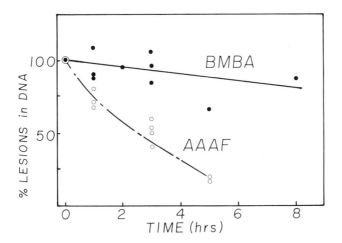

Fig. 3. Loss of radioactive AAAF or BMBA lesions from the DNA
of RAJI cells. Cells were treated at 37°C with concentrations of
[^{14}C]AAAF or [^{3}H]BMBA which gave approximately equal numbers of
lesions in the DNA. Following treatment, the cells were incubated
for the times indicated, harvested and the DNA was prepared and
purified by CsCl centrifugation. The experiments were performed
at concentrations of [^{3}H]BMBA of 0.2, 0.5 and 2 µg/ml and at concentrations of [^{14}C]AAAF of 25, 50 and 100 µg/ml. The number of
the lesions in the DNA immediately after treatment (t = 0) was
taken as 100% for each concentration used (Unpublished data of
P. Karran).

markedly slowed and isotope incorporated by residual semi-conservative synthesis remains in the growing point region. Since the
growing point contains single-stranded regions, isotope incorporated
by replicative synthesis will adhere to the column. In contrast,
isotope incorporated by repair synthesis will occur in both native
and replicating regions of the DNA and the native region will be
eluted by NaCl. After corrections for pool size are made, the
specific repair activity induced by any particular treatment can
be calculated from the radioactivity and absorbancy of the NaCl
eluate from a BND-cellulose column.

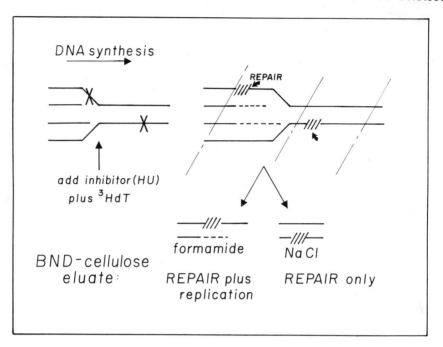

Fig. 4. The BND-cellulose method for the measurement of
excision repair.

We have shown that after treatment with alkylating agents the
NaCl eluate from the BND-cellulose column contains only isotope
incorporated by repair synthesis as demonstrated by experiments in
which cells were incubated with bromodeoxyuridine and hydroxyurea
after treatment with MMS, AAAF, or BMBA. In all cases isotope
was incorporated only into molecules of light buoyant density
(Scudiero *et al.*, 1975). Cells derived from an individual with
XP are unable to carry out excision type repair of AAAF as measured
with the BND-cellulose column (Fig. 5). XP cells have been reported
to repair X-ray induced damage (Kleijer *et al.*, 1970) and the repair
of MMS damage, like X-ray induced damage does not require the UV-
incision enzyme (Reiter and Strauss, 1965). The rate of repair as
measured by our method is proportional to the dose of compound
with which the cells are treated (Fig. 6). Furthermore, rough
calculations of the number of nucleotides incorporated per lesion
give values compatible with those obtained by other methods, particularly the ingenious technique of flash photolysis devised by
Regan and Setlow (1974).

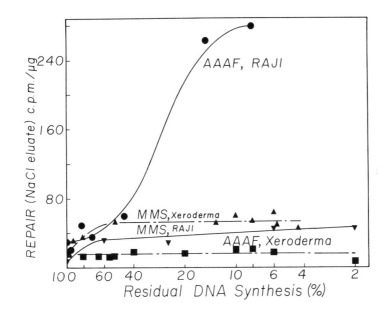

Fig. 5. DNA repair as a function of residual synthesis for xeroderma pigmentosum cells. RAJI and XP cells were preincubated with 10 mmol hydroxyurea for 30 min. They were then incubated for 60 min with drug, 10 mmol hydroxyurea and [^{3}H]dT (10 µCi/ml; 13 Ci/mmol). The cells were harvested and lysed and the sheared sample passed through a BND-cellulose column. Inhibition of DNA synthesis by drug was measured in the absence of hydroxyurea (Scudiero *et al.*, 1975). ● RAJI cells treated with AAAF, ■ Xeroderma pigmentosum treated with AAAF, ▼ RAJI cells treated with MMS, ▲ Xeroderma pigmentosum treated with MMS.

Using the flash photolysis technique, Regan and Setlow (1974) showed that there are two modal repair responses to DNA damage. The first, which they call "large patch" repair is characteristic of UV-irradiation-induced damage and involves the addition of up to 100 nucleotides per lesion. The second mode, "small patch repair", is characteristic of X-irradiation and involves the substitution of the order of three or four bases. Chemical agents can be classified as inducing large or small patch repair; AAAF induces UV-like large patch repair, MMS induces small patch, X-ray-like repair. We think this difference can be seen in the

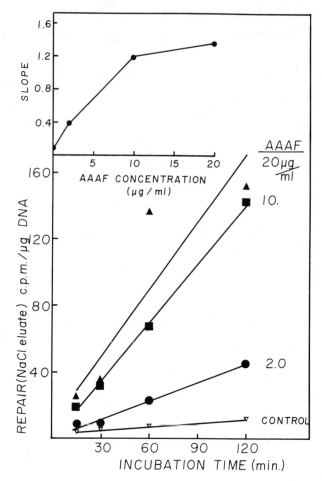

Fig. 6. DNA repair as a function of incubation time. RAJI cells were preincubated for 30 min with 10 mmol hydroxyurea. They were then incubated in medium with 10 mmol hydroxyurea, [³H]dT (10 μCi/ml, 13 Ci/mmol), and AAAF for the indicated times. Cells were harvested, lysed, and passed through BND-cellulose. Regression lines were calculated from the data. ∇ Control, ● Treated with 2.0 μg/ml AAAF, ■ Treated with 10.0 μg/ml AAAF, ▲ Treated with 20.0 μg/ml AAAF. Insert Fig. 6. The slope of the regression lines in Fig. 7 plotted as a function of AAAF concentration (Scudiero *et al.*, 1975).

shape of the dose-response curve for repair after treatment with chemicals (Fig. 7) since the specific activity of repair is always (in growing cells) considerably greater for AAAF than for MMS.

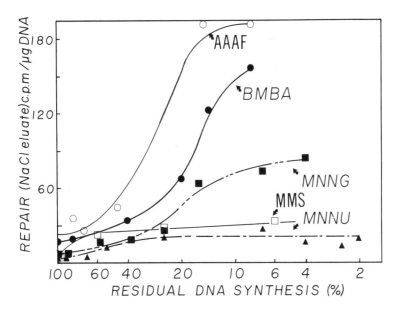

Fig. 7. DNA repair as a function of residual synthesis after
treatment with five inhibitory drugs. RAJI cells were preincubated
with 10 mmol hydroxyurea for 30 min. They were then incubated for
60 min with drug, 10 mmol hydroxyurea, and [³H]dT (10 µCi/ml, 13
Ci/mmol). The cells were harvested and lysed and the sheared
sample passed through a BND-cellulose column. Inhibition of DNA
synthesis by drug was measured in the absence of hydroxyurea
(Fig. 1). Repair is measured as the specific activity of the DNA
in the 1.0 M NaCl eluate of a BND-cellulose column (CPM/µg of DNA).
● BMBA, ■ MNNG, ▲ MNNU, o AAAF, □ MMS (Scudiero *et al.*, 1975).

        Compounds like MNNG give specific activities of repair per
lethal event intermediate between the values obtained with compounds like MMS and AAAF which we use as paradigms of small and
large patch-inducing agents. This intermediate nature is under-
standable considering that MNNG produces a variety of reaction
products, some of which can be considered as small-patch and others,
such as O^6-methylguanine [produced at 25 times the level found with
MMS (Lawley, 1974a)], are likely to be large-patch inducing.
Although we have not yet tested a large variety of compounds, we
think that our technique can serve as a rapid method for determining whether particular compounds produce a variety of reaction
products, since compounds which induce repair values intermediate

between MMS and AAAF are likely to be those which produce a variety
of reaction products.

The distinction of large and small patch repair by the BND-
cellulose method requires that the enzymes which carry out repair
and which provide the substrates for nucleotide incorporation be
in excess, so that the rate at which bases can be added is not a
limiting step. This requirement is probably met by growing cells
but such enzymes may be limiting in cells that are in an extended
G_0 state (Table 5). Although large-patch inducing agents produce
much higher specific repair activities when tested in growing cells
such as the human lymphoblastoid cell line RAJI, there is no such
distinction between large- and small-patch inducing agents in non-
stimulated human peripheral blood lymphocytes (Table 5). Once
stimulated, the lymphocytes behave like other growing cell systems.
This finding implies that although a lesion may induce incision,
the amount of excision depends on the level of polymerase and other
repair enzymes in the system. Alternatively, the measurement
utilizing thymidine may be limited by the low levels of thymidine
kinase in non-growing cells or by both polymerase and kinase or by
the presence of large pools of thymidylic acid in the cells. The
stability of lesions in brain tissue (Goth and Rajewsky, 1974) is
possibly related to the nature of the cell system in which DNA
synthesis does not normally occur and in which the level of replication and repair enzymes may be very low. The failure to repair
rapidly may be related to the great sensitivity of the lymphocytes
to radiation and to radiomimetic chemicals.

Growing cells carry out DNA repair in the region of the DNA
growing point and also in the bulk of the DNA. These two regions
are biologically differentiated in bacteria by their differential
sensitivity to particular mutagens (Cerdá-Olmedo et al., 1968).
MNNG and MNNU also produce more mutations in the growing point
region than in the bulk of the DNA (Hince and Neal, 1974). This
selectivity seems to obtain also for DNA repair.

Although MMS, BMBA, and AAAF induce equal specific repair
activities at growing points and in the bulk of the DNA, treatment
with MNNU and particularly with MNNG results in higher specific
repair activities in the formamide eluate of the BND-cellulose
column (Table 6). These experiments are carried out as follows:
Repair is allowed to occur in the presence of hydroxyurea and BrdUrd.
The cell lysates are then passed through BND-cellulose and the NaCl
fraction (representing the bulk DNA) and the formamide fraction
(representing the growing point regions and any degradation products
containing extensive single-stranded regions) are collected (Fig.
4). We usually pool the eluates of several columns to make possible the determination of the DNA in the growing point region by
its absorbancy after alkaline CsCl gradient centrifugation. The
DNA from both fractions is then centrifuged through alkaline CsCl

Table 5. Excision Repair in Human Peripheral Blood Lymphocytes
and in Burkitt's Lymphoma (RAJI) Cells*

Cell type	Treat-ment	Residual DNA synthesis	Repair (cpm/μg in the NaCl eluate)	
			Observed	Corrected for zero dose incorporation and to 13 Ci/mmol
RAJI	AAAF	15	263.8	236.4
	MMS	5	46.9	38.9
Stimulated HPBL	AAAF	24	197.8	45.8
	MMS	14	97.2	17.4
Non-stimu-lated HPBL	AAAF	--	15.5	3.7
	MMS	--	42.5	11.3

*Repair was measured as [^{3}H]dT incorporated radioactivity in
the NaCl eluate from BND-cellulose. Cells were incubated with
isotope for 1 h in the presence of either MMS (132 μg/ml) or AAAF
(10 μg/ml). RAJI was treated in the exponential growth phase.
Human peripheral blood lymphocytes (HPBL) were treated, non-
stimulated 24 h after harvest or stimulated 72 h after the addition of the mitogen, concanavalin A (10 μg/ml). HPBL were incubated with [^{3}H]dT of 46 Ci/mmol; RAJI was incubated with [^{3}H]dT
of 13 Ci/mmol (Unpublished data of D. Scudiero and A. Norin).

gradients to separate any BrdUrd incorporated by semi-conservative
replication from analog incorporated by repair, and the specific
radioactivity of the light DNA strands is determined. Comparisons
of such measurements show that the DNA isolated from the growing
point region after MNNG treatment has about four times the specific
activity of the bulk DNA (Table 6). At the very least these observations show that MNNG behaves differently than the other compounds
tested. At most the results indicate that there is more intense
MNNG-induced repair activity in the growing point regions or in
cells in S phase.

These observations point out the possible functional differentiation of DNA for reaction with alkylating agents. Not only is
it necessary to know the adducts which are possible, but it is also
necessary to recognize that particular portions of the DNA may be
specially reactive or may produce particular reaction products.
We have not been able to determine the relative reactivity of
growing points and of bulk DNA in whole cells because at the dose
of MNNG required to fix a measurable amount of radioactivity at

Table 6. Repair in the Bulk DNA and at the Growing Point
(Unpublished data of N. Scudiero)

Treatment	Specific repair activity (cpm/μg DNA) in BND-cellulose:						Ratio: (b)/(a)
	NaCl eluate (a)			Formamide eluate (b)			
	Expt.	Value	Av.-control	Expt.	Value	Av.-control	
None	1	1.1		1	3.8		
(Control)	2	1.4		2	4.6		
	3	1.3		3	2.8		
MMS	1	14.4		1	22.8		
(275 μg/ml)	2	15.4	13.6	2	17.8	14.5	1.1
	3	15.0		3	14.0		
BMBA	1	27.8		1	23.2		
(2.0 μg/ml)	2	24.3	23.5	2	22.2	18.4	0.8
	3	22.2		3	21.0		
AAAF	1	47.7		1	44.5		
(20 μg/ml)	2	35.3	40.1	2	35.4	35.6	0.9
	3	41.1		3	38.1		
MNNU	1	11.8		1	22.9		
(100 μg/ml)	2	10.8	9.7	2	23.6	19.9	2.1
	3	10.5		3	24.4		
MNNG	1	14.0		1	68.8		
(20 μg/ml)	2	26.9	18.4	2	101.6	73.4	4.0
	3	18.1		3	60.9		

the specific activity of the [^{3}H]MNNG we have been able to prepare
there was degradation, producing an excess of DNA eluting with
formamide. When DNA from growing cells was isolated and treated
in vitro with [^{3}H]MNNG under conditions which were comparable to
the concentrations used in the *in vivo* experiments to induce
measurable repair (Table 4) there was no measurable degradation
and no difference in the reactivity of the growing point and bulk
DNA regions. We therefore conclude, tentatively, that the increased
repair at the growing point may be due to either the concentration
of repair enzymes in this region or to the special reactivity of
the region so that some particular adduct which is excised in large
patches tends to be formed at growing points.

4. POST-REPLICATION REPAIR

The biologically important lesion for carcinogenesis and
mutagenesis should not block DNA synthesis irrevocably nor should

it cause cell death since the mutant or precancerous cell is important only insofar as it multiplies and leaves progeny. Therefore,
the significant lesion must be one which permits cell division and,
insofar as the determinative processes occur in the DNA, the lesion
must permit division with altered DNA replication. It is now almost
standard to compare this altered replication with the bacterial
replication which occurs in the presence of pyrimidine dimers in
organisms unable to excise such lesions and which is called post-
replication repair (Rupp and Howard-Flanders, 1968). There are a
number of post-replication repair pathways controlled by different
genes (Clark, 1973) and certain of these pathways have been identified as "error prone" because excision defective strains of bacteria
have high induced mutation frequencies (Witkin and George, 1973) and
because particular mutants unable to carry out certain reactions
of post-replication repair are mutagen stable and do not produce
mutants on treatment with lethal doses of mutagenic agents (Radman,
1974). There is evidence that mammalian cells similarly unable to
excise damage may be supersensitive to some mutagenic agents (Maher
and McCormick, 1975). Such lines can survive small fluences of
UV light [sufficient to produce about 110,000 cyclobutane-type
thymine dimers per cell (Cleaver, 1970)] and must be able to synthesize DNA since they produce progeny. At the same time they are
unable to remove the lesion.

The process in mammalian cells is the physiological equivalent
of bacterial recombinational repair. However, actual recombination
between parental and daughter DNA strands does not occur in mammalian
cells (Lehmann, 1972) as it does in bacteria (Rupp et al., 1971).
The process has therefore been described as one in which DNA replication "jumps over" the lesions which block DNA synthesis leaving
unreplicated, single-stranded gaps. These single-stranded regions
are then presumably filled by some caffeine-sensitive replication
process (Lehmann and Kirk-Bell, 1974). A simplistic model for the
gap filling process assumes that after some delay, a nucleotidyl
transferase type reaction adds nucleotides in a random fashion
until the lesion is bridged, after which normal semi-conservative
replication might occur. This hypothesis has the advantage of
accounting for the "error prone" nature of the synthesis since the
random nucleotide addition would result in numerous transitions
and transversions. On the other hand, the mechanism would result
in too many errors. A case against extensive single-stranded
regions in cells undergoing post-replication repair has been put
by Scudiero and Strauss (1974) and by Painter (1974) who summarizes
the reasons for thinking that gaps do not occur in mammalian cells
and that the base damage acts as a block to DNA replication for a
relatively long time.

We wish to suggest a mechanism for post-replication repair in
mammalian cells (Fig. 8). This model, developed by N.P. Higgins
in this laboratory, utilizes the known biochemical reactions of

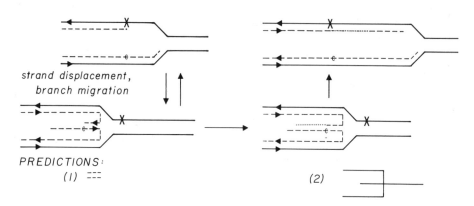

Fig. 8. A model for post-replication repair in mammalian cells (N.P. Higgins, personal communication).

strand displacement and branch migration to account for the synthesis of a complement of the damaged region by a "copy choice" mechanism. DNA synthesis, blocked on one strand by a lesion is presumed to proceed past this point on the undamaged template until the three stranded structure produced makes further unwinding of the helix impossible (Fig. 8). Displacement of the newly synthesized strands then restores the lesion to a double-stranded state where, we note, excision repair is possible as suggested previously (Scudiero and Strauss, 1974; Kato and Strauss, 1974). A four-pronged fork results, consisting of three normal double-stranded molecules and one prong in which both strands are newly synthesized. One of these strands contains a copy of the damaged region which is in a single-stranded condition (Fig. 8). This single-stranded region serves as a template for DNA synthesis and by making a complement of the copy of the damaged region the lesion is effectively bridged. Synthesis can then continue along both DNA strands.

The model leads to at least two predictions. First, we predict a small region in which both strands are newly synthesized (Fig. 8). If alkylated cells were incubated in BrdUrd immediately after treatment, one would expect to observe a small fraction of doubly substituted DNA fragments appearing long before a second round of cellular DNA synthesis could be expected. Such doubly substituted fragments would appear as material of high density (Heavy-Heavy) in neutral CsCl gradients. We have observed such fragments formed within 4 h after the start of incubation of MMS-treated HEp.2 cells in BrdUrd (Fig. 9) but until the development of this model we were unable to account for their appearance. The Heavy-Heavy DNA observed can be rebanded in CsCl and only about ten per cent can be degraded by single-strand specific nucleases.

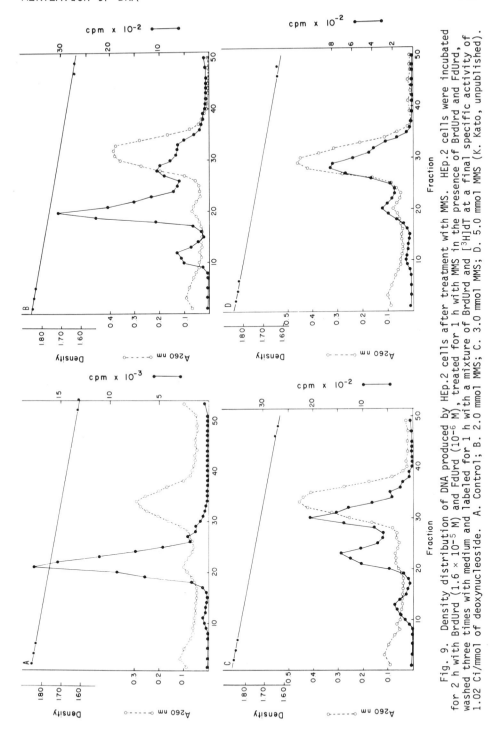

Fig. 9. Density distribution of DNA produced by HEp.2 cells after treatment with MMS. HEp.2 cells were incubated for 2 h with BrdUrd (1.6 × 10⁻⁵ M) and FdUrd (10⁻⁶ M), treated for 1 h with MMS in the presence of BrdUrd and FdUrd, washed three times with medium and labeled for 1 h with a mixture of BrdUrd and [³H]dT at a final specific activity of 1.02 Ci/mmol of deoxynucleoside. A. Control; B. 2.0 mmol MMS; C. 3.0 mmol MMS; D. 5.0 mmol MMS (K. Kato, unpublished).

Second, we predict the occurrence of four-pronged forks as described above. Such structures are seen in the intermediate density fraction (Kato and Strauss, 1974) of BrdUrd-substituted DNA from MMS-treated HEp.2 cells (Fig. 10). This fraction contains replicating molecules. Our electron micrography requires quantitation to show that the structures observed are not due to a random superposition of strands but the results with HEp.2 cells treated with MMS have prompted us to continue these studies with an XP lymphoblastoid line treated with AAAF in which post-replication recovery should be the dominant reaction. We think the model is particularly attractive because it utilizes the biochemical reactions presumed to play a role in normal genetic recombination (Meselson and Radding, 1975). Our mechanism should be "error free"--some other factor is required to account for the generation of errors.

5. CONCLUSION

If mutagenesis and carcinogenesis are closely related, the ability of a compound or a physical agent to alter DNA is a necessary requirement for carcinogenic action, since mutation requires a change in the DNA structure. However, as has been discussed above (Section 2), chemical demonstration of a reaction product or even a series of reaction products with DNA is only a start towards identifying the biologically significant lesion. In some cases biological experiments have been successful in correlating particular chemical lesions with particular biological effects, but it is not at all certain that the minor reaction product implicated is the necessary cause of the biological effect.

The excision repair system probably serves as an indicator of the importance of particular adducts in the DNA. Recognition by the excision enzymes is a sign that the DNA structure has been deformed sufficiently to result in a perturbed DNA replication. One may consider DNA repair as an analog of the immune response-- in fact, similar questions can be asked: How is it that organisms have developed systems to protect themselves from compounds they have not encountered in the course of evolution? How is it that excision repair is well developed in human cells but poorly developed in adult rodents (Klimer, 1966)?

It is very likely that some sort of generalized DNA deformation is recognized by the excision repair system and it is possible that this same deformation results in pathological change, or error, when the replication complex passes over it before excision. In my opinion it is this process of replication while the lesion remains in the DNA which deserves the greatest degree of attention. Although excision repair in human cells may be useful dosimeter for the determination of potential hazard, the hazard itself is the replication process which occurs while the lesion is still in

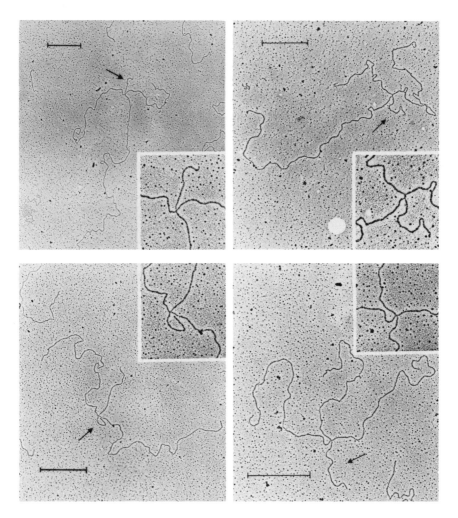

Fig. 10. Electron micrographs of four-pronged replication
forks found in the intermediate density region of CsCl gradients
of DNA from alkylated cells. Grids were prepared using the aqueous
spreading technique of Davis *et al.* (1971), stained with uranyl
acetate and shadowed with Pt:Pd(80:20). Arrows indicate short
fourth prong representing displaced strands. Scale indicate 1 μ.
Inserts, magnified branch points. Data of Karen Kato (unpublished).

the DNA. A good deal of experience in the study of bacterial
mutation can be summarized by the statement that damage in the DNA
is "fixed" by the passage of the replication complex past the point
of the lesion. It is the molecular nature of the events which
occur during such passage that are probably critical to both

carcinogenesis and to mutagenesis and it is this process which must be understood.

Acknowledgment. The research of the author reported here was supported in part by grants from the National Institutes of Health (GM 07816), (AI-12116), The University of Chicago Cancer Research Center (CA 14599-02) and the U.S. Energy Research and Development Administration [AT(11-1) 2040]. I am particularly indebted to Karen Kato, Peter Karran, N. Pat Higgins, Allen Norin and Dominic Scudiero for permission to utilize previously unpublished data.

References

Auerbach, C., and Robson, J., 1946, Chemical production of mutations, *Nature* 157:302.

Auerbach, C., and Robson, J., 1947, The production of mutation by chemical substances, *Proc. Roy. Soc. Edn. B.* 62:271-283.

Bannon, P., and Verly, W., 1972, Alkylation of phosphates and stability of phosphate triesters in DNA, *Eur. J. Biochem.* 31:103-111.

Brookes, P., and Lawley, P., 1961, The reaction of mono- and difunctional alkylating agents with nucleic acids, *Biochem. J.* 80:496-503.

Cerdá-Olmedo, E., Hanawalt, P., and Guerola, N., 1968, Mutagenesis of the replication point by nitrosoguanidine: map and pattern of replication of the *Escherichia coli* chromosome, *J. Mol. Biol.* 33:705-719.

Clark, A., 1973, Recombination deficient mutants of *E. coli* and other bacteria, *Annu. Rev. Genet.* 7:67-86.

Cleaver, J., 1970, DNA repair and radiation sensitivity in humans (Xeroderma pigmentosum) cells, *Int. J. Radiat. Biol.* 18:557-565.

Coyle, M., McMahon, M., and Strauss, B., 1971, Failure of alkylated HEp2 cells to replicate newly synthesized DNA, *Mutat. Res.* 12:427-440.

Craddock, V., 1973, The pattern of methylated purines formed in DNA of intact and regenerating liver of rats treated with the carcinogen dimethylnitrosamine, *Biochim. Biophys. Acta* 312: 202-210.

Craddock, V., 1975, Effect of a single treatment with the alkylating carcinogens dimethylnitrosamine diethylnitrosamine and methyl methanesulfonate, on liver regenerating after partial hepatectomy. II. Alkylation of DNA and inhibition of DNA replication, *Chem. Biol. Interactions* 10:323-332.

Cramer, J., Miller, J., and Miller, E., 1960, N-hydroxylation: A new metabolic reaction observed in the rat with the carcinogen 2-acetyl aminofluorene, *J. Biol. Chem.* 235:885-888.

Davis, R., Simon, M., and Davidson, N., 1971, Electron microscope heteroduplex methods for mapping regions of base sequence homology in nucleic acids, *Methods in Enzymology* 21:413-428.

Dipple, A., Brookes, P., Mackintosh, D., and Rayman, M., 1971,
    Reaction of 7-bromomethyl benz (α) anthracene with nucleic
    acids, polynucleotides and nucleosides, *Biochemistry* 10:4323-
    4330.
Freese, E., 1971, Molecular mechanisms of mutations, *Chemical
    Mutagens* 1:1-56.
Geiduschek, E.P., 1961, "Reversible" DNA, *Proc. Nat. Acad. Sci.
    USA* 47:950-955.
Goth, R., and Rajewsky, M., 1974, Persistence of O^6-ethylguanine
    in rat brain DNA; Correlation with nervous system-specific
    carcinogenesis by ethylnitrosourea, *Proc. Nat. Acad. Sci.
    USA* 71:639-643.
Hadi, S., and Goldthwait, D., 1971, Endonuclease II of *Escherichia
    coli* degradation of partially depurinated deoxyribonucleic
    acid, *Biochemistry* 10:4986-4994.
Hill, R., 1958, A radiation-sensitive mutant of *Escherichia coli*,
    Biochim. Biophys. Acta 30:636-637.
Hince, T., and Neale, S., 1974, A comparison of the mutagenic
    action of the methyl and ethyl derivatives of nitrosamides
    and nitrosamidines on *Escherichia coli*, *Mutat. Res.* 24:383-387.
Kato, K., and Strauss, B., 1974, Accumulation of an intermediate
    in DNA synthesis by HEp2 cells treated with methyl methanesul-
    fonate, *Proc. Nat. Acad. Sci. USA* 71:1969-1973.
Kleijer, W., Lohman, P., Mulder, M., and Bootsma, D., 1970, Repair
    of X-ray damage in DNA of cultivated cells from patients
    having Xeroderma pigmentosum, *Mutat. Res.* 9:517-523.
Klimek, M., 1966, Thymine dimerization in L-strain mammalian cells
    after irradiation with ultraviolet light and the search for
    repair mechanisms, *Photochem. Photobiol.* 5:603-607.
Lawley, P., 1973, Reaction of N-methyl-N-nitrosourea (MNUA) with
    ^{32}P-labeled DNA: evidence for formation of phosphotriesters,
    Chem. Biol. Interactions 7:127-130.
Lawley, P., 1974a, Some chemical aspects of dose-response relation-
    ships in alkylation mutagenesis, *Mutat. Res.* 23:283-295.
Lawley, P., 1974b, Alkylation of nucleic acids and mutagenesis, *in*
    "Molecular and Environmental Aspects of Mutagenesis" (L. Prakash,
    F. Sherman, M. Miller, C. Lawrence, and H. Taber, eds.), pp. 17-
    33, C. Thomas, Springfield.
Lawley, P., and Brookes, P., 1963, Further studies on the alkyla-
    tion of nucleic acids and their constituent nucleotides,
    Biochem. J. 89:127-138.
Lawley, P., and Orr, D., 1970, Specific excision of methylation
    products from DNA of *Escherichia coli* treated with N-methyl-
    N'-nitro-N-nitrosoguanidine, *Chem. Biol. Interactions* 2:154-157.
Lawley, P., and Shah, S., 1972, Reaction of alkylating mutagens and
    carcinogens with nucleic acids: detection and estimation of a
    small extent of methylation at O-6 of guanine in DNA by methyl
    methanesulphonate *in vitro*, *Chem. Biol. Interactions* 5:286-
    288.

Lawley, P., and Shah, S., 1973, Methylation of DNA by ^{3}H-^{14}C-methyl-labeled N-methyl-N-nitrosourea--evidence for transfer of the intact methyl group, *Chem. Biol. Interactions* 7:115-120.

Lawley, P., and Thatcher, C., 1970, Methylation of deoxyribonucleic acid in cultured mammalian cells by N-methyl-N'-nitro-N-nitro-soguanidine, *Biochem. J.* 116:693-707.

Lehmann, A., 1972, Post replication repair of DNA in ultraviolet-irradiated mammalian cells, *J. Mol. Biol.* 66:319-337.

Lehmann, A., and Kirk-Bell, S., 1974, Effects of caffeine and theophylline on DNA synthesis in unirradiated and UV-irradiated mammalian cells, *Mutat. Res.* 26:73-82.

Lieberman, M., and Dipple, A., 1972, Removal of bound carcinogen during DNA repair in non-dividing human lymphocytes, *Cancer Res.* 32:1855-1860.

Lindahl, T., and Nyberg, B., 1972, Rate of depurination of native DNA, *Biochemistry* 11:3610-3618.

Ljungquist, S., and Lindahl, T., 1974, A mammalian endonuclease specific for apurinic sites in double-stranded deoxyribonucleic acid. I. Purification and general properties, *Biol. Chem.* 249:1530-1535.

Loveless, A., 1969, Possible relevance of 0-6 alkylation of deoxy-guanosine to mutagenicity of nitrosamines and nitrosamides, *Nature* 223:206-208.

Magee, P., 1969, *In vivo* reactions of nitroso compounds, *Annu. N.Y. Acad. Sci.* 163:717-729.

Maher, V., and McCormick, J., 1975, Effect of DNA repair on the cytotoxicity and on the frequency of mutations induced in normal human skin fibroblasts and in strains of Xeroderma pigmentosum by ultraviolet irradiation and by chemical carcinogens. Abstr. Int. Symp. "Protein and Other Adducts to DNA: Their Significance to Aging, Carcinogenesis and Radiation Biology," Williamsburg, Virginia, May 2-6, 1975.

Meselson, M., and Radding, C., 1975, A general model for genetic recombination, *Proc. Nat. Acad. Sci. USA* 72:385-361.

Miller, E., and Miller, J., 1969, Studies on the mechanism of activation of aromatic amine and amide carcinogens to ultimate carcinogenic electrophilic reactants, *Annu. N.Y. Acad. Sci.* 163:731-750.

Miller, J., Cramer, J., and Miller, E., 1960, The N- and ring-hydroxylation of 2-acetylaminofluorene during carcinogenesis in the rat, *Cancer Res.* 20:950-962.

Nicoll, J., Swann, P., and Pegg, A., 1975, Effect of dimethylnitro-samine on persistence of methylated guanines in rat liver and kidney DNA, *Nature* 254:261-262.

O'Connor, P., Margison, G., and Craig, A., 1975, Phosphotriesters in rat liver deoxyribonucleic acid after the administration of the carcinogen N N-dimethylnitrosamine *in vivo, Biochem. J.* 145:475-482.

Painter, R., 1974, DNA damage and repair in eukaryotic cells, *Genetics* 78:139-148.

Prakash, L., and Strauss, B., 1970, Repair of alkylation damage: stability of methyl groups in *Bacillus subtilis* treated with methyl methanesulfonate, *J. Bacteriol.* 102:760-766.

Radman, M., 1974, Phenomenology of an inducible mutagenic DNA repair pathway in *Escherichia coli*: SOS repair hypothesis, *in* "Molecular and Environmental Aspects of Mutagenesis" (L. Prakash, F. Sherman, M. Miller, C. Lawrence, and H. Taber, eds.), pp. 128-140, C. Thomas, Springfield.

Regan, J., and Setlow, R., 1974, Two forms of repair in the DNA of human cells damaged by chemical carcinogens and mutagens, *Cancer Res.* 34:3318-3325.

Reiter, H., and Strauss, B., 1965, Repair of damage induced by a monofunctional alkylating agent in a transformable, ultra-violet-sensitive strain of *Bacillus subtilis, J. Mol. Biol.* 14:179-194.

Robbins, J., Kraemer, K., Lutzner, M., Festoff, B., and Coon, H., 1974, Xeroderma pigmentosum. An inherited disease with skin sensitivity, multiple cutaneous neoplasms, and abnormal DNA repair, *Annu. Intern. Med.* 80:221-248.

Roberts, J., Pascoe, J., Plant, J., Sturrock, J., and Crathorn, A., 1971, Quantitative aspects of the repair of alkylated DNA in cultured mammalian cells. I. The effect on HeLa and chinese hamster cell survival of alkylation of cellular macromolecules, *Chem. Biol. Interactions* 3:29-47.

Rupp, W., and Howard-Flanders, P., 1968, Discontinuities in the DNA synthesized in an excision-defective strain of *E. coli* following ultraviolet irradiation, *J. Mol. Biol.* 31:291-304.

Rupp, W., Wilde, C., Reno, D., and Howard-Flanders, P., 1971, Exchanges between DNA strands in ultraviolet irradiated *E. coli, J. Mol. Biol.* 61:25-44.

Scudiero, D., Henderson, E., Norin, A., and Strauss, B., 1975, The measurement of chemically-induced DNA repair synthesis in human cells by BND-cellulose chromatography, *Mutat. Res.* (in press).

Scudiero, D., and Strauss, B., 1974, Accumulation of single-stranded regions in DNA and the block to replication in a human cell line alkylated with methyl methanesulfonate, *J. Mol. Biol.* 83:17-34.

Setlow, R.B., and Carrier, W., 1964, The disappearance of thymine dimers from DNA: an error-correcting mechanism, *Proc. Nat. Acad. Sci. USA* 51:226-231.

Shooter, K., Howse, R., and Merrifield, R., 1974, Reaction of alkylating agents with bacteriophage R17: biological effects of phosphotriester formation, *Biochem. J.* 137:313-317.

Stacey, K., Cobb, M., Cousens, S., and Alexander, P., 1958, The reactions of the "radiomimetic" alkylating agents with macro-molecules *in vitro, Annu. N.Y. Acad. Sci.* 68:682-701.

Strauss, B., 1974, Repair of DNA in mammalian cells, *Life Sci.* 15: 1685-1693.

Trosko, J., Chang, C., Yotti, L., and Chu, E.H.Y., 1975, Mutageni-
     city of cancer-promoting agents in cultured chinese hamster
     cells. Abstr. Int. Symp. "Protein and Other Adducts to DNA:
     Their Significance to Aging, Carcinogenesis and Radiation
     Biology," Williamsburg, Virginia, May 2-6, 1975.
Venitt, S., and Tarmy, E., 1972, The selective excision of arylal-
     kylated products from the DNA of *Escherichia coli* treated with
     the carcinogen 7-bromomethyl benz (α) anthracene, *Biochim.*
     Biophys. Acta 287:38-51.
Whitelock, O., 1958, Comparative clinical and biological effects
     of alkylating agents, *Annu. N.Y. Acad. Sci.* 68:657-1266.
Witkin, E., and George, D., 1973, Ultraviolet mutagenesis in *polA*
     and *uvrA polA* derivatives of *Escherichia coli* B/r: Evidence
     for an inducible error-prone repair system, *Genetics Suppl.*
     73:91-108.
Zimmerman, F., 1971, Genetic aspects of carcinogenesis, *Biochem.*
     Pharmacol. 20:985-995.

PHOTOAFFINITY LABELING OF PROTEINS AND MORE COMPLEX RECEPTORS

Barry S. Cooperman

Department of Chemistry, University of Pennsylvania

Philadelphia, Pa. 19174

1.   INTRODUCTION

In the past several years affinity labeling has emerged as a powerful method for studying ligand-receptor interactions. The logic of an affinity labeling experiment (Singer, 1967) is described in Eq. (1)-(3). A reactive group, X (electrophilic or photolabile), is attached to the natural ligand, L. If the resulting modified ligand L̃X retains high affinity for the native ligand receptor site and forms a non-covalent complex, R.L̃X, [Eq. (1)], then, at low L̃X concentration, covalent attachment via the reaction in Eq. (2) , a first order process, will proceed at a much faster rate than attachment via the reaction in Eq. (3), a second order process, and specific attachment to the ligand site will be achieved.

$$R + L'X \quad \xrightleftharpoons \quad R.L'X \qquad\qquad\qquad\qquad (1)$$

$$R.L'X \quad \xrightarrow{\hspace{3cm}} \quad R-L' + X \qquad \text{affinity labeling} \qquad (2)$$

$$R + L'X \quad \xrightarrow{\hspace{3cm}} \quad R-L' + X \qquad \text{non-specific labeling} \qquad (3)$$

Affinity labeling has been most frequently applied in studies directed toward mapping the ligand binding site. When the receptor is relatively small, such as a single protein, the experiment is usually directed toward placing the covalently labeled amino acid(s) within the primary structure of the protein. With more complex receptors, such as membranes or ribosomes, resolution to a much coarser level is often sufficient, the usual goal being to identify the proteins on regions of RNA which are labeled. Labeled receptors can also provide useful information about functional aspects of ligand-receptor interaction. Affinity labels can be designed so as to incorporate physical probes, such as fluorescent groups, chromopores, or stable free radicals, which can then be used to monitor conformational changes. For receptors such as allosteric enzymes, studying the effects of simple covalent occupancy of an effector site can lead to interesting results, and, in a quite general way, the labeling pattern itself can be a sensitive indicator of structure. It is worth noting that these two applications place different requirements on the affinity labeling process, in the sense that functional studies frequently require stoichiometric labeling of sites, whereas mapping studies can often be done on sites labeled to a minor extent, if an affinity labeling reagent of sufficiently high specific radioactivity is available.

In Section 2 the problems involved in interpreting affinity labeling results, and the properties of several different types of reagents which have been used in photoaffinity labeling studies are discussed. In Section 3 brief summaries of photoaffinity labeling studies published from the beginning of 1974 through the first part of 1975 are presented, the literature on photoaffinity labeling through the end of 1973 having been previously reviewed by Knowles (1972) and Creed (1974).

2.   PHOTOAFFINITY LABELING-PROCEDURES AND REAGENTS

2.1.   Electrophilic and Photoaffinity Labeling

If we admit that an actual ligand-receptor interaction may take place at several sites, and that what is meant by specific interaction is that the ligand is bound to one site much more tightly

than to others, then once it is found that an affinity labeling
reagent incorporates covalently into the receptor, we can assess
the accuracy of an affinity labeling experiment on the basis
of how closely the extent of covalent labeling of different
sites reflects the relative amounts of the different noncovalent
complexes in solution. Earlier reviews, which dealt mainly
with electrophilic labeling, have discussed the importance of demonstrating three points in this connection (Singer, 1967; Shaw,
1970). First, that the reagent forms a non-covalent complex prior
to covalent bond formation, second, that this complex mimics that
found with the normal ligand, and third that covalent bond formation
is quantitatively correlated to a loss of reversible binding sites
for native ligand. The first of these points can be demonstrated
by a number of standard techniques and the second is usually tested
by examining whether the natural ligand blocks either non-covalent
binding or covalent incorporation of the affinity label. The third
point is often difficult to demonstrate, since it not only requires
that a high fraction of receptor sites be labeled, but also that
there be a reliable quantitative assay for natural ligand binding.
With electrophilic affinity labels one often obtains high yields of
receptor labeling, but with photoaffinity labels the yields are
frequently quite low, reflecting an intrinsic problem arising from
the reaction of the photogenerated species with solvent. Iterative
methods have been devised for increasing the yields to stoichiometric
levels (Cooperman and Brunswick, 1973; Rosenstein and Richards, 1972),
but these involve the use of high light fluences and thus will only
be applicable in cases where there is no significant receptor damage
during the course of photolysis. Because of the difficulties mentioned above, and because it is possible to map sites labeled in
low yield, the third point is unfortunately often simply left unde-
monstrated. However, it is important to recognize that even the
successful demonstration of all three points would not unequivocally
establish the accuracy of an affinity labeling experiment, since
the first two examine the non-covalent binding of the affinity labeling reagent, while demonstration of the third leaves open the possibility that label covalently bound to a site different from the true
(i.e., tightest) receptor site blocks natural ligand binding by steric
interference or allosteric effects.

Given the inherent difficulty of verifying the accuracy of
affinity labeling, and the wide choice of reactive groups which can
be attached to a natural ligand, it is important to consider what
criteria an affinity labeling reagent must meet in order to maximize
the probability that it will yield accurate results. There are
basically two: first, that the reagent be totally non-selective in
its covalent reactions with receptor, or second, that the reagent
be generated while non-covalently bound to receptor and have a short
enough lifetime and a broad enough reactivity that covalent reaction
at the site(s) of generation will take place at a rate fast compared
to equilibration among sites. If neither condition is met, then

labeling patterns will reflect not only the relative affinities of different sites for the affinity labeling reagent, but also the relative reactivities of different sites toward the reagent.

These considerations emphasize the major weaknesses of electrophilic affinity labeling reagents since not only do electrophiles require nucleophiles for reaction, but also a given electrophile may react specifically with a particular nucleophile [e.g., bromoacetyl with sulfhydryl, aryl diazonium ion with phenols, etc. (Vallee and Riordan, 1969)], and in general electrophilic centers cannot be generated *in situ* (although see Walsh *et al.*, 1972) and react relatively slowly with nucleophiles. By contrast, photolabile reagents have the advantages that on irradiation they give rise to reactive species *in situ*, and that many of these species have very short lifetimes and are often much less selective toward covalent bond formation than electrophiles. As we shall see in Sections 2.2-2.4, none of the photolabile reagents used currently are ideal, but they are clearly superior to electrophilic reagents and there are real prospects for reagent improvement through further systematic studies correlating selectivity and reactivity with structure.

This superiority, first pointed out and exploited by Westheimer and his co-workers (Singh *et al.*, 1962) has prompted the current widespread utilization of the photoaffinity labeling technique which is, however, not without problems of its own. We have already alluded to the problem of low yields. There are additionally two other problems which up until the present have been largely ignored, but which should receive more attention as our sophistication in the use of this technique increases. The first is that destruction of a receptor may be taking place during the course of the photolabeling experiment. This is so even when irradiation is at wavelengths where receptor doesn't absorb because of the possibility of photosensitized destruction by the photolabile ligand (Section 2.5) and raises the question of whether the labeling patterns obtained reflect native or altered receptor structure. This problem can be addressed directly by examining the labeling pattern obtained as a function of light fluence, since light-induced conformational changes in the receptor should be reflected by changes in the labeling pattern. The second is the problem of elucidating the photochemical mechanism giving rise to incorporation. The importance of this problem is that confidence in the accuracy of a photolabeling experiment depends in large measure on knowledge of the properties of the labeling species. It must be acknowledged that given the chemical complexity of most receptors and the consequent possibilities for internal energy transfer, it is doubtful that the labeling mechanism can be elucidated in detail. One approach is to identify the exact chemical nature of the covalent bond formed between label and receptor, but this has proven to be very difficult for simple systems (for example, Hexter and Westheimer 1971a,b: Shafer *et al.*, 1966; Bridges and Knowles, 1974; Hew *et al.*, 1973; Cannon *et al.*, 1974), and is probably hopeless for more complex ones. However, it is in principle

possible (though it has not as yet been done) to determine the identity of the species responsible for absorbing the radiation leading
to incorporation by determining the action spectrum for incorporation.
In addition, for photolabile reagents such as α-diazocarbonyls or
azides, which on photolysis irreversibly lose nitrogen in high quantum
yield reactions to give carbenes and nitrenes, respectively, (see
Section 2.2) it has been possible to separately pre-photolyze the
diazo or azide reagent with a light fluence just high enough for
complete nitrogen loss, and to then measure the effect of pre-photo-
lysis on subsequent photo-incorporation into receptor. The finding
that incorporation is lost or substantially reduced has been taken
as providing strong evidence that incorporation proceeds via carbene
or nitrene formation, rather than via photoactivation of some other
portion of the molecule or via insertion of activated receptor into
the labeling reagent.

The procedures we have discussed so far for confronting the
problems involved in interpreting the results of a photoaffinity
labeling experiment can considerably increase our confidence in the
accuracy of labeling results, but obviously fall short of providing
a method of absolute verification. One additional procedure which
is therefore highly desirable is to derivatize a ligand with several
different photolabile groups and compare the labeling results obtained with each derivative. Common labeling patterns would constitute strong evidence that the true binding site has been identified, since differences in the specificities of the photogenerated
species should prevent common artifactual results. Divergent patterns would at least show that the results were problematical. A
decision as to which pattern was most likely to be correct would
have to be made on the basis of how much information was available
on the accuracy of each of the photolabeling experiments as determined by the procedures discussed above.

2.2. α-Carbonyl Carbenes and Aryl Nitrenes

The two reagents most frequently used to date in photoaffinity
affinity labeling experiments have been α-diazocarbonyls and aryl
azides (Knowles, 1972). On photolysis these reagents give rise to
α-carbonyl carbenes and aryl nitrenes, respectively. Both of these
reagents display broad spectra of reactivity (Smith, 1970; Baron *et
al.*, 1973) including insertion into C-H bonds, which will be present
at all sites (Fig. 1,2). Moreover, both can be generated while non-
covalently bound to receptor, if equilibration is allowed to proceed
prior to photolysis. They are thus clearly superior to electrophilic
reagents although each has limitations. Aryl nitrenes are relatively
long-lived ($t_{1/2}$, ~10^{-3}s) and quite selective with respect to C-H insertion (phenyl nitrene inserts into tertiary C-H bonds more than
100 times faster than into primary C-H bonds) so it certainly does
not meet the first criterion set forth in Section 2.1, and except

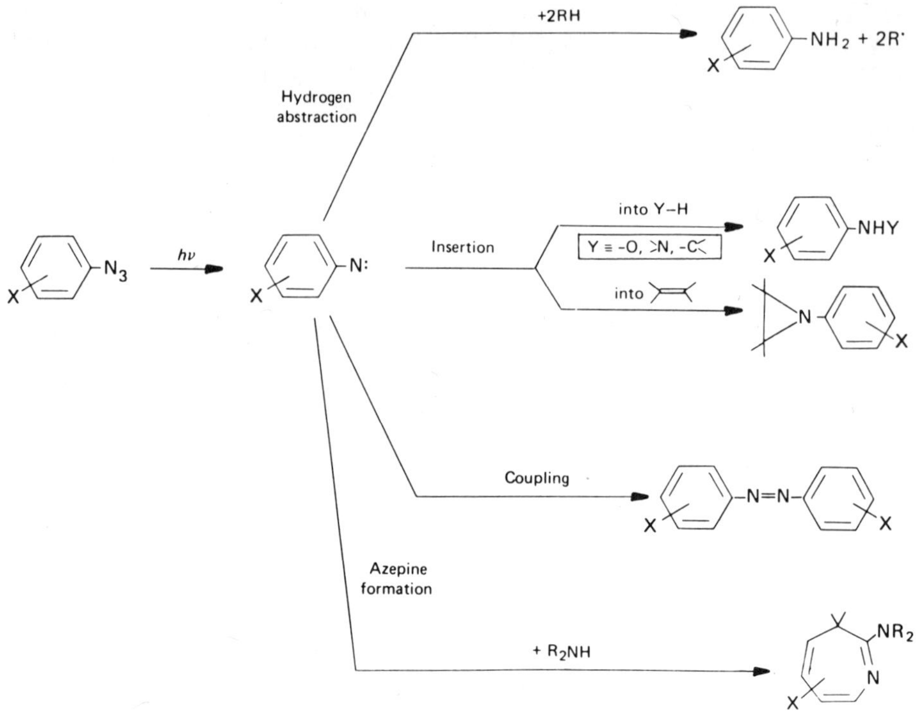

Fig. 1. Products from aryl azide photolysis. X refers to any
substituent.

for very tight binding sites does not meet the second criterion
either. These problems with the use of aryl nitrenes are very
clearly demonstrated by two recent experiments. Richards *et al*.
(1974) (Section 3.1.1) found that, on photolysis, 2,4-dinitrophenol
azide incorporates into tyrosines 33 and 88 of the heavy chain of
mouse myleoma protein 460. Making the assumption that these residues are homologous with residues in the human myleoma protein
NEW, whose structure has been determined by X-ray diffraction, these
two tyrosines must be 23 Å from one another, i.e., too far apart to
be contact residues at a single binding site. It is unclear which
tyrosine is at the tight site and which is at a secondary site.
Staros and Richards (1974) and Staros *et al*. (1974) have made use
of the relative stability of aryl nitrenes to advantage in studying
the topology of red cell membranes. α-Carbonyl carbenes are much
less selective toward bond insertion, and presumably quite a bit
shorter-lived [although little rate data are available (Closs, 1975)]
and are thus clearly superior reagents in these respects. They are,
however, subject to Wolff rearrangement leading to ketene formation,
and this electrophilic species has the problems of selectivity discussed above. It should be pointed out that for both aryl nitrenes

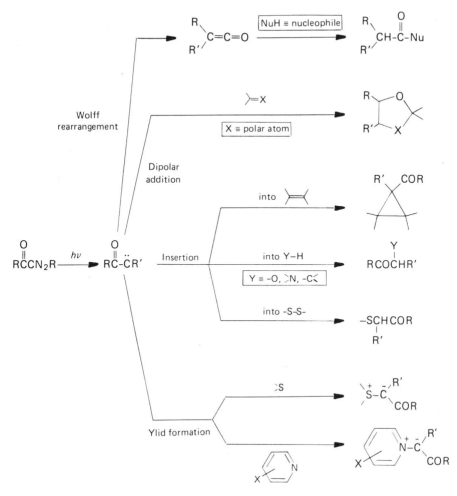

Fig. 2. Products from α-carbonyl diazo compound photolysis.

and α-carbonylcarbenes, appropriate structural modifications and
choice of photolysis conditions can at least partially correct the
deficiencies described above. Thus, electron withdrawing groups
attached to aryl nitrenes increase nitrene reactivity and presumably
also decrease selectivity (although the latter point has not really
been tested), whereas substituents such as carbethoxy and trifluoro-
methyl attached to the carbene carbon decrease the extent of Wolff
rearrangement (Vaughan, 1970), as does photolysis via triplet sensitization (Hixon and Hixon, 1972). In addition, labeling by a reagent which is sufficiently long-lived to equilibrate between receptor and solution can be suppressed through appropriate use of
scavengers (Ruoho *et al.*, 1973), although scavengers will not always
be able to suppress equilibration of reagent between sites which

occurs intramolecularly. Suitably substituted aryl azides have strong absorption above 400 nm, and can thus be photolyzed to nitrenes at wavelengths where photoinduced conformational changes in most receptors should be minimal (although see Section 2.5). α-Carbonyl diazo compounds have two absorption maxima, a very intense one at 250-270 nm with an extinction coefficient of the order of 10^4, and a broad weak one, centered at about 350 nm, with an extinction coefficient of the order of 10-40. In cases where the length of time required for photolysis is unimportant, it is possible to photolytically generate carbenes at the longer wavelength, with little expected damage to the receptor. However, it is important to realize that the combination of a high α-carbonyl diazo compound extinction coefficient and a high quantum yield for carbene generation will frequently make it possible to efficiently generate carbenes with fluences of short wavelength (e.g., 254 nm) radiation which are insufficient to cause major structural damage to the receptor and that furthermore carbenes generated at the shorter wavelength are more reactive and thus more desirable as labeling reagents (Cooperman and Brunswick, 1973).

Phosphoryl azides and aryl diazirenes are examples of reagents which, though similar to those discussed above, might prove superior in photoaffinity labeling experiments. Breslow et al. (1974) have found that phosphoryl nitrenes react exclusively via direct bond insertion processes (no rearrangement) with very low selectivity toward tertiary versus primary C-H insertion. Smith and Knowles (1973) have found that on irradiation in hexane at >300 nm, 3-phenyl-3H-diazirine decomposes rapidly, partially via phenyldiazomethane formation and partially via a direct, but as yet unelucidated, fragmentation. Although no applications of either of these reagents has been reported as yet, one may anticipate such work in the future.

2.3. Conjugated Ketones

Conjugated and especially aryl ketones have also been used as photoaffinity labeling reagents by several groups (Martyr and Benisek 1973; Galardy et al., 1974; Glover et al., 1974; E. Kuechler, persona communication and perhaps Ruoho and Kyte, 1974). Ketones containing γ C-H bonds undergo characteristic 1,5 hydrogen shifts to yield both cleavage and cyclization products, via the mechanism shown in Fig. 3 (Wagner, 1971). As pointed out by Breslow et al. (1973) the requirement for hydrogen transfer via a six-membered ring is an entropic one, and an analogous hydrogen transfer could take place in a noncovalent complex if the hydrogen atom donor and acceptor were properl aligned, resulting in a covalent bond formation between ligand and receptor. It is thus possible to use what is known about the cyclization reaction to assess the potential of conjugated ketones as labeling reagents. The rate of hydrogen abstraction is very sensitive to the substituents on the γ-C, the relative reactivities of

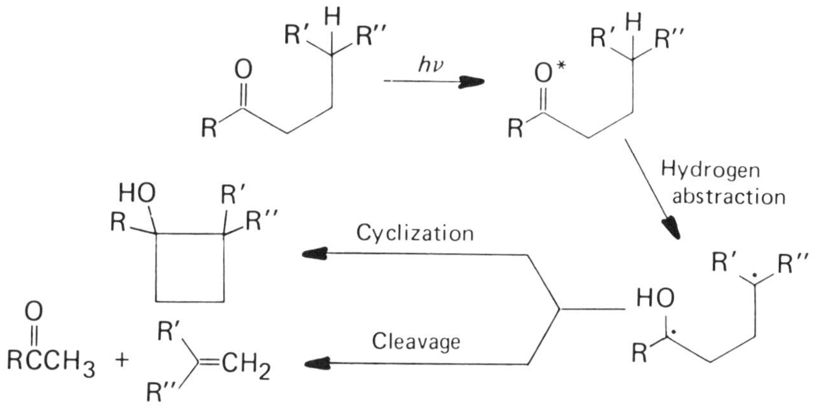

Fig. 3.   Products from photolysis of ketones with γ C-H bonds.

tertiary primary C-H bonds being approximately 200, so that these reagents, like nitrenes, do not meet the first criterion mentioned in Section 2.1. On the other hand, the absolute rates of both hydrogen abstraction and subsequent cyclization or cleavage are extremely rapid, with rate constants greater than 10^6 s^{-1} for the slowest systems, so that the second criterion mentioned in Section 2.1 may well be met in most cases. The major difficulty in using aryl ketones appears to be that the net rate of covalent bond formation is slow compared to other relevant photochemical reactions, such as amino acid destruction. One approach to solving this problem is to use those aryl ketones with high absorption maxima at wavelengths >300 nm, such as benzophenone (Galardy *et al.*, 1974). Another approach would be to use those aryl ketones, such as α-diketones and α,α-dimethyl ketones, which have been shown in studies on ketones with γ C-H bonds to suppress cleavage in favor of cyclization (Wagner, 1971). With conjugated ketones covalent labeling may proceed via processes other than that described above, such as via ketene formation (Turro *et al.*, 1972), but as discussed above, labeling via this species could be suppressed by performing photolyses in buffers containing nucleophilic scavengers.

2.4.   Other Photolabile Groups

Other reagents for which there is direct or indirect evidence of photoincorporation into receptors are listed in Table 1. In most of the cases cited the photochemistry of the process or processes leading to incorporation has not been defined so that it is difficult to assess how accurately the covalent incorporation pattern reflects the non-covalent binding situation.

Table 1. Photoincorporation via Reagents Other Than Azides, Diazo
Compounds, or Conjugated Ketones.

Ligands	Receptor	Irradiation Wavelength (nm)	Reference
Z-Ala-Ala-pNO$_2$Phe-OH	chymotrypsin	365	1
chloramphenicol	ribosomes	>300	2
4-thiouridine triphosphate	RNA polymerase	254	3
poly rU	ribosomes	254	4
DNA	DNA polymerase	254	5
poly dA.dT	RNA polymerase	254	6
fd-DNA	gene 5 protein	254	7
tRNA^{Tyr}	Tyr-tRNA synthetase	254	8
tRNA^{Phe}	Phe-tRNA synthetase	>300	9
puromycin	ribosomes	254,350	10
3'-5'-c-AMP	lamb testis extract	254	11
N^6-butyryl c-AMP	erythrocyte ghost	254	12
IdUrd	thymidine kinase	254	13
BrdUrd-DNA	RNA, histones, polylysine, polyarginine	243,313	14
	lac repressor DNA polymerase RNA polymerase c-AMP binding protein	254	15
pyridoxal phosphate	glutamate dehydrogenase	unfiltered	16
	aspartate transcarbamylase	>300	17
triarylethylenes	rate uterine cytosol	254,>315	18
fluorescein	ribonuclease	>400	19
	RNA	>400	19
	bovine serum albumin	>400	19
acridine orange		>400	19
methylene blue		>400	19

1. Escher and Schwyzer, 1974; 2. Sonenberg *et al.*, 1974; 3. Frischauf
and Scheit, 1973; 4. Schenkman *et al.*, 1974; 5. Markovitz, 1972;
6. Strniste and Smith, 1974; 7 Anderson *et al.*, 1974; 8. Schoemaker
and Schimmel, 1974; 9. Budker *et al.*, 1974; 10. Cooperman *et al.*,

Table 1. (contd.)

1975: 11. Antonoff and Ferguson, 1974; 12. Guthrow *et al.*, 1973;
13. Cysyk and Prusoff, 1972; 14. Weintraub *et al.*, 1974; 15. Lin
and Riggs, 1974; 16. Hucho *et al.*, 1973; 17. Greenwell *et al.*, 1973;
18. Katzenellenbogen *et al.*, 1974; 19. Brandt *et al.*, 1974.

2.5. Site Directed Inactivation

It has been known for some time that dyes such as methylene
blue and Rose Bengal can sensitize amino acid residues in proteins
towards photooxidation, and in an analogous but more specific manner,
chromophoric ligands have been shown to inactivate receptor sites
in the absence of covalent bonding via a photosensitization process
(Knowles, 1972). Recent examples of this type of experiment are
the inactivation of RNAse by thio-UMP (Sawada, 1974) and of thymidine phosphorylase by 5-iodouracil (Vortek, 1975).

3. PHOTOAFFINITY LABELING STUDIES

3.1. Applications to Isolated Proteins

3.1.1. *Antibodies*. Richards and his co-workers (Lifter *et al.*,
1974), in an extension of their earlier work, have mapped the amino
acid residues photochemically labeled in the heavy chain of the mouse
IgA myeloma protein 460 by 2,4-dinitrophenyl-1-azide. These were
found to be principally tyrosines 33 and 88. There is evidence,
based on Edman degration results, that tyrosine 88 may undergo reaction at more than one position, and the authors suggest nitrene
insertion at the α carbon as a possibility. In an accompanying
article (Richards *et al.*, 1974), the photoaffinity labeling results
with 2,4-dinitrophenyl-1-azide and 2,4-dinitrophenylalanine diazoketone are compared with results obtained by electrophilic affinity
labels (see Section 2.2). Cannon *et al.*, (1974) have used 2,4-dini-
trophenyl-1-azide and 2,4-dinitrophenyl-ε-aminocaproyl diazoketone
to photoaffinity label isoelectrofocussed fractions from a dini-
trophenyl (Dnp) antibody preparation. Using the azide reagent, and
a mass spectral analysis of Nagarse digested antibody chains, they
have tentatively identified alanine as a primary site of labeling
in the heavy chain of one fraction, and phenylalanine and histidine
in the heavy chain of another. The distribution of label in fractions labeled with the diazo reagent were polydisperse and mass
spectral analysis was not possible. However, with this reagent
widely differing heavy/light labeling ratios were obtained for different fractions (ranging from 5.6 to 0.12), suggesting that the
typical heavy/light ratio of between two and four obtained in affinity labeling experiments on anti-Dnp antibodies represents an

average over homogeneous sites which are themselves labeled essentially exclusively on either the H or L chain. Fisher and Press
(1974) have used the photoaffinity label ε-(4-azido-2-nitrophenyl)-
L-lysine, [ε-Nap-lysine] introduced by Fleet *et al.* (1972) to map
the combining regions of both anti-Nap and anti-Dnp antibodies.
They found the labeling ratio of heavy/light chains in anti-Nap
antibody to be 3.3-5.0, and localized 80% of the heavy chain labeling to two hypervariable regions, positions 29-34 and 95-114. The
heavy/light ratio agrees with the results of Fleet *et al.* (1972),
but in contrast to the earlier work which placed 13% of the label
on positions 92 and 93 of the heavy chain, in the current paper
no more than 1% of the label is found in this region. This difference may be due to differences in the rabbit allotype used for
antisera preparation. Smith and Knowles (1974) have compared the
results obtained in photoaffinity labeling experiments on anti-Nap
antibody using ε-Nap-lysine and ε-isoNap-lysine [ε-(5-azido-2-nitro-
phenyl)-L-lysine]. They found, as expected, that ε-Nap-lysine both
binds more tightly and covalently labels more extensively than ε-
isoNap-lysine. Furthermore, the heavy/light labeling ratios obtained
with the two reagents differ, and although there is a sub-population
of antibodies that will form non-covalent complexes with both, the
antibodies covalently labeled by each reagent appear to fall into
two mutually exclusive groups. These differences are taken as
evidence for the specificity of the photoaffinity labeling method.

3.1.2. *Chymotrypsin.* The first application of photochemical
probes was in a study of the enzyme chymotrypsin (Singh *et al.*,
1962; Shafer *et al.*, 1966; Hexter and Westheimer, 1971a,b) and in
the past year it has been used as a test protein for the detailed
investigation of aspects of the photoaffinity labeling technique.
Thus, Bridges and Knowles (1974) have prepared p-azido[^{14}C]cinnamoyl-
α-chymotrypsin and have partially characterized products arising
from its photolysis. They find that 60% of the label is retained
on photolysis and subsequent de-acylation, presumably due to covalent
bond formation by the nitrene, and that 80% of the label is localized
in the C-chain. Attempts to further characterize the products were
not pursued, because of the finding that radioactivity was spread
over several different peptides. However, there was some evidence
that a major site of labeling occurred in the region asparagine-204
to arginine-230, which contains much of the aromatic binding locus
of α-chymotrypsin and would thus be expected to be in contact with
the photogenerated nitrene. Glover *et al.* (1974) have alkylated
methionine 192 of α-chrymotrypsin with both phenacyl and naphthacyl
bromide. On irradiation (>300 nm) of the radioactive phenacyl derivative, approximately 60% of the label comes off the enzyme and
40% is retained. No products have been characterized, but it is
suggested that at least some of the retained label may be attributed
to covalent reactions with neighboring amino acid residues, by
either carbene insertion or Norrish Type II hydrogen abstraction.
Escher and Schwyzer (1974) have conducted photoaffinity labeling

experiments on α-chrymotrypsin (at 365 nm) with tri-peptides of
general structure Z-Ala-Ala-Phe(X)-OH, where X = H(1); pNO_2(2); pN_3
(3); mN_3(4); oNO_2,pN_3(5). Compounds 2-5 all gave reasonably efficient affinity labeling, which seems to indicate, somewhat surpris-
ingly, that, at least in this case, the nitrophenyl group is about
as effective as a photolabeling reagent as the azidophenyl group.
The photochemistry of aromatic nitro compounds has been reviewed by
Morrison (1969) and one possibility for the labeling reaction is the
photocycloaddition of the nitrophenyl moiety to a nearby double bond.

   3.1.3. *Other Proteins*. Galardy *et al*. (1974) have synthesized
a series of aryl azide and aryl ketone derivatives of pentagastrin,
a pentapeptide which binds to the exocrine cells of guinea pig pan-
creas, and tested them for their ability to photoaffinity label
bovine serum albumin. The aryl azides and a benzophenone derivative
were found to label protein at rates which were fast compared with
amino acid destruction, thus demonstrating their utility as photoaffinity labeling reagents. However, an acetophenone derivative,
though labeling protein, did so at a rate which was comparable to
amino acid destruction, thus limiting its usefulness. Labeling by
one derivative, 4-azidobenzoylpentagastrin, was found to be spread
over much of the protein, and this was attributed either to the relatively weak binding of this ligand to albumin ($K_a = 3 \times 10^3$ M^{-1})
or to the presence of more than one binding site. The authors also
describe some useful model photochemistry, demonstrating addition
of both acetophenone and benzophenone to the α carbon of N-acetyl-
glycine methyl ester on photolysis in solution.

   Brandt *et al*. (1974) have shown that several dyes, including
fluorescein, methylene blue, and acridine orange, will photoincorporate into proteins on irradiation at wavelengths >400 nm. Two
systems were studied in detail, ribonuclease-fluorescein and bovine
serum albumin-fluorescein. Incorporation appears to be at least
partially oxygen dependent and is completely inhibited by cysteine
(5mM). Although chromatographic analysis of a tryptic digest of
labeled albumin showed fluorescein spread over many peptides, one
small peptide, probably located near position 130, was labeled to
a notably high extent, providing some evidence for specificity in
the labeling process, especially as this peptide is not highly
labeled in a comparable experiment with denatured albumin (in 6 M
urea). Despite this result, use of these dyes as photoaffinity
labels is highly questionable, since the quantum yield for incorporation is much lower than the quantum yields for competing photoinduced process, such as amino acid destruction, protein aggregation,
and, in the case of ribonuclease, loss of enzymatic activity.

3.2. Applications to Complex Systems

3.2.1 *Ribosomes*. Cantor and his co-workers (Hsuing and Cantor,

1974; Hsuing *et al.*, 1974) have used two different aryl azide derivatives of Phe-tRNA^{Phe}, N-p-[2-nitro-4-azidophenoxyl]-phenylacetyl
and N-2[2-nitro-4-azidophenyl]-glycyl as photoaffinity reagents for
the *E. coli* ribosome. Both derivatives are good analogs of N-acetyl
Phe-tRNA^{Phe}; the non-covalent binding of each to ribosomes is stimulated by poly U and each participate in peptide bond formation with
puromycin. Three different types of photolabeling experiments were
carried out. In the first, the non-covalent complex of radioactive
reagent with ribosomes is photolyzed. In the second, the same non-
covalent complex made with non-radioactive reagent is photolyzed
and radioactive Phe-tRNA is added under conditions favoring peptide
bond formation. In the third, non-radioactive reagent and radioactive Phe-tRNA are first added to the ribosomes and the complete
reaction mixture is then photolyzed. The latter two experiments
would be expected to specifically label functional ribosome-tRNA
complexes since radioactive incorporation can only take place as a
result of peptide bond formation. This approach is especially apt,
given the general difficulty that ribosomal heterogeneity poses for
mapping experiments, and particularly in this work in view of the
very low yields of covalent bond formation obtained. [As estimated
by this reviewer from the published data, only 1-2% of the non-covalently bound aryl azide tRNA is covalently incorporated under
conditions of high excess of ribosomes over aryl azide tRNA]. Both
reagents in all three experiments label chiefly the protein fraction
of the 50S subunit, and, as expected, the protein labeling pattern
is more specific in the second and third experiments than in the
first. The currently accepted model for ribosome action posits two
binding sites for tRNA, an amino acyl tRNA or peptidyl acceptor site,
known as the P site. The second experiment should reflect labeling
by dipeptidyl tRNA in the P site and the third should reflect labeling by dipeptidyl tRNA in the A site, so the result that L11 and
L18 are the major labeled proteins obtained in the second and third
experiments using either reagent is taken by the authors as evidence
that the peptide end of tRNA moves little as a result of peptide
bond formation.

       In a related experiment, Kuechler and his co-workers (1975)
have shown that N-(3-benzophenonyl)-propionyl Phe-tRNA^{Phe} also
photoaffinity labels ribosomes, but in contrast to the results discussed above, almost all of the labeling is found in the 23S RNA,
which agrees with the findings of Bispink and Matthaei (1973), who
photoaffinity labeled ribosomes with N-(ethyl-2-diazomalonyl)-Phe-
tRNA^{Phe}. The reasons for the qualitative differences in labeling
pattern found by the latter two groups and Cantor's group (Hsuing
and Cantor, 1974; Hsuing *et al.*, 1974) are not clear. One possible
interpretation is that the 3'-end of tRNA is in a site made up of
both protein and RNA, and the different results obtained reflect
small differences in the orientation and chemical specificity of
the photogenerated species.

Schwartz and Ofengand (1974) have alkylated the thiouridine of
E. coli tRNA ^{Val} with both phenacyl and p-azidophenacyl bromide.
Both tRNA derivatives are essentially as active as native tRNA in
a number of assays (amino acid acceptor activity, binding to the
ribosomal P site, elongation factor Tu (EFTu)-dependent binding to
the A site, EFTu-GTP ternary complex formation, valine donation in
polypeptide synthesis). Photolysis of the p-azidophenacyl tRNA-
ribosome complex, with the tRNA in the P site, results in covalent
labeling all of which is located in 16S RNA. Preliminary experiments
are reported for photolysis of p-azidophenacyl tRNA in the A site,
giving different labeling patterns. Photolysis of the phenacyl tRNA-
ribosome complex gave no covalent binding. The light fluence used
in photolabeling (>305 nm, maximum at 350 nm) appears not to damage
the ribosomes, at least as measured by their ability to bind Val-
tRNA. Maason and Möller (1974) have shown that the 4-azidophenyl-
β-phosphate ester of guanosine diphosphate (GDP) functions as an
inhibitor of GDP binding to 50S ribosomes and examined the labeling
pattern of 50S proteins obtained on photolysis of the presumed 50S
ribosome-GDP ester complex in the presence and absence of fusidic
acid. In both cases a rather non-specific labeling pattern is found,
but if the labeling obtained in the absence of fusidic acid is sub-
tracted from that obtained in its presence, L5, L11, L18 and L30 are
found to be the major proteins differentially labeled. Photolysis
of the 70S ribosome-GDP ester complex affords similar results with
little labeling of 30S proteins observed.

Several groups have reported experiments using unmodified ribosomal ligands as potential photoaffinity reagents. Cooperman *et al.*
(1975) have demonstrated that both puromycin and the photolabile
derivative N-ethyl-2-diazomalonyl puromycin are incorporated into
both the protein and RNA portions of ribosomes on irradiation at
254 nm. Puromycin incorporation proceeds at least partially via a
saturation process as a function of puromycin concentration, providing evidence for affinity labeling, and L23 is shown to be by
far the major protein labeled, although several other proteins are
labeled significantly above background. N-Ethyl-2-diazomalonyl
puromycin has a much weaker affinity for ribosomes than puromycin,
and there is no evidence that incorporation proceeds via affinity
labeling, although the derivative is demonstrated to be an inhibitor of two ribosomal assays. The labeling pattern obtained with
the derivative differs markedly from that seen with puromycin, S14
and S18 being the major labeled proteins. Sonnenberg *et al.* (1974)
have found that chloramphenicol will also photoincorporate into 50S
ribosomes (>300 nm) and that there is a concomitant partial loss in
the peptidyl transferase activity of the ribosomes. These two processes may not be directly linked, since added erythromycin has the
effect of protecting the peptidyl transferase activity while at the
same time increasing chloramphenicol incorporation. More than 80%
of incorporation is into protein, but no specific labeling pattern
was discerned in either the absence or presence of erythromycin.

The photochemistry underlying incorporation is unexplained, but this reviewer is tempted to speculate, on the basis of the results of Escher and Schwyzer (1974) (Section 3.1.2), that the p-NO$_2$ phenyl moiety in chloramphenicol is responsible for the observed incorporation. Irradiation (254 nm) of a 70S-poly U complex has been found by Schenkman et al., (1974) to lead to virtually exclusive incorporation of poly U into the 30S subunit, where it appears to label both proteins and 16S RNA. In an essentially identical experiment, Fiser et al., (1975a) have localized the label in the 30S protein fraction to protein S1. This is in accord with earlier results in which, on irradiation (330 nm), poly 4-thio U was found to label mostly S1, with smaller amounts found in S18 and S21 (Fiser et al., 1974; 1975b).

3.2.2. *Protein-Nucleic Acid Interactions*. It has been known for some time (Smith, 1975) that proteins will cross-link to DNA, both *in vivo* and *in vitro*, on ultraviolet irradiation, and in recent years several groups have used this cross-linking as a way of probing protein-nucleic acid interactions.

One approach has been to form cross-links using the photoreactivity of natural nucleic acids. Markovitz (1972) demonstrated that UV (254 nm) irradiation of a DNA polymerase-DNA complex results in the covalent cross-linking of DNA to protein. Cross-linking requires prior complex formation, as shown by the effects of high salt (0.5 M NaCl) which blocks both processes. Other experiments with DNA polymerase and a series of homopolymer pairs led to the conclusion that cross-linking was not highly base specific. In a similar study Strniste and Smith (1974) cross-linked RNA polymerase to poly d(A-T)-d(A-T) and found the rate of cross-linking to be biphasic as a function of light fluence, with the first phase proceeding much more rapidly than the second. Schimmel and his coworkers (Schoemaker and Schimmel, 1974; Schimmel et al., This Volume) have used 254 nm irradiation to cross-link tRNA's to their respective tRNA synthetases. The cross-linking reaction is specific in the sense that cross-linking is achieved only with synthetase-tRNA pairs that form strong non-covalent complexes, and, for a given pair, the pH dependence of cross-linking parallels that of complex formation. Those parts of the tRNA involved in cross-linking have been identified by comparison of tRNAse fragments of native and cross-linked tRNA. For example, for *E. coli* tyrosyl-tRNA synthetase-tRNA$_2$[Tyr], cross-linking takes place to only 3 out of 14 fragments (located in the second helical region, the anticodon loop, and the extra loop). Konigsberg and his co-workers (Anderson et al., 1975; Nakashima and Konigsberg 1975) have cross-linked (254 nm) bacteriophage fd gene 5 protein to single stranded fd DNA. The specificity of this reaction is indicated by the finding that under similar conditions little cross-linking is found to coat protein or protein A, both of which are coded for by fd DNA. Using [^{32}P] labeled DNA, and a combination of several DNAse and protease digestions followed by paper

electrophoresis, a single peptide (positions 29-34 of gene 5 protein) was found to be covalently attached to DNA. Within this
peptide it appears that cysteine-33 is the only amino acid linked
to DNA.

There are two major difficulties with the use of unmodified
nucleic acids for cross-linking. The first is that since, in
general,* no especially photolabile groups are present, photochemical reactions other than those leading to cross-linking may be
taking place at rates comparable or greater than the cross-linking
rate, so that the complex that is cross-linked might have a geometry
which is substantially different than that of the natural complex.
Indeed, evidence for important UV-induced damage accompanying cross-
linking has been reported in some of the above-cited studies (Anderson *et al.*, 1975; Markovitz, 1972). The second is that the photochemistry leading to cross-linking will be very hard to determine,
making it difficult to evaluate the results in terms of the two
criteria discussed in Section 2.1.

A second approach has been to introduce photolabile groups
into the nucleic acid and carry out cross-linking with the resulting modified nucleic acids. Thus, Budker *et al.*, (1974), in work
similar to that of Schwartz and Ofengand (see Section 3.2.1.), have
alkylated the thiouracil(thioUra) of *E.coli* tRNA^{Phe} with both
iodoacetamide and N-(p-azidophenyl)-iodoacetamide and examined the
effect of irradiating Phe-tRNA synthetase in the presence of unmodified tRNA^{Phe} and of each of the two modified tRNAs. The rates
of photoinduced synthetase inactivation are in the order N-(p-azidophenyl)-carboxamido-tRNA^{Phe} > unmodified tRNA^{Phe} > carboxamido
tRNA^{Phe}, which presumably reflects the photoreactivity order azide
>thioUra (Frischauf and Scheit, 1973) > alkylated thioUra. If the
inactivation rates reflect rates of incorporation, use of the aryl
azide tRNA derivative should permit cross-linking to the synthetase
at much lower light fluences, and consequently, with less photo-
damage, than the use of unmodified tRNA, as in Schimmel's experiments. Since it is possible to specifically modify tRNA at several
positions, the entire locus of tRNA binding to the synthetase could
be mapped by preparing a suitable series of photolabile derivatives.

With DNA there is no clear strategy for specific modification,
and the approach has been to introduce photolability by substituting
5-bromodeoxyuridine (BrdUrd) for thymidine (dThd). Photolysis of
BrdUrd leads to debromination and production of reactive uracilyl
radicals, which can cross-link to protein. Weintraub (1974) showed
that on UV irradiation BrdUrd-DNA effectively cross-links to proteins
which it binds non-covalently (histones, polylysine, polyarginine,

---

*Of course in some cases, such as thioUra containing tRNA's,
the natural nucleic acids themselves have highly photolabile groups.

RNA polymerase), but not to proteins with which it does not bind (trypsin, RNAse A), and that with histones the cross-linking procedure was much faster (>10 x) with BrdUrd-DNA than with natural DNA. In fact, using light of 313 nm confers an additional 5-fold specificity for BrdUrd-DNA (reflecting the red shifted UV spectrum of BrdUrd as compared with dThd). Similar results have been reported by Lin and Riggs (1974) for cross-linking *lac* repressor to BrdUrd-substituted *lac* operator, and for cross-linking DNA polymerase, RNA polymerase, and cyclic AMP binding protein to BrdUrd-DNA. Interestingly, both groups report that the extent of cross-linking is rather insensitive to added thiols. Ogata (1975) has recently begun an effort to extend the work of Lin and Riggs (1974) by mapping the regions of repressor involved in cross-linking.

Introduction of BrdUrd certainly increases the efficiency of protein-DNA cross-linking, and, since cross-linking parallels non-covalent complex formation, this technique is valuable for demonstrating a specific binding interaction (Lin and Riggs, 1974). Its utility for exploring the microscopic details of DNA-protein (e.g., contact residues) is more questionable. Although it does offer the advantage of defining the species responsible for cross-linking, placement of BrdUrd all over the DNA does nothing to solve the problem discussed above of competing non-cross-linking reactions and in some cases may actually make the problem worse. One way of obtaining a more defined cross-linking process would be to introduce photolabile groups into the protein, rather than into the DNA, but so far this approach has not been utilized.

3.2.3. *Other Complex Systems.* Haley and Hoffman (1974) have used 8-azido ATP to photoaffinity label (254 nm) ATP receptor sites on human erythrocyte ghost membranes. 8-Azido ATP is found to be a substrate for both the Na, K-ATPase and the Mg-ATPase of the ghosts. On photolysis, 8-azido ATP incorporation was found to parallel ATPase inactivation. Incorporation takes place specifically into a few of the erythrocyte proteins and is completely abolished in the presence of ATP. The authors cite several other studies in progress using 8-azide-adenine analogs and conclude that these appear to be potent reagents for probing nucleotide binding sites. Hanstein and Hatefi (1974) have photoincorporated 2-azido-4-nitrophenol into mitochondria. The dependence of incorporation on concentration of aryl azide suggests covalent labeling of both specific and non-specific sites. In accord with this, some uncouplers of oxidative phosphorylation inhibit incorporation only partially and the labeling pattern of mitochondrial proteins shows at best only partial specificity. Rudnick *et al.,* (1975) have shown that photolysis of bacterial membrane vesicles in the presence of the photolabile lactose transport inhibitor, 2-nitro-4-azidophenyl-1-thio-β-D-galactopyranoside, leads to an irreversible inactivation of lactose transport (but not amino acid transport) which is lactate dependent. No affinity labeling studies are presented, but such

studies would certainly seem worthwhile for this system. Ruoho and
Kyte (1974) have shown that both 4'-(ethyl 2-diazomalonyl)cymarin
and 4'-(ethyl-2-chloromalonyl)cymarin photoaffinity label (254 nm)
the large peptide chain in microsomal (Na^+ + K^+) ATPase, leaving
the small chain unlabeled. Incorporation is more efficient with
the chloromalonyl compound, and this unexplained result makes it
uncertain to what extent incorporation of the diazo compound is
dependent on carbene formation. A possible explanation, offered
by this reviewer, is that the incorporation of the chloromalonyl
derivative, and perhaps some of the incorporation of the diazo compound, is due to the α,β unsaturated γ-lactone in cymarin. Antonoff
and Ferguson (1974) have reported that unmodified 3',5'-cyclic AMP
(cAMP) is photoincorporated into trichloroacetic acid precipitable
material from lamb testis extracts. Evidence that incorporation
proceeds via an affinity labeling process comes from the observations
that covalent incorporation and non-covalent binding show the same
concentration dependence, and that incorporation and binding are
specifically decreased by N^6-butyryl-cAMP and cIMP, but not by
adenosine, AMP, ADP, etc. The underlying photochemistry behind the
process is not understood, but the authors suggest that their findings might be related to the earlier result noted by Guthrow *et al.*,
(1973) that N^6-butyryl cAMP can be photoincorporated into erythrocyte
ghost membranes on irradiation at 254 nm. The authors mention briefly
that cGMP also photoincorporates into extracts. Katzenellenbogen
et al., (1974) have studied the ability of a large series of photosensitive estrogens or antiestrogens to non-covalently bind, and on
photolysis (254 nm and >315 nm) irreversibly inactivate, estrogen
receptors in rat uterine cytosol. They found no clear correlation
between binding affinity and inactivation efficiency. Although
several diazo and azide derivatives both bind and irreversibly inactivate, the most potent irreversible inactivators are a class of
triarylethylene antiestrogens. The authors discuss the relative
merits of irreversible photolabile groups (azide and diazo) as opposed to photoexcitable groups (aromatic ketones, triarylethylenes)
in photoaffinity labeling studies. No incorporation studies are
reported, since radioactive compounds were not available. In related work, Wolff *et al.*, (1975) have demonstrated that several
21-diazo steroids compete, though weakly, for aldosterone binding
sites in rat kidney slices, and for corticosterone binding sites in
rat plasma, and have presented preliminary evidence that one of them,
9α-bromo-21-diazo-21-deoxycorticosterone can be photoincorporated
into plasma protein.

Hixon *et al.*, (1975) have synthesized an azide derivative of
ethidium bromide and shown that it is incorporated into DNA *in vitro*,
on photolysis with visible light. They also present evidence for
photoincorporation of the azide into DNA in yeast cells *in vivo*,
with mitochondrial rather than nuclear DNA being labeled selectively,
based mainly on changes in the UV absorption spectrum and the melting curve of DNA isolated from photolyzed cells. However, a more

convincing demonstration will require a radioactive derivative, which is not presently available.

3.3. Photolabile Reagents as Topological Probes

Richards and his co-workers (Staros and Richards, 1974; Staros *et al.*, 1974) have made use of the relatively long lifetime of aryl nitrenes, which is detrimental to affinity labeling studies, to advantage in studying the disposition of proteins in the erythrocyte membrane. They have synthesized a hydrophilic aryl azide, N-(4-azido-2-nitrophenyl)-2-amino-ethylsulfonate which on photolysis in the presence of erythrocyte ghost membranes successfully incorporates into all of the proteins and glycoproteins in the membrane. By contrast, the corresponding experiment on intact erythrocyte cells, to which the reagent is impermeable, showed a more selective labeling pattern, and this difference was attributed to the inaccessibility of proteins on the inner face of the intact membrane to the reagent. Labeling patterns obtained with resealed ghosts differed from those obtained with intact erythrocytes which was taken as evidence for important structural differences between the membranes. Although the aim of the study was to utilize a general modification reagent which showed no binding specificity and was thus a pure topological probe, in fact some proteins are labeled preferentially, particularly one which has been associated with the anion channel, so that it appears that their reagent is acting as both a topological probe and an affinity label.

Klip and Gitler (1974) have followed a similar approach to label sarcoplasmic reticulum vesicles, but from within the lipid core of the membrane, by using two hydrophobic azides, 1-azidonaph-thalene and 1-azido-4-iodobenzene. The results with both reagents were the same -- approximately 90% of the photoincorporated reagent was found in the fatty acid fraction and the remainder in membrane-bound protein, and evidence was presented that at least some of the protein labeling took place from within the core.

4. FINAL REMARKS

This review and the two reviews which precede it (Knowles, 1972; Creed, 1974) provide ample evidence that photoaffinity labeling is a generally useful technique for studying ligand-receptor interactions, particularly with respect to mapping the site of ligand binding to a complex target. Given the widespread interest in such information, one may expect a continued expansion in the use of this technique in the future. Several years ago it was regarded as a considerable achievement when covalent labeling with a photoaffinity label was obtained. With the results of a large number of experiments now in hand, it has become increasingly clear that the difficul part of such an experiment is not in obtaining covalent labeling but rather in showing what the labeling really means. Hopefully, this review will spur efforts in this direction.

References

Anderson, E., Nakashima, Y., and Konigsberg, W., 1975, Photo-induced cross-linkage of gene-5 protein and bacteriophage fd DNA, *Nucleic Acids Res.* 2:361-371.

Antonoff, R., and Ferguson, Jr., J.J., 1974, Photoaffinity labeling with cyclic nucleotides, *J. Biol. Chem.* 249:3319-3321.

Baron, W.J., DeCamp, M.R., Henrick, M.A., Jones, Jr., M., Levin, R.H., and Sohn, M.B., 1973, Carbenes from diazo compounds *in* "Carbenes" (M. Jones, Jr., and R.A. Moss, eds.), Vol. I, pp. 1-151, Wiley-Interscience, New York.

Bispink, L., and Matthaei, H., 1973, Photoaffinity labeling of 23S RNA in *E.coli* ribosomes with poly (U)-coded ethyl-2-diazomalonyl phenylalanyl-tRNA, *FEBS Lett.* 37:291-294.

Brandt, J., Fredriksson, M., and Anderson, L.-O., 1974, Coupling of dyes to biopolymers by sensitized photooxidation affinity labeling of a binding site in bovine serum albumin, *Biochemistry* 13:4758-4764.

Breslow, R., Baldwin, S., Flechtner, T., Kalicky, P., Liu, S., and Washburn, W., 1973, Remote oxidation of steroids by photolysis of attached benzophenone groups, *J. Amer. Chem. Soc.* 95:3251-3262.

Breslow, R., Feiring, A., and Herman, F., 1974, Intramolecular insertion reactions of phosphoryl nitrenes, *J. Amer. Chem. Soc.* 96:5937-5939.

Bridges, A.J., and Knowles, J.R., 1974, An examination of the utility of photogenerated reagents by using α-chymotrypsin, *Biochem. J.* 143:663-668.

Budker, V.G., Knorre, O.G., Kravchenko, U.Va., Lavrik, O. II, Nevinsky, G.A., and Teplova, N.M., 1974, Photoaffinity reagents for modification of amino acyl-tRNA synthetases, *FEBS Lett.* 49:159-162.

Cannon, I.E., Woodward, D.K., Woehler, M.E., and Lovins, R.E., 1974, Affinity labeling of isoelectrofocused fractions from a DNP antibody preparation with the photoactive labels 2,4-dinitrophenyl-1-azide and 2,4-dinitrophenyl-ϵ-aminocaproyldiazoketone, *Immunology* 26:1183-1194.

Closs, G.L., 1975, Application of physical methods to the study of carbene reactions in solution, *in* "Carbenes", (R.A. Moss, and M. Jones, Jr., eds), Vol. II, pp. 159-183, Wiley-Interscience, New York.

Cooperman, B.S., and Brunswick, D.J., 1973, On the photoaffinity labeling of rabbit muscle phosphofructokinase with $0^{2'}$-(ethyl-2-diazomalonyl)adenosine 3':5'-cyclic monophosphate, *Biochemistry* 12:4079-4084.

Cooperman, B.S., Jaynes, Jr., E.N., Brunswick, D.J., and Luddy, M.A., 1975, On the photoincorporation of puromycin and N-(ethyl-2-diazomalonyl)-puromycin into *E. coli* ribosomes, *Proc. Nat. Acad. Sci. USA* 72 (in press).

Creed, D., 1974, Photochemical probes for biological interactions, *Photochem. Photobiol.* 19:459-462.

Cysyk, R., and Prusoff, W.H., 1972, Alteration of ultraviolet sensitivity of thymidine kinase by allosteric regulators, normal substrates, and a photoaffinity label, 5-iodo-2'deoxy-uridine, a metabolic analog of thymidine, *J. Biol. Chem.* 247: 2522-2532.

Escher, E., and Schwyzer, R., 1974, p-Nitrophenylalanine-p-azido-phenylalanine, m-azidophenylalanine, and o-nitro-p-azido-phenylalanine as photoaffinity labels, *FEBS Lett.* 46:347-350.

Fiser, I., Margaritella, P., and Kuechler, E., 1975a, Photoaffinity reaction between polyuridylic acid and protein S1 on the *E. coli* ribosome, *FEBS Lett.* 52:281-283.

Fiser, I., Scheit, K.H., Stöffler, G., and Kuechler, E., 1974, Identification of protein S1 at the messenger RNA binding site of *E.coli* ribosome, *Biochem. Biophys. Res. Commun.* 60:1112-1118.

Fiser, I., Scheit, K.H., Stöffler, G., and Kuechler, E., 1975b, Proteins at the mRNA binding site of the *E.coli* ribosome, *FEBS Lett.*, In Press.

Fisher, C.E., and Press, E.M., 1974, Affinity labeling of the binding site of rabbit antibody-evidence for the involvement of the hypervariable regions of the heavy chain, *Biochem. J.* 139:135-149.

Fleet, G.W.J., Knowles, J.R., and Porter, R.R., 1972, The antibody site-labeling of a specific antibody against the photo-precursor of an aryl nitrene, *Biochem. J.* 128:499-508.

Frischauf, A.M. and Scheit, K.H., 1973, Affinity labeling of *E.coli* RNA polymerase with substrate and template analogs, *Biochem. Biophys. Res. Commun.* 53:1227-1233.

Galardy, R.E., Craig, L.C., Jamieson, J.D., and Printz, M.P., 1974, Photoaffinity labeling of peptide hormone binding sites, *J. Biol. Chem.* 249:3510-3518.

Glover, G.I., Mariano, P.S., Wilkinson, T.J. Hildreth, R.A., and Lowe, T.W., 1974, Photofragmentation and photoaffinity labeling of phenacyl and naphthacyl α-chymotrpsins, *Arch. Biochem. Biophys.* 162:73-83.

Greenwell, P., Jewett, S.L., and Stark, G.R., 1973, Aspartate transcarbamylase from *E.coli*. The use of pyridoxal 5'phosphate as a probe in the active site, *J. Biol. Chem.* 248:5994-6001.

Guthrow, C.E., Rasmussen, H., Brunswick, D.J., and Cooperman, B.S., 1973, Specific photoaffinity labeling of the adenosine 3':5'-cyclic monophosphate receptor in intact ghosts from human erythrocytes, *Proc. Nat. Acad. Sci. USA*, 70:3344-3346.

Haley, B.E., and Hoffman, J.F., 1974, Interactions of a photo-affinity ATP analog with cation-stimulated adenosine triphosphatases of human red cell membranes, *Proc. Nat. Acad. Sci.*

USA 71:3367-3371.

Hanstein, W.G., and Hatefi, Y., 1974, Characterization and locali-
    zation of metochondrial uncoupler binding sites with an un-
    coupler capable of photoaffinity labeling, *J. Biol. Chem.*
    249:1356-1362.

Hexter, C.S., and Westheimer, F.H., 1971a, Intermolecular reaction
    during photolysis of diazoacetyl α-chymotrypsin, *J. Biol.
    Chem.* 246:3928-3933.

Hexter, C.S., and Westheimer, F.H., 1971b, S-carboxymethylcysteine
    from the photolysis of diazoacyl trypsin and chymotrypsin,
    J. Biol. Chem. 246:3924-3928.

Hew, C-L., Lifter, J., Yoshioka, M., Richards, F.F., and Konigsberg,
    W.H., 1973, Affinity labeled peptides obtained from the com-
    bining region of protein 460. Light chain labeling patterns
    using dinitrophenyl based photoaffinity labels, *Biochemistry*
    12:4685-4689.

Hixon, S.C., White, Jr., W.E., and Yielding, K.L., 1975, Selective
    covalent binding of an ethidium analog to mitochondrial DNA
    with production of petite mutants in yeast by photoaffinity
    labeling, *J. Mol. Biol.* 92:319-329.

Hixson, S.S., and Hixson, S.H., 1972, The photochemistry of s-methyl
    diazothioacetate, *J. Org. Chem.* 37:1279-1280.

Hsiung, N., and Cantor, C.R., 1974, A new simpler photoaffinity
    analogue of peptidyl tRNA, *Nucleic Acids Res.* 1:1753-1762.

Hsiung, N., Reines, S.A., and Cantor, C.R., 1974, Investigation of
    the ribosomal peptidyl transferase center using a photoaffinity
    label, *J. Mol. Biol.* 88:841-855.

Hucho, F., Markau, U., and Sund, H., 1973, Studies of glutamate
    dehydrogenase characterization of histidine residues involved
    in the activity and association photoactivated labelling with
    pyridoxal 5'-phosphate, *Eur. J. Biochem.* 32:69-75.

Katzenellenbogen, J.A., Johnson, Jr., H.J., Carlson, K.E., and
    Myers, H.N., 1974, Photoreactivity of some light-sensitive
    estrogen derivatives. Use of an exchange assay to determine
    their photointeraction with the rat uterine estrogen binding
    protein, *Biochemistry* 13:2986-2994.

Klip, A., and Gitler, C., 1974, Photoactive covalent labeling of
    membrane components from within the lipid core, *Biochem.
    Biophys. Res. Commun.* 60:1155-1162.

Knowles, J.R., 1972, Photogenerated reagents for biological receptor-
    site labeling, *Accounts Chem. Res.* 5:155-160.

Lifter, J., Hew, C.L., Yoshioka, M., Richards, F.F., and Konigsberg,
    W.H., 1974, Affinity-labeled peptides obtained from the com-
    bining region of myeloma protein 460. I. Heavy-chain-labeling
    patterns using dinitrophenyl azide photoaffinity label,
    Biochemistry 13:3567-3571.

Lin, S.-Y, and Riggs, A.D., 1974, Photochemical attachment of *lac*
    repressor to bromodeoxyuridine-substituted *lac* operator by
    ultraviolet irradiation, *Proc. Nat. Acad. Sci. USA*, 71:947-951.

Maasen, J.A., and Möller, W., 1974, Identification by photo-affinity labeling of the proteins in *Escherichia coli* ribosomes involved in elongation factor G-dependent GDP binding, *Proc. Nat. Acad. Sci. USA* 71:1277-1280.

Markovitz, A., 1972, Ultraviolet light-induced stable complexes of DNA and DNA polymerase, *Biochim. Biophys. Acta* 281:523-534.

Martyr, R.J., and Benisek, W.F., 1973, Affinity labeling of the active sites Δ^5-ketosteroid isomerase using photoexcited natural ligands, *Biochemistry* 12:2172-2178.

Morrison, H.A., 1969, The photochemistry of the nitro and nitroso groups *in* "The Chemistry of the Nitro and Nitroso Groups," (H. Feurer, ed.). pp. 165-213, Interscience, New York.

Nakashima, Y., and Konigsberg, W., 1975, Photo-induced cross-linkage of gene 5 protein and bacteriophage fd DNA, Abstr. Int. Symp. "Protein and Other Adducts to DNA: Their Significance to Aging, Carcinogenesis and Radiation Biology," Williamsburg, Virginia, May 2-6, 1975.

Ogata, R., 1975, Affinity labeling of the operator binding site on the *lac* repressor, Abstr. Int. Symp. "Protein and Other Adducts to DNA: Their Significance to Aging, Carcinogenesis and Radiation Biology," Williamsburg, Virginia, May 2-6, 1975.

Richards, F.F., Lifter, J., Hew, C.L., Yoshioka, M., and Konigsberg, W.H., 1974, Photoaffinity labeling of the combining region of myeloma protein 460. II. An interpretation of the labeling patterns, *Biochemistry* 13:3572-3575.

Rosenstein, R.W., and Richards, F.F., 1972, Synthesis of a photo-activate menadione (VIT K.). Affinity label in its reaction with a menadione-binding myeloma protein, *J. Immunol.* 108: 1467-1469.

Rudnick, G., Kaback, H.R., and Wiel, R., 1975, Photoinactivation of the β-galactoside transport system in *Escherichia coli* membrane vesicles with 2-nitro-4-azidophenyl-1-thio-β-d-galactopyranoside, *J. Biol. Chem.* 250:1371-1375.

Ruoho, A.E., Kiefer, H., Roeder, P.E., and Singer, S.J., 1973, The mechanism of photoaffinity labeling, *Proc. Nat. Acad. Sci. USA,* 70:2567-2571.

Ruoho, A., and Kyte, J., 1974, Photoaffinity labeling of the ouabain-binding site on ($Na^+ + K^+$) adenosinetriphosphatase, *Proc. Nat. Acad. Sci. USA,* 71:2352-2356.

Sawada, F., 1974, Kinetics of 4-thiouridylate-sensitized photoin-activation of ribonuclease A, *Photochem, Photobiol.* 20:523-526.

Schenkman, M., Ward, D.C., and Moore, P.B. 1974, Covalent attachment of a messenger RNA to the *Escherichia coli* ribosome, *Biochim. Biophys. Acta,* 353:503-508.

Schoemaker, H.J., and Schimmel, P.R., 1974, Photo-induced joining of a transfer RNA with its cognate amino acyl-transfer RNA synthetase, *J. Mol. Biol.* 84:503-513.

Schwartz, I., and Ofengand, J., 1974, Photo-affinity labeling of tRNA binding sites in macromolecules. I. Linking of the phenacyl-p-azide of 4-thiouridine in (*Escherichia coli*) valyl-tRNA to 16S RNA at the ribosomal P site, *Proc. Nat. Acad. Sci. USA* 71:3951-3955.

Shafer, J., Baronowsky, P., Laursen, R., Finn, F., and Westheimer, F.H., 1966, Products from the photolysis of diazoacetyl chymotrypsin, *J. Biol. Chem.* 241:421-427.

Shaw, E., 1970, Chemical modification by active-site directed reagents, *Enzymes* 1:91-146.

Singer, S.J., 1967, Covalent labeling of active sites, *Adv. Protein Chem.* 22:1-54.

Singh, A., Thornton, E.R., and Westheimer, F.H., 1962, The photolysis of diazoacetyl chymotrypsin, *J. Biol. Chem.* 237:PC 3006.

Smith, K.C., 1975, The radiation-induced addition of proteins and other molecules to nucleic acids, *in* "Photochemistry and Photobiology of Nucleic Acids" (S.Y. Wang, ed.), Academic Press, New York (in press).

Smith, P.A.S., 1970, Aryl nitrenes and formation of nitrenes by rupture of heterocyclic rings, *in* "Nitrenes" (W. Lwowski, ed.), pp. 99-162, Wiley-Interscience, New York.

Smith, R.A.G., and Knowles, J.R., 1974, The utility of photo-affinity labels as 'mapping' reagents. A study of sub-populations of a specific rabbit antibody by using structually related photoaffinity reagents, *Biochem. J.* 141:51-56.

Sonenberg, N., Zamir, A., and Wilchek, M., 1974, A photo induced reaction of chloramphenicol with *E. coli* ribosomes: covalent binding of the antibiotic and inactivation of peptidyl transferase, *Biochem. Biophys. Res. Commun.* 59:693-696.

Staros, J.V., and Richards, F.M., 1974, Photochemical labeling of the surface proteins of human erythrocytes, *Biochemistry* 13:2720-2726.

Staros, J.V., Haley, B.E., and Richards, F.M., 1974, Human erythrocytes and resealed ghosts, a comparison of membrane topology, *J. Biol. Chem.* 249:5004-5007.

Strniste, G.F., and Smith, D.A., 1974, Induction of stable linkage between the deoxyribonucleic acid dependent ribonucleic acid polymerase and $d(A-T)_n \cdot d(A-T)_n$ by ultraviolet light, *Biochemistry* 13:485-493.

Turro, N.J., Dalton, C.J., Dawes, R., Farrington, G., Harltala, R., Morton, D., Niemczyk, M., and Schore, N., 1972, Molecular photochemistry of alkanones in solution: α-cleavage, hydrogen abstraction, cycloaddition, and sensitization reactions, *Accounts Chem. Res.* 5:92-101.

Vallee, B.L., and Riordan, J.F., 1969, Chemical approaches to the properties of active sites of enzymes, *Annu. Rev. Biochem.* 38:733-794.

Vaughan, R., 1970, Diazo esters as bifunctional inhibitors. A method for marking the hydropholic binding sites of enzymes, Ph.D. Thesis, Harvard University.

Vortek, P., 1975, Enhanced photoinactivation of thymidine phosphorylase by halogenated reactants accompanied by changes in physical properties of the enzyme. Abstr. Int. Symp. "Protein

and Other Adducts to DNA: Their Significance to Aging, Carcinogenesis and Radiation Biology," Williamsburg, Virginia, May
2-6, 1975.
Wagner, P.J., 1971, Type II. Photoelimination and photocyclization
of ketones, *Accounts Chem. Res.* 4:168-177.
Walsh, C.T., Schonbrunn, A., Lockridge, O., Massey, V., and Abeles,
R.H., 1972, Inactivation of a flavoprotein, lactate oxidase,
by an acetylenic substrate, *J. Biol. Chem.* 247:6004-6006.
Weintraub, H., 1974, The assembly of newly replicated DNA into
chromatin, *Cold Spring Harbor Symp. Quant. Biol.* 38:247-256.
Wolff, M.E., Feldman, D., Catsoulacos, P., Funder, J.W., Hancock,
C., Amano, Y., and Edelman, I.S., 1975, Steroidal 21-diazo
ketones: photogenerated corticosteroid receptor labels,
Biochemistry 14:1750-1759.

CHEMICALLY AND METABOLICALLY INDUCED DNA ADDUCTS: RELATIONSHIP TO

CHEMICAL CARCINOGENESIS

Charles Heidelberger

McArdle Laboratory for Cancer Research, University of

Wisconsin, Madison, Wisconsin 53706

1.   INTRODUCTION

It is clearly impossible within the assigned scope to give a complete literature review and overview of this enormous field. Therefore, it is inevitable that this chapter will reflect my own biases, interests, and research. In the literature citations, emphasis will be placed on reviews, but important original papers will be covered.

In 1947 the Miller's made the epoch-making discovery that hepatocarcinogenic aminoazo dyes were covalently bound to the proteins from the livers of rats following feeding in the diet (Miller and Miller, 1947). This initial discovery has led to an avalanche of similar findings with all classes of chemical carcinogens that have been properly studied. In the case of polycyclic aromatic hydrocarbon (PAH) carcinogens, covalent binding to mouse skin proteins was demonstrated following local application by means of fluorescence (Miller, 1951) and radiochemical techniques (Wiest and Heidelberger, 1953). This binding, in direct proportion to the carcinogenic activity of the hydrocarbon, is to a specific protein, termed the h-protein (Abell and Heidelberger, 1962), which has been isolated and purified to homogeneity (Tasseron *et al.*, 1970; Sarrif *et al.*, 1975). It is not identical to ligandin, a cytoplasmic liver protein that binds many ligands, and its function is now under intense investigation.

In 1961 we reported for the first time that carcinogenic hydrocarbons are also bound covalently to mouse skin DNA and RNA following local application (Heidelberger and Davenport, 1961), and this was followed by much more work, indicating that PAH are bound to DNA to an extent roughly correlating with their carcinogenic activities (Brookes and Lawley, 1964; Brookes, 1966; Goshman and Heidelberger, 1967; Brookes and Heidelberger, 1969). Such binding of PAH to nucleic acids and proteins is in accord with the electronic theories of the Pullman's (Pullman and Pullman, 1955, 1969). The covalent binding to DNA has also been observed with all classes of chemical carcinogens that have been properly studied (see reviews by: Magee and Barnes, 1967; Miller, 1970; Heidelberger, 1970a, b, 1973a, 1975; Irving, 1973; Miller and Miller, 1974; Kriek, 1974; Brookes, 1975).

Wünderlich *et al.* (1971/1972) observed that diethylnitrosamine alkylates mitochondrial DNA to a considerably greater extent than nuclear DNA. It has been shown in cell cultures and on mouse skin that PAH bind covalently to both replicating and non-replicating DNA (Yuspa *et al.*, 1969/1970; Yuspa and Bates, 1970; Bowden *et al.*, 1974a).

As a result of all the work cited thus far, it has become axiomatic and generally accepted that the process of carcinogenesis is initiated as a result of the covalent interaction of the chemical carcinogen and some cellular macromolecule. As can be seen from the emphasis at this meeting, many people believe that DNA is the primary target of chemical carcinogen action, which implies that carcinogenesis results from a somatic mutation. The relationship between the processes of carcinogenesis and mutagenesis will be discussed below. Suffice it to say that at present it is not proved that DNA is the molecular target of chemical carcinogens.

A major advance in studying the mechanisms of chemical carcinogenesis has been the development of quantitative systems for obtaining malignant transformation of cells in culture. These systems involve the use of early passage hamster embryo cells (Berwald and Sachs, 1965; DiPaolo *et al.*, 1969), lines of C3H mouse prostate fibroblasts (Chen and Heidelberger, 1969), lines of BALB/3T3 mouse embryo fibroblasts (DiPaolo *et al.*, 1972; Kakunaga, 1973), lines of C3H mouse embryo fibroblasts, known as 10T1/2 (Reznikoff *et al.*, 1973a, b); long-passage rat embryo fibroblasts (Freeman *et al.*, 1973); and leukemia virus-infected mouse embryo cells (Rhim *et al.*, 1974). All the above work has been done with fibroblasts. There is currently considerable activity and some success at transforming epithelial cells, but the systems have not yet been made quantitative

The field of chemical carcinogenesis in cell cultures has been reviewed (Casto and DiPaolo, 1973; Heidelberger, 1973b, 1974, 1975), and the use of these systems for studies of metabolic activation will be described below.

2. COVALENT BINDING OF ALKYLATING AGENTS TO DNA

Since Dr. Bernard Strauss (This Volume) will discuss in some detail the reactions of simple alkylating agents with DNA and the possible relationship of DNA repair and carcinogenesis, only cursory attention will be given here to the covalent binding of these simple alkylating agents to DNA. This field was largely initiated and developed by Lawley, who has reviewed it (Lawley, 1966, 1972, and in an American Chemical Society Monograph, in press).

It is well known that the most reactive base in DNA towards alkylating agents is guanine, which has the highest degree of nucleo-philicity. Most of the simple methylating agents react primarily with the N-7 nitrogen of guanine, which leads to the lability of the glycosidic bond and results in depurination of the DNA at the alkylated site. This can produce single-strand breaks of the DNA and frameshift mutations. Bifunctional alkylating agents, such as nitrogen mustard, can form cross-links between the N-7's of guanines that are located either on the same strand or on opposite strands of the DNA. It is believed that the latter cross-linking, which prevents the movement of DNA and RNA polymerases down the DNA double helix, is responsible for the cancer chemotherapeutic action of the nitrogen mustards. In addition to the N-7 of guanine, other sites of simple alkylation of DNA are N-3 of adenine and the N-3 of cytosine (Lawley, 1965).

It has been found that β-propiolactone, which is a chemically reactive skin carcinogen, also alkylates the N-7 of guanine (Colburn *et al.*, 1965) and is bound *in vivo* to mouse skin DNA, RNA, and proteins (Colburn and Boutwell, 1968). β-Propiolactone also pro-duces DNA protein complexes, which is most appropriate to one of the topics of this meeting (Nietert *et al.*, 1974), and furthermore it produces intermolecular cross-linking of *E. coli* and lambda phage DNA molecules followed by fragmentation (Kubinski and Szybalski, 1975).

Returning to the alkylation of guanine by simple methylating and ethylating agents, Loveless (1969) drew attention to the fact that O-6-alkyl guanines are also formed, which are unstable to the usual methods of strong acid hydrolysis of the DNA used for the analysis of alkylated bases. He further suggested that the occur-rence in DNA of O-6 alkylated (but not N-7) guanines could result in base-transition mutants (Fig. 1). Magee and Barnes (1967) had found no correlation between the extent of *in vivo* methylation of

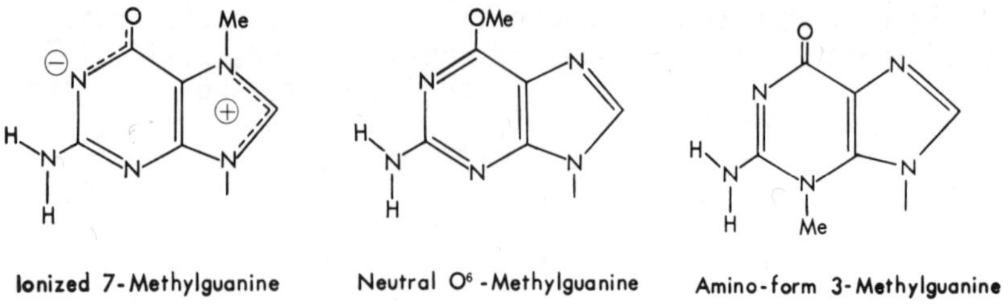

Ionized 7-Methylguanine   **Neutral O⁶-Methylguanine**   **Amino-form 3-Methylguanine**

Fig. 1. Possible mutagenic effects produced by mis-pairing of the products of the alkylation of guanine (Lawley, 1972).

the N-7 of guanine and the biological activities of carcinogenic and noncarcinogenic methylating agents. N-methyl-N'-nitro-N-nitrosoguanidine (MNNG), a powerful mutagen and carcinogen, reacts directly with DNA guanine in a thiol catalyzed reaction; the intracellular thiol concentration determined the amount of DNA alkylation in cultured cells (Lawley and Thatcher, 1970). Lawley (1972) has also adduced evidence that the strongly carcinogenic methylating agents, such as nitrosomethylurea, react by an S_{N1} mechanism, whereas the less carcinogenic compounds such as methyl methane sulfonate react by S_{N2} mechanisms. Similarly, it was observed that the former compounds produce more 0-6-methyl guanine than do the latter (Lawley and Shah, 1972). By the use of a double-labeled precursor, it was demonstrated that the methyl group of MNNG is transferred intact to both the N-7 and 0-6 of guanine (Lawley and Shah, 1973). Some evidence for phosphotriester formation was obtained following the reaction of MNNG with DNA, but the significance of this reaction to biological effects is presently unknown (Lawley, 1973). The details of nucleic acid base methylations under various conditions have been reviewed (Lawley, 1972).

Although this impinges somewhat on Dr. Strauss' territory (Strauss, This Volume), it might be worth mentioning that we could find no correlation between the production and repair of single-stranded breaks in the DNA of 10T1/2 cells and malignant transformation produced by MNNG in asynchronous (Peterson *et al.*, 1974a) and synchronized (Bertram and Heidelberger, 1974; Peterson *et al.*, 1974b) cells.

In vivo studies suggest that the retention of 0-6-methylated or ethylated DNA in target tissues is associated with carcinogenesis. Craddock (1973) found for the first time that 0-6-methyl guanine was present in liver DNA following *in vivo* administration of the carcinogenic dimethylnitrosamine (DMN), but not following the non-carcinogenic methyl methane sulfonate. This was found independently (O'Connor *et al.*, 1973), and the 0-6-methyl guanine was excised from the DNA at a more rapid rate than was N-7-methyl guanine, indicating that there is a specific repair process in liver for O-6-alkylated DNA. Ethylnitrosourea (ENU) has considerable carcinogenic specificity for nervous tissue as compared to liver, and Goth and Rajewsky (1972) found no correlation between the tissue contents of N-7-ethylguanine and the carcinogenic effect, but did find a much longer retention time of O-6-ethyl guanine in brain than in liver (Goth and Rajewsky, 1974). All the above studies suggest that alkylation at the O-6 of guanine is more likely to be associated with carcinogenesis than N-7 alkylation.

3. METABOLIC ACTIVATION OF CARCINOGENS

As emphasized above, all chemical carcinogens that have been properly studied are bound covalently to cellular macromolecules, and this interaction is thought to be responsible for the initiation of carcinogenesis. However, with the exception of the alkylating agents including nitrosamides, most chemical carcinogens do not react chemically with these macromolecules in the test tube. Therefore, it is necessary that most chemical carcinogens be metabolically converted into chemically reactive compounds. This concept of metabolic activation was first discovered and enunciated by the Miller's, who have drawn the additional generalization that the activated or ultimately carcinogenic forms all react as electrophilic reagents, that is, they seek out relatively negatively charged centers in the target molecules. This conclusion points to a least common denominator of reactivity from the bewildering variety of chemical structures of chemical carcinogens (Miller and Miller, 1966, 1967, 1974; Miller, 1970). This concept is illustrated in Fig. 2 which also points out that the activated ultimate carcinogenic form is subject to various competing reactions, including detoxification.

The pioneer work that led to this generalization stemmed from the observations by the Miller's and their colleagues that N-hydroxylation of 2-acetylaminofluorene (AAF) occurred metabolically by means of microsomal enzymes. The N-hydroxy derivative is considered to be a proximal carcinogenic form, but is not chemically reactive *per se*. It is further converted in rat liver to a highly reactive O-sulfate ester, which does react directly with DNA, RNA, and proteins, as illustrated in Fig. 3. A very important contribution was the discovery that the bulky AAF residue is covalently attached to the C-8 of guanine, instead of the N-7 and O-6 positions that are preferred by the simple alkylating agents. Binding to proteins has been identified as being primarily to methionine to form a sulfonium salt (Fig. 3) (Miller, 1970; Miller and Miller, 1966, 1967, 1974). Very recently, evidence has been obtained that the hepatocarcinogenic aminoazo dyes are also N-hydroxylated to an electrophilic form that reacts with the C-8 of guanine in the nucleic acids. In these studies, the N-benzoyloxy compounds were

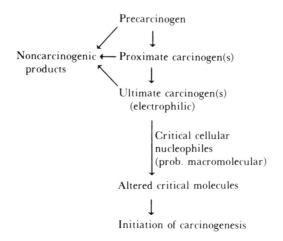

Fig. 2. General scheme for the metabolic activation and detoxification of chemical carcinogens (Miller and Miller, unpublished).

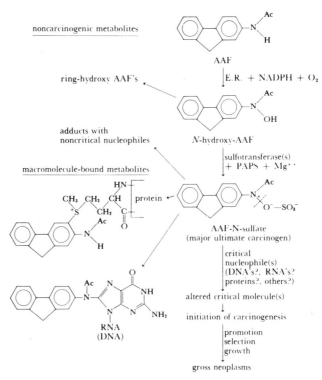

Fig. 3. Metabolic activation in rat liver of 2-acetylamino-fluorene (Miller and Miller, 1974).

used as chemically reactive models, and produced tumors at the site of local injections (Lin *et al.*, 1975a, b; Wislocki *et al.*, 1975).

Dimethyl and diethylnitrosamines also require metabolic activation by microsomal enzymes before they alkylate DNA guanine (Magee and Barnes, 1967; Krüger, 1972); it was shown in a classical experiment that the methyl group is transferred intact and that diazomethane is not an intermediate (Lijinsky *et al.*, 1968). The insidious nature of nitrosamines as likely environmental carcinogens stems from the findings that they are produced from secondary amines and sodium nitrite (a widely used food preservative) in the stomach (Mirvish, 1972) and give rise to stomach tumors (Sander *et al.*, 1972).

The metabolic activation of PAH carcinogens has been the subject of extensive recent investigations. The following kinds of active intermediates have been suggested: epoxides (arene oxides) (reviews: Heidelberger, 1972, 1973a, b, 1975; Sims and Grover, 1974; Jerina and Daly, 1974), free radicals (Nagata *et al.*, 1968, 1974; Lesko *et al.*, 1971; Ts'o *et al.*, 1974; Ts'o *et al.*, This Volume), one-electron oxidation to give radical cations (Wilk and Girke, 1969; Fried, 1974; Cavaliere and Auerbach, 1974; Blackburn *et al.*, 1974), and the 6-hydroxymethylation of benzo[a]pyrene (Flesher and Sydnor, 1973; Sloane and Davis, 1974). Since Dr. Ts'o (This Volume) will do justice to the free radical mechanism, I choose to concentrate on the epoxide (arene oxide) mechanism of activation, for which there is the most evidence at present. This, however, does not mean that other mechanisms of metabolic activation of PAH are excluded. It should be stated at the outset that the structure of "the" active epoxide (if, indeed, there is only one for each PAH) or the structure of epoxide-DNA adducts have not yet been conclusively elucidated.

The clearest demonstration of the necessity for the metabolic activation of PAH came from the simultaneous and independent discoveries that incubation of PAH with rat liver microsomes, followed by the addition of exogenous DNA, led to covalent binding of the PAH to DNA (Grover and Sims, 1968; Gelboin, 1969). It was well-known from the work of Boyland and Sims that PAH are metabolized into phenols, *trans*-dihydrodiols, and glutathione conjugates in whole rats, rat livers, and rat liver microsomes. Boyland (1950) suggested that an epoxide was the most likely intermediate in these reactions (Fig. 4). Later, with the recognition that the electrophilic character of epoxides qualified them to be potential activated metabolites, it was found that K-region epoxides bound covalently to DNA and proteins in the test tube (Grover and Sims, 1970) and in cultured cells (Grover *et al.*, 1971a). Moreover, epoxides have been isolated as intermediates in the microsomal hydroxylation to the phenols of naphthalene (Jerina *et al.*, 1970), dibenz[a,h]anthracene

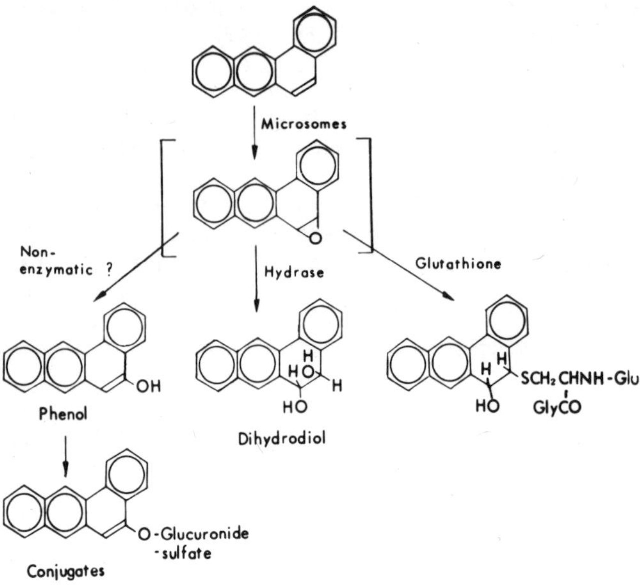

Fig. 4.   Scheme for the metabolic activation and metabolism of benz[a]anthracene (Heidelberger, 1972).

(Selkirk *et al.*, 1971), and pyrene and benzo[a]pyrene (Grover *et al.*, 1972).

In our laboratory and others' it had been shown that PAH were metabolized by a variety of cells in culture to water-soluble derivatives and were also bound to cellular DNA, RNA, and proteins (Huberman *et al.*, 1971b; Kuroki and Heidelberger, 1971; Duncan *et al.*, 1969; Duncan and Brookes, 1970, 1972; Brookes and Duncan, 1971). We also found (Fig. 5) that the K-region epoxides of benz[a]anthracene and dibenz[a,h]anthracene were bound to DNA, RNA, and proteins of transformable mouse prostate fibroblasts more than were the corresponding parent hydrocarbons, dihydrodiols, and phenols (Kuroki *et al.*, 1971/1972), again indicating that epoxides could be the proximal or ultimate carcinogens. It was reported that epoxides reacted more rapidly and to a greater extent with polynucleotides containing guanine, suggesting a chemical similarity with other alkylating agents and carcinogens, but the nature of the interaction was not determined (Swaisland *et al.*, 1974a). Preliminary evidence also suggested that PAH are bound covalently both to purine and pyrimidine bases of DNA in cultured hamster embryo cells (Jones *et al.*, 1973).

Although some epoxides that were tested as carcinogens on mouse skin were less active than the parent hydrocarbons, it

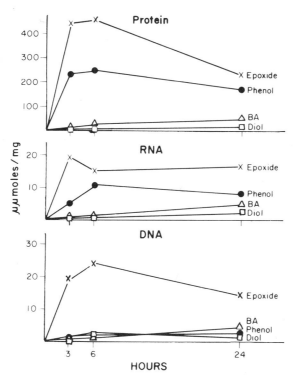

Fig. 5. Binding of benz[a]anthracene (BA) and K-region derivatives to the DNA, RNA, and proteins of cultured mouse prostate
cells (Kuroki *et al.*, 1971/1972).

appeared worthwhile to test their effects on oncogenic transformation of cultured cells. This we did in collaboration with Grover
and Sims, and found that K-region epoxides were considerably more
active than the parent unsubstituted hydrocarbons, phenols, *cis*-
and *trans*-dihydrodiols at producing malignant transformation of
mouse prostate and hamster embryo cells (Grover *et al.*, 1971b;
Marquardt *et al.*, 1972; Huberman *et al.*, 1972). However, the K-
region epoxides of methylated PAH did not appear to be more active
than the parent hydrocarbons at producing malignant transformation
of mouse prostate fibroblasts (Marquardt *et al.*, 1974). These
studies all demonstrate clearly that K-region epoxides of PAH ful-
fill all the necessary requirements for being ultimately carcinogenic forms of PAH, including carcinogenic activity in cell cultures.

The microsomal enzyme system that carries out the epoxidation
reaction is bound to the membranes of the endoplasmic reticulum
and is referred to as the mixed-function oxidase or aryl hydrocarbon hydroxylase (AHH) system. It requires NADPH and molecular

oxygen and involves cytochrome P450 or P448; it is ordinarily considered to be primarily a detoxification system, so that it is an
irony of nature that it activates a variety of chemical carcinogens, including PAH, aromatic amines, nitrosamines, aflatoxins,
etc. The enzyme is also induced by various polycyclic compounds
or by barbiturates, which act at two different sites. A review of
this field is beyond the scope of this chapter. The induction of
AHH is under strict genetic control, since the induction of hepatic
AHH of several strains of mice segregates as an autosomal dominant
trait (Nebert and Gielen, 1972). Determination of the inducibility
of AHH in cultured human lymphocytes has indicated that the human
population falls into three groups of low, medium, and high inducibility (Kellermann *et al.*, 1973a), and that the majority of individuals suffering from lung cancer fall into the groups with the
higher levels of inducibility (Kellermann *et al.*, 1973b). This
raises the exciting prospect that it may be possible to identify
individuals at risk before they develop their chemically-induced
cancers.

It can be seen from Fig. 4 that whether a PAH is or is not
carcinogenic under a given circumstance is rather complicated, and
is the resultant of a series of reactions: the formation of the
epoxide by AHH, the state of inducibility of AHH, the solubility
of the epoxide in the microsomal lipid membrane, the availability
of target macromolecules, the nonenzymatic rearrangement of the
epoxide to the phenol, the microsomal conversion of the epoxide
into biologically inert *trans*-dihydrodiols by the inducible enzyme,
epoxide hydrase (review: Oesch, 1973), and the conversion by
soluble enzymes into glutathione conjugates. Because of this
complexity, it is not surprising that conflicting results on the
effects of manipulating some of these variables on carcinogenesis
have been obtained in various laboratories.

In cultured mouse prostate fibroblasts we have found that
malignant transformation by methylcholanthrene (MCA) was enhanced
by prior induction of AHH and was inhibited by the inhibition of
AHH with 7,8-benzoflavone. Cocultivation with a lethally-irradiated
"feeder layer" of mouse embryo cells, which retain AHH activity,
enhanced transformation produced by MCA. These experiments clearly
show that activation of MCA by AHH is required in order for these
cells to be transformed (Marquardt and Heidelberger, 1972). In *in
vivo* experiments with mouse skin carcinogenesis, it was found that
7,8-benzoflavone inhibited AHH, skin tumor formation, and binding
of 7,12-dimethylbenz[a]anthracene (DMBA) to DNA (Kinoshita and
Gelboin, 1972; Bowden *et al.*, 1974b). Similar relationships have
been observed with some carcinogenic cyclopentaphenanthrone derivatives (Coombs *et al.*, 1975).

There has been some question as to whether highly reactive
epoxides could find their way to the putative nuclear target before

being inactivated by various ubiquitous cellular nucleophiles.
Consequently, a preliminary report is of considerable interest
that PAH are bound covalently to DNA by purified rat liver nuclei
obtained from MCA-induced rats (Rogan and Cavaliere, 1974).

The enzymatic degradation of DNA following application of
various labeled PAH and derivatives and the partial chromatographic
separation of the uncharacterized degradation products have been
intensively used to gain some insight into the nature of the activated intermediate that binds to the DNA. It was found that similar
chromatographic peaks were obtained from mouse skin and from mouse
and human embryo cells treated with tritiated 7-methylbenz[a]-
anthracene (Baird and Brookes, 1973), but that the peaks of the
products of the DNA digest were different from those obtained after
direct treatment of DNA with 7-bromomethylbenz[a]anthracene and the
K-region epoxide of 7-methylbenz[a]anthracene (Baird *et al.*, 1973).
Moreover, it was found that the peaks obtained after treatment of
mouse embryo cells with benzo[a]pyrene (BP) were different from
those found after reaction of the K-region epoxide of BP with DNA.
The conclusion was drawn that the K-region epoxide is not an intermediate in the binding of BP to DNA (Baird *et al.*, 1975). Using
the same techniques, it was found that the peaks obtained following
treatment of mouse embryo cells with benz[a]anthracene (BA) were
the same as the peaks obtained following direct reaction of DNA with
the product of microsomal incubation of the 7,8-dihydrodiol of BA
(Swaisland *et al.*, 1974b). Similarly, the same peaks were obtained
following incubation of mouse embryo cells with BP and the direct
reaction of DNA with the product of the microsomal reaction of the
7,8-dihydrodiol of BP (Sims *et al.*, 1974). The interpretation of
these experiments was that both hydrocarbons were activated first
by the epoxidation of the non-K-region 7,8-double bond, conversion
by epoxide hydrase to the 7,8-dihydrodiol, followed by epoxidation
of the 9,10 bond; the latter compound was postulated to be the
active intermediate in binding of these hydrocarbons to DNA (Fig.
6). In further support of this notion, a highly reactive and uncharacterized epoxide was synthesized from the 7,8-dihydrodiol of
BP, reacted with DNA, and found to give the same peak (Sims *et al.*,
1974). It need hardly be emphasized that such interpretations, based
on the isolation of unknown and uncharacterized degradation products that comigrate in one chromatographic system with the equally
uncharacterized peak obtained from the reaction of DNA with an
uncharacterized epoxide or with the uncharacterized product of
microsomal reaction with a partially characterized dihydrodiol,
are hazardous in the extreme. No firm conclusions can be reached
until all the aforementioned intermediates, products, and degradation products have been unambiguously separated, characterized,
and their exact chemical structures determined. Hopefully, such
work is in progress in several laboratories.

An interesting approach to the structure of the PAH-DNA adduct

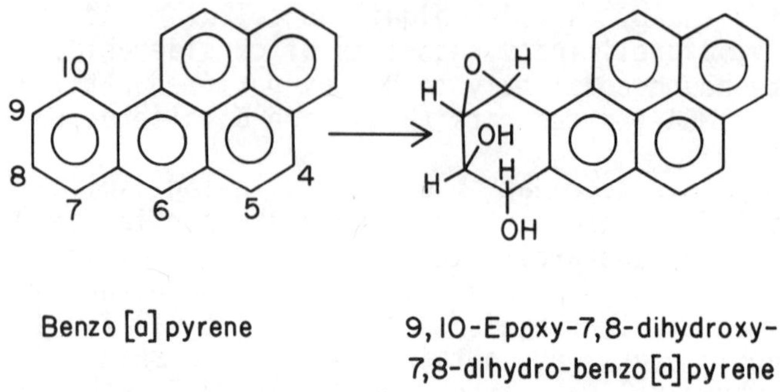

Benzo [a] pyrene   9, 10-Epoxy-7,8-dihydroxy-
                          7,8-dihydro-benzo[a]pyrene

Fig. 6.   Putative metabolic conversion of benzo[a]pyrene to
the compound postulated to bind to DNA (Sims *et al.*, 1974).

involves the development of a very highly sensitive spectrofluori-
meter, which can detect the presence of a few hydrocarbon moieties
bound to intact DNA without the necessity for degradation. It was
found when 7-methyl-BA-5,6-epoxide was reacted with DNA that the
bound hydrocarbon moiety was hydroaromatic, as expected; however,
the product of the treatment of hamster embryo cells with the
parent hydrocarbon was completely aromatic (Daudel *et al.*, 1973,
1974). This need not, however, exclude an epoxide as an intermediate in the binding process, and it will be interesting to
await further results using this powerful method.

Finally, it has been found that the very potent hepatocarcinogen, aflatoxin B_1, is activated via a 2,3-epoxide (Swenson *et al.*,
1973).

Thus, a convincing case can be constructed to indicate that
epoxides (of as yet unknown structure) are ultimately carcinogenic
forms of PAH. It will be interesting to find out whether equally
convincing cases can be offered for the other mechanisms of activation that have been proposed.

4.   CONSEQUENCES OF THE BINDING OF BULKY CARCINOGENS TO DNA

In a classical series of investigations, Weinstein and Grunberger (1974) have determined the conformational and structural
modifications produced in DNA and RNA as a result of substitution
of AAF residues following reaction of N-acetoxy-AAF with the macromolecules in the test tube. In a computer-generated model they
demonstrated with a simple dinucleoside monophosphate, ApG, that
the substitution of the bulky AAF residue at the C-8 of the guanine
forced the conformation around the glycosidic bond from the normal
anti to the syn conformation. This, when applied to macromolecules,

produces a result quite distinct from intercalation, and was termed
the "base-displacement" model (Fig. 7) (Nelson *et al.*, 1971). The
evidence for this was adduced by circular dichroism and nuclear
magnetic resonance.

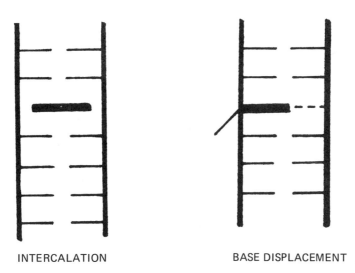

INTERCALATION   BASE DISPLACEMENT

Fig. 7. Comparison of intercalation and base-displacement
models of AAF-substitution of DNA. The AAF residue is depicted as
the heavy line (Weinstein and Grunberger, 1974).

In studies of tRNA modification and structure, it was found
that attachment of an AAF residue to a codon containing G in the
triplet led to loss of ability to function in codon recognition,
and when the substituted G was adjacent to the codon the coding
capacity was reduced; this effect was limited to the adjacent base
only (Grunberger and Weinstein, 1971). When formylmethionine tRNA
was allowed to react with N-acetoxy-AAF in low concentration, substitution occurred only at one G-residue in a single-stranded
region of the dihydrouridine loop, as shown in Fig 8 (Fujimura *et
al.*, 1972). By contrast, the simple methylating agent, MNNG,
alkylates the guanines in tRNA at random (Pegg, 1973).

The effects of the substitution of AAF residues on calf thymus
DNA led to a lowering of the melting temperature, a decreased viscosity (intercalation would produce an increased viscosity), and a
decreased hybridization of ribosomal RNA to the DNA; these observations are best interpreted on the basis that the AAF modification
produces localized denaturation of the double-stranded molecule,
which is consistent with the base-displacement model (Levine *et
al.*, 1974). Additional physical studies by Fuchs and Daune (1972)

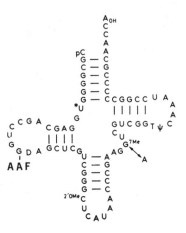

Fig. 8.   Substitution of a single AAF residue on formylmethio-
nine-tRNA (Fujimura *et al.*, 1972).

also led to the conclusion that the modified base was shifted out
of the double helix and that the AAF residue was inserted (Fig. 7).

Some of the biological consequences of the base displacement
model are indicated schematically in Fig. 9, where the means of
producing base substitutions, frameshift, and small deletion mutants,
such as we actually found in bacteriophage T4 treated with N-acetoxy-
AAF (Corbett *et al.*, 1970), are depicted. In addition to mutagenesis
DNA substitution leads to effects on polymerase action (see below),
and substitution of various RNA's could lead to effects on codon
recognition, which could affect cell regulation and possibly block
translation (Weinstein and Grunberger, 1974). The effects of AAF
substitution on DNA repair will be considered below.

The effects of AAF-substitution of template DNA on DNA and RNA
polymerases have been studied. The DNA isolated from livers of rats
fed AAF had a lower template activity for bacterial RNA polymerase
than the controls, and when the DNA was treated directly with N-
acetoxy-AAF template activity was abolished, whereas there was a
negligible effect on DNA polymerase (Troll *et al.*, 1968). The
inactivation by N-acetoxy-AAF of template activity for RNA polymerase occurred at levels of substitution too low to have an effect
on the melting temperature (Zieve, 1973). When bacteriophage T7
DNA was modified with N-acetoxy-AAF and used as a template for
purified *E. coli* RNA polymerase, the rate and extent of RNA synthesis were inhibited, but not its initiation. Since shorter RNA
chain lengths were found with increasing substitution, it was concluded that AAF substitution causes premature termination of the
RNA chains (Millette and Fink, 1975). Rats partially hepatectomized

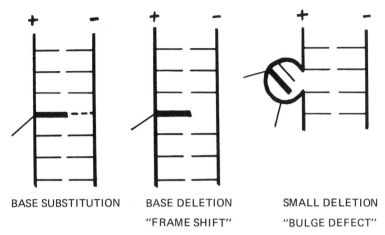

Fig. 9. Mutagenic consequences of base-displacement in DNA by AAF-substitution; the AAF residue is depicted as the heavy line (Levine *et al.*, 1974).

and then treated with N-hydroxy-AAF were used to furnish the source of liver DNA, which was used as a template for the nucleolar and nucleoplasmic RNA polymerases from rat liver; the latter polymerase, which is probably responsible for the synthesis of mRNA, was inhibited and not the former. The liver DNA treated with N-acetoxy-AAF did not have reduced template activity for the nucleoplasmic RNA polymerase, leading to the conclusion that the inhibition was produced by AAF modification of some nucleoprotein, rather than of the DNA (Glazer *et al.*, 1975). Thus, it is evident that the effects of AAF substitution on RNA polymerase are complicated, and further work is required to fully elucidate the mechanism of action.

5. REPAIR OF DNA SUBSTITUTED WITH BULKY CARCINOGENS

The repair of DNA substituted by simple alkylating agents has been reviewed by Strauss (This Volume). I will examine briefly the effects of substitution of DNA with bulky carcinogenic molecules on its repair.

The impetus responsible for the activity in this field came from the important discovery by Cleaver (1968) that cells from humans afflicted by xeroderma pigmentosum (XP), a disease of photosensitivity of the skin leading to multiple carcinomas, are defective in excision repair of the DNA and cannot excise the thymine dimers. The tremendous amount of work on the repair processes for photochemical damage to DNA in mammalian cells has been reviewed (Cleaver, 1974).

     Stich and his colleagues have carried out important studies
on DNA repair as measured by unscheduled thymidine incorporation
in arginine deprived human skin fibroblasts obtained from normal
and XP individuals. It was found that damage induced by the carcinogenic 4-nitroquinoline-N-oxide (NQO) was repaired in normal, but
not in XP cells, whereas MNNG damage was repaired equally well in
both types of cells (Stich and San, 1971). DNA repair synthesis
was then examined in Syrian hamster cells treated with 30 derivatives of NQO, and a good correlation was found between the extent
of repair synthesis provoked and the carcinogenic activities of
the compounds (Stich *et al.*, 1971). A more extensive study of DNA
repair in XP cells revealed that there was an excellent correlation between the lack of repair of NQO damage in XP cells and the
increased lethality produced in these cells by NQO. This was in
complete analogy to their finding of lack of UV repair and increased
UV lethality in XP cells. However, MNNG produced repair and
lethality in XP cells comparable to that found in the normal cells
(Stich *et al.*, 1973). When XP cells were treated with N-acetoxy-
AAF, a decreased repair replication was observed in XP as compared
to normal cells. When several XP cell lines were compared there
was a parallel between the amount of repair replication produced
by NQO and UV radiation (Stich *et al.*, 1972). Impaired repair of
N-acetoxy-AAF treated XP cells was found independently by Setlow
and Regan (1972), who used a different technique that involves
incorporation of 5-bromodeoxyuridine, photolysis, and alkaline
sucrose gradient sedimentation. Furthermore, it was found that
the damage induced by the K-region epoxide of benz[a]anthracene
was not repaired as well by XP as by normal cells, and that the
compound was much more cytotoxic to the XP cells (Stich and San,
1973).

     All the above studies demonstrate that DNA damaged by bulky
carcinogens is repaired poorly by XP cells, in complete analogy
with UV-induced damage, whereas no difference in repair of MNNG
damage was found between normal and XP cells. This fits in with
the categories of "long" (UV type) and "short" (ionizing and
methylating type) forms of DNA repair produced in mammalian cells
by chemical carcinogens and mutagens (Regan and Setlow, 1974). It
seems likely, in accord with the "base displacement" model of
Grunberger and Weinstein (see above), that the bulky carcinogens
produce regions of local denaturation in the DNA that are recognized
by the excision endonucleoase that is deficient in XP cells. Finally
the apparently good correlation between the carcinogenic activities
of chemicals and the repair that they induce provides evidence
that repair may be involved in chemical carcinogenesis and consequently that DNA may be the macromolecular target of chemical carcinogens.

     Somewhat unrelated to the topic of repair, but germane to the
subject of this symposium, is the finding that NQO and its

derivatives produce scission of a DNA-protein complex in L-cells
(Andoh *et al.*, 1975).

6. RELATIONSHIPS BETWEEN MUTAGENESIS AND CARCINOGENESIS

About ten years ago it appeared that there was almost an
inverse correlation between the processes of mutagenesis and carcinogenesis: most powerful carcinogens were not mutagenic in
bacterial or bacteriophage systems, and many powerful mutagens
were not carcinogenic. This was in the era before metabolic activation had been discovered, and of course, microorganisms lack the
microsomal enzymes that carry out the metabolic activation. Now
the situation is quite different. In every case properly studied,
metabolically activated forms of chemical carcinogens are mutagenic
in one or more test systems. However, it is still true that the
powerfully mutagenic base analogs and acridine dyes are not carcinogenic. This subject has been critically reviewed by Miller
and Miller (1971). It is far beyond the scope of this chapter to
review this field completely, so I will concentrate on a few
examples that are most pertinent to my present subject.

First let me consider direct-acting carcinogens, excluding
simple alkylating agents. Maher *et al.* (1968) found that *B. subtilis*
transforming DNA treated with N-acetoxy-AAF and N-benzoyloxy-MAB
was inactivated and also mutated. We studied the induction by N-
acetoxy-AAF and β-propiolactone of mutations in bacteriophage T4
and found that both compounds produced all of the following types
of mutations: base-pair transitions, frameshifts, small deletions,
and large deletions (Corbett *et al.*, 1970). We also found that
epoxides of PAH were very active at producing mutations at the
HGPRT locus in cultured Chinese hamster cells (Fig. 10); the parent
hydrocarbons and other derivatives were inactive (Huberman *et al.*,
1971). Ames *et al.* (1972) found that epoxides of PAH are active in
strains of *Salmonella typhimurium* that detect primarily frameshift
mutants.

Considerable effort has been expended on developing systems
for the measurement of mutagenesis by compounds requiring metabolic
activation. The host-mediated assays cannot be discussed here.
One of the most promising systems has been developed by Ames and
his colleagues, which is becoming a widely-used method to screen
for environmental mutagens. They have developed a number of tester
strains of *Salmonella typhimurium* that are highly sensitive in
detecting mutations. They found that the test compounds could be
activated by treatment with suitably fortified rat liver microsomes
and then become mutagenic to the bacteria. A good preliminary
correlation has emerged between the mutagenic activity of the
microsome-activated compounds and their carcinogenic activities
(Ames *et al.*, 1973). With this technique mutagenic activity was

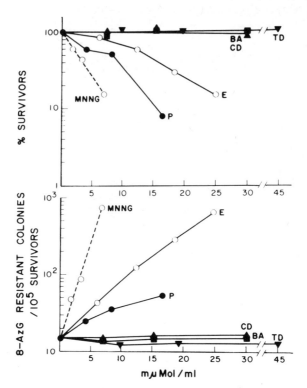

Fig. 10.   Cytotoxicity and mutagenicity at the HGPRT locus to
Chinese hamster V-79 cells by MNNG, benz[a]anthracene (BA) and its
K-region phenol (P), epoxide (E), *cis*-dihydrodiol (CD), and *trans*-
dihydrodiol (TD) (Huberman *et al.*, 1971a).

detected in cigarette smoke condensates (Kier *et al.*, 1974). It
has also been used to study the urinary metabolites of AAF; the
urines with or without microsomal treatment are applied to the test
bacteria and mutations are scored (Durston and Ames, 1974). An
excellent correlation was found between the microsome-activated
mutations produced by 7 PAH and their carcinogenic activities in
the TA-1538, but not in the TA-1537, tester strains of *Salmonella
typhimurium*. The reason for this discrepancy is not known (Teranishi
et al., 1975). A somewhat similar approach was used to study the
activation of dimethyl and diethylnitrosamines by incubating them
with slices of various tissues and measuring the mutagenic activity
of extracts with *Salmonella typhimurium*, with or without additional
liver microsomal activation. There was a reasonably good correlation between the production of mutagenic metabolites and the susceptibility of the tissue to *in vivo* carcinogenesis (Bartsch *et
al.*, 1975).

In order to study metabolic activation and mutagenesis in mammalian cells, which may be more pertinent to the problem of carcinogenesis than mutagenesis in bacteria, two approaches have been used. Huberman and Sachs (1974) have used Chinese hamster V79 cells, which do not activate unreactive carcinogens, and have cocultivated them with lethally irradiated rodent cells that do activate PAH. With this system they produced forward mutagenesis at the HGPRT locus with BP, MCA, and DMBA. Whether or not other classes of chemical carcinogens will be activated by such feeder layers remains to be determined. The other approach has been carried out in our laboratory, also using Chinese hamster V79 cells, in which activation is produced by a liver microsomal preparation similar to that of Ames *et al*. (1973). No cytotoxicity or mutations were produced in the absence of the microsomal system with PAH, DMN, DAB, β-naphthylamine, or aflatoxin B_1. However, all of these diverse carcinogens on incubation with the microsomal preparation were cytotoxic and mutagenic to these mammalian cells (Krahn and Heidelberger, 1975). This promises to be a useful system for pre-screening of environmental mutagens, although it is more expensive and time-consuming than the bacterial system.

One interesting conclusion that can be drawn from these studies is that the metabolically activated mutagenic compounds are sufficiently stable to emerge from the microsomal membrane, enter the tester cell, enter the nucleus of the tester cell, and react with the DNA.

In looking over the situation at present I have reached the following viewpoint. All known metabolically active forms of chemical carcinogens are mutagenic, but not all mutagens are carcinogens. So there is a good but not perfect correlation between the processes of mutagenesis and carcinogenesis. Even if the correlation was perfect, however, it would constitute no proof that carcinogenesis is the result of a somatic mutation. Carcinogenesis could still result from some perpetuated effect on gene expression, such as a derepression (Pitot and Heidelberger, 1963) or aberrant differentiation (Pierce, 1974). The proof or disproof of the somatic mutation mechanism of chemical carcinogenesis must await new and critical experiments, which hopefully will soon be performed. However, even if cancer is not caused by somatic mutation, the closeness of the correlation between the two processes allows mutagenesis testing in proper systems to be a very useful pre-screen for environmental hazards.

Acknowledgment. I greatly appreciate the valuable assistance of Patricia F. Boshell in the preparation of this manuscript.

References

Abell, C.W., and Heidelberger, C., 1962, The interaction of carcinogenic hydrocarbons with tissues. VIII. Binding of tritium-
labeled hydrocarbons to the soluble proteins of mouse skin,
Cancer Res. 22:931-946.

Ames, B.N., Durston, W.E., Yamasaki, E., and Lee, F.D., 1973, Carcinogens are mutagens: A simple test system combining liver
homogenates for activation and bacteria for detection, *Proc.
Nat. Acad. Sci. USA* 70:2281-2285.

Ames, B.N., Sims, P., and Grover, P.L., 1972, Epoxides of carcinogenic polycyclic hydrocarbons are frameshift mutagens, *Science*
176:47-49.

Andoh, T., Ide, T., Saito, M., and Kawazoe, Y., 1975, Breakage of
a DNA-protein complex induced by 4-nitroquinoline 1-oxide,
4-nitropyridine 1-oxide, and their derivatives in cultured
mouse fibroblasts, *Cancer Res.* 35:521-527.

Baird, W.M., and Brookes, P., 1973, Isolation of the hydrocarbon-
deoxyribonucleoside products from the DNA of mouse embryo cells
treated in culture with 7-methylbenz[a]anthracene, *Cancer Res.*
33:2378-2385.

Baird, W.M., Dipple, A., Grover, P.L., Sims, P., and Brookes, P.,
1973, Studies on the formation of hydrocarbon deoxyribonucleoside products by the binding of derivatives of 7-methylbenz-
[a]anthracene to DNA in aqueous solution and in mouse embryo
cells in culture, *Cancer Res.* 33:2386-2392.

Baird, W.M., Harvey, R.G., and Brookes, P., 1975, Comparison of the
cellular DNA-bound product of benzo[a]pyrene with the products
formed by the reaction of benzo[a]pyrene-4,5-oxide with DNA,
Cancer Res. 35:54-57.

Bartsch, H., Malaveille, C., and Montesano, R., 1975, *In vitro* metabolism and microsome-mediated mutagenicity of dialkylnitros-
amines in rat, hamster, and mouse tissues, *Cancer Res.* 35:644-
651.

Bertram, J.S., and Heidelberger, C., 1974, Cell cycle dependency
of oncogenic transformation induced by N-methyl-N'-nitro-N-
nitrosoguanidine in culture, *Cancer Res.* 34:526-537.

Berwald, Y., and Sachs, L., 1965, *In vitro* transformation of normal
cells into tumor cells by carcinogenic hydrocarbons, *J. Nat.
Cancer Inst.* 35:641-661.

Blackburn, G.M., Flavell, A.J., and Thompson, M.H., 1974, Oxidative
and photochemical linkage of diethylstilbestrol to DNA *in
vitro, Cancer Res.* 34:2015-2019.

Bowden, G.T., Shapas, B.G., and Boutwell, R.K., 1974a, The binding
of 7,12-dimethylbenz[a]anthracene to replicating and non-
replicating DNA in mouse skin, *Chem.-Biol. Interactions* 8:
379-394.

Bowden, G.T., Slaga, T.J., Shapas, B.G., and Boutwell, R.K., 1974b,
     The role of aryl hydrocarbon hydroxylase in skin tumor initia-
     tion by 7,12-dimethylbenz[a]anthracene and 1,2,5,6-dibenz-
     anthracene using DNA binding and thymidine-^{3}H incorporation
     into DNA as criteria, *Cancer Res.* 34:2634-2642.
Boyland, E., 1950, The biological significance of metabolism of
     polycyclic compounds, *Symp. Biochem. Soc.* 5:40-54.
Brookes, P., 1966, Quantitative aspects of the reaction of some
     carcinogens with nucleic acids and the possible significance
     of such reactions in the process of carcinogenesis, *Cancer
     Res.* 26:1994-2003.
Brookes, P., 1975, Covalent interaction of carcinogens with DNA,
     Life Sciences 16:331-344.
Brookes, P., and Duncan, M.E., 1971, Carcinogenic hydrocarbons and
     human cells in culture, *Nature* 234:40-43.
Brookes, P., and Heidelberger, C., 1969, Isolation and degradation
     of DNA from cells treated with tritium-labeled 7,12-dimethyl-
     benz[a]anthracene: studies on the nature of the binding of
     this carcinogen to DNA, *Cancer Res.* 29:157-165.
Brookes, P., and Lawley, P.D., 1964, Evidence for the binding of
     polynuclear aromatic hydrocarbons to the nucleic acids of
     mouse skin: relation between carcinogenic power of hydro-
     carbons and their binding to deoxyribonucleic acid, *Nature*
     202:781-784.
Casto, B.C., and DiPaolo, J.A., 1973, Virus, chemicals and cancer,
     Prog. Med. Virol. 16:1-47.
Cavaliere, E., and Auerbach, R., 1974, Reactions between activated
     benzo[a]pyrene and nucleophilic compounds, with possible
     implications on the mechanism of tumor initiation, *J. Nat.
     Cancer Inst.* 53:393-397.
Chen, T.T., and Heidelberger, C., 1969, Quantitative studies on the
     malignant transformation of mouse prostate cells by carcino-
     genic hydrocarbons *in vitro, Int. J. Cancer* 4:166-178.
Cleaver, J.E., 1968, Defective repair replication of DNA in *Xeroderma
     pigmentosum, Nature* 218:652-656.
Cleaver, J.E., 1974, Repair processes for photochemical damage in
     mammalian cells, *Adv. Radiat. Biol.* 4:1-75.
Colburn, N.H., and Boutwell, R.K., 1968, The binding of β-propio-
     lactone to mouse skin DNA, RNA, and protein, *Cancer Res.*
     28:653-660.
Colburn, N.H., Richardson, R.G., and Boutwell, R.K., 1965, Studies
     of the reaction of β-propiolactone with deoxyguanosine and
     related compounds, *Biochem. Pharmacol.* 14:1113-1118.
Coombs, M.M., Bhatt, T.S., and Vose, C.W., 1975, The relationship
     between metabolism, DNA binding, and carcinogenicity of 15,
     16-dihydro-11-methylcyclopenta[a]phenanthrene-17-one in the
     presence of a microsomal enzyme inhibitor, *Cancer Res.* 35:
     305-309.

Corbett, T.H., Heidelberger, C., and Dove, W.F., 1970, Determination
    of the mutagenic activity to bacteriophage T4 of carcinogenic
    and noncarcinogenic compounds, *Mol. Pharmacol.* 6:667-679.
Craddock, V.M., 1973, The pattern of methylated purines formed in
    DNA of intact and regenerating liver of rats treated with the
    carcinogen dimethylnitrosamine, *Biochim. Biophys. Acta* 312:
    202-210.
Daudel, P., Croisy-Delcey, M., Alonso-Verduras, C., Duquesne, M.,
    Jacquignon, P., Markovits, P., and Vigny, P., 1974, Etude par
    fluorescence d'acides nucléiques extraits de cellules en
    cultures traitées par le méthylbenzo[a]anthracène, *C.R. Acad.
    Sci. Paris* 278:2249-2252.
Daudel, P., Croisy-Delcey, M., Jacquignon, P., and Vigny, P.,
    1973, Sur la structure d'un complexe résultant de l'action
    d'un époxyde aromatique polycyclique sur un acid désoxyribo-
    nucléique, *C.R. Acad. Sci. Paris* 277:2437-2439.
DiPaolo, J.A., Donovan, P., and Nelson, R.L., 1969, Quantitative
    studies of *in vitro* transformation by chemical carcinogens,
    J. Nat. Cancer Inst. 42:867-874.
DiPaolo, J.A., Takano, K., and Popescu, N., 1972, Quantitation of
    chemically induced neoplastic transformation of BALB 3T3 cell
    lines, *Cancer Res.* 32:2686-2695.
Dipple, A., Lawley, P.D., and Brookes, P., 1968, Theory of tumour
    initiation by chemical carcinogens: dependence on structure
    of ultimate carcinogen, *Europ. J. Cancer* 4:493-506.
Duncan, M.E., and Brookes, P., 1970, The relation of metabolism to
    macromolecular binding of the carcinogen benzo[a]pyrene by
    mouse embryo cells in culture, *Int. J. Cancer* 6:496-505.
Duncan, M.E., and Brookes, P., 1972, Metabolism and macromolecular
    binding of dibenz[a,c]anthracene and dibenz[a,h]anthracene
    by mouse embryo cells in culture, *Int. J. Cancer* 9:349-352.
Duncan, M., Brookes, P., and Dipple, A., 1969, Metabolism and bind-
    ing to cellular macromolecules of a series of hydrocarbons by
    mouse embryo cells in culture, *Int. J. Cancer* 4:813-819.
Durston, W.E., and Ames, B.N., 1974, A simple method for the detec-
    tion of mutagens in urine: studies with the carcinogen 2-
    acetylaminofluorene, *Proc. Nat. Acad. Sci. USA* 71:737-741.
Flesher, J.W., and Sydnor, K.L., 1973, Possible role of 6-hydroxy-
    methylbenzo[a]pyrene as a proximate carcinogen of benzo[a]-
    pyrene and 6-methylbenzo[a]pyrene, *Int. J. Cancer* 11:433-437.
Freeman, A.E., Weisburger, E.K., Weisburger, J.H., Wolford, R.G.,
    Maryak, J.M., and Huebner, R.J., 1973, Transformation of cell
    cultures as an indication of the carcinogenic potential of
    chemicals, *J. Nat. Cancer Inst.* 51:799-808.
Fried, J., 1974, One-electron oxidation of polycyclic aromatics as
    a model for the metabolic activation of carcinogenic hydro-
    carbons, *in* "Chemical Carcinogenesis" (P.O.P. Ts'o and J.A.
    DiPaolo, eds.), Part A, pp. 197-215, Marcel Dekker, New York.

Fuchs, R., and Daune, M., 1972, Physical studies on deoxyribonucleic acid after covalent binding of a carcinogen, *Biochemistry* 11: 2659-2666.

Fujimura, S., Grunberger, D., Carvajal, G., and Weinstein, I.B., 1972, Modifications of ribonucleic acid by chemical carcinogens. Modification of *E. coli* formylmethionine transfer ribonucleic acid with N-acetoxy-2-acetylaminofluorene, *Biochemistry* 11:3629-3635.

Gelboin, H.V., 1969, A microsome-dependent binding of benzo[a]pyrene to DNA, *Cancer Res.* 29:1272-1276.

Glazer, R.I., Glass, L.E., and Menger, F.M., 1975, Modification of hepatic ribonucleic acid polymerase activities by N-hydroxy-2-acetylaminofluorene and N-acetoxy-2-acetylaminofluorene, *Mol. Pharmacol.* 11:36-43.

Goshman, L.M., and Heidelberger, C., 1967, Binding of tritium-labeled polycyclic hydrocarbons to DNA of mouse skin, *Cancer Res.* 27:1678-1688.

Goth, R., and Rajewsky, M.F., 1972, Ethylation of nucleic acids by ethylnitrosourea-1-^{14}C in the fetal and adult rat, *Cancer Res.* 32:1501-1505.

Goth, R., and Rajewsky, M.F., 1974, Persistence of 06-ethylguanine in rat-brain DNA: correlation with nervous system-specific carcinogenesis by ethylnitrosourea, *Proc. Nat. Acad. Sci. USA* 71:639-643.

Grover, P.L., Forrester, J.A., and Sims, P., 1971a, Reactivity of the K-region epoxides of some polycyclic hydrocarbons towards the nucleic acids and protein of BHK21 cells, *Biochem. Pharmacol.* 20:1297-1302.

Grover, P.L., Hewer, A., and Sims, P., 1972, The formation of K-region epoxides as microsomal metabolites of pyrene and benzo-[a]pyrene, *Biochem. Pharmacol.* 21:2713-2726.

Grover, P.L., and Sims, P., 1968, Enzyme-catalysed reactions of polycyclic hydrocarbons with deoxyribonucleic acid and protein *in vitro, Biochem. J.* 110:159-160.

Grover, P.L., and Sims, P., 1970, Interactions of the K-region epoxides of phenanthrene and dibenz[a,h]anthracene with nucleic acids and histone, *Biochem. Pharmacol.* 19:2251-2259.

Grover, P.L., Sims, P., Huberman, E., Marquardt, H., Kuroki, T., and Heidelberger, C., 1971b, *In vitro* transformation of rodent cells by K-region derivatives of polycyclic hydrocarbons, *Proc. Nat. Acad. Sci. USA* 68:1098-1101.

Grunberger, D., and Weinstein, I.B., 1971, Modifications of ribonucleic acid by chemical carcinogens. III. Template activity of polynucleotides modified by N-acetoxy-2-acetylaminofluorene, *J. Biol. Chem.* 246:1123-1128.

Heidelberger, C., 1970a, Studies on the cellular and molecular mechanisms of hydrocarbon carcinogenesis, *Europ. J. Cancer* 6:161-172.

Heidelberger, C., 1970b, Chemical carcinogenesis, chemotherapy: cancer's continuing core challenges. G.H.A. Clowes Memorial Lecture, *Cancer Res.* 30:1549-1569.

Heidelberger, C., 1972, *In vitro* studies on the role of epoxides in carcinogenic hydrocarbon activation, *in* "Topics in Chemical Carcinogenesis" (W. Nakahara, S. Takayama, T. Sugimura, and S. Odashima, eds.), pp. 371-386, discussion, pp. 387-388, University of Tokyo Press, Tokyo, Japan.

Heidelberger, C., 1973a, Current trends in chemical carcinogenesis, *Fed. Proc.* 32:2154-2161.

Heidelberger, C., 1973b, Chemical oncogenesis in culture, *Adv. Cancer Res.* 18:317-366.

Heidelberger, C., 1974, Cell culture studies on the mechanisms of hydrocarbon oncogenesis, *in* "Chemical Carcinogenesis" (P.O.P. Ts'o and J.A. DiPaolo, eds.), Part B, pp. 457-462, Marcel Dekker, New York.

Heidelberger, C., 1975, Chemical carcinogenesis, *Annu. Rev. Biochem.* 44:79-121.

Heidelberger, C., and Davenport, G.R., 1961, Local functional components of carcinogenesis, *Acta Unio Internat. Contra Cancrum* 17:55-63.

Huberman, E., Aspiras, L., Heidelberger, C., Grover, P.L., and Sims, P., 1971a, Mutagenicity to mammalian cells of epoxides and other derivatives of polycyclic hydrocarbons, *Proc. Nat. Acad. Sci. USA* 68:3195-3199.

Huberman, E., Kuroki, T., Marquardt, H., Selkirk, J.K., Heidelberger, C., Grover, P.L., and Sims, P., 1972, Transformation of hamster embryo cells by epoxides and other derivatives of polycyclic hydrocarbons, *Cancer Res.* 32:1391-1396.

Huberman, E., and Sachs, L., 1974, Cell-mediated mutagenesis of mammalian cells with chemical carcinogens, *Int. J. Cancer* 13: 326-333.

Huberman, E., Selkirk, J.K., and Heidelberger, C., 1971b, Metabolism of polycyclic aromatic hydrocarbons in cell cultures, *Cancer Res.* 31:2161-2167.

Irving, C., 1973, Interaction of chemical carcinogens with DNA, *Methods Cancer Res.* 7:189-244.

Jerina, D.M., and Daly, J.W., 1974, Arene oxides: a new aspect of drug metabolism, *Science* 185:573-582.

Jerina, D.M., Daly, J.W., Witkop, B., Zaltman-Nirenberg, P., and Udenfriend, S., 1970, 1,2-Naphthalene oxide as an intermediate in the microsomal hydroxylation of naphthalene, *Biochemistry* 9:147-155.

Jones, P.A., Gevers, W., and Hawtrey, A.O., 1973, Evidence for the binding of the carcinogen 3-methylcholanthrene to both the purine and the pyrimidine bases of hamster fibroblast deoxyribonucleic acid, *Biochem. J.* 135:375-378.

Kakunaga, T., 1973, A quantitative system for assay of malignant transformation by chemical carcinogens using a clone derived from BALB/3T3, *Int. J. Cancer* 12:463-473.

Kellermann, G., Luyten-Kellermann, M., and Shaw, C.R., 1973a, Genetic variation of aryl hydrocarbon hydroxylase in human lymphocytes, *Am. J. Human Genet.* 25:327-331.

Kellermann, G., Shaw, C.R., and Luyten-Kellermann, M., 1973b, Aryl hydrocarbon hydroxylase inducibility and bronchogenic carcinoma, *New England J. Med.* 289:934-937.

Kier, L.D., Yamasaki, E., and Ames, B.N., 1974, Detection of mutagenic activity in cigarette smoke condensates, *Proc. Nat. Acad. Sci. USA* 71:4159-4163.

Kinoshita, N., and Gelboin, H.V., 1972, Aryl hydrocarbon hydroxylase and polycyclic hydrocarbon tumorigenesis: effect of the enzyme inhibitor 7,8-benzoflavone on tumorigenesis and macromolecule binding, *Proc. Nat. Acad. Sci. USA* 69:824-828.

Krahn, D.F., and Heidelberger, C., 1975, Microsome-mediated mutagenesis in Chinese hamster cells by chemical oncogens, *Proc. Am. Assoc. Cancer Res.* 16:74.

Kriek, E., 1974, Carcinogenesis by aromatic amines, *Biochim. Biophys. Acta* 355:177-203.

Krüger, F.W., 1972, New aspects in metabolism of carcinogenic nitrosamines, *in* "Topics in Chemical Carcinogenesis" (W. Nakahara, S. Takayama, T. Sugimura, and S. Odashima, eds.), pp. 213-232, University of Tokyo Press, Tokyo, Japan.

Kubinski, H., and Szybalski, E.H., 1975, Intermolecular linking and fragmentation of DNA by β-propiolactone, a monoalkylating carcinogen, *Chem.-Biol. Interactions* 10:41-55.

Kuroki, T., and Heidelberger, C., 1971, The binding of polycyclic aromatic hydrocarbons to the DNA, RNA, and proteins of transformable cells in culture, *Cancer Res.* 31:2168-2176.

Kuroki, T., Huberman, E., Marquardt, H., Selkirk, J.K., Heidelberger, C., Grover, P.L., and Sims, P., 1971/1972, Binding of K-region epoxides and other derivatives of benz[a]anthracene and dibenz[a,h]anthracene to DNA, RNA, and proteins of transformable cells, *Chem.-Biol. Interactions* 4:389-397.

Lawley, P.D., 1966, Effects of some chemical mutagens and carcinogens on nucleic acids, *Progr. Nucleic Acid Res. Mol. Biol.* 5:89-131.

Lawley, P.D., 1972, The action of alkylating mutagens and carcinogens on nucleic acids: N-methyl-N-nitroso compounds as methylating agents, *in* "Topics in Chemical Carcinogenesis" (W. Nakahara, S. Takayama, T. Sugimura, and S. Odashima, eds.), pp. 237-256, University of Tokyo Press, Tokyo, Japan.

Lawley, P.D., 1973, Reaction of N-methyl-N-nitrosourea (MNUA) with ^{32}P-labelled DNA: evidence for formation of phosphotriesters, *Chem.-Biol. Interactions* 7:127-130.

Lawley, P.D., and Shah, S., 1972, Methylation of RNA by the carcinogens, dimethyl sulphate, N-methyl-N-nitrosourea, or N-methyl-N'-nitro-N-nitrosoguanidine: Comparisons of analyses at the base and nucleoside levels, *Biochem. J.* 128:117-132.

Lawley, P.D., and Shah, S.A., 1973, Methylation of DNA by ^{3}H-^{14}C-methyl-labelled N-methyl-N-nitrosourea - evidence for transfer of the intact methyl group, *Chem.-Biol. Interactions* 7:115-120.

Lawley, P.D., and Thatcher, C.J., 1970, Methylation of deoxyribonucleic acids in cultured mammalian cells by N-methyl-N'-nitro-N-nitrosoguanidine, *Biochem. J.* 116:693-707.

Lesko, S.A., Hoffman, H.D., Ts'o, P.O.P., and Maher, V.M., 1971, Interaction and linkage of polycyclic hydrocarbons to nucleic acids, *Progr. Mol. Subcell. Biol.* 2:347-370.

Levine, A.F., Fink, L.M., Weinstein, I.B., and Grunberger, D., 1974, Effect of N-2-acetylaminofluorene modification on the conformation of nucleic acids, *Cancer Res.* 34:319-327.

Lijinsky, W., Loo, J., and Ross, A.E., 1968, Mechanism of alkylation of nucleic acids by nitrosodimethylamine, *Nature* 218:1174-1175.

Lin, J.-K., Miller, J.A., and Miller, E.C., 1975a, Structures of hepatic nucleic acid-bound dyes in rats given the carcinogen N-methyl-4-aminoazobenzene, *Cancer Res.* 35:844-850.

Lin, J.-K., Schmall, B., Sharpe, I.D., Miura, I., Miller, J.A., and Miller, E.C., 1975b, N-Substitution of carbon 8 in guanosine and deoxyguanosine by the carcinogen N-benzyloxy-N-methyl-4-aminoazobenzene *in vitro*, *Cancer Res.* 35:832-843.

Loveless, A., 1969, Possible relevance of O-6 alkylation of deoxyguanosine to mutagenicity and carcinogenicity of nitrosamines and nitrosamides, *Nature* 223:206-207.

Magee, P.N., and Barnes, J.M., 1967, Carcinogenic nitroso compounds, *Adv. Cancer Res.* 10:163-246.

Maher, V.M., Miller, E.C., Miller, J.A., and Szybalski, W., 1968, Mutations and decreases in density of transforming DNA produced by derivatives of the carcinogens 2-acetylaminofluorene and N-methyl-4-aminoazobenzene, *Mol. Pharmacol.* 4:411-426.

Marquardt, H., and Heidelberger, C., 1972, Influence of "feeder cells" and inducers and inhibitors of microsomal mixed-function oxidases on hydrocarbon-induced malignant transformation of cells derived from C3H mouse prostate, *Cancer Res.* 32:721-725.

Marquardt, H., Kuroki, T., Huberman, E., Selkirk, J.K., Heidelberger, C., Grover, P.L., and Sims, P., 1972, Malignant transformation of cells derived from mouse prostate by epoxides and other derivatives of polycyclic hydrocarbons, *Cancer Res.* 32:716-720.

Marquardt, H., Sodergren, J.E., Sims, P., and Grover, P.L., 1974, Malignant transformation *in vitro* of mouse fibroblasts by 7,12-dimethylbenz[a]anthracene and 7-hydroxymethylbenz[a]anthracene and by their K-region derivatives, *Int. J. Cancer* 13:304-310.

Miller, E.C., 1951, Studies on the formation of protein-bound derivatives of 3,4-benzpyrene in the epidermal fraction of mouse skin, *Cancer Res.* 11:100-108.

Miller, E.C., and Miller, J.A., 1947, The presence and significance of bound aminoazo dyes in the livers of rats fed p-dimethylaminoazobenzene, *Cancer Res.* 7:468-480.

Miller, E.C., and Miller, J.A., 1966, Mechanisms of chemical carcinogens: nature of proximate carcinogens and interactions with macromolecules, *Pharmacol. Rev.* 18:806-838.

Miller, E.C., and Miller, J.A., 1971, The mutagenicity of chemical carcinogens: correlations, problems, and interpretations, *in* "Chemical Mutagens: Principles and Methods for their Detection" (A. Hollaender, ed.), Vol. 1, pp. 83-119, Plenum Press, New York.

Miller, E.C., and Miller, J.A., 1974, Biochemical mechanisms of chemical carcinogenesis, *in* "The Molecular Biology of Cancer" (H. Busch, ed.), pp. 377-402, Academic Press, New York.

Miller, J.A., 1970, Carcinogenesis by chemicals: an overview. G.H.A. Clowes Memorial Lecture, *Cancer Res.* 30:559-576.

Miller, J.A., and Miller, E.C., 1967, The metabolic activation of carcinogenic aromatic amines and amides, *Progr. Exp. Tumor Res.* 11:273-301.

Millette, B.L., and Fink, L.M., 1975, The effect of modification of T7 DNA by the carcinogen N-2-acetylaminofluorene: Termination of transcription *in vitro*, *Biochemistry* 14:1426-1432.

Mirvish, S.S., 1972, Studies on N-nitrosation reactions: Kinetics of nitrosation, correlation with mouse feeding experiments, and natural occurrence of nitrosable compounds (ureides and guanidines), *in* "Topics in Chemical Carcinogenesis" (W. Nakahara, S. Takayama, T. Sugimura, and S. Odashima, eds.), pp. 279-294, University of Tokyo Press, Tokyo, Japan.

Nagata, C., Inomata, M., Kodama, M., and Tagashira, Y., 1968, Electron spin resonance study on the interaction between chemical carcinogens and tissue components. III. Determination of the structure of the free radical produced either by stirring 3,4-benzopyrene with albumin or incubating it with liver homogenates, *Gann* 59:289-298.

Nagata, C., Tagashira, Y., and Kodama, M., 1974, Metabolic activation of benzo[a]pyrene: significance of the free radical, *in* "Chemical Carcinogenesis" (P.O.P. Ts'o and J.A. DiPaolo, eds.), Part A, pp. 87-111, Marcel Dekker, New York.

Nebert, D.W., and Gielen, J.W., 1972, Genetic regulation of aryl hydrocarbon hydroxylase induction in the mouse, *Fed. Proc.* 31:1315-1325.

Nelson, J.H., Grunberger, D., Cantor, C.R., and Weinstein, I.B., 1971, Modification of ribonucleic acid by chemical carcinogens. IV. Circular dichroism and proton magnetic resonance studies of oligonucleotides modified with N-2-acetylaminofluorene, *J. Mol. Biol.* 62:331-346.

Newman, M.S., and Olson, D.R., 1974, A new hypothesis concerning the reactive species in carcinogenesis by 7,12-dimethylbenz-[a]anthracene. The 5-hydroxy, 7,12-dimethylbenz[a]anthracene-7,12-dimethylbenz[a]anthracene-5(6H)-one equilibrium, *J. Am. Chem. Soc.* 96:6207-6208.

Nietert, W.C., Kellicutt, L.M., and Kubinski, H., 1974, DNA-protein complexes produced by a carcinogen, β-propiolactone, *Cancer Res.* 34:859-864.

O'Connor, P.J., Capps, M.J., and Craig, A.W., 1973, Comparative studies of the hepatocarcinogen N-N-dimethylnitrosamine *in vivo*: reaction sites in rat liver DNA and the significance of their relative stabilities, *Brit. J. Cancer* 27:153-166.

Oesch, F., 1973, Mammalian epoxide hydrases: Inducible enzymes catalysing the inactivation of carcinogenic and cytotoxic metabolites derived from aromatic and olefinic compounds, *Xenobiotica* 3:305-340.

Pegg, A.E., 1973, Alkylation of transfer RNA by N-methyl-N-nitro-sourea and N-ethyl-N-nitrosourea, *Chem.-Biol. Interactions* 6:393-406.

Peterson, A.R., Bertram, J.S., and Heidelberger, C., 1974a, DNA damage and its repair in transformable mouse fibroblasts treated with N-methyl-N'-nitro-N-nitrosoguanidine, *Cancer Res.* 34:1592-1599.

Peterson, A.R., Bertram, J.S., and Heidelberger, C., 1974b, Cell cycle dependency of DNA damage and repair in transformable mouse fibroblasts treated with N-methyl-N'-nitro-N-nitroso-guanidine, *Cancer Res.* 34:1600-1607.

Pierce, G.B., 1974, Cellular heterogeneity of cancers, *in* "Chemical Carcinogenesis" (P.O.P. Ts'o and J.A. DiPaolo, eds.), Part B, pp. 463-472, Marcel Dekker, New York.

Pitot, H.C., and Heidelberger, C., 1963, Metabolic regulatory circuits and carcinogenesis, *Cancer Res.* 23:1694-1700.

Pullman, A., and Pullman, B., 1955, Electronic structure and car-cinogenic activity of aromatic molecules, *Adv. Cancer Res.* 3:117-169.

Pullman, A., and Pullman, B., 1969, A quantum chemist's approach to the mechanism of chemical carcinogenesis, *in* "Physico-Chemical Mechanisms of Carcinogenesis" (E. Bergmann and B. Pullman, eds.), The Jerusalem Symposia on Quantum Chemistry and Biochemistry, Vol. 1, pp. 9-24, The Israeli Academy of Sciences and Humanities, Jerusalem.

Regan, J.D., and Setlow, R.B., 1974, Two forms of repair in the DNA of human cells damaged by chemical carcinogens and mutagens, *Cancer Res.* 34:3318-3325.

Reznikoff, C.A., Bertram, J.S., Brankow, D.W., and Heidelberger, C., 1973a, Quantitative and qualitative studies of chemical trans-formation of cloned C3H mouse embryo cells sensitive to post-confluence inhibition of cell division, *Cancer Res.* 33:3239-3249.

Reznikoff, C.A., Brankow, D.W., and Heidelberger, C., 1973b, Establishment and characterization of a cloned line of C3H mouse embryo cells sensitive to postconfluence inhibition of division, *Cancer Res.* 33:3231-3238.

Rhim, J.S., Park, D.K., Weisburger, E.K., and Weisburger, J.H., 1974, Evaluation of an *in vitro* assay system for carcinogens based on prior infection of rodent cells with nontransforming RNA tumor virus, *J. Nat. Cancer Inst.* 52:1167-1173.

Rogan, E.G., and Cavaliere, E., 1974, 3-Methylcholanthrene-inducible binding of aromatic hydrocarbons to DNA in purified rat liver nuclei, *Biochem. Biophys. Res. Commun.* 58:1119-1126.

Sander, J., Bürkle, G., and Schweinsberg, F., 1972, Induction of tumors by nitrite and secondary amines or amides, *in* "Topics in Chemical Carcinogenesis" (W. Nakahara, S. Takayama, T. Sugimura, and S. Odashima, eds.), pp. 297-310, University of Tokyo Press, Tokyo, Japan.

Sarrif, A.M., Bertram, J.S., Kamarck, M., and Heidelberger, C., 1975, The isolation and characterization of polycyclic hydrocarbon-binding proteins from mouse liver and skin cytosols, *Cancer Res.* 35:816-824.

Selkirk, J.A., Huberman, E., and Heidelberger, C., 1971, An epoxide is an intermediate in the microsomal metabolism of the chemical carcinogen, dibenz[a,h]anthracene, *Biochem. Biophys. Res. Commun.* 43:1010-1016.

Setlow, R.B., and Regan, J.D., 1972, Defective repair of N-acetoxy-2-acetylaminofluorene-induced lesions in the DNA of *Xeroderma pigmentosum* cells, *Biochem. Biophys. Res. Commun.* 46:1019-1024.

Sims, P., and Grover, P.L., 1974, Epoxides in polycyclic aromatic hydrocarbon metabolism and carcinogenesis, *Adv. Cancer Res.* 20:166-274.

Sims, P., Grover, P.L., Swaisland, A., Pal, K., and Hewer, A., 1974, Metabolic activation of benzo[a]pyrene proceeds by a diol-epoxide, *Nature* 252: 326-328.

Sloane, N.H., and Davis, T.K., 1974, Hydroxymethylation of the benzene ring. Microsomal hydroxymethylation of benzo[a]-pyrene to 6-hydroxymethylbenzo[a]pyrene, *Arch. Biochem. Biophys.* 163:46-52.

Stich, H.F., and San, R.H.C., 1971, Reduced DNA repair synthesis in *Xeroderma pigmentosum* cells exposed to the oncogenic 4-nitroquinoline 1-oxide and 4-hydroxyaminoquinoline 1-oxide, *Mutat. Res.* 13:279-282.

Stich, H.F., and San, R.H.C., 1973, DNA repair synthesis and survival of repair deficient human cells exposed to the K-region epoxide of benz[a]anthracene, *Proc. Soc. Exp. Biol. Med.* 142:155-158.

Stich, H.F., San, R.H.C., and Kawazoe, Y., 1971, DNA repair synthesis in mammalian cells exposed to a series of oncogenic and non-oncogenic derivatives of 4-nitroquinoline 1-oxide, *Nature* 229:416-419.

Stich, H.F., San, R.H.C., and Kawazoe, Y., 1973, Increased sensi-
    tivity of *Xeroderma pigmentosum* cells to some chemical car-
    cinogens and mutagens, *Mutat. Res.* 17:127-137.
Stich, H.F., San, R.H.C., Miller, J.A., and Miller, E.C., 1972,
    Various levels of DNA repair synthesis in *Xeroderma pigmentosum*
    cells exposed to the carcinogens N-hydroxy and N-acetoxy-2-
    acetylaminofluorene, *Nature New Biol.* 238:9-10.
Swaisland, A.J., Grover, P.L., and Sims, P., 1974a, Reactions of
    polycyclic hydrocarbon epoxides with RNA and polyribonucleo-
    tides, *Chem.-Biol. Interactions* 9:317-326.
Swaisland, A.J., Hewer, A., Pal, K., Keysell, G.R., Booth, J.,
    Grover, P.L., and Sims, P., 1974b, Polycyclic hydrocarbon
    epoxides: the involvement of 8,9-dihydro-8,9-dihydroxybenz-
    [a]anthracene 10,11-oxide in reactions with the DNA of benz-
    [a]anthracene-treated hamster embryo cells, *FEBS Lett.* 47:
    34-38.
Swenson, D.H., Miller, J.A., and Miller, E.C., 1973, 2,3-Dihydro-
    2,3-dihydroxy-aflatoxin B_1: an acid hydrolysis product of an
    RNA-aflatoxin B_1 adduct formed by hamster and rat liver
    microsomes *in vitro, Biochem. Biophys. Res. Commun.* 53:1260-
    1267.
Tasseron, J.G., Diringer, H., Frohwirth, N., Mirvish, S.S., and
    Heidelberger, C., 1970, Partial purification of soluble pro-
    tein from mouse skin to which carcinogenic hydrocarbons are
    specifically bound, *Biochemistry* 9:1636-1644.
Teranishi, K., Hamada, K., and Watanabe, H., 1975, Quantitative
    relationship between carcinogenicity and mutagenicity of
    polyaromatic hydrocarbons in *Salmonella typhimurium* mutants,
    Mutat. Res. 31:97-102.
Troll, W., Belman, L., Berkowitz, E., Chmielewicz, Z.F., Ambrus,
    J.H., and Bardos, T.J., 1968, Differential responses of DNA
    and RNA polymerase to modifications of the template rat liver
    DNA caused by action of the carcinogen acetylaminofluorene
    in vivo and *in vitro, Biochim. Biophys. Acta* 157:16-24.
Ts'o, P.O.P., Caspary, W.J., Cohen, B.I., Leavitt, J.C., Lesko, S.A.,
    Lorentzen, R.J., and Schechtman, L.M., 1974, Basic mechanisms
    in polycyclic hydrocarbon carcinogenesis, *in* "Chemical Carcino-
    genesis" (P.O.P. Ts'o and J.A. DiPaolo, eds.), Part A, pp. 113-
    147, Marcel Dekker, New York.
Weinstein, B., and Grunberger, D., 1974, Structural and functional
    changes in nucleic acids modified by chemical carcinogens, *in*
    "Chemical Carcinogenesis" (P.O.P. Ts'o and J.A. DiPaolo, eds.),
    pp. 217-235, Marcel Dekker, New York.
Wiest, W.G., and Heidelberger, C., 1953, The interaction of carcino-
    genic hydrocarbons with tissue constituents. I. Methods,
    Cancer Res. 13:246-249; II. 1,2,5,6-Dibenzanthracene-9,10-
    C^{14} in skin, *Cancer Res.* 13:250-254; III. 1,2,5,6-Dibenz-
    anthracene-9,10-C^{14} in the submaxillary gland, *Cancer Res.*
    13:255-261.

Wilk, M., and Girke, W., 1969, Radical cations of carcinogenic alternant hydrocarbons, amines and azo dyes, and their reactions with nucleobases, *in* "Physico-Chemical Mechanisms of Carcinogenesis" (E. Bergmann and B. Pullman, eds.), The Jerusalem Symposia on Quantum Chemistry and Biochemistry, Vol. 1, pp. 91-105, The Israeli Academy of Sciences and Humanities, Jerusalem.

Wislocki, P.G., Miller, J.A., and Miller, E.C., 1975, The carcinogenic and electrophilic activities of N-benzoyloxy derivatives of N-methyl-4-aminoazobenzene and related dyes, *Cancer Res.* 35:880-885.

Wünderlich, V., Tetzlaff, I., and Graffi, A., 1971/1972, Studies on nitrosodimethylamine: preferential methylation of mitochondrial DNA in rats and hamsters, *Chem.-Biol. Interactions* 4:81-89.

Yuspa, S.H., and Bates, R.R., 1970, The binding of benz[a]anthracene to replicating and nonreplicating DNA in cell culture, *Proc. Soc. Exp. Biol. Med.* 135:732-734.

Yuspa, S.H., Eaton, S., Morgan, D.L., and Bates, R.R., 1969/1970, The binding of 7,12-dimethylbenz[a]anthracene to replicating and nonreplicating DNA in cell culture, *Chem.-Biol. Interactions* 1:223-233.

Zieve, F.J., 1973, Effects of the carcinogen N-acetoxy-2-fluorenylacetamide on the template properties of deoxyribonucleic acid, *Mol. Pharmacol.* 9:658-669.

INVOLVEMENT OF RADICALS IN CHEMICAL CARCINOGENESIS

Paul O.P. Ts'o, James C. Barrett, William J. Caspary,

Stephen A. Lesko, Ronald J. Lorentzen, and Leonard M.

Schechtman

Department of Biochemical and Biophysical Sciences

Division of Biophysics, The Johns Hopkins University

Baltimore, Maryland 21205

1. INTRODUCTION

Chemical carcinogens comprise a large and structurally diverse

group of synthetic and naturally occurring compounds. It appears
almost axiomatic that such compounds must react with tissue components in order to induce neoplastic transformation. With the
exception of the carcinogenic alkylating agents, most chemical
carcinogens are not reactive *per se* and must be converted to
reactive forms either chemically or metabolically. Data are
emerging to indicate that electrophilic reactants are the ultimate
form of most, if not all, chemical carcinogens (Miller, 1970). The
proximate forms of a number of chemical carcinogens might be con-
vertible to free radicals, i.e., electrophilic reactants, and suggest a possible role for the free radical in carcinogenesis. The
presence of free radicals in tobacco smoke has been demonstrated
(Lyons and Spence, 1960; Bluhm *et al.*, 1971) and the increased
incidence of lung cancer in cigarette smokers based on epidemiological studies is well known. The chemical and metabolic conversion of a number of chemical carcinogens to free radicals and the
interaction of these radicals with DNA will be described in this
communication.

2.   FORMATION OF FREE RADICALS FROM CHEMICAL CARCINOGENS

2.1. Mild Chemical Oxidation of Aromatic Polycyclic Hydrocarbons

Electron paramagnetic response (EPR) studies in our laboratory
have shown the presence of benzo(a)pyrene [B(a)P] radicals (Fig. 1)
induced by I_2 at 25°C and measured in frozen solutions of benzene,
methanol, and cyclohexane (Caspary *et al.*, 1973). The steady-state
concentration of B(a)P radicals in benzene was reached within 1 min
upon addition of I_2 and remained constant for at least 2 h. The
maintenance of constant steady-state radical concentrations was
also observed with other hydrocarbons in this system. The highest
steady-state concentration of radicals found in solutions of B(a)P
was about 10% and the formation of these radicals was critically
dependent on I_2 concentration (Table 1). The differences in radical concentration in the various solvents at similar I_2 concentration appears to be a result of complex formation between I_2 and
benzene as well as different reaction rates of the radicals in
methanol.

The steady-state radical concentration of the B(a)P radicals
in benzene was not reduced by the introduction of methanol, iso-
propanol, acetaldehyde, and water, or by bubbling nitrogen gas
through the system. The B(a)P radical concentration, however,
was drastically reduced upon introduction of substituted adenosine
or guanosine (substituted at the ribose hydroxyl groups to increase
solubility in benzene). Many nitrogenous compounds, such as
imidazole, purine, pyrimidine, pyridine, aniline, and nucleosides
could quench the B(a)P radical signal in methanol. The extent of

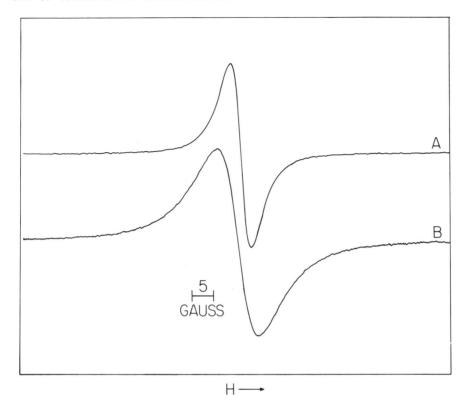

Fig. 1.   EPR spectra of B(a)P (A) and MCA (B) when mixed with I_2 in benzene and quick frozen in liquid nitrogen. Spectra taken at -25°C using a hydrocarbon concentration of 5×10^{-4} M and I_2 concentration of 5×10^{-3} M. Modulation amplitude, 1.66 gauss; microwave power, 5 mW (From Caspary *et al.*, 1973).

quenching was proportional to the nucleoside concentration; at low nucleoside concentration adenosine was slightly more effective as a quencher than gunaosine.

The steady-state radical concentration of 14 hydrocarbons formed in the presence of I_2 have been investigated by EPR (Table 2). In general, the carcinogenic compounds such as B(a)P, 7,12-dimethyl-benz(a)anthracene (DMBA), 3-methylcholanthrene (MCA), and dibenzo(a,h)pyrene had a much higher concentration of radicals than the noncarcinogenic compounds, such as B(e)P, benz(a)anthracene, pyrene, anthracene, picene, dibenz(a,c)anthracene, naphthalene, and naphthacene, etc. The steady-state radical concentrations of these compounds did not correlate well with their ionization potentials, though the compounds having low ionization potentials

Table 1. Formation of B(a)P Radicals in Different Solvents and
Iodine Concentrations*

Iodine concentration (M)	Benzene (-25°C)	Cyclohexane (-25°C)	Methanol (-120°C)
	Radical concentration (M × 10⁶)		
2.5×10^{-1}	20	-	-
5×10^{-2}	19	-	18
2.5×10^{-2}	20	20	18
5×10^{-3}	3	17	15
2.5×10^{-3}	0	19	6
5×10^{-4}	0	11	0
2.5×10^{-4}	-	6	
2×10^{-4}	-	7	-

*B(a)P at 2×10^{-4} M. Accuracy ±10% (From Caspary *et al.*, 1973).

Table 2. Comparison of Ionization Potential and Steady State
Radical Concentration of Various Polycyclic Hydrocarbons in
Benzene*

Compound	Carcino-genicity	Ioniza-tion potential	% Hydrocar-bon found as radical
Naphthalene	-	8.12-8.16	0
Picene	-	7.62-7.75	0
Benzo(e)pyrene	-	7.60-7.73	2.5 ± 1.0
Pyrene	-	7.58-7.72	2.7
Dibenz(a,c)anthracene	-	7.43-7.60	0.2
Dibenz(a,h)anthracene	+	7.42-7.58	0
Benz(a)anthracene	-	7.35-7.53	0.5
Anthracene	-	7.23-7.43	0
Benzo(a)pyrene	++	7.15-7.37	11 ± 1
Perylene	-	6.83-7.11	7.4
Dibenzo(a,h)pyrene	+++	6.75-7.04	12.5
Napthacene	-	6.64-6.95	3.0
7,12-Dimethylbenz(a)anthracene	++++	-	9.0
3-Methylcholanthrene	++	-	17.0

*Hydrocarbon concentration was 2×10^{-4} M and I_2 concentration was 5×10^2 M (From Caspary *et al.*, 1973).

did tend to yield higher concentrations of radicals (Table 2).

In 1960, Szent-Györgi *et al.* reported the existence of radicals of several carcinogenic polycyclic hydrocarbons, as well as several other compounds, when activated by I_2.

It was not unexpected that the steady-state concentrations of radicals produced by the 12 hydrocarbons so far investigated was not correlated with the ionization potentials of these compounds (Table 2). Since the radical concentration measured is governed by the balance between rate of formation and rate of decay, a compound, such as naphthacene which has the lowest ionization potential, may not yield the highest steady-state concentration of radicals if the radical also has a high rate of decay. One may expect, however, that if the initiation process in hydrocarbon carcinogenesis is related to the chemical reaction with these radicals, then the hydrocarbon which yields a high steady-state concentration of radicals will have carcinogenic activity, especially when this radical is chemically reactive to biologically active substances (such as nitrogenous compounds) but is stable in aqueous medium. By and large, this expectation was verified though not with perfect correlation among the 14 compounds so far investigated. Hopefully, this study may lead to a convenient and reliable procedure for screening for the carcinogenic potential of polycyclic hydrocarbons.

As for the mechanism of the formation of B(a)P radicals, the general reaction scheme (Fig. 2), based on a proposal constructed by Jeftic and Adams (1970) from an electrochemical oxidation study on B(a)P and from observations in this and other laboratories, appears to be applicable. According to this scheme, the radical species induced by I_2 presumably would be the cation radical, the first intermediate depicted in the oxidation scheme. Unfortunately, this assumption has not been verified in the I_2 induced reaction because of the lack of hyperfine structure in the radical signal observed.

Fried (1974) was able to obtain an EPR signal by oxidizing DMBA in acetone-water with ammonium ceric nitrate, a one-electron oxidant. He proposed that the signal was indicative of a radical cation intermediate formed in the oxidation of DMBA, viz. that of 7,12-dimethylenebenz(a)anthracene.

2.2. Formation of the 6-oxo-B(a)P Radical in Enzymic Reactions and by Other Oxidative Mechanisms

The environmental carcinogen, B(a)P, is metabolized by microsomal mixed function oxidases to a number of identifiable products (Holder *et al.*, 1974; Selkirk *et al.*, 1974; Rasmussen and Wang,

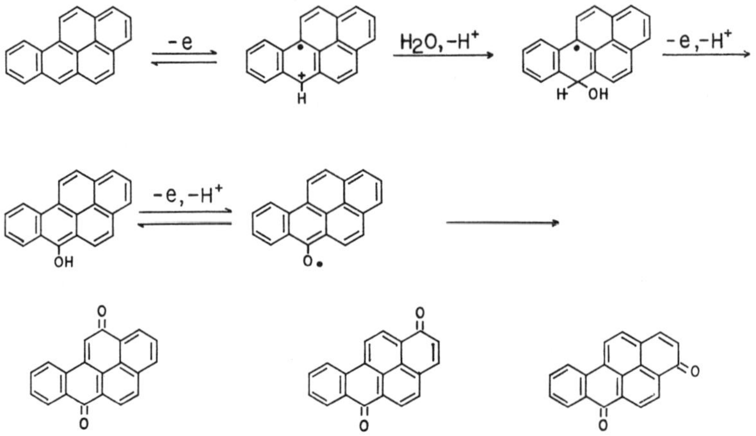

Fig. 2.   General reaction scheme proposed for the oxidation of B(a)P to B(a)P diones (From Jeftic and Adams, 1970; Lorentzen *et al.*, 1975).

1974). The six position of B(a)P is chemically more reactive than the other sites on the hydrocarbon (Cavalieri and Clavin, 1971; Jeftic and Adams, 1970) but 6-OH-B(a)P often is not reported as a metabolite although its formation has been implied by the detection of the 6-OH-B(a)P glucuronide *in vivo* (Falk *et al.*, 1962). Nagata *et al.* (1968, 1974) demonstrated that 6-OH-B(a)P can be detected in the metabolism of B(a)P in rat liver homogenate, as well as in mouse and rat skin homogenates, via its phenoxy radical, 6-oxo-B(a)P. This observation has been confirmed and extended by our laboratory (Lesko *et al.*, 1975).

Upon incubation of B(a)P in uninduced rat liver homogenates fortified with a NADPH-generating system at 37°C a metabolite was formed which gave rise spontaneously to an EPR signal. The metabolite and the radical were extracted quantitatively into benzene in which they were relatively stable. The metabolite also could be quantitatively converted to the radical by shaking with aqueous solutions of 2,6-dichloroindophenol or $K_3Fe(CN)_6$. The latter compound, however, was not selective in its action and would also oxidize 3-OH-B(a)P to its oxo radical. The EPR measurement of the quantity of radical was done in benzene after the extracted solution had been taken to dryness under vacuum and redissolved in a small volume. The EPR signal obtained with B(a)P was identical to that extracted after incubating 6-OH-B(a)P in fortified rat liver homogenates (Fig. 3) and has been identified as the 6-oxo-B(a)P radical by its characteristic hyperfine structure (Nagata *et al.*, 1968; Lorentzen *et al.*, 1975). Identical hyperfine spectra were obtained before and after oxidation with 2,6-dichloroindophenol.

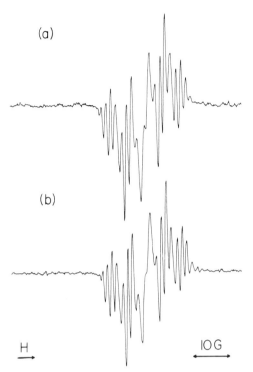

(a)

(b)

H →   IOG

Fig. 3. EPR spectra of 6-oxo-B(a)P radicals in benzene solutions measured at room temperature after extensive sparging with nitrogen. The radicals were obtained by incubating B(a)P or 6-OH-B(a)P at 37°C in fortified rat liver homogenates, after which they were extracted into benzene. The extracted products in benzene were oxidized by shaking with aqueous solutions of 2,6-dichloro-indophenol. (a) B(a)P; (b) 6-OH-B(a)P (From Lesko *et al*., 1975).

No EPR signal was seen when B(a)P or cofactors were eliminated from the incubation mixture or when the homogenate was heated at 65°C for 10 min. These observations indicate that the oxidation of B(a)P to 6-OH-B(a)P was enzymic in nature. Figure 4 shows the effect of protein concentration on radical production. Increasing amounts of homogenate resulted in higher concentrations of 6-oxo-B(a)P radical being produced. Kinetics of 6-oxo-B(a)P radical formation in liver homogenates showed an initial increase peaking at 14-15 min followed by a rapid decline to a low concentration at 20 min which persisted up to at least 40 min (Fig. 5).

B(e)P, a structural and noncarcinogenic analog of B(a)P, did not give an EPR signal when incubated 10, 20, or 40 min in a rat liver homogenate under conditions in which B(a)P was converted to

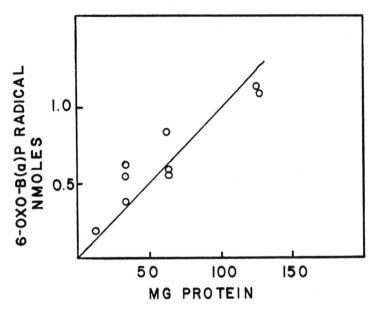

Fig. 4.   Dependence of 6-oxo-B(a)P radical formation from
B(a)P on the amount of rat liver homogenate present in incubation
mixture. B(a)P concentration was 0.14 mM. Radical concentration
was measured after oxidation of metabolite in benzene by shaking
with aqueous 2,6-dichloroindophenol (From Lesko *et al.*, 1975).

a radical. No EPR signal was seen even after shaking the benzene
extract with aqueous $K_3Fe(CN)_6$. Incubation of the strongly carcinogenic dibenzo(a,h)pyrene did give rise spontaneously to an EPR
signal after incubation for 10 or 30 min. The EPR signal in benzene
was a singlet and no hyperfine structure could be detected even
after extensive sparging with N_2.

Figure 6 shows the kinetics of 6-OH-B(a)P in rat liver homogenates. At each experimental point, unreacted 6-OH-B(a)P was
quantitatively converted to 6-oxo-B(a)P radical with $K_3Fe(CN)_6$ and
total radical concentration was measured by EPR. The decay of
6-OH-B(a)P in rat liver homogenates showed first order kinetics
with a rate constant of 0.29 min^{-1}. The half-life of 6-OH-B(a)P
in this system was about 2.4 min. The rate of degradation of 6-OH-
B(a)P was not decreased by either elimination of the NADPH-generating
system or by heating the homogenate at 65°C for 10 min, thus indicating that this reaction was nonenzymic in nature.

The products formed by incubating 6-OH-B(a)P in rat liver
homogenates were extracted into benzene and isolated by aluminum
oxide chromatography (Lorentzen *et al.*, 1975). The data show that

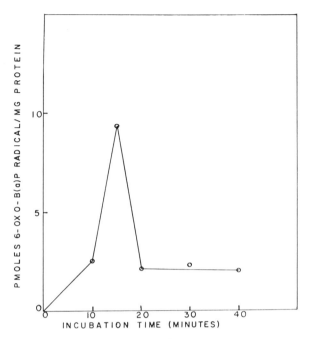

Fig. 5. Kinetics of 6-oxo-B(a)P radical production from the incubation of B(a)P at 37°C in fortified female ACI rat liver homogenates. B(a)P concentration was 0.68 mM (From Lesko *et al.*, 1975).

6-OH-B(a)P was oxidized in this system and the following were the only products detected after 40 min of incubation: 6,12-B(a)P dione (15%), 1,6-B(a)P dione (41%), and 3,6-B(a)P dione (44%).

The metabolic pathway of B(a)P to 6-OH-B(a)P and beyond can be schematically represented as follows:

$$B(a)P \xrightarrow{k_1} 6\text{-OH-B(a)P} \xrightarrow{k_2} 6\text{-oxo-B(a)P radical}$$

$$6\text{-oxo-B(a)P radical} \xrightarrow{k_3} products.$$

Our results indicate that the procedures used to extract the radical from the homogenate allowed some air oxidation of the 6-OH-B(a)P to the radical. Consequently, the observed concentrations of the 6-oxo-B(a)P radical extracted into benzene were not reliable estimates of the amount of radical in the homogenate and were variable from experiment to experiment. In contrast, the quantity of the 6-oxo-B(a)P radical measured in the benzene extract *after* the 2,6-dichloroindophenol oxidation was consistent and reliable. The ease of oxidation of 6-OH-B(a)P to 6-oxo-B(a)P radical suggests that the rate constant of this conversion (k_2) in the homogenate

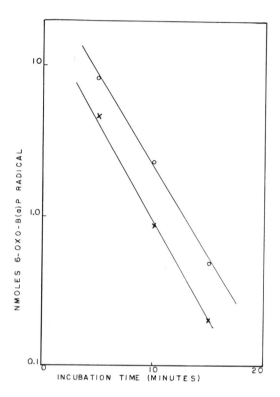

Fig. 6.   Kinetics of 6-OH-B(a)P degradation in fortified
Sprague-Dawley male liver homogenates at 37°C, measured after
$K_3Fe(CN)_6$ oxidation.   Initial 6-OH-B(a)P concentration 5.3 µM (x);
6.1 µM (o) (From Lesko *et al.*, 1975).

may be substantially greater than k_3, the rate constant describing
the disappearance of radical. This notion was supported by the
kinetics of oxidation of synthetic 6-OH-B(a)P in rat liver homogenate. The rate of formation of the 6-oxo-B(a)P radical was too
rapid to be observed in one minute whereas its decay could be
monitored over a 15 min period. If k_2 is substantially greater
than k_3 (5-fold or more), as was observed in the autoxidation of
6-OH-B(a)P in ethanol-buffer solution, then k_2 can be ignored and
the reaction approximated by the following scheme:

$$B(a)P \xrightarrow{k_1} R \xrightarrow{k_3} Products,$$

where (R) = [6-OH-B(a)P] + [6-oxo-B(a)P radical], that is, the
radical concentration after oxidation by 2,6-dichloroindophenol.
The concentration of (R) at any given time can be quantitatively
described by the following equation:

$$\frac{d(R)}{dt} = k_1 - k_3(R) \tag{1}$$

which is a homogeneous linear differential equation. This differential equation can be solved to yield the value of the zero-order rate constant k_1 at time t, when (R) and k_3 can be independently measured as shown in equation (2):

$$k_1 = \frac{(R) \cdot k_3}{(1-e^{-k_3 t})} \tag{2}$$

The k_3 value of 0.29 min^{-1} was measured with synthetic 6-OH-B(a)P and described above. The average values for the rate constant, k_1, per mg of protein for 6-OH-B(a)P formation in the early period of incubation as calculated from equation (2) and the measurements of (R) are 2.8 × 10^{-9} and 1.5 × 10^{-9} mol $liter^{-1}$ min^{-1} for Sprague-Dawley and ACI rats, respectively. As shown in Fig. 5, these values would decrease rapidly after about a 12-15 min period of incubation.

Using these rate constants we were able to estimate the percentage of B(a)P metabolism proceeding through the 6-OH-B(a)P pathway by comparison with the initial rate of total B(a)P metabolism. The total metabolism of $[^3H]$B(a)P was determined by measuring the release of tritium from the site of hydroxylation on the substrate catalyzed by the aryl hydrocarbon hydroxylase system (Hayakawa and Udenfriend, 1973). The percentage of metabolism proceeding through 6-OH-B(a)P was about 18% for female Sprague-Dawley rats and about 20% for female ACI rats. The reaction rates were measured at relatively high substrate concentration to ensure zero-order kinetics.

Ioki et al. (1974) have obtained the 6-oxo-B(a)P radical by reacting B(a)P in benzene with trifluoroacetic acid plus H_2O_2 or Fenton's reagent (Fe^{++} + H_2O_2). The 6-oxo-B(a)P radical has also been produced by photoirradiation of B(a)P in organic solvents (Inomata and Nagata, 1972). Forbes and Robinson (1968) have obtained a free radical by heating B(a)P to 220°C in vacuum. The EPR spectrum they observed was similar to that obtained with the 6-oxo-B(a)P radical.

2.3. Autoxidation of 6-OH-B(a)P and 6-oxo-B(a)P Radical

We have synthesized 6-OH-B(a)P from B(a)P using modifications of the procedure of Fieser and Hershberg (1939). In aqueous buffer-ethanol (1:1) solutions synthetic 6-OH-B(a)P was autoxidized to a mixture of three stable B(a)P diones, 6,12-; 1,6-; and 3,6-, plus a small amount of an unidentified paramagnetic, violet-colored material (Lorentzen et al., 1975). In this reaction, O_2 was

reduced to H_2O_2 and probably to other reactive reduced oxygen
species as well. The half-life of 6-OH-B(a)P in air saturated
aqueous-ethanol (1:1) was about 45 min at 22°C. A free radical
(Fig. 3) derived from 6-OH-B(a)P by one electron oxidation, the
6-oxo-B(a)P radical, is most likely an obligatory intermediate in
the autoxidation as indicated by its kinetics of formation and
decay (Lorentzen *et al.*, 1975). Figure 7 presents the time course
of the observed concentrations of free-radicals during autoxidation
of 6-OH-B(a)P in buffer-ethanol (1:1) solution. The observed free
radical signal at the later stages of the autoxidation was a mixture of the signal of the 6-oxo-B(a)P radical and the singlet
signal of an unidentified radical present in the violet-colored
material described above, and which persisted after the decay of
the 6-oxo-B(a)P radical. In the first 3-4 h of the autoxidation,
the EPR signal was mainly that of the 6-oxo-B(a)P radical. The
6-oxo-B(a)P radical could be produced quantitatively in benzene by
oxidation with aqueous $K_3Fe(CN)_6$ and isolated in the absence of
oxygen. Like 6-OH-B(a)P, this isolated free radical was autoxidized in aqueous buffer-ethanol solutions and yielded identical
products.

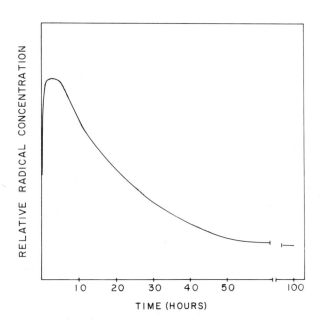

Fig. 7. Relative concentration of radicals during the autoxidation of 6-OH-B(a)P (0.52 mM) in pH 7 ethanol-Na phosphate buffer
(1:1, v/v) at 22°C (From Lorentzen *et al.*, 1975).

2.4. Formation of Radicals from Various Kinds of Chemical Carcinogens

N-Hydroxylation appears to be a necessary metabolic activation step for carcinogenic activity of aromatic amines and amides (Miller and Miller, 1969). The proximate carcinogen N-hydroxy-N-2-acetylaminofluorene (N-OH-AAF) was readily converted by $K_3Fe(CN)_6$ into an unstable nitroxide radical (Bartsch *et al.*, 1971). The radical underwent disproportionation in organic and aqueous solutions to yield 2-nitrosofluorene and N-acetoxy-N-2-acetylamino-fluorene (N-AcO-AAF). The same oxidation could also be achieved with horseradish peroxidase and H_2O_2 (Bartsch and Hecker, 1971). The proximate form of 4-nitroquinoline-1-oxide, 4-hydroxyaminoquino-line-1-oxide, was converted to a free radical in organic solvents and in alkaline aqueous solution (Nagata *et al.*, 1966). Proximate forms of 2-napthylamine, 2-amino-1-naphthol and 1- and 2-hydroxy-aminonaphthalenes, could be converted to radicals under physiolog-ical conditions (Nagata *et al.*, 1969). N-Methyl-N'-nitro-N-nitrosoguanidine gave an EPR signal when stirred in buffered aqueous solution at pH 3 to 6 (Nagata *et al.*, 1972). The mechanism for radical formation is not clear in all cases but N-hydroxy derivatives of aromatic amines and amides were rather easily con-verted to free radicals.

3. INTERACTION OF DNA WITH CHEMICAL CARCINOGENS

3.1. Polycyclic Hydrocarbon-DNA Adducts Formed by Chemical Activation

The previous section documented the formation of free radicals from carcinogenic polycyclic hydrocarbons by mild oxidation with I_2 or $H_2O_2 + Fe^{++}$. In this section we will describe the formation of DNA-polycyclic hydrocarbon adducts induced by such oxidants. The procedure that has been established for determining covalent linkage is as follows:

When DNA was precipitated from an aqueous solution containing a [³H]B(a)P-DNA physical complex by ethanol, and the precipitate was washed repeatedly with ethanol, about 99.7% of the physically-bound hydrocarbon could be extracted (Ts'o and Lu, 1964; Lesko *et al.*, 1969). However, with [³H]B(a)P was covalently linked to DNA, it could no longer be removed by precipitation and extraction with organic solvent. The possibility of a mere exchange of tritium between the [³H]hydrocarbon and DNA was excluded when no radio-activity was found in the extracted DNA from a reaction mixture containing [³H]water instead of [³H]B(a)P (Rapaport and Ts'o, 1966).

In order to show that the chemical complex was not contaminated by any [³H]B(a)P reaction products insoluble in organic solvents, solutions of washed chemical complex were analyzed by physico-chemical techniques. It could be demonstrated that under the influence of a force field (electrical or centrifugal), or in a system of molecular-sieve chromatography, that the movement of [³H]B(a)P was coincident with the movement of DNA. These findings provide a strong argument that the [³H]B(a)P assayed after the washing procedure was actually attached to DNA.

Finally the [³H]B(a)P-DNA chemical complex could be enzymatically hydrolyzed and examined by sucrose gradient electrophoresis and other chromatographic techniques. However, we have not excluded the possibility that attachment of polycyclic hydrocarbons to DNA would inhibit complete enzymic degradation. Demonstrating that electrophoretic migration of [³H]B(a)P resulted from attachment to the hydrolytic products of DNA provided conclusive proof of a covalent linkage.

Table 3 shows the percentage of [³H]B(a)P or [³H]B(e)P that became nonextractable from DNA after reaction with I_2 or H_2O_2 + Fe^{++} (Lesko *et al.*, 1969). Table 3 also shows the specificity of chemical complex formation and the influence of the conformational states of DNA when hydrocarbons were activated with I_2 and H_2O_2. Both reactions were specific in two respects: carcinogenic B(a)P reacted with DNA to a much greater extent than noncarcinogenic B(e)P; with B(a)P, the extent of the reaction was much higher for denatured DNA than for native DNA. The [³H]B(a)P-DNA chemical complexes induced by iodine and H_2O_2 were examined by sucrose gradient electrophoresis and gel filtration chromatography before and after enzymic degradation to prove covalent binding.

The extent of DNA degradation produced by these chemical reactions has been examined. No diminution in sedimentation coefficient of DNA was found after the iodine reaction. However, CsCl density gradient sedimentation as well as UV hyperchromicity studies on heat or alkaline denatured B(a)P-DNA revealed that a considerable portion of the DNA (up to 40%) became cross-linked upon reaction with the B(a)P in the iodine induced reaction (Maher *et al.*, 1971). On the other hand, there was a reduction in the sedimentation coefficient of DNA after reaction with B(a)P in a H_2O_2-$FeCl_2$ system. The data suggested the occurrence of chain scission of DNA by the hydroxyl or perhydroxyl radicals (Rhaese and Freese, 1968; Massie *et al.*, 1972).

We have been able to improve the reaction yield of the iodine system by conducting the reaction in a solution composed of 0.01 M phosphate buffer (pH 6.8)-ethanol (1:1 v/v), where the concentration of I_2 and B(a)P can be substantially increased (DNA, 4×10^{-4} M; [³H]hydrocarbon, 2.5×10^{-5} M; I_2, 5×10^{-3} M). After two

Table 3. Percentage of Physically Bound [^{3}H]B(a)P and B(e)P that
Becomes Chemically Linked to DNA in Reactions Induced by Iodine
and H$_2$O$_2$ in HMP*

| | Iodine[†] | H$_2$O$_2$[‡] | |
		10^{-2} M Citrate	10^{-3} M FeCl$_2$
		Native DNA	
Benzo(a)pyrene	10.5	4.5	15.5
Benzo(e)pyrene	1.0	2.0	3.0
		Denatured DNA	
Benzo(a)pyrene	31.5	15.0	40.0
Benzo(e)pyrene	1.0	1.0	2.0

*HMP, 10^{-2} M phosphate buffer, pH 6.8. Physical complexes
contained about one hydrocarbon per 1000-3000 nucleotides.
[†]I$_2$ concentration was 10^{-4} M; reaction at 23°C for 2 h.
[‡]H$_2$O$_2$ concentration was 1.5 × 10^{-2} M; reaction at 37°C for
24 h (From Lesko *et al.*, 1969).

Table 4. Extent and Efficiency of Adduct Formation upon Incubation
of 6-OH-B(a)P with SB 19 *B. subtilis* DNA in 10^{-2} Na Phosphate-
Ethanol Buffer (1:1, pH 7.5) at Room Temperature*

Hours incubation	Base/B(a)P	Efficiency of conversion
	Native DNA	
16	13,000	1/2500
40	10,000	1/2000
	Denatured DNA	
16	2,600	1/500
40	1,550	1/300

*Hydrocarbon/base, 1.5; DNA concentration, 3.8 × 10^{-4} M (From
Ts'o *et al.*, 1974).

sequential reactions, about 3.2 molecules of [^{3}H]B(a)P have been
linked per 10^3 bases of mouse DNA (Hoffmann *et al.*, 1970). The
specificity of the iodine-induced covalent linkage of polycyclic
hydrocarbons to DNA was maintained in the ethanol-phosphate buffer
system, i.e., the carcinogenic hydrocarbons [B(a)P, DMBA MCA] are
4 to 14-fold more reactive than their noncarcinogenic analogs
[B(e)P, and benz(a)anthracene]. The extraction procedure had to
be improved because of the increase in hydrocarbon concentration.

The new procedure involved the removal of iodine by chloroform extraction, the removal of the unbound hydrocarbons by phenol extraction, and the removal of water-soluble tritium by dialysis.

The base specificity of the chemically-induced covalent linkage of polycyclic hydrocarbons to nucleic acids was examined using hompolynucleotide and their double-stranded complexes as model systems (Hoffmann *et al.*, 1970). The reaction with [^{3}H]B(a)P was indeed base specific with poly G being more reactive than the other polynucleotides in the iodine system. This was true even when poly G was complexed with poly C in a double helical conformation. When [^{3}H]B(a)P was activated in a H_2O_2/Fe^{++} system, the hydrocarbon was bound preferentially to purine polynucleotides with poly G still being the most reactive.

In order to exclude the possibility of tritium exchange between [^{3}H]B(a)P and poly G and to further substantiate the existence of a covalent linkage, the following experiment was performed (Hoffmann *et al.*, 1970). Poly G was reacted with B(a)P containing a mixture of [^{3}H] and [^{14}C] labeled hydrocarbons in a ratio of 18:1. After precipitation and washing, the isolated B(a)P-poly G complex was found to contain radioactivity with a [^{3}H]/[^{14}C] ratio of 15:1. The finding completely excluded the possibility that the radioactivity associated with nucleic acids, in experiments using only [^{3}H]B(a)P, could have originated from tritium exchange. The reduction of [^{3}H]/[^{14}C] ratio was equivalent to a loss of about 16% of the tritium of [^{3}H]B(a)P in reacting with poly G. Formation of a covalent bond between [^{3}H]B(a)P and poly G should remove at least one hydrogen atom (therefore, also the corresponding amount of tritium) from the hydrocarbon. If the [^{3}H]B(a)P was labeled randomly with the tritium, the loss of tritium should be 8.3%. Further oxidation or non-random labeling could lead to a greater percentage of loss as observed.

The radical cation of B(a)P has been proposed as the intermediate in the reaction of B(a)P with pyridine or nucleic acid bases in a solid phase system activated by I_2 vapor (Rochlitz, 1967; Wilk and Girke, 1969). The 6-benzo(a)pyrenyl-pyridinium adduct reported by Rochlitz (1967) in the solid phase system was also found by us in our B(a)P-pyridine-I_2-aqueous system (Hoffmann *et al.*, 1970). The chemical mechanism for the reaction induced by hydroxyl radical in the H_2O_2-Fe^{++} system did not appear to be identical to that induced by I_2 in that a product other than the 6-benzo(a)pyrenyl-pyridinium salt was found in the B(a)P-pyridine-aqueous H_2O_2-Fe^{++} system. This was not surprising since Ioki *et al.* (1974) obtained the 6-oxo-B(a)P radical from B(a)P by oxidation with H_2O_2-Fe^{++} and this radical was probably the intermediate in adduct formation. The adduct obtained with the H_2O_2-Fe^{++} system had different fluorescence, chromatographic and electrophoretic properties than the 6-benzo(a)pyrenyl pyridinium salt.

A high extent of covalent linkage of carcinogenic polycyclic hydrocarbon free radicals, produced indirectly by irradiation of I_2, to DNA has been reported (Pascal *et al.*, 1971). B(a)P, MCA, and dibenz(a,h)anthracene free radicals formed adducts with DNA to the extent of one to five hydrocarbons per 1000 bases while the reaction of noncarcinogens was not measureable. The 6-benzo(a)-pyrenyl-pyridinium adduct has been reported upon anodic oxidation of B(a)P in the presence of pyridine (Blackburn and Will, 1974). This suggests that the radical cation of B(a)P was formed by electrochemical oxidation of B(a)P as depicted in the scheme of Jeftic and Adams (1970) shown in Fig. 2.

3.2. Reaction of a Labile Metabolite, 6-OH-B(a)P, with DNA

The isolation of covalent adducts between DNA and [³H]B(a)P from *in vivo* systems (Brookes and Lawley, 1964; Goshman and Heidelberger, 1968; Prodi *et al.*, 1970; Carlassare *et al.*, 1972) indicated an enzymic basis for the chemical interaction. The covalent linkage of [³H]B(a)P and other tritiated polycyclic hydrocarbons to DNA has been reported after incubation of these materials in the presence of rat liver microsomes (Gelboin, 1969; Grover and Sims, 1968).

As described earlier, 6-OH-B(a)P is a major metabolite of B(a)P and is easily and readily converted to the 6-oxo-B(a)P radical by O_2 in aqueous-ethanol solution. When synthetic 6-OH-[³H]B(a)P and DNA were dissolved in phosphate buffer-ethanol and incubated for 40 h at 23°C (Table 4), a small portion of the 6-OH-B(a)P became covalently linked to DNA with a concomitant decay of most of the 6-OH-B(a)P to a mixture of quinones as indicated by efficiency of conversion [DNA-linked B(a)P versus quinones].

As shown in Table 4, the reaction of 6-OH-B(a)P with denatured DNA was much more extensive than with the native DNA. A reaction with poly A and poly G (both at 4×10^{-4} M concentration) was carried out with a ratio of 6-OH-B(a)P/base of 1.6 under the same conditions as that shown in Table 4. The amount of 6-OH-B(a)P reacted was the same for both poly A and poly G and was to the extent of one B(a)P per 450 bases with an efficiency of conversion of one adduct formed per 880 quinones produced. Figure 8 demonstrates that the kinetics of the covalent linkage of 6-OH-B(a)P to poly A were comparable to the life time of the 6-oxo-B(a)P radical in solution (Ts'o *et al.*, 1974).

In these reactions, the quinones and other possible byproducts were removed from the nucleic acid by repeated extraction with phenol and then with ether to remove the phenol, a procedure similar to that described for iodine reaction. The nucleic acid was then dialyzed against 10^{-2} M Na phosphate buffer (pH 7) to

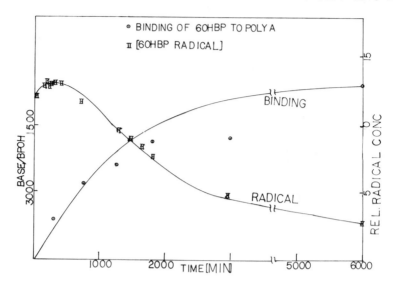

Fig. 8.   Comparison of the kinetics of the 6-oxo-B(a)P radical
and of the covalent binding of [³H]6-OH-B(a)P to poly A at room
temperature in ethanol-Na phosphate buffer (1:1, pH 7). Hydro-
carbon/base, 1:1; poly A concentration, 5×10^{-4} M in nucleotide.
Radical concentration is measured by comparing peak heights of the
6-oxo-radical and a standard. After 3000 min, the 6-oxy radical
concentration has diminished to zero. After 3000 min the radical
observed shows a singlet spectrum whose peak height is measured
and included in the graph. Between 2000 and 3000 min a combination of singlet and 6-oxy radical multiplet is observed (From Ts'o
et al., 1974).

remove water-soluble radioactive contaminants. Covalent attachment was proved by enzymic degradation of the DNA-[³H]6-OH-B(a)P
and by showing that electrophoretic migration of hydrocarbon
(measured by radioactivity) resulted from attachment to hydrolytic
products of DNA as described earlier.

    Native T7 DNA also was reacted with 6-OH-B(a)P both at 23°
and 37°C and with an input ratio of 6-OH-B(a)P/base of 2.9. As
shown in Fig. 9, after 23 h at 37°C, one 6-OH-B(a)P was linked to
about 420 bases in the T7 DNA. The yield was higher at 37° than
at 23°C. Introduction of higher DNA concentration (from 20 µg
to 85 µg/0.1 ml) in the reaction mixture for a given concentration
of 6-OH-B(a)P (50 µg/0.1 ml), decreased the ratio of B(a)P/base
of the product as expected, but not proportionally. The increase
in DNA concentration also increased the efficiency of binding of
6-OH-B(a)P to DNA versus its conversion to quinones from 1/1000
to 2.5/1000.

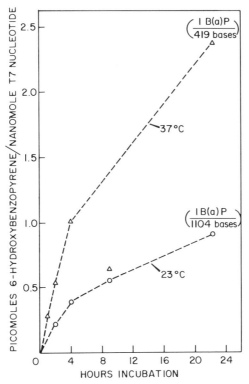

Fig. 9. Kinetics of covalent binding of [³H]6-OH-B(a)P to T7 DNA in 2 × 10⁻² M Tris buffer-ethanol (1:1, pH 7.9). Hydrocarbon/base, 2.9:1; DNA concentration, 6.5 × 10⁻⁴ M in nucleotide (From Ts'o *et al.*, 1974).

Incubation of T7 DNA with 6-OH-B(a)P under the conditions described above to obtain a B(a)P-DNA adduct with a B(a)P/base ratio of 1:400 resulted in considerable degradation of the DNA (3 to 9 double-strand breaks per genome). B(a)P-DNA adducts with lower B(a)P/base ratios (1:2000-4000) still had 10-20 single-strand breaks per genome as measured by alkaline sedimentation. These strand breaks were probably caused by H_2O_2 or other reduced oxygen species generated during autoxidation of 6-OH-B(a)P. H_2O_2 and hydroxyl radical generators are known to cause DNA strand breakage (Rhaese and Freese, 1968; Massie *et al.*, 1972). We have found that addition of EDTA (0.01 to 1 mM) to the reaction mixture would completely inhibit the production of single-strand breaks induced in DNA by 6-OH-B(a)P autoxidation but it also inhibited adduct formation by at least 50% or more.

The mechanism by which adduct formation takes place during

the autoxidation of 6-OH-B(a)P is unknown at present. The 6-oxo-B(a)P radical may be the species that reacts directly with DNA, although other electrophilic intermediates in the oxidation to quinones may also be potentially reactive towards this macromole-cule.

3.3.   Reaction of Various Other Radicals with DNA

As described in the section on free radical formation, the N-hydroxy derivatives of many aromatic amines and amides are easily converted to free radicals. N-AcO-AAF was formed from the disproportionation of a nitroxide radical formed by oxidation of N-OH-AAF. N-AcO-AAF has been shown to react efficiently with the C-8 of guanine in DNA (Miller, 1970). This reactivity may be a special case, untypical of N-acetoxy-N-arylacetamides, arising from the rapid transition of the N-2-fluorenyl-N-acetyl nitrenium ion from a relatively high-energy singlet (non-radical) state to a triplet (radical) ground state (Scribner and Naimy, 1973). The ability of N-AcO-AAF to decolorize a stable free radical was closely related to the adduct-forming ability of this compound. However, this adduct-forming ability was not correlated with local carcinogenicity (Scribner *et al.*, 1970) and thus the propensity for radical formation and reactivity with nucleic acid guanine could be a process that competes with a reaction necessary to initiate carcinogenesis or it may be lethal to many cells that would otherwise be transformed by N-AcO-AAF (Scribner and Naimy, 1973).

Exposure of bacteria to the carcinogen N-hydroxyurethan resulted in cell death and the lethal effect was accompanied by degradation of the cellular DNA (Mullinix and Rosenkrantz, 1971). Two types of reactions take place between DNA and N-hydroxyurethan *in vitro* (Mullinix *et al.*, 1973). The predominant reaction involved degrada-tion of DNA, presumably through scissions of phosphodiester bonds and was blocked by scavengers of free radicals. The second reaction involved modifications of deoxycytidine and it was also blocked by scavengers of free radicals. It appears that an intermediate, ethoxycarbonylurethan, arising from the oxidation of hydroxyurethan was involved in the reactions with DNA.

4.   CONCLUSIONS

In the above discourse, the conversion of a number of chemical carcinogens to free radicals which react with DNA either directly, to yield adducts or indirectly, to cause polynucleotide chain scission, has been described. The exact nature of the adducts formed between such radicals and DNA is not known at present with the exception of N-AcO-AAF, which reacts with DNA to yield

N-deoxyguanosin-8-yl-AAF as one product. It appears that autoxida-
tions in general and of certain phenolic compounds, in particular
6-OH-B(a)P, are capable of producing all of the reactive species
derived from the reduction of molecular oxygen (e.g., hydroxyl
radical, superoxide radical and excited state singlet molecular
oxygen) and which are known to degrade DNA (Lorentzen *et al.*,
1975).

There is evidence for the involvement of radicals in neoplastic
transformation. Synthetic 6-OH-B(a)P which spontaneously forms
the 6-oxo-B(a)P radical in solution has been shown to induce *in
vitro* morphological transformation of Syrian hamster embryo fibroblasts (Schechtman *et al.*, 1974). There was a close similarity in
the dose responses on the morphological transformation of these
cells by B(a)P and 6-OH-B(a)P after 24 h of exposure within the
dose range of 0.01 to 3 µg/ml. However, a much shorter time was
required to reach maximal transformation efficiency with 6-OH-
B(a)P as compared to B(a)P (2 versus 24 h). This lends credence
to the premise that the labile metabolite, 6-OH-B(a)P, is a proximate or ultimate carcinogen of B(a)P. Using EPR spectroscopy,
6-OH-B(a)P was shown to be a major metabolite of B(a)P in rat
liver homogenates (Lesko *et al.*, 1975).

The radical scavenger, cysteamine-HCl, has been shown to
markedly decrease the number of transformed foci when DMBA was
added to mouse fibroblasts without any reduction in carcinogen-
induced toxicity (Marquardt *et al.*, 1974). *In vivo*, this agent
did not affect DMBA-induced necrosis in Sprague-Dawley rats but
it did markedly reduce the number of mammary tumors. Thus, it
appears that the toxic and oncogenic effects induced by DMBA are
due to two different metabolites and suggest that the oncogenic
activity may be mediated by a radical. Antioxidants have been
used in various studies to reduce chromosomal breaks (Shamberger
et al., 1973) and to decrease neoplasia incidences (Wattenberg,
1973).

The nature of the critical cellular target involved in interaction with chemical carcinogens is still a matter of conjecture.
Since most, if not all, chemical carcinogens are mutagenic, many
investigators feel that some alteration in DNA is essential for
oncogenic activity. This hypothesis has been examined in our laboratory with the use of 5-bromodeoxyuridine (BrdUrd) which is
selectively incorporated into DNA in place of its analog thymidine. Irradiation of BrdUrd-DNA at 313 nm results in single-
strand breaks (Hutchinson, 1973). A uracilyl radical, formed by
the photochemical dissociation of the bromine atom in BrdUrd,
extracts a hydrogen atom from the deoxysugar of the nucleotide on
the 5' side of the BrdUrd substitution with a concomitant single
strand. Our preliminary results have shown that irradiation above
300 nm of Syrian hamster cells that have incorporated BrdUrd into

their DNA resulted in morphological transformation of the cells
under conditions where treatment with BrdUrd or light only failed
to produce such changes. Demonstrating that these morphologically
aberrant cells will produce tumors *in vivo* should lend support to
the hypothesis that DNA may be the critical cellular target for
chemical carcinogens.

One of the current trends in the study of chemical carcinogenesis, and one that should be examined much more extensively in
the future, is the attempt to isolate and identify metabolites
that will covalently link with DNA and produce adducts which are
identical to those formed when the parent compound is administered
in vivo or added to transformable cell systems. Since such compounds should by nature be labile, we feel that EPR spectroscopy
should be a very promising tool for detecting the presence of these
metabolites in biologic systems. Using EPR spectroscopy, Nagata
et al. (1974) detected enzymic activity in the nucleus capable of
converting considerable amounts of B(a)P to the 6-oxo-B(a)P radical, thereby enabling an active metabolite to be formed in the
area of the genetic material. The development of techniques to
increase the sensitivity of EPR spectrometers would be valuable
for investigating radicals in chemical carcinogenesis. With an
increase in sensitivity it may be possible to detect the formation
of specific radicals from carcinogens in cellular systems and the
fate of such radicals could then be followed. Hopefully, the radical interaction could be followed to a specific biologic endpoint,
e.g., morphological transformation.

Acknowledgment. This research was supported in part by Atomic
Energy Commission Contract No. AT (11-1)-3280 and by National
Cancer Institute Grant No. CA 13370-05. W.J. Caspary is a post-
doctoral fellow of the National Cancer Institute.

References

Bartsch, H., and Hecker, E., 1970, On the metabolic activation of
    the carcinogen N-hydroxy-N-2-acetylaminofluorene. III.
    Oxidation with horseradish peroxidase to yield 2-nitroso-
    fluorene and N-acetoxy-N-2-acetylaminofluorene, *Biochim.
    Biophys. Acta* 237:567-578.
Bartsch, H., Traut, M., and Hecker, E., 1970, On the metabolic
    activation of N-hydroxy-N-2-acetylaminofluorene. II. Simul-
    taneous formation of 2-nitrosofluorene and N-acetoxy-N-2-
    acetylaminofluorene from N-hydroxy-N-2-acetylaminofluorene
    via a free radical intermediate, *Biochim. Biophys. Acta*
    237:556-566.
Blackburn, G., and Will, J., 1974, Bonding of benzo(a)pyrene to
    nitrogen heterocycles by anodic oxidation, *J.C.S. Chem. Commun.*
    1974:67-68.

Bluhm, A., Weinstein, J., and Sousa, J., 1971, Free radicals in tobacco smoke, *Nature* 229:500.

Brookes, P., and Lawley, P., 1964, Evidence for the binding of polynuclear aromatic hydrocarbons to the nucleic acids of mouse skin: Relation between carcinogenic power of hydrocarbons and their binding to deoxyribonucleic acid, *Nature* 202:781-784.

Carlassare, F., Antonello, C., Baccichetti, F., and Malfer, P., 1972, On the binding of benzo(a)pyrene to DNA "*in vivo*", *Z. Naturforsch.* 27b:200-202.

Caspary, W., Cohen, B., Lesko, S., and Ts'o, P., 1973, Electron paramagnetic resonance study on iodine induced radicals of benzo(a)pyrene and other polycyclic hydrocarbons, *Biochemistry* 12:2649-2656.

Cavalieri, E., and Calvin, M., 1971, Molecular characteristics of some carcinogenic hydrocarbons, *Proc. Nat. Acad. Sci. USA* 68:1251-1253.

Falk, H.L., Kotin, P., Lee, S., and Nathan, A., 1962, Intermediary metabolism of benzo(a)pyrene in the rat, *J. Nat. Cancer Inst.* 28:699-724.

Fieser, L., and Hershberg, E., 1939, The orientation of 3,4-benzpyrene in substitution reactions, *J. Amer. Chem. Soc.* 61:1565-1574.

Forbes, W., and Robinson, J., 1968, Possible formation of an azuline-type radical obtained on heating 3,4-benzpyrene, *Nature* 217:550-551.

Fried, J., 1974, One-electron oxidation of polycyclic aromatics as a model for the metabolic activation of carcinogenic hydrocarbons, *in* "Chemical Carcinogenesis," Part A (P. Ts'o and J. DiPaolo, eds.), pp. 197-215, Marcel Dekker, New York.

Gelboin, H., 1969, A microsome-dependent binding of benzo(a)pyrene to DNA, *Cancer Res.* 29:1272-1276.

Goshman, L., and Heidelberger, C., 1967, Binding of tritium labeled polycyclic hydrocarbons to DNA of mouse skin, *Cancer Res.* 27:1678-1688.

Grover, P., and Sims, P., 1968, Enzyme-catalyzed reactions of polycyclic hydrocarbons with deoxyribonucleic acid and protein *in vitro*, *Biochem. J.* 110:159-160.

Hayakawa, T., and Udenfriend, S., 1972, A simple radioisotope assay for microsomal aryl hydroxylase, *Anal. Biochem.* 51:501-509.

Hoffmann, H., Lesko, S., and Ts'o, P., 1970, Chemical linkage of polycyclic hydrocarbons to DNA and polynucleotides in aqueous solution and in a buffer-ethanol solvent system, *Biochemistry* 9:2594-2604.

Holder, G., Yagi, H., Dansette, P., Jerina, D., Levin, W., Lu, A., and Conney, A., 1974, Effects of inducers and epoxide hydrase on the metabolism of benzo(a)pyrene by liver microsomes and a reconstituted system: analysis by high pressure liquid chromatography, *Proc. Nat. Acad. Sci. USA* 71:4356-4360.

Hutchinson, F., 1973, The lesions produced by ultraviolet light

in DNA containing 5-bromouracil, *Quart. Rev. Biophys.* 6:201-246.
Inomata, M., and Nagata, C., 1972, Photoinduced phenoxy radical of
    3,4-benzopyrene, *Gann* 63:119-130.
Ioki, Y., Kodama, M., Tagashira, Y., and Nagata, C., 1974, Oxygena-
    tion of benzo(a)pyrene in a model system using trifluoroacetic
    acid and hydrogen peroxide, *Gann* 65:379-380.
Jeftic, L., and Adams, R., 1970, Electrochemical oxidation pathways
    of benzo(a)pyrene, *J. Amer. Chem. Soc.* 92:1332-1337.
Lesko, S., Caspary, W., Lorentzen, R., and Ts'o, P., 1975, Enzymic
    formation of 6-oxo-benzo(a)pyrene radical in rat liver homo-
    genates from carcinogenic benzo(a)pyrene, *Biochemistry* 14:3978-
    3984.
Lesko, S., Ts'o, P., and Umans, R., 1969, Interaction of nucleic
    acids. V. Chemical linkage of 3,4-benzpyrene to deoxyribo-
    nucleic acid in aqueous solution, *Biochemistry* 8:2291-2298.
Lorentzen, R., Caspary, W., Lesko, S., and Ts'o, P., 1975, The
    autoxidation of 6-hydroxylbenzo(a)pyrene and 6-oxo-benzo(a)-
    pyrene radical, reactive metabolites of benzo(a)pyrene,
    Biochemistry 14:3970-3977.
Lyons, M., and Spence, J., 1960, Environmental free radicals, *Brit.*
    J. Cancer 14:703-708.
Maher, V., Lesko, S., Straat, P., and Ts'o, P., 1971, Mutagenic
    action, loss of transforming activity and inhibition of DNA
    template activity *in vitro* caused by the chemical linkage of
    carcinogenic polycyclic hydrocarbons to DNA, *J. Bacteriol.*
    108:202-212.
Marquardt, H., Sapozink, M., and Zedeck, M., 1974, Inhibition by
    cysteamine-HCl of oncogenesis induced by 7,12-dimethylbenz(a)-
    anthracene without affecting toxicity, *Cancer Res.* 34:3387-
    3390.
Massie, H., Samis, H., and Baird, M., 1972, The kinetics of degra-
    dation of DNA by H_2O_2, *Biochim. Biophys. Acta* 272:539-548.
Miller, J., 1970, Carcinogenesis by chemicals: an overview, G.H.A.
    Clowes Memorial Lecture, *Cancer Res.* 30:559-576.
Miller, J., and Miller, E., 1969, Metabolic activiation of carcino-
    genic aromatic and N-hydroxy-esterification and its relation-
    ship to ultimate carcinogens as electrophilic reactants, *in*
    "The Jerusalem Symposia on Quantum Chemistry and Biochemistry.
    Physiochemical Mechanisms of Carcinogenesis," Vol. I (E.
    Bergman and B. Pullman, eds.), pp. 237-261, Israel Academy of
    Sciences and Humanities, Jerusalem.
Mullinix, K., and Rosenkrantz, H., 1971, Effects of N-hydroxyurethan
    on viability and metabolism of *Escherichia coli, J. Bacteriol.*
    105:556-564.
Mullinix, K., Rosenkrantz, S., Carr, H., and Rosenkrantz, H., 1973,
    Reaction between DNA and N-hydroxyurethan, *Biochim. Biophys.*
    Acta 312:1-13.
Nagata, C., Inomata, M., Kodama, M., and Tagashira, Y., 1968,
    Electron spin resonance study on the interaction between the
    chemical carcinogens and tissue components. III. Determination

of the structure of the free radical produced either by stirring 3,4-benzopyrene with albumin or incubating it with liver
homogenates, *Gann* 59:289-298.

Nagata, C., Ioki, Y., Inomata, M., and Imamura, A., 1969, Electron
spin resonance study on the free radicals produced from carcinogenic aminonaphthaols and N-hydroxyaminonaphthalenes,
Gann 60:509-522.

Nagata, C., Kataoka, N., Imamura, A., Kawazoe, Y., and Chihara, G.,
1966, Electron spin resonance study on the free radical produced from 4-hydroxyaminoquinoline-1-oxide and its significance in carcinogenesis, *Gann* 57:323-335.

Nagata, C., Nakadate, M., Ioki, Y., and Imamura, A., 1972, Electron
spin resonance study on the free radical production from N-
methyl-N'-nitro-N-nitrosoguanidine, *Gann* 63:471-481.

Nagata, C., Tagashira, Y., and Kodama, M., 1974, Metabolic activation of benzo(a)pyrene: significance of the free radical, *in*
"Chemical Carcinogenesis," Part A (P. Ts'o and J. DiPaolo, eds.),
pp. 87-111, Marcel Dekker, New York.

Pascal, Y., Pochon, F., and Michelson, A., 1971, Free radical mediated linkage of carcinogenic hydrocarbons to polynucleotides,
Biochimie 53:365-368.

Prodi, G., Rocchi, P., and Grilli, S., 1970, Binding of 7,12-
dimethylbenz(a)anthracene and benzo(a)pyrene to nucleic acids
and proteins of organs of rats, *Cancer Res.* 30:1020-1023.

Rapaport, S., and Ts'o, P., 1966, Interaction of nucleic acids.
III. Chemical linkage of the carcinogen 3,4-benzpyrene to
DNA induced by X-ray irradiation, *Proc. Nat. Acad. Sci. USA*
55:381-387.

Rasmussen, R., and Wang, I., 1974, Dependence of specific metabolism
of benzo(a)pyrene on the inducer of hydroxylase activity,
Cancer Res. 34:2290-2295.

Rhaese, H., and Freese, E., 1968, Chemical analysis of DNA alterations. I. Base liberation and backbond breakage of DNA and
oligodeoxyadenylic acid induced by hydrogen peroxide and
hydroxylamine, *Biochim. Biophys. Acta* 155:476-490.

Rochlitz, J., 1967, Neue reaktionen der carcinogenen kohlenwasser-
stoffe. II, *Tetrahedron* 23:3043-3048.

Schechtman, L., Lesko, S., Lorentzen, R., and Ts'o, P., 1974, A
cellular system for the study of the chemical reactivity and
transforming ability of benzo(a)pyrene and its derivatives,
Proc. Amer. Assoc. Cancer Res. 15:66.

Scribner, J., Miller, J., and Miller, E., 1970, Nucleophilic substitution on carcinogenic N-acetoxy-N-arylacetamides, *Cancer
Res.* 30:1570-1579.

Scribner, J., and Naimy, W., 1973, Reactions of esters of N-hydroxy-
2-acetamidophenanthrene with cellular nucleophiles and the
formation of free radicals upon decomposition of N-acetoxy-
N-arylacetamides, *Cancer Res.* 33:1159-1164.

Selkirk, J., Croy, R., Roller, P., and Gelboin, H., 1974, High-
pressure liquid chromatographic analysis of benzo(a)pyrene

metabolism and covalent binding and the mechanism of action of 7,8-benzoflavone and 1,2-epoxy-3,3,3-trichloropropane, *Cancer Res.* 34:3474-3480.

Shamberger, R., Baughman, F., Kalchert, S., Willis, C., and Hoffman, G., 1973, Carcinogen-induced chromosomal breakage decreased by antioxidants, *Proc. Nat. Acad. Sci. USA* 70:1461-1463.

Szent-Gyorgyi, A., Isenberg, I., and Baird, S., 1960, On the electron donating properties of carcinogens, *Proc. Nat. Acad. Sci. USA* 46:1444-1449.

Ts'o, P., Caspary, W., Cohen, B., Leavitt, J., Lesko, S., Lorentzen, R., and Schechtman, L., 1974, Basic mechanisms in polycyclic hydrocarbon, *in* "Chemical Carcinogenesis," Part A (P. Ts'o and J. DiPaolo, eds.), pp. 113-147, Marcel Dekker, New York.

Ts'o, P., and Lu, P., 1964, Interaction of nucleic acids. II. Chemical linkage of the carcinogen 3,4-benzpyrene to DNA induced by photoirradiation, *Proc. Nat. Acad. Sci. USA* 51:272-280.

Wattenberg, L., 1973, Inhibition of chemical carcinogen-induced pulmonary neoplasia by butylated hydroxyanisole, *J. Nat. Cancer Inst.* 50:1541-1544.

Wilk, M., and Girke, W., 1969, Radical cations of carcinogenic alternant hydrocarbons, amines and azo dyes, and their reactions with nucleo bases, *in* "The Jerusalem Symposia on Quantum Chemistry and Biochemistry. Physiochemical Mechanisms of Carcinogenesis," Vol. I (E. Bergman and B. Pullman, eds.), pp. 91-105, Israel Academy of Sciences and Humanities, Jerusalem.

ROLE OF DNA REPAIR IN MUTATION AND CANCER PRODUCTION

James E. Trosko and Chia-Cheng Chang

Department of Human Development, College of Human

Medicine, Michigan State University, East Lansing,

Michigan 48824

1. INTRODUCTION

The somatic mutation theory of carcinogenesis was postulated long before there was knowledge of the molecular structure of genetic material, the physical, chemical and/or biological nature of carcinogens, or the nature of the interaction between cellular DNA and the carcinogenic agents (Boveri, 1929). The concept was originally introduced to account for two of the many observations of neoplastic growth; (a) the unlimited variety of tumor types, and (b) the fact that, after cell division, the daughter cells maintain their neoplastic properties.

Subsequently, new observations and advances in a variety of disciplines (e.g., virology, molecular biology, and cytology) have helped to spawn several other theories, as well as strengthen the mutation theory of carcinogenesis (Markert, 1968; Temin, 1971; Klein, 1972; Koller, 1972; Comings, 1973). Basically, the theories can be classified into those which assume that (a) certain types of mutations [on the gene, chromosome or chromosome set levels (Court-Brown, 1962)] increase the probability that the normal cell will transform into a neoplastic cell (Comings, 1973) and (b) the neoplastic state has nothing to do with the mutagenic alteration of the original cell's genome.

In recent years, rather than viewing these as conflicting theories, attempts have been made to unify these into a broader paradigm. Since the neoplastic state is a phenotypic expression of the genome of the tumor cells, it seems only reasonable to assume that the phenotypic expression of the tumor cells could be the result of the alteration of gene activity by either mutagenesis or gene repression or derepression. Viewed in this manner, various viral theories (provirus, oncogene, and protovirus) and the muta- tion theory of cancer are seen, not so much as mutually exclusive and conflicting theories, but as complementary components of a unified theory. Several recent attempts have tried to view car- cinogenesis in this way (Potter, 1972; Cleaver, 1973; Temin, 1974; Fischinger and Haapala, 1974; Trosko and Chu, 1975).

In this article, evidence for the theory of somatic mutations as one mechanism of carcinogenesis will be reviewed. The role of DNA repair as one mechanism responsible for mutagenesis will be examined. Moreover, we will examine the role of DNA adducts as initiators of errors in DNA replication and/or DNA repair, and of gene repression or derepression.

2.   THE NATURE AND NURTURE OF MUTAGENESIS AND CARCINOGENESIS

2.1.   Genetic and Environmental Predisposition

How often is the question "Is cancer inherited?" used? The fact that the question continues to be asked means the basic con- cept of the role of genes is not fully understood by those who asked the question. Every biological trait ("normal" or "abnormal") is the result of an interaction of genetic and environmental factors (nature and nurture, not nature versus nurture) (Lynch and Kaplan, 1974; Trosko and Chu, 1975). Cancer, as an "abnormal" trait, is

not inherited, but only the genetic material that sets the individual's range of potential reactions is (i.e., the qualitative
and quantitative nature of reactions to different environmental
influences).

Figure 1 illustrates the concept that the genetic information
locked in the DNA molecules of the zygote must constantly interact
with various environmental factors throughout development. Development of the individual will be "normal" or "abnormal" depending
upon the unique genetic-environmental interactions. DNA molecules,
which are able to code genetically for functional, structural or
metabolic needs of organisms, might be exposed to unfavorable
environmental factors which inhibit the genetic expression (e.g.,
mutagens, gene repressors, enzyme inhibitors, etc.). Alternatively,
at the other extreme, some genes are unable to code for normal
functioning structures or metabolic needs in the prevailing, or in
most known, environments.

In the following discussion of the nature and nurture model
of carcinogenesis, we will postulate that there are at least three
functional classes of genetic and environmental predisposing factors
to cancer--genes and environmental agents involved (a) in carcinogenic initiation; (b) in the replication, repair and read-out of
DNA; and (c) in tumor promotion. Within this conceptual framework,
understanding the influence of genetic variation in certain drug-
metabolizing enzymes on carcinogenic predispositions (Conney,
1973) might provide means to predict the consequences of environmental stimulators or inhibitors of normal drug-metabolizing enzymes
on carcinogenesis. Moreover, syndromes such as xeroderma pigmentosum, which genetically predisposes the individual to cancer in
"normal" environments of some chemicals and UV light (Cleaver, 1973),
could provide information on the mechanisms by which abnormal
environments (inhibitors of "error-free" DNA repair enzymes) predispose "normal" individuals to cancer. Genetic deficiencies in
immunological mechanisms, which also predispose individuals to
cancer (Penn, 1974), can conceivably aid in understanding how normal
biological processes, such as ageing, or some environmental conditions, such as immunological suppressant drugs, also predispose
individuals to cancer (Penn and Starzl, 1972).

2.2. Mutagenesis

Since the genetic information of mammals resides in a hierarchy
of DNA units [e.g., whole cells, haploid sets of chromosomes, single
chromosomes (possible operator and structural subunits), and nucleo-
tides], (Edwards, 1974), it ought to be clear that mechanisms which
cause change (mutation) and the rate by which this change occurs
(mutation rate) are specific to each level of the hierarchy. We
will restrict our discussion primarily to gene mutations. Gene

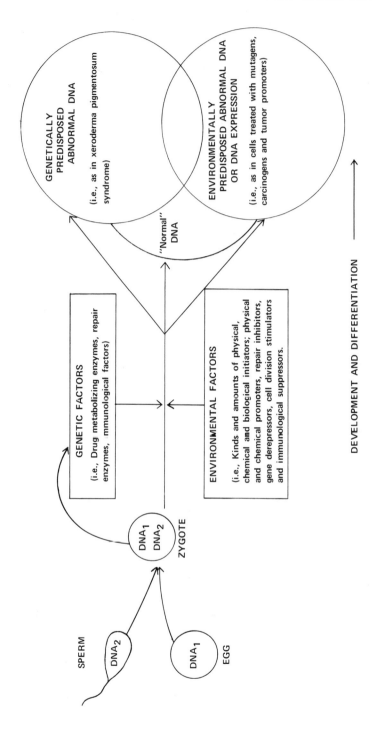

Fig. 1. The "nature and nurture" model for genetic and environmental predispositions to cancer (From Trosko and Chu, 1975).

mutation, by definition, is the alteration of information locked in the nucleotide composition and sequence in DNA. The types of mutation include substitution, insertion or deletion of nucleic acid bases, which lead either to a change of information (missense mutation) or to incomplete or no information (nonsense mutation). It is possible to account for the mutagenic effect of many chemical adducts on the basis of their *in vitro* reactions with DNA (Freese, 1963). Moreover, studies in bacteria indicate that mutagenesis is a complex enzymatic process, involving several genes and enzyme systems (Witkin, 1969; Kondo, 1974). In the case of mammals, complete analysis of the effect of physical or chemical treatments of DNA will require knowledge of the developmental influences on the metabolic response of an organism to the potential alterations of the DNA molecules, as well as its ability to respond enzymatically to such alterations.

2.3.   Carcinogenesis

Carcinogenesis, particularly skin tumor induction, has been considered as a process consisting of at least, two basic steps, *initiation* followed or accompanied by *promotion* (Berenblum, 1954; Boutwell, 1974). On the molecular level, carcinogenic initiation is thought to involve the stable alteration of DNA molecules by carcinogens (physical, chemical or viral-proviruses and/or proto-viruses) (Fig. 2). Most, if not all, carcinogens interact with DNA, directly or indirectly, and most physical and chemical carcinogens are mutagens (Miller and Miller, 1971; Ames *et al.*, 1973). Agents which in some manner enhance the process of tumor formation when administered after the initiating agent would be considered as promoters (Berenblum, 1954; Boutwell, 1974). In the strictest sense, promoters would not be carcinogenic by themselves.

Restricting, for the moment, our discussion of the molecular basis for the permanent alteration of DNA during the initiation phase of carcinogenesis by physical or chemical agents, initiation would be then viewed as the interaction of a carcinogen which forms an adduct with DNA. If the adduct to DNA leads to a structural alteration in the DNA molecule, then based on the bacterial model (Kondo, 1974; Witkin, 1975), the alteration could act as a signal (1) to repair the DNA to its original condition, (2) to replicate past an unexcised lesion, (3) to repair excision gaps in an error-prone manner, (4) to repair daughter-strand gaps opposite unexcised lesions via an "error-prone" postreplication repair synthesis, or (5) to repair via a recombinational repair system. If similar mechanisms are found in mammalian systems, then the observations that carcinogens are mutagens might be relevant to the somatic mutation hypothesis of carcinogenesis and that one mode of initiation would be through mutagenesis.

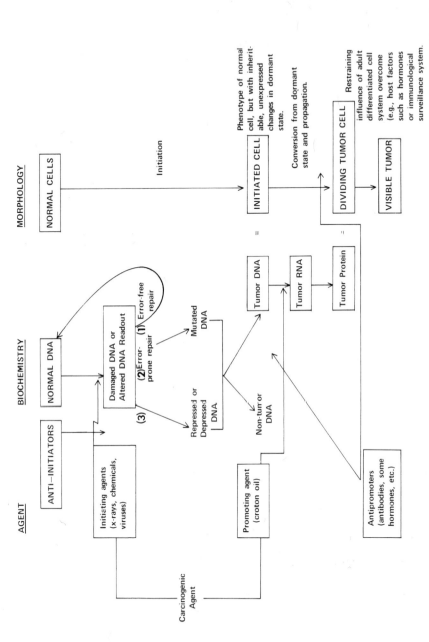

Fig. 2. A heuristic model of carcinogenesis. Carcinogenesis is conceived as a two-staged process involving initiation (altering DNA information) and promotion (proliferation of cells with altered DNA information). Genetic factors can influence carcinogenesis on the level of anti-initiation (drug metabolizing enzymes), on the level of DNA repair or replication, and on the level of anti-promoters (e.g., genetic deficiencies of the immuno-surveillance system) (modified after Boutwell, 1974) (From Trosko and Chu, 1975).

Since experimental mutagenesis by pure chemical agents was
first reported in 1944 by Auerbach and Robson, mechanisms of action
of chemical, as well as physical agents, are beginning to be understood as leading to "mutation fixation" or to heritable changes
in the genetic material (Drake, 1969). The physical and chemical
basis of mutation has enhanced the acceptance of the somatic mutation theory of carcinogenesis as an intellectually satisfying theory
for the mechanism of chemical carcinogenesis (Clayton, 1962).

If mutagenesis is one mechanism for carcinogenic initiation,
then the potential carcinogenicity of an agent is the result of a
direct reaction of the carcinogen with a biological target molecule,
probably DNA in most cases. The manner of illucidating this hypothesis may be approached by at least three types of studies: (1)
studies to explore the nature of interactions between the carcinogen and biological molecules; (2) studies of the DNA-carcinogen
complex on DNA replication and repair; and (3) studies using biological test systems for assaying the mutagenicity of carcinogens.

Considerable progress has been made in the past decade leading
to the observation that many chemical carcinogens are not active
as such but require metabolic conversion *in vivo* to active forms.
Furthermore, in a number of cases, positive correlations have been
obtained between the level of protein- or nucleic acid-carcinogen
interactions and the likelihood of tumor development. Mainly through
the work of J.A. Miller and E.C. Miller (see review, 1971), it was
concluded that most, if not all, chemical carcinogens either are
strong electrophilic (i.e., containing relatively-electron deficient forms) reactants as administered or are converted to potent
electrophilic reactants *in vivo*. This generalization not only
provides a unified view for the action of structurally diverse
chemical carcinogens, but also predicts some uniformity in the
sites on the cellular macromolecules susceptible to their attack.

As electrophiles or potential electrophiles, the carcinogens
have common nucleophilic targets, which include the guanine,
adenine, and cytosine bases and tertiary phosphate groups of the
nucleic acids, as well as methionine, cysteine, tyrosine, and
histidine in proteins. This broad spectrum of chemical reactivity
between electrophilic carcinogens and biological macromolecules
has been demonstrated both *in vitro* and *in vivo*. Nevertheless,
the knowledge of chemical reactions does not necessarily lead to
an understanding of the ensuing biological processes, such as mutation induction or tumor formation and development. At best, it
might be possible to establish some correlation between the chemical reactivity of a carcinogen, its carcinogenicity, and mutagenicity. It should be noted, however, that such a correlation cannot
be expected to be complete. As pointed out by Malling and Chu
(1974), the following factors could conceivably affect any attempted
correlation between carcinogenicity and mutagenicity of chemical

compounds. First, a number of carcinogens or procarcinogens are
almost water-insoluble and may have to be tested in systems both
remote from the site and different from the type of cells in which
tumors occur. Second, promoters may change intracellular or inter-
cellular conditions permitting preneoplastic cells to develop into
tumors, but may not be mutagenic by themselves. Third, many carcinogens require metabolic activation in the mammals to become
reactive electrophiles. Hence, tests without the proper activation may not reveal their mutagenicity. Finally, lack of demonstrable mutagenicity could also result from an efficient repair
of altered DNA.

Despite these uncertainties and limitations, it is remarkable
that considerable inroads have been made in the past several years
to establish the mutagenic properties of a host of known chemical
carcinogens. This is due largely to the development of biological
test systems for this purpose (Hollaender, 1971, 1973). The biological materials employed have ranged from bacteriophage, bacteria,
fungi, higher plants, insects, mammalian cells in tissue culture to
intact laboratory mammals. When structurally related chemical
potent carcinogens, weak carcinogens, and noncarcinogens were
tested in these systems, it became abundantly clear that there is
a positive correlation between carcinogenicity and mutagenicity of
most chemical compounds tested. Furthermore, these studies have
led to the conclusion that certain chemical carcinogens must be
metabolically activated before their biological function becomes
manifest (c.f., Miller and Miller, 1971; Malling and Chu, 1974).
Metabolic activation of "procarcinogens" or potential mutagens can
be achieved experimentally either (1) chemically by Udenfriend's
oxidation system, (2) metabolically by liver microsomes, or (3) in
host-mediated assays (Malling and Chu, 1974).

Several hypotheses have been advanced for the promotion phase
of carcinogenesis on the molecular, biochemical and cellular levels.
Cell proliferation and epidermal hyperplasia are among the more
conspicuous effects of promoters (Ryser, 1971), as well as induction
of inflammation and influx of leukocytes (Iversen and Eversen, 1962;
Frei and Stephens, 1968). However, not all agents which stimulate
cell proliferation have tumor-promoting activity (Raick, 1973).
Some promoters have been demonstrated to stimulate DNA, RNA, protein phospholipid and non-histone nuclear protein synthesis (Paul
and Hecker, 1969; Baird *et al.*, 1971; Dierks-Ventling and Jost,
1974). Raick (1973) has advanced a hypothesis, based on the
observation that promoter-treated cells appear to develop to a
less differentiated phenotype, that the tumor-promoter acts by
altering the phenotype expression of variant, but quiescent or
repressed, initiated cells which are present in the cell population.

On the molecular level, some tumor promoters have been shown

to interact with cell membranes (Sivak and Van Duuren, 1971).
Gaudin *et al.* (1972) have demonstrated that tumor promoters tested
in their studies can inhibit the unscheduled or excision repair
of carcinogen-induced DNA damage. They have advanced the hypothesis that the tumor promotion could be due to the direct inhibition of the excision repair process. Two important observations
which are not accounted for in their hypothesis are (1) the tumor-
promoting potential of many chemicals exists many months after
the application of short half-lived carcinogens (Boutwell, 1974),
and (2) most of the repair that is going to occur in any given
cell (far less than 100% in most mammalian cells tested) takes
place within 24 h (Regan *et al.*, 1968; Edenberg and Hanawalt, 1973).
Other serious objections to their observations, which will be
discussed later, have been recently made (Cleaver and Painter, 1975).

In summary, although it is by no means explicitly known what
the exact molecular events are which lead to the initiation and
promotion phases of carcinogenesis, it does seem that (1) since
most carcinogens, if not all, interact with DNA; and (2) since
many of these altered DNA molecules are substrates of various
types of DNA replication and repair enzymes, mutagenesis might
be one important mode of carcinogenic initiation (the other being
gene derepression). As will be seen later, tumor promotion might
be the mitotic stimulator of cells whose genes have been mutated
during the initiation phase, or whose genes have been either repressed or derepressed.

2.4. Genetic Basis for Mutagenesis and Carcinogenesis

The molecular mechanisms which lead to mutations at each of
the hierarchical genetic levels in mammals are poorly understood
at this time, particularly those at levels above the structural
gene level. It is clear from studies on organisms, such as bacteria,
maize, yeast, *Drosophila* and human beings, that there are genetic
factors which influence mutation rates and frequencies of gene
mutations, chromosome breaks, chromosome partitioning and replication (Green, 1973; Mohn and Wurgler, 1972).

A number of bacterial systems have been found which modify
damaged DNA in biologically significant ways so as to give us some
insight into the mutation and carcinogenic processes. For example,
(1) microorganisms separated by a single mutational step differ in
their radiation sensitivity (Hill, 1958; Witkin, 1947); (2) it is
also possible to demonstrate definite chemical changes in DNA after
doses of UV light, within the biological dose range, and to show
that the resulting photoproducts are important in producing certain biological effects associated with irradiation (Setlow and
Carrier, 1964); (3) furthermore, nonsensitive wild type organisms
are able to remove UV-produced lesions from their DNA and this

removal can permit the growth of the organism which would otherwise be inactivated (Boyce and Howard-Flanders, 1964; Setlow and
Carrier, 1964). Mutant strains for several of the different repair
enzymes found in bacteria have led to the concept of genetic control of "error-free" versus "error-prone" DNA repair mechanisms
(Witkin, 1969; Kondo, 1974).

In human beings, several clinical syndromes, among which are
xeroderma pigmentosum (XP), dyskeratosis congenita, Fanconi's
anemia, ataxia telangiectasia, Werner's, Bloom's, Chediak-Higashi,
and Down's syndromes, have genetic predispositions to cancer, as
well as to other specific syndrome anomalies. In the case of the
XP syndrome, which is characterized by hypersensitivity of the
skin to solar radiation and high incidence of multiple carcinomas,
the cells from these individuals, *in vitro*, are more sensitive to
UV radiation than are normal cells (Cleaver, 1970) and lack of
the ability to excise pyrimidine dimers (Cleaver and Trosko, 1970;
Setlow *et al.*, 1969). Fibroblast cells from patients with XP also
contain low levels of photoreactivating enzyme in comparison to
normal cells (Sutherland *et al.*, 1975). XP cells are also susceptible to chromosome breakage in adenovirus type 12 (Stich *et al.*,
1974), as well as to radiation-induced chromosome breaks (Parrington *et al.*, 1971).

Several hypotheses have been advanced to explain the mechanism
of carcinogenesis in XP individuals (1) increased mutation rates
(both point and chromosomal); (2) induction of oncogenic viruses
by low UV doses; and (3) increased malignant transformation of UV-
damaged cells by viruses (Cleaver, 1973). As pointed out by Cleaver,
these might not be mutually exclusive hypotheses. The defect of
excision repair in XP cells is similar to that in *uvr⁻ (hcr⁻)* bacterial mutants, which have elevated UV-induced mutation rates
(Witkin, 1969). V.M. Maher (personal communication) has observed
that UV radiation and chemical carcinogen-induced mutation frequencies of XP cells are higher than those found in normal fibroblasts.
Moreover, studies (Sasaki, 1973) with 4-nitroquinoline 1-oxide,
which induced non-repairable lesions in the DNA of XP cells, indicate that this chemical induces many chromosome aberrations in
XP cells. XP cells, treated with methylmethanesulfonate (MMS),
can repair the MMS-damaged DNA without manifesting significant
chromosome damage (Sasaki, 1973).

Sasaki and Tonomura (1973) have shown that cells from patients
with Fanconi's anemia are more susceptible to chromosome breakage
caused by DNA cross-linking agents than normal cells. Poon *et al.*
(1974) have reported that these cells from Fanconi's anemia patients,
who are characterized by a high incidence of neoplasms and high
frequence of spontaneous and chemically-induced chromosome breaks
in their cells, might have a defect in the exonuclease step in
excision repair.

It is well known that the spontaneous mutation rates differ greatly with the type of mutation and organism when rates are calculated per gene and per generation (per replication, cell division or sexual generation) (Propping, 1972; Neal, 1971). Since observed mutation rates depend on several factors: (1) the primary rate of damage or error formation; (2) the efficacy of replication and repair; and (3) the probability of detection of an altered phenotype (Drake, 1969), these heritable species specific spontaneous rates reflect, in large part, the extent to which many genes are involved in determining these rates.

In higher organisms, genes which influence the mutability of other genes were discovered by McClintock (1951) in maize and Demerec (1941) in *Drosophila*. Several "mutator" genes have been observed in human beings which predispose these individuals to a susceptibility to chromosomal breakage and rearrangement. As mentioned previously, recessive genes inherited in Fanconi's anemia, Bloom's syndrome, xeroderma pigmentosum and ataxia telengiectasia influenced the karotype of cells from these homozygous individuals (Passarge, 1972).

The addition of a single chromosome, such as the Down's syndrome trisomy, also produces chromosome instability in the affected individual. Down's syndrome cells are more susceptible to SV40 virus transformation (Young, 1971). When chromosomes from lymphocytes of normal and Down's syndrome individuals were compared prior to and after measles infection (Higurashi *et al.*, 1973), the number of breaks in Down's cells infected with the measles virus were significantly higher than that found in normal cells. *In vitro* susceptibility to chromosomal aberrations produced by ionizing radiation (Sasaki and Tonomura, 1969; Higurashi and Conen, 1973) and chemical carcinogens (O'Brien *et al.*, 1971) was also increased.

The molecular basis for the "mutator-influence" of certain genes and chromosomes in the cancer-prone human individuals is not yet understood for most of these syndromes. However, defects in DNA repair enzymes appear to be associated with XP, Hutchinson-Gilford (progeria), and Fanconi's anemia syndrome (Cleaver, 1969; Setlow *et al.*, 1969; Epstein *et al.*, 1973; Poon *et al.*, 1974). It is not known at present whether the lack of DNA repair enhances the carcinogenic process (1) by increasing the rate of gene mutations (of structural or regulator genes), some of which could influence the transformation of a normal cell to a cancer cell (Trosko and Chu, 1975), (2) by causing chromosome breaks which could also influence the transformation process (Comings, 1973), (3) by rendering the cell more susceptible to various viral modes of transformation (Fischinger and Haapala, 1974), or (4) by derepressing genes (Hart and Trosko, 1975). Along these lines, it is of interest to note that DeMars (1972) has shown that a fibroblast cell strain of a patient with Fanconi's anemia did not render any higher gene mutation frequencies at this hypoxanthine-guanine phosphoribosyltransferase (HG-PRT) locus.

If we assume mutagenesis in mammalian systems is similar to that process found in bacterial systems, we could predict that, along with certain DNA repair enzymes, enzymes involved in the initiation of DNA damage, prevention of DNA damage, as well as enzymes involved in the replication and segregation of DNA and chromosomes (Conney, 1973; Kondo, 1974; Kouri *et al.*, 1974; Miller and Miller, 1971; Trosko and Hart, 1975) will influence the mutation rates in mammals. There is a growing amount of evidence that there are many such genes (Lynch and Kaplan, 1974).

The work of the Miller's (1971) indicates that there are species and sex-influenced genes and enzymes which metabolize chemicals which can damage DNA molecules. Conney (1973) has observed that genetically influenced high and low levels of aryl hydrocarbon hydroxylase inducibility in human lymphocytes were correlated with high and low incidences of lung cancers in cigarette smokers (Kellermann *et al.*, 1973). Conney further hypothesized that genetic variation in this drug metabolizing enzyme will determine the level of DNA damage. Such genetic variation in this enzyme has been found in rats by Kouri (1974). It remains to be shown in these cases of genetically-altered metabolizing enzyme levels whether the mutation rates of the affected cells, *in vivo*, are different from other cells.

Heston (1974) has reviewed the topic of the "genetics of cancer" and has clearly demonstrated that many other genes could influence other mechanisms of carcinogenesis (e.g., viral induced carcinogenesis). In his review, genes in a wide variety of organisms (animals and plants, invertebrates and vertebrates, mammals and non-mammals) were predisposed to various forms of cancers when exposed to a wide range of known environmental agents (e.g., UV light, oncogenic viruses, proviruses, etc.).

These forementioned "genetic" syndromes dealing with drug metabolism, DNA repair, chromosome "mutability", as well as those associated with hormone imbalances and immunological deficiencies, indicate that the ultimate appearance of a tumor is the end result of a cell having escaped the many genetic regulatory mechanisms on the molecular, biochemical, cellular and physiological levels (Potter, 1973). Moreover, these syndromes strongly implicate mutagenesis as one mode of carcinogenesis.

3. DNA DAMAGE AND ITS REPAIR

3.1. Initiation of DNA Damage

Since there is ample evidence indicating that the nature of
the DNA lesion can determine the nature of the enzymatic mechanism(s)
responsible for the repair, it is important that we understand the
nature of the damage incurred in DNA molecules after organisms have
been exposed to various environmental mutagens and carcinogens.
For example, XP cells, which are unable to repair UV light-induced
pyrimidine dimers (Cleaver, 1969; Setlow and Regan, 1969; Cleaver
and Trosko, 1970) or N-acetoxy-2-acetylaminofluorene-induced DNA
damage (Setlow and Regan, 1972), or 4-nitroquinoline 1-oxide (Stich
et al., 1971) base damage in DNA, are apparently able to repair
X ray or N-methyl-N-nitro-N-nitrosoguanidine (MNNG)-induced single-
strand breaks (Cleaver, 1971). Fibroblast cells from patients with
the Hutchinson-Gilford (progeria) syndrome can repair UV-induced
DNA damage (Cleaver, 1970) but apparently are unable to repair
gamma-ray-induced DNA single-strand breaks (Epstein et al., 1973;
however, see Regan and Setlow, 1974).

In eukaryotic organisms, the role of DNA repair in mutagenesis
and carcinogenesis is influenced by many genetic and environmental
factors. In other words, the species, tissue, cell type, stage
of cell cycle, developmental stage and individual genetic variation will affect both the amount of damage and repair of DNA.
Genetic factors influencing detoxifying or metabolizing enzyme
activities will influence the level of initial chemical-induced
DNA damage, as well as determine both the types and rates of DNA
repair enzymes. Based on observations that high and low levels of
aryl hydrocarbon hydroxylase inducibility in human lymphocytes
were correlated with high and low incidences of lung cancer in
cigarette smokers (Kellermann et al., 1973), Conney (1973) hypothesized that genetic variation in this drug metabolizing enzyme
will determine the level of potential carcinogen-induced DNA damage.
Kouri et al. (1974) have shown that a genetic strain of mice which
has high inducibility of aryl hydrocarbon hydroxylase is significantly more sensitive to 3-methylcholanthrene-induced tumorigenesis
than a non-inducible strain. These studies, as well as those of
the Miller's (1971), indicate that many such genetic variations
could influence the initiation phase of mutagenesis and carcinogenesis by controlling the amount of DNA damage.

Conceptually, one ought to be able to increase or decrease
the ability of a potential mutagen or carcinogen to damage DNA by
environmentally inhibiting or stimulating drug metabolizing enzymes
or by adding agents which selectively compete with DNA as a substrate for these mutagens and carcinogens. It has been demonstrated that antioxidants, such as butylated hydroxyanisole, can

reduce the potential of a carcinogen to induce chromosome breaks (Shamberger *et al.*, 1973) and to induce tumor formation (Wattenberg, 1973). Although the molecular basis of the antimutagenic and anticarcinogenic properties of these compounds are not yet known, it has been implied that they act on an anti-initiation level by inducing drug metabolizing enzymes (Commings and Walton, 1973).

3.2. Repair of DNA Damage

The interaction of mutagens and most, if not all, carcinogens with DNA leads to alterations in the structure of the DNA molecule. If these alterations of structure lead to impairment of function, the cell must repair the lesion or suffer the consequences of impaired function. Lesions, such as those which have been identified and discussed in This Volume, are those which (1) are associated with altered bases, such as UV-induced pyrimidine dimers (Setlow and Setlow, 1972), X ray-induced thymine damage (Cerutti, 1974) or chemical-induced base damage, such as alkylated DNA (Scudiero and Strauss, 1974); (2) are identified as single- or double-strand breaks in the DNA helix (Lett and Sun, 1970; Corry and Cole, 1968); (3) lead to depurination of DNA (Verly *et al.*, 1974); (4) comprise DNA protein cross-links (Habazin and Han, 1970; Todd and Han, This Volume); and (5) form cross-links with the DNA molecules (Smith, This Volume).

Although a plethora of studies on the repair of some of these various lesions in mammalian cells exist (see reviews, Painter, 1974; Hart and Trosko, 1975) we can only speculate on the specific consequences of the repair or non-repair of each type of lesion on the initiation phase of carcinogenesis. "Excision" repair of damaged DNA has been measured via a variety of techniques in a number of mammalian systems (Rasmussen and Painter, 1964; Regan *et al.*, 1968; Regan and Setlow, 1974; Wilkins, 1973). It has yet to be demonstrated, directly, whether the "excision" repair mechanisms are "error-free" mechanisms as seems to be the case in bacterial systems (Witkin, 1969). Within limits of the techniques used, Lieberman and Poirier (1974) have shown that excision repair in normal human fibroblasts appears to be "error-free" on the chemical level. Moreover, Meltz and Painter (1973) and Lieberman and Poirier (1974) have shown many types of repetitive and unique sequences are repairable or partially repairable after carcinogen-induced damage. The observation that fibroblast cells from XP patients, which lack excision repair, have higher carcinogen-induced mutation frequencies at the HG-PRT locus (Maher, loc. cit.) is indirect evidence of the "error-free" nature of excision repair.

If one assumes that lesions, unrepaired via an "error-free" excision mechanism, could be responsible for the initiation phase of carcinogenesis, then there are several potential mechanisms which might give rise to either mutagenesis, gene derepression or viral transformation. The long-term binding of carcinogens to DNA (Goth and Rajewsky, 1974) might be responsible for errors in DNA replication (Sirover and Loeb, 1974). Alternatively, post replication repair of gaps formed in daughter strands opposite unexcised lesions (Lehmann, 1974) might lead to errors in gap-filling. At this time, since there is a challenge to the interpretation of the post replication repair phenomenon (Painter, 1974), the understanding of the mutation process will probably depend on the use of post replication repair mutants. The observation that certain variant strains of XP fibroblasts might be "post replication" repair mutants could aid in this task (Lehmann et al., 1975).

The repair of DNA single-strand breaks, in and of itself, appears not to be correlated with carcinogen-induced biological damage (Peterson et al., 1974). However, the presence of single-strand breaks, as a result of no repair or of incomplete repair, might provide openings for virus insertion (Stich et al., 1971), as well as initiate error-prone repair mechanisms.

Since the use of the photoreactivation phenomenon has provided valuable insights to the mutagenic process in bacteria (Setlow, 1966), evidence obtained by using the same approach in eukaryotic systems, appears to be consistent with the hypothesis that mutagenesis does play a role in carcinogenesis. With the demonstration of the photoreactivating enzyme activity in many eukaryotic systems (Cook, 1970), including certain cells from higher mammals and human beings (Sutherland et al., 1975), it might be possible to characterize the role of pyrimidine dimers and other adducts in UV-induced mutagenesis and carcinogenesis. Hart and Setlow (1974) have demonstrated that UV-induced neoplastic transformation of cells from the fish, Poecilia formosa, could be reduced by post treatment with photoreactivating (PR) light. Their interpretation of PR-reduction of tumor formation in fish is based on the in situ photomonomerization of UV-induced pyrimidine dimers. By inference, the disappearance of the pyrimidine dimers removes potential lesions leading to gene or chromosomal mutations (or viral insertion or activation).

If DNA repair mechanisms lead to chromosome breaks and rejoining (Strauss et al., 1972; Wolff et al., 1974) and if chromosome breaks also contribute to the transformation process (Comings, 1973), then the use of the photoreactivation phenomenon to study the mechanism of transformation is possible. Since there is reason to believe that lesions in DNA molecules can lead to chromosome aberrations (Kilhman, 1971), one would expect that both the repair or the interference of the repair of these lesions would modify both the frequency of chromosome aberrations and the transformation frequencies. For example, Griggs and Bender (1973) have shown that Xenopus cells, which have the ability to photoreactivate UV-induced pyrimidine dimers, have lower UV-induced chromatid-type aberrations after

PR-treatment. Moreover, Kato (1974) has shown that the UV-induced sister chromatid exchanges in rat kangaroo cells were significantly reduced when the cells were post treated with photoreactivating light.

Since the only UV-induced lesion in DNA that is known to be reversible by photoreactivation is the pyrimidine dimer, it seems reasonable to assume that the lesion signals a particular repair mechanism which could lead to chromosome aberrations. Evidence which tends to support that idea has been reported by Wolff *et al.* (1974). They were able to show that UV-induced sister chromatid exchanges appear to be caused only by persistent lesions (presumably including pyrimidine dimers) which pass through the S phase of the cell cycle. This observation, similar to the one on colony-formation in UV-irradiated mouse L cells (Domon and Rauth, 1969), was interpreted as being the result of non-excised lesions in template DNA affecting damage in newly synthesized DNA which is repaired via a post replication mechanism. With observations which have been interpreted as an inducible repair system in bacteria, Witkin (1975) has introduced a caution to the interpretation of the photoreversibility of induced mutations. In essence, she points out that the UV-induced pyrimidine dimer might be necessary for the induction of the mutagenic repair system, and therefore for all mutagenesis resulting from its error-prone activity, whatever the nature of the lesions causing the error at the actual site of the mutation. Whether or not an inducible DNA repair enzyme(s) is triggered by certain DNA lesions in mammalian cells, has yet to be determined. However, observations made by Lytle *et al.* (1974) on UV-enhanced reactivation of *Herpes* virus in human tumor cells might be consistent with the hypothesis that an inducible repair enzyme can be found in certain mammalian cells. The observation that the fractionation of UV doses, when part or all of the S-phase occurs between fractions, leads to increased cell survival in some mammalian cells (Todd *et al.*, 1969; Humphrey *et al.*, 1970), although subject to other interpretations, would be consistent with an inducible post-replication repair hypothesis.

4. FACTORS INFLUENCING DNA REPAIR

4.1. Developmental Factors

4.1.1. *Chromatin*. In higher organisms which depend on differential gene action for the production of specialized cells, the nuclear protein-DNA complexes, which influence DNA transcription and DNA replication during the cell cycle and development, appear to influence the nature of DNA repair and, by inference, mutagenesis and carcinogenesis. Since the eukaryotic chromosome is distinguished from the bacterial chromosome by the nuclear protein complexes it

contains (e.g., histones and acidic "residual" proteins), and since
it is known that, at any given moment in time, the chromosome has
two distinct but variable regions (euchromatic and heterochromatic
regions), it stands to reason that the initiation of DNA damage
and the repair of that damage might be different in these regions.
Hewish and Burgoyne (1973) have shown that nuclear proteins can
regulate the sites of endonuclease activity in rat liver nuclei.
Silverman and Mirsky (1973) have shown that nuclear proteins can
limit the accessibility of DNA polymerase. Wilkins and Hart (1974)
have shown directly that chromatin does inhibit excision repair in
human cells. The biological consequences of differential production and repair of lesions in euchromatic and heterochromatic regions
of the chromosomes with mutagens on the mutagenic and carcinogenic
processes will have to be tested.

    4.1.2. *Differentiation and DNA Repair.* Since it is assumed
that the process of differentiation involves not only the appearance
of new structures and functions in the developing eukaryote, but
also the physical repression and derepression of DNA via nuclear
protein mediators, DNA repair studies in differentiating systems
might give us a picture of the possible complex relationship between
DNA repair and mutagenesis. For example, Darzynkiewicz (1971) has
shown that phytohemagglutinin stimulation of lymphocytes, which
involves the stimulation of RNA and DNA synthesis and cell division, increased the rate of unscheduled DNA repair synthesis.
Darzynkiewicz and Chelmicha-Szorc (1972) have shown that during
erythropiesis, repression of DNA synthesis in red blood cells is
accompanied by a depression of unscheduled DNA synthesis. When
cells of dormant and active erythrocytes are fused both semiconservative DNA synthesis and unscheduled DNA repair synthesis occurs.
Along these same lines, Gledhill and Darzynkiewicz (1973) have
demonstrated unscheduled DNA repair synthesis decreases as cells
progress through spermatogenesis in rats.

    Hahn and his coworkers (1971) and Stockdale (1971) demonstrated
quantitative changes in unscheduled DNA repair synthesis in rat and
chick embryo muscle cells, respectively. As the cells differentiate
from the myeloblast to fully developed muscle fibers, there was a
reduction (up to 50% of the nondifferentiated levels) in unscheduled
DNA synthesis. Since cancer cells are characterized by a marked
change in the state of differentiation from the tissue of origin,
one might predict an alteration of DNA repair capacities to be
found in these cells. Huang *et al.* (1972) observed that cells
from patients suffering with chronic lymphocytic leukemia have
increased excision repair compared to lymphocytes from normal
patients. Satoh and Yamamoto (1972) have observed that HeLa cells
carrying Sendai virus were more resistant than HeLa cells to several
chemical carcinogens, and they interpreted their data as indicating
that Sendai-carrying HeLa cells have more effective, nonexcision
type of DNA repair. Lytle *et al.* (1974) also showed that UV

reactivation of UV-irradiated *Herpes* virus occurred in a human tumor
cell line (HeLa) and its Sendai virus-carrier culture, HeLa (HVJ),
but not in a nontransformed embryonic lung culture. Moreover,
Hellman *et al.* (1974) have demonstrated UV reactivation in rat
mammary tumor cells but not in rat embryo cultures. It appears, in
these limited cases at least, that the differentiation or transformation state of a cell influences the DNA repair capacity. If
certain DNA repair enzymes influence mutation rates, then experiments to test the effect of differentiation and mutagenesis will
have to be performed.

4.2.   Development, DNA Repair and Ageing

If DNA repair and somatic mutagenesis are related, then developmental influences of DNA repair would be expected to modify the
somatic mutation rates. Consequently, if somatic mutagenesis is
responsible for some carcinogenic and ageing events, then we would
expect a corresponding effect of development on these levels.
Development, in effect, could be interpreted as "programming" a
cell's senescence and eventual "self-destruction".

Since "chromatization" of DNA on the molecular level is somehow responsible for cellular and tissue differentiation during
development (Stein *et al.*, 1974), the forementioned observations
would indicate that normal development does influence DNA repair.
To illustrate this general phenomenon, repair studies performed on
embryonic and established cells in culture suggest that certain
repair enzyme activities are modified either by gene inactivation
(and activation) or by enzyme modification. The first attempt to
detect excision repair in rodent cells (Trosko *et al.*, 1965;
Klimek, 1966; Steward and Humphrey, 1966; Horikawa *et al.*, 1968)
suggested very little, if any, excision repair in Chinese hamster,
mouse L and other rodent cells. These studies were performed on
transformed cells grown *in vitro*. Ruth Ben-Ishai (1974) reported
excision repair in mouse embryo cells and its subsequent repression
in established mouse cell lines. Moreover, although excision repair
could be detected in early passages of these primary cell lines
from mouse embryos, excision repair gradually disappeared within a
few later passages. No excision of DNA damage could be detected
in early passages if primary cells were derived from "old" embryos.
Hart *et al.* (1975) have noticed a similar phenomenon in the long-
lived mouse, *P. leucopus*; however the degree of repression of
excision repair which occurs at 19 days post conception is less
severe.

Goldstein (1971) has observed that very late-passage human
fibroblasts had a slightly reduced amount of unscheduled DNA
synthesis than did early or intermediate passage cells. Painter
et al. (1973) also observed a slight decrease of repair replication

in late passage WI-38 cells. Hart and Setlow (1974) have recently demonstrated an interesting correlation between the initial rate and the maximum level of unscheduled DNA synthesis in several types of fibroblasts *in vitro* and the life-span of the species. They offered a hypothesis which states that different species have more or less efficient repair mechanisms which excise lesions from DNA. As a given individual of a certain species accumulates more damage per unit DNA, they speculate that there would be a rapid deterioration of the fidelity of transcription and translation which, could, together with other molecular, cellular and physiological factors, account for the shortened life-span in organisms which have lower levels of excision repair. Consistant with this hypothesis, Hart *et al*. (1975) have also observed that in two similar species, *Mus musculus* and *Peromycus leucopus*, with different life-spans, the longer-lived species demonstrated greater excision repair of UV-induced damage.

A series of experiments have been reported which relate to the accumulation of damage in DNA of older cells. Price *et al*. (1971) and Modak and Price (1971) have observed that old tissues of mice acted as better primers for DNA synthesis than young tissues. The observations were interpreted as the result of DNA from old cells having larger numbers of strand breaks which acted as initiation sites than DNA from younger cells. Karran and Ormerod (1973) have reported that DNA of young red cells had fewer alkali-labile bonds (single-strand breaks) than DNA from old ones. Furthermore, old rat muscle cells did not repair single-strand breaks as young ones. However, Wheeler and Lett (1972) and Wheeler *et al*. (1973) have shown that in unreplaced, non-dividing cells such as rabbit retinal and dog neuronal cells, ionizing radiation-induced DNA breaks were repaired as well as in fibroblast cells.

It has been reported that fibroblasts from individuals suffering from Hutchinson-Gilford syndrome (progeria or premature ageing) appear to be defective in the ability to rejoin DNA strands, but were able to perform normal repair replication after UV irradiation (Epstein *et al*., 1973). The mechanism by which the non-repair of DNA manifests itself in cellular, physiological or organism ageing (e.g., increased mutation rates) will have to be determined.

To put all of these observations into another perspective, a speculative hypothesis linking DNA repair, mutagenesis, carcinogenesis and ageing is proposed. First, the eukaryotic chromosome can be functionally viewed as containing three units (Fig. 3): (1) those derepressed regions being expressed or transcribed; (2) those repressed regions capable of being derepressed in an adaptive response of the cell to some stimulus; and (3) those repressed regions of the chromosome that, in a particular cell type will never, under normal conditions, be transcribed. Since there is

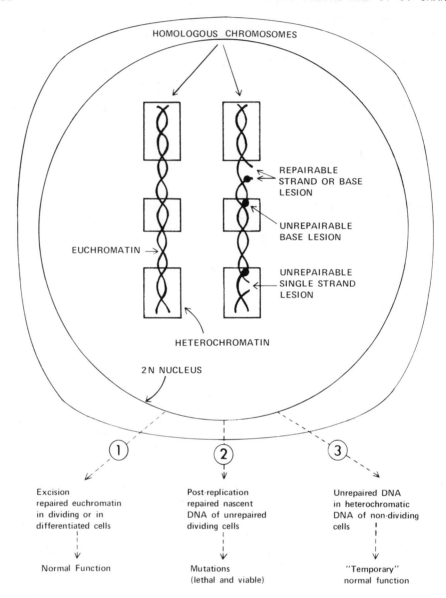

Fig. 3. Diagrammatic representation of the speculated role of chromosomal protein on differential damage and repair in the DNA of eukaryotic chromosomes (From Trosko and Chu, 1975).

evidence that chromosomal proteins can inhibit repair (Wilkins and Hart, 1974) and the phytohemagglutinin-stimulation (presumably causing derepression) enhances repair (Darzynkiewicz, 1971), one would surmise that the DNA in the derepressed regions (region 1) might be readily accessible to the repair enzymes while the DNA in region 2 would be less accessible but eventually repairable. The permanently repressed regions might be completely inaccessible to the repair enzymes and it is here that damaged DNA may persist or even accumulate. A model for ageing based on the differential repair of damaged DNA has been proposed by Yielding (1974). Support for such a hypothesis can be inferred from the work of Hart and Setlow (1974). There is also evidence that both UV and X ray-induced chromosome breaks in human chromosomes are not randomly dispersed throughout the chromosomes (Holmberg and Jonasson, 1973; Roman and Bobrow, 1973). If X ray-induced DNA breaks are responsible for chromsome breaks, then differential repair, rather than differential damage apparently would be responsible (Lett and Sun, 1970). One possible interpretation is that these lesions are inaccessible to repair.

Hart *et al.* (1975) have postulated that, together with the ability of an organism to maintain the genetic fidelity via DNA repair systems, the redundancy of genetic information for vital functions within the genome will contribute to the rate modifying factors in the ageing process. They further postulate that the unrepaired or incorrectly repaired DNA damage can be reflected in (1) transcription of erroneous RNA; (2) synthesis of non-functional enzymes; (3) cessation of transcription; or (4) alteration of gene expression (gene repression or derepression).

In any given non-dividing cell, only those regions of DNA which are responsible for providing information to maintain the development and metabolic state of that cell would be repaired by a relatively error-free type repair enzyme. Many of the lesions in the repressed regions, if not repaired, will not interfere with the functioning of this non-dividing cell. Following treatment with mutagenic agents, different cell types with quantitatively different excision repair capacities (Bootsma *et al.*, 1970; Setlow *et al.*, 1972) repair the DNA accessible to repair enzymes to different extents. However, no matter how high a cell's repair capacity, unrepaired lesions will still exist in chromatin inaccessible to repair enzymes. Upon stimulation of cell division, which might occur minutes or months after initiation of damage, DNA synthesis and concomitant derepression in DNA are triggered, where upon nascent DNA is made off of an unrepaired or incompletely repaired template. One would predict that mutagenic and carcinogenic frequencies would be higher in cells that enter DNA synthesis shortly after DNA damage than those that have more time to repair damage. Such evidence does exist (Hennings *et al.*, 1973). Nascent DNA would be made with gaps which might subsequently be repaired by an error-prone gap-filling process misnamed post replication repair. In this context, repair only means that the gap was filled, for the cell is certainly not repaired or rendered normal. The errors produced (e.g., point mutations or chromosome aberrations) could result in either no adverse effect on the cell, death or a mutated expression that could, among other things, ultimately give rise to a cancer or senescence of a cell.

Probably more than any factor which distinguishes mutagenesis in mammalian systems from lower organisms, and that which probably links DNA repair, mutagenesis and ageing, the influence of developmental differentiation processes, which could cause differential repair, on mutation frequencies is paramount. Clearly, if mutations can result in the repair of damage in rarely dividing, or non-dividing cells, these could contribute to the abnormal functioning of the cell.

4.3. Environmental Factors

It is intuitively obvious that environmental factors influence mutagenesis and carcinogenesis (Harris, 1970). The specific mechanisms by which each environmental factor acts with various genetic elements in mammalian cells have not yet been delineated. Along with the genetic tools to measure DNA repair mechanisms and their possible relationship to mutagenesis, we can utilize the fact that genetic information, in order to be functional, must be modulated by proper environmental factors (in this case, either in the expression of the gene, in the synthesis or in the functioning of DNA repair enzymes). If we assume for the moment that DNA repair is responsible for some of the mutation fixation in eukaryotic cells, it should be obvious that environmental agents which cause the initiation and repair of DNA damage, as well as those which stimulate or inhibit drug metabolizing and DNA repair enzymes, are those which influence mutagenesis and, by inference, carcinogenesis. One can study the influence of DNA repair mechanisms on mutagenesis by using environmental means. By using as biological endpoints, mutations (point, chromosome aberrations, etc.), cell survival and potentially-mutation related phenomena (ageing or cancer), a variety of external conditions or chemicals which sensitize or act synergistically with known mutagens would be candidates for potential inhibitors of DNA repair or DNA replication mechanisms. Alternatively, chemicals suspected or known to inhibit enzymatic functions needed for DNA repair or replication (e.g., endonuclease or DNA polymerase inhibitors) should be examined for the mutation-modifying potential.

Caffeine and butylated hydroxytoluene, which have been shown to have anti-tumor activities under certain conditions, as well as phorbol esters and 17-β-estradiol, which are known tumor promoters, are known to influence, in one fashion or another, the level of DNA damage, its repair, or its expression in mammalian systems.

Caffeine has been known to increase the killing of UV-irradiated bacteria and to modify the frequency of mutations recovered (Witkin, 1969). The mechanism of caffeine sensitization to UV damage in bacteria has been attributed to the inhibition of an "error-free" excision repair of pyrimidine dimers (Lumb et al., 1968), and the forced "error-prone" repair of the unexcised pyrimidine dimers. In mutagen-treated mouse L and Chinese hamster cells, but not human cells, caffeine decreases the colony-forming ability (Kihlman et al., 1973; Walker and Reid, 1971; Wilkinson, Kiefer and Nias, 1970). Kihlman et al. (1973) have demonstrated the potentiating effect of post-treatment of caffeine on chromosome aberrations induced by UV radiation and chemical mutagens in plants and several mammalian cells. However, caffeine does not inhibit excision repair, unscheduled DNA synthesis or repair replication (Regan et al., 1968; Cleaver, 1969), but does inhibit a post replication type of repair in several non-human mammalian cell lines (Cleaver and Thomas, 1969; Lehmann, 1972; Trosko and Chu, 1973) and in some XP fibroblast cells (Lehmann, 1975).

Caffeine is ineffective in the induction of auxotrophic mutants in Chinese hamster cells (Kao and Puck, 1969); although it can induce chromsome aberrations in mammalian cells at high concentrations (Kuhlmann et al., 1968). Trosko and Chu (1973) have found that a non-toxic concentration of caffeine lowers the frequency of forward mutations to 8-azaguanine resistance in UV-irradiated Chinese hamster cells under the same conditions which inhibit post replication repair. Arlett and Harcourt (1972), using a similar protocol, found that caffeine reduced the UV-induced mutation frequency only if it was present during the entire post-irradiation period. Roberts and Sturrock (1973), using N-methyl-N-nitrosourea to initiate DNA damage have, however, found that although caffeine potentiates the loss of colony-forming ability, it raises, rather than lowers, the mutation frequency of the survivors. They also interpret their results as indicating that caffeine inhibits a post replication repair mechanism. Although at first glance, both results and inferred mechanisms seem contradictory (Fox, 1974), it might be that these two mutagens induce lesions which are repaired by different excision repair mechanisms such as those described by Regan and Setlow (1974).

To emphasize the possible relationship between DNA repair and biological consequences (e.g., chromosome aberrations, point mutations and carcinogenesis), the observations that caffeine inhibits the post replication repair of UV damage but not excision repair in rodent cells, and that it lowered UV-induced mutation frequencies, allow one to predict that caffeine would act as an anticarcinogen in rodents, if (1) post replication repair is "error-prone" and (2) mutagenesis is responsible for some carcinogenic events. Recently, Zajdela and Latarjet (1973), and Rothwell (1974) have shown that caffeine post treatment reduces the frequency of

UV-induced skin tumors in mice. However, since caffeine has many
effects on the cell [e.g., inhibits cyclic AMP phosphodiesterase
(Sutherland and Rall, 1958), membrane permeability (Weber, 1968)
and induces G_1 arrest in exponentially growing cells (Walters
et al., 1974)], it is quite fortuitous at this time to suggest
that caffeine acts only at the DNA repair level.

Conceptually, it should be possible to increase or decrease
the ability of a potential mutagen to damage DNA by environmentally
inhibiting or stimulating drug metabolizing enzymes or by adding
agents which selectively compete with DNA as a substrate for these
mutagens. It has been demonstrated that anti-oxidants such as
butylated hydroxytoluene and butylated hydroxyanisole can reduce
the potential of mutagens and carcinogens to induce chromosome
breaks (Shamberger et al., 1973), and to induce tumor-formation
(Wattenberg, 1973).

Although the molecular bases of the anti-mutagenic and anti-
carcinogenic properties of these compounds are not yet known, it
has been implied that they act by inducing drug-metabolizing enzymes
which prevent damage to DNA molecules (Commings and Walton, 1973).
If the anti-carcinogenic potential of butylated hydroxytoluene
resides in its ability to prevent induced gene mutations, it is
tempting to speculate that its mechanism of action might reside
in its ability to prevent DNA damage. Moreover, if somatic mutations also contribute to the ageing process (Failla, 1958;
Szilard, 1959; Trosko and Chu, 1975; Sinex, 1974; Trosko and Hart,
1975), one would expect butylated hydroxytoluene to protect against
induced "premature" ageing. It would appear that the anti-oxidant
properties of compounds, such as butylated hydroxytoluene, which
can help prolong the mean life span of mice by as much as 45%
(Comfort and Youhotsky-Gore, 1971; Kohn, 1971) are consistent with
the free radical theory of ageing in mammals (Gordon, 1974).

Another class of chemicals, the tumor promoters, also appears
to modify the biological consequences of known carcinogens. For
example, croton oil constituents, such as phorbol myristate acetate,
and hormones, such as 17-β-estradiol, which are powerful tumor
promoters, have been shown to inhibit carcinogen induced unscheduled
DNA synthesis (Gaudin et al., 1972). Since environmental inhibition of excision repair of DNA should, in principle, lead to identical consequences of genetic inhibition of DNA repair, one would
predict that, based on observed higher mutation frequencies found
in excision-deficient E. coli mutants or higher cancer predispositions in XP individuals, inhibition of excision repair by phorbol
ester and 17-β-estradiol in mammalian cells would lead to higher
frequencies of induced mutations.

Cleaver and Painter (1975) have challenged the hypothesis of
Gaudin et al. (1972) that the mechanism of co-carcinogenesis is

dependent on the ability of a tumor promoter to inhibit excision repair of DNA damage. They have demonstrated that, at the concentrations of co-carcinogens previously reported to inhibit excision repair of DNA, there was as much, or more, inhibition to normal DNA synthesis. The inference drawn from their work is that, since there was no evidence that co-carcinogens are specific inhibitors to DNA repair, these compounds probably do not act as tumor promoters via their ability to cause DNA repair errors. Chang *et al.* (1975) have shown that, although phorbol myristate acetate does seem to enhance the frequency of UV-induced mutations at relatively high UV doses, 17-β-estradiol does not appear to do so. Although the evidence at present is limited, it does seem safe to conclude that there might be various mechanisms of tumor promotion. As previously mentioned, since many, if not all tumor promoters, under particular conditions, seem to stimulate DNA and nucleoprotein synthesis via different mechanisms *in vivo*, one might speculate that phorbol esters and 17-β-estradiol act as tumor promoters on previous initiated cells by derepressing mutated genes controlling cell division, or by forcing error-prone replication or repair of persistent lesions in repressed regions of DNA of quiescent cells.

5. GENE MODULATION IN PHENOTYPIC EXPRESSION AND CARCINOGENESIS

Stable heritable phenotypic changes in animal cells can arise from mutational events such as errors in DNA repair and replication, as well as from epigenetic processes which underlie cellular differentiation. In animal somatic cell cultures, mutant cells, which exhibit altered gene products, have been well characterized (Albrecht *et al.*, 1972; Chan *et al.*, 1972; Secher *et al.*, 1973; Beaudet *et al.*, 1973; Thompson *et al.*, 1973; Sharp *et al.*, 1973; Chasin *et al.*, 1974). Equally clear is the existence of phenotypic changes caused by epigenetic processes. These types of changes can be detected from the induction (Schneider and Weiss, 1971) or extinction (Darlington *et al.*, 1974) of certain gene products in hybrids formed between two different types of cells. They are also inferred from the failure to find expected differences in mutation rates at different ploidy levels of frog or Chinese hamster cells (Harris, 1973; Mezger-Freed, 1974).

In the cancer-prone genetic syndromes of Bloom's, Down's, Fanconi's and ataxia-telangiectasia, there are high frequencies of chromosomal breakage (German, 1965; Hecht, 1966; Sasaki and Nonomura, 1973; Higurashi and Conen, 1973; Chagant *et al.*, 1974). Chromosome breaks and rearrangements are capable of inducing a "position effect". The influence of a specific type of position effect on the expression of a specific gene has been speculated to induce the expression of certain types of cancer (Comings, 1973).

The sorting out of true genetic mutants from other stable phenotypic changes is of practical importance in detecting various environmental mutagens and in the use of mutagenesis as a means to study gene regulation and carcinogenesis. At present, three different approaches have been exploited to detect or differentiate phenotypically-identical variants:

a) Cell fusion:
        The existing cellular control system may be interrupted by virus-mediated cell fusion which introduces new regulatory elements, as well as chromosome breaks and rearrangements (Sun *et al.*, 1974). The re-expression of rat and mouse genes for hypoxanthine: guanine phosphoribosyltransferase was detected in human-rat and mouse-chick hybrids (Croce *et al.*, 1973; Bakay *et al.*, 1973). The deficiency of isocitrate dehydrogenase in Chinese hamster galactose-negative mutants can also be corrected by a human gene(s) located on chromosome A-2 in human-hamster hybrid cells (Sun *et al.*, 1975). Other regulatory elements were also found in cell hybrids (Kao and Puck, 1972; Shows and Ruddle, 1968).

b) Karyotypic stability and mutagenic specificity:
        Two classes of 6-thioguanine resistant mutants are differentiated by several criteria. Those with no demonstratable qualitative difference in gene products are associated with karyotypic disturbance, high reversion rates, low plating efficiency and non-inducibility by mutagenic treatment (Terz, 1974). The reverse characteristics are true for the second class of mutants.

c) Combination of mutation systems:
        The phenotypic expression of 6-thioguanine resistance in mammalian cells can conceivably result from mutations at the structural gene level or from the non-expression of the hypoxanthine-guanine phosphoribosyltransferase gene. Therefore, both mutagens and agents which specifically cause gene repressions are effectively in inducing 6-thioguanine resistant phenotypes. The phenotype of ouabain resistance is due to the alteration of the structural gene for the Na^+/K^+ ATPase or its related protein component on the membrane. Since the expression of the gene is required for cell survival and the non-expression of the gene does not contribute to ouabain resistance, the frequency of ouabain resistant mutants can conceivably be enhanced by a mutagen but not by agents which inactivate the expression of the gene (Fig. 4).

Chang *et al.* (1975) have tested the effect of tumor promoters on mutations at both the HG-PRT and Na^+/K^+ ATPase loci in cultured

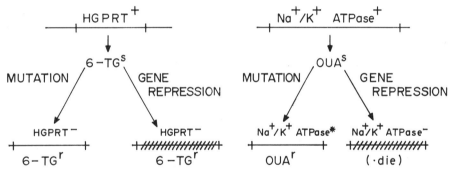

Fig. 4. Scheme illustrating the potential use of the combination of mutation assay systems to differentiate between structural
gene mutations and gene modulation. Mutagens which cause the defect
or absence of the activity of HG-PRT (hypoxanthine: guanine phosphoribosyltransferase) would increase 6-thioguanine resistant
mutants. Mutagens can also increase ouabain resistant mutants if
certain types of mutations are induced, namely those which influence conformation or the active site for ouabain-building, but
not the enzymatic activity of Na^+/K^+ ATPase. Compounds which cause
gene repression would result in the non-expression of the gene
for HG-PRT and therefore increase the frequency of 6-thioguanine
resistant phenotypes. Gene repression, however, would not modify
the frequency of cells resistant to ouabain, since the non-expression of the gene would cause the death of the cell.

Chinese hamster cells. The results (Table 1) indicate that the mutagen, UV light, did increase mutation frequencies at both loci.
Treatment with phorbol myristate acetate increased the recovery of
6-thioguanine resistant colonies but not ouabain resistant colonies.
The data seem to indicate that phorbol myristate acetate induced
gene repression, rather than causing structural gene mutations.
The results from these studies also indicated that non-cytotoxic
levels of phorbol ester (1 μg/ml) slightly inhibited unscheduled
DNA synthesis and also significantly increased the frequency of
UV-induced mutations. Although this observation is consistent
with the concept of an error-free versus an error-prone DNA repair
mechanism, we do not believe that the tumor promoter potential
of phorbol myristate acetate resides in its ability to inhibit
excision repair. Rather, since phorbol ester tumor promotion can
occur weeks and months after DNA damage, we feel the tumor potential of the molecule resides in its derepression and mitogenic
activity (Trosko *et al.*, 1975). Moreover, the study of 17-β-
estradiol indicates that the hormone is unable to increase UV-
induced mutations, but that it can induce stable heritable phenotypic changes by itself (Chang *et al.*, 1975).

Table 1. Survival and Frequency of Mutations After UV Irradiation
          and Phorbol Myristate Acetate (PMA) Treatment

Selective agent	UV fluence (ergs/mm^2)	PMA (1 μg/ml)	% Survival	No. of mutants	Mutations per 10^6 survivors
6-Thioguanine	0[a]*	-	108	19	5.89
(10 μg/ml)	0[b]	+	104	52	16.63**
	200[c]	-	8	10	14.51
	200[d]	+	5	28	57.72**
Ouabain	0[e]	-	108	33	5.12
(1 mM)	0[f]	+	104	35	5.58
	200[g]	-	8	314	113.87
	200[h]	+	5	450	231.91**

*Number of cells and plates (9 cm) used: a, b = 3 × 10^6/30;
c, d = 9 × 10^6/30; e, f = 6 × 10^6/30; g, h = 36 × 10^6/18.
**Mutation frequencies of phorbol myristate acetate treated
cells compared to control cells with same selective agent and at
equivalent fluences of UV light were highly significant, P <1%
[Statistical test was done by the method of W.L. Stevens, J.
Genet. 43:301-307 (1942)].

Although the molecular mechanism for gene regulation in eukaryotic cells is not well understood at present (Davidson and Britten,
1973), it would not be unreasonable to speculate that there are several means to alter the expression of a structural gene. A mutation in the regulator segment could result in the derepression (or
repression) of a structural gene. Possibly, the activation of
integrated viral information, or the insertion and activation of
viral DNA, due to the consequence of DNA repair of the eukaryotic
host DNA, might lead to altered structural gene activity. Alternatively, the non-repair of DNA lesions in the regulatory region
of DNA might conceivably modify the expression of a structural gene.
Viewed in this manner, the consequence of faulty or non-repair of
various DNA adducts might be either (or both) a mutation in a structural or regulator gene or a derepression of a structural gene.

6. EVOLUTIONARY PERSPECTIVE OF SOMATIC MUTAGENESIS

The human being consists of both somatic and germinal tissue.
In essence, mutations on the germ level are the grist for evolution's mill. Organisms live in a constantly changing environment;
consequently, every species has had to produce mutant variants
that would be adaptable to a new environment that is hostile to the

"non mutant". From this perspective, limited mutations in the germ level are of selective advantage. We must recall (1) that genes of each mammal potentially contribute to the development of that organism (genes of the soma) and to the overall development of the species (germinal genes); (2) each organism must have mechanisms to maintain the integrity of the genetic information in order to insure normal function and (3) both unaltered and altered genes are passed on in both somatic and germ tissue.

Von Borstel (1969) has postulated that enzyme systems which act on DNA, such as DNA polymerases and certain DNA repair enzymes, are the principal sources of spontaneous mutations. Such mechanisms, which allow for some errors in the production of germ cells, place the rate of mutation itself under genetic control and subject to natural selection. Kaplan (1972) has further postulated that the level of the average mutation frequency is adjusted to the generation time by Darwinian selection. When mutations occur too rarely, the genetic adaptation to environmental changes is hampered and the species will die out. When they become too frequent, the rate of reproduction in a normal milieu is decreased due to too many injuries by mutations.

However, since genes and chromosomes in the somatic tissue are not refractory to environmental damage, DNA repair and mutagenesis also must take place (Fig. 5). Since mutations can be induced in human somatic cells (Albertini and DeMars, 1973), we have some reason to believe that they can be the result of "error-prone" repair mechanisms. If we assume that some somatic mutations contribute to the carcinogenic and ageing processes, both cancer and ageing might be the somatic "price" individual organisms have to pay for the germinal mutations which could contribute to the survival of the species (DeGrouchy, 1973) (the "Yin-Yang" hypothesis of cancer and ageing, Fig. 6).

This hypothesis ultimately would have to explain, among other things, two observations linking carcinogenesis with the ageing process: First, normal cells, grown in cell cultures as fibroblasts have a finite life span, whereas transformed or cancer cells, *in vitro*, can proliferate indefinitely (Hayflick, 1965). Second, as one gets older, the probability of cancer increases (Dorn and Cutler, 1959).

As an explanation for the increase of tumor frequency with age, as well as the high frequencies of tumors in genetically deficient individuals, or in individuals with drug-depressed immune systems, the concept of immunological surveillance has been advanced (Burnet, 1970). This hypothesis suggests that growth of neoplasms (promotion of initiated, but latent precancerous cells) is prevented by a complex combination of factors preventing the mitosis of initiated cells and the immunological destruction of some of those that do

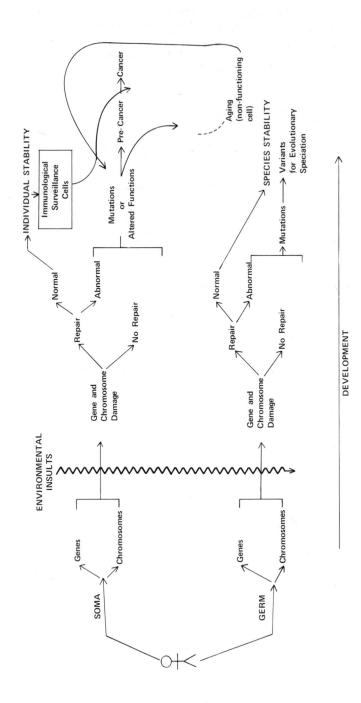

Fig. 5. A speculative model relating faulty DNA repair on the germ and soma levels with evolution, cancer and ageing. Thus, mutated cells, resulting from DNA damage, which have a tumor potential, are held in check only as long as cells of the immunological surveillance system function properly. In time, non-repaired lesions accumulate in all cells, including those of the immunological surveillance system. Thus, the "ageing" of the surveillance cells, due to the non-repair of DNA lesions, allows mutated somatic cells, on stimulation, to develop into tumors (From Trosko and Chu, 1975).

divide. In this sense, the immunological surveillance system can
be viewed as one of several "anti-promoters" (Fig. 2). Other anti-
promoters might be hormones which repress mitosis. Further, it
suggests that the cellular immune response should decline with age.
Evidence does exist which supports the prediction that the immune
surveillance cells are not "immune" to the ageing process. Immunological competence, measured several ways, of lymphocytes from old
persons were shown to be depressed compared with the response of
lymphocytes from young persons (Weksler and Hutteroth, 1974).

Barnhill and Yielding (1974) have proposed a model for antibody diversity based on somatic mutations. Since the cells of
immunological surveillance systems, themselves, are not "immune"
to the ageing process, one might predict the decline of the immunological competency of cells is related to a decrease in some kind
of DNA repair competency during development. Supporting this idea
are the series of reports which demonstrate that DNA repair is
modulated by genetic factors influencing development and differentiation in eukaryotic organisms (Darzynkiewicz, 1971; Hahn *et al.*,
1971; Wilkins and Hart, 1974). One would also predict that not
only would more tumors appear due to the non-functioning (ageing)
of the immunological surveillance cells, but also to the increase in
mutations. Assuming mutagenesis is responsible for some carcinogenic events, Ebbesen (1974) has produced data that support the
preceding hypothesis. He was able to show that ageing increases
susceptibility of mouse skin to chemical carcinogenesis, independent of the general immune status.

TAO OF DNA REPAIR

or

YIN—YANG OF CANCER AND AGING

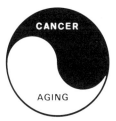

"Tao produces both renewal and decay, but is neither renewal or decay.
It causes being and non-being, but is neither being or non-being. Tao
assembles and it destroys, . . ."   Readings from Chuang Tzu, xxii

Fig. 6. A symbolic representation of the hypothesis which
encompasses cancer and ageing as natural consequences of somatic
mutagenesis brought about by faulty DNA repair.

Orgel has presented an "error catastrophe" theory of ageing (1963, 1973) which features an accumulation of random errors in amino acid sequences of proteins. Errors occurring in proteins involved in protein synthesis would be expected to lead to the "ageing" of cells. Holliday and his co-workers (1972, 1974) have shown that altered enzymes, as well as an increased mutation frequency, are characteristic in senescent cells when compared to young cells. Petes *et al.* (1972) have shown that the rate of DNA chain elongation in senescent cells was slower than in non-senescent cells. One possible explanation for the slower rate of DNA elongation is that a proportion of the enzyme molecules required for DNA replication is defective in senescent cells. Consistent with that explanation, Goldstein and Singal (1974) were able to demonstrate that three diverse gene products (2 surface-related antigens and G-6PD, a cytoplasmic enzyme) were markedly abnormal in cultured cells from Werner's syndrome (a hereditary disease of accelerated ageing). Holliday *et al.* (1974) also have demonstrated a similar protein anomaly in Werner's syndrome.

It would appear that if somatic mutagenesis is the result of defective repair, caused in part by programmed developmental constraints on "error-free" repair, then cancer and ageing might be the biological consequence. Cancer might be the result of a limited number of mutations (and derepressions) affecting the cell's ability to divide and escape the immunological surveillance system. Ageing might be the result of a large number of general mutations affecting any cell's ability to carry on normal metabolic functions.

Acknowledgment. The authors' research was supported by a grant (CA 13048-04) from the National Cancer Institute. Manuscript was written while J.E.T. was a Career Development Awardee of the Public Health Service (IK4 CA 24,085-04). The secretarial assistance of Ms. Sue Milton is gratefully acknowledged.

References

Albertini, R.J., and DeMars, R., 1973, Detection and quantification of X-ray-induced mutation in cultured, diploid human fibroblasts, *Mutat. Res.* 18:199-224.

Albrecht, A., Biedler, J., and Hutchison, D., 1972, Two different species of dihydrofolate reductase in mammalian cells differentially resistant to amethopterin and methasquin, *Cancer Res.* 32:1539-1546.

Ames, B.N., Durston, W.E., Yamasaki, E., and Lee, F.D., 1973, Carcinogens are mutagens: A simple test system combining liver homogenates for activation and bacteria for detection, *Proc. Nat. Acad. Sci. USA* 70:2281-2285.

Arlett, C., and Harcourt, S., 1972, The induction of 8-azaguanine-resistant mutants of cultured Chinese hamster cells by ultraviolet light, *Mutat. Res.* 61:301-306.

Auerbach, C., and Robson, J.M., 1944, Production of mutations by allyl isothiocyanate, *Nature* 154:81.

Baird, W.M., Sedgwick, J.A., and Boutwell, R.K., 1971, Effects of phorbol and four diesters of phorbol on the incorporation of tritiated precursors into DNA, RNA, and protein into mouse epidermis, *Cancer Res.* 31:1434-1439.

Bakay, B., Croce, C.M., Koprowski, H., and Nyhan, W.L., 1973, Restoration of hypoxanthine phosphoribosyltransferase activity in mouse IR cells after fusion with chick-embryo fibroblasts, *Proc. Nat. Acad. Sci. USA* 70:1998-2002.

Barnhill, C.W., and Yielding, K.L., 1974, A model for antibody diversity based on non-conservative DNA synthesis errors, *J. Theor. Biol.* 43:197-209.

Beaudet, A., Roufa, D., and Caskey, C., 1973, Mutations affecting the structure of hypoxanthine-guanine phosphoribosyltransferase in cultured Chinese hamster cells, *Proc. Nat. Acad. Sci. USA* 70:320-324.

Ben-Ishai, R., and Peleg, L., 1974, Excision repair in primary mouse embryo cells and its decline in progressive passages and in established cell lines, Abstr. ICN-UCLA Winter Conf. on *Molecular Mechanisms for the Repair of DNA*, Squaw Valley, California, February 24-March 1, 1974.

Berenblum, I., 1954, A speculative review: The probable nature of promoting action and its significance in the understanding of the mechanism of carcinogenesis, *Cancer Res.* 14:471-477.

Bootsma, D., Mulder, M.P., Pot, F., and Cohen, J.A., 1970, Different inherited levels of DNA repair replication in xeroderma pigmentosum cell strains after exposure to ultraviolet irradiation, *Mutat. Res.* 9:507-516.

Boutwell, R.K., 1974, The function and mechanism of promoters of carcinogenesis, *in* "CRC Critical Reviews in Toxicology," pp. 419-443, Chemical Rubber Company, Cleveland.

Boveri, T., 1929, "The Origin of Malignant Tumors," The Williams and Wilkins Company, New York.

Boyce, R., and Howard-Flanders, P., 1964, Release of ultraviolet light-induced thymine dimers from DNA in *E. coli* K-12, *Proc. Nat. Acad. Sci. USA* 51:293-300.

Burnet, F.M., 1970, "Immunological Surveillance," Pergamon Press, Ltd., Oxford.

Cerutti, P.A., 1974, Effects of ionizing radiation on mammalian cells, *Naturwiss.* 61:51-59.

Chagant, R.S.K., Schomberg, S., and German, J., 1974, A many fold increase in sister chromatid exchanges in Bloom's syndrome lymphocytes, *Proc. Nat. Acad. Sci. USA* 71:4508-4512.

Chan, V., Whitmore, G., and Siminovitch, L., 1972, Mammalian cells with altered forms of RNA polymerase II, *Proc. Nat. Acad. Sci. USA* 69:3119-3123.

Chang, C.C., Trosko, J.E., Yotti, L., and Chu, E.H.Y., 1975, Muta-
    genicity of cancer-promoting agents in cultural Chinese hamster
    cells, *Abstr. Environm. Mutagen Soc. Meetings*, Miami.
Chasin, L., Feldman, A., Konstam, M., and Urlaub, G., 1974, Rever-
    sion of a Chinese hamster cell auxotrophic mutant, *Proc. Nat.
    Acad. Sci. USA* 71:718-722.
Clayton, D.B., 1962, "Chemical Carcinogens," Little, Brown, Inc.,
    Boston.
Cleaver, J.E., 1969, A human disease in which an initial stage of
    DNA repair is defective, *Proc. Nat. Acad. Sci. USA* 63:428-435.
Cleaver, J.E., 1970, DNA repair and radiation sensitivity in human
    (xeroderma pigmentosum) cells, *Int. J. Radiat. Biol.* 18:557-
    565.
Cleaver, J.E., 1970, DNA damage and repair in light-sensitive human
    skin disease, *J. Invest. Dermatol.* 54:181-195.
Cleaver, J.E., 1971, Repair of alkylation damage in ultraviolet
    sensitive (xeroderma pigmentosum) human cells, *Mutat. Res.*
    12:453-462.
Cleaver, J.E., 1973, Xeroderma pigmentosum, DNA repair and carcino-
    genesis, *in* "Current Research in Oncology" (C.B. Anfinsen, ed.),
    pp. 15-43, Academic Press, New York.
Cleaver, J.E., and Painter, R.B., 1975, Absence of specificity in
    inhibition of DNA repair by DNA binding agents, cocarcinogens,
    and steroids in human cells, *Cancer Res.* 35:1773-1778.
Cleaver, J.E., and Thomas, E.H., 1969, Single strand interruptions
    in DNA and the effects of caffeine on Chinese hamster cells
    irradiated with ultraviolet light, *Biochem. Biophys. Res.
    Commun.* 36:203-208.
Cleaver, J.E., and Trosko, J.E., 1970, Absence of excision of ultra-
    violet-induced cyclobutane dimers in xeroderma pigmentosum,
    Photochem. Photobiol. 11:547-550.
Comfort, A., Youhotosky-Gore, I., and Pathmanathan, K., 1971, Effect
    of ethoxyquin on the longevity of C3H mice, *Nature* 229:254-255.
Comings, D.E., 1973, A general theory of carcinogenesis, *Proc. Nat.
    Acad. Sci. USA* 70:3324-3328.
Commings, R.B., and Walton, M.F., 1973, Modification of the acute
    toxicity of mutagenic and carcinogenic chemicals in the mouse
    by prefeeding with antioxidants, *Fd. Cosmet. Toxicol.* 11:547-
    553.
Conney, A.H., 1973, Carcinogen metabolism and human cancer, *N. Eng.
    J. Med.* 289:971-973.
Cook, J.S., 1970, Photoreactivation in animal cells, *Photophysiology*
    5:191-233.
Corry, P.M., and Cole, A., 1968, Radiation-induced double-strand
    scission of the DNA of mammalian metaphase chromosomes, *Radiat.
    Res.* 36:528-543.
Court Brown, W.M., 1962, Role of genetic change in neoplasia, *Brit.
    Med. J.* 1:961-964.
Croce, C.M., Bakay, B., Nyhan, W.L., and Koprowski, H., 1973, Re-
    expression of the rat hypoxanthine phosphoribosyltransferase

gene in rat-human hybrids, *Proc. Nat. Acad. Sci. USA* 70:2590-2594.

Darlington, G., Bernard, H., and Ruddle, F., 1974, Human serum albumin phenotype activation in mouse hepatoma-human leukocyte cell hybrids, *Science* 185:859-862.

Darzynkiewicz, Z., 1971, Radiation induced DNA synthesis in normal and stimulated human lymphocytes, *Exp. Cell Res.* 69:356-360.

Darzynkiewicz, Z., and Chelmicha-Szorc, E., 1972, Unscheduled DNA synthesis in hen erythrocyte nuclei reactivated in heterokaryons, *Exp. Cell Res.* 74:131-139.

Davidson, E., and Britten, R., 1973, Organization, transcription, and regulation in the animal genome, *Quart. Rev. Biol.* 48:565-613.

De Grouchy, J., 1973, Cancer and the evolution of species: a ransom, *Bio. Med.* 18:6-8.

DeMars, R., 1972, in Concluding Remarks; F. Vogel, *Humangenetik* 16:178-180.

Demerec, M., 1941, Unstable genes in Drosophila, *Cold Spring Harbor Symp. Quant. Biol.* 9:145-150.

Dierks-Ventling, C., and Jost, J.-P., 1974, Effect of 17-β-estradiol on the synthesis of non-histone nuclear proteins in chick liver, *Eur. J. Biochem.* 50:33-48.

Domon, M., and Rauth, A.M., 1969, The effects of caffeine on ultraviolet irradiated mouse L cells, *Radiat. Res.* 39:207-221.

Dorn, H.F., and Cutler, S.J., 1959, Morbidity from cancer in the United States, *Public Health Monogr.* No. 56:1.

Drake, J., 1969, Comparative rates of spontaneous mutation, *Nature* 221:1132.

Ebbensen, P., 1974, Ageing increases susceptibility of mouse skin to DMBA carcinogenesis independent of general immune status, *Science* 183:217-218.

Edenberg, H.J., and Hanawalt, P.C., 1973, The time course of DNA repair replication in ultraviolet irradiated HeLa cells, *Biochim. Biophys. Acta* 324:206-217.

Edwards, J.H., 1974, The mutation rate in man, *Prog. Med. Genet.* 10:1-17.

Epstein, J., Williams, J.R., and Little, J., 1973, Deficient DNA repair in human progeroid cells, *Proc. Nat. Acad. Sci. USA* 170:977-981.

Failla, G., 1958, The ageing process and carcinogenesis, *Annu. N.Y. Acad. Sci.* 71:1124-1140.

Fischinger, P.J., and Haapala, D.K., 1974, Oncoduction. A unifying hypothesis of viral carcinogenesis, *Immun. Cancer. Progr. Exp. Tumor Res.* 19:1-22.

Fox, M., 1974, The effect of post-treatment with caffeine on survival and UV-induced mutation frequencies in Chinese hamster and mouse lymphoma cells in vitro, *Mutat. Res.* 24:187-204.

Freese, E., 1963, Molecular mechanism of mutations, *in* "Molecular Genetics" (J.H. Taylor, ed.), Part I, pp. 207-269, Academic Press, New York.

Frei, J.V., and Stephens, P., 1968, The correlation of promotion of tumor growth and of induction of hyperplasia in epidermal two-stage carcinogenesis, *Brit. J. Cancer* 22:83-92.

Gaudin, D., Gregg, R., and Yielding, K., 1972, Inhibition of DNA repair by co-carcinogens, *Biochem. Biophys. Res. Commun.* 48: 945-949.

German, J., Archibald, R., and Bloom, D., 1965, Chromosomal breakage in a rare and probably genetically determined syndrome in man, *Science* 148:506-507.

Gledhill, B., and Darzynkiewicz, Z., 1973, Unscheduled synthesis of DNA during mammalian spermatogenesis in response to UV irradiation, *J. Exp. Zool.* 183:375-382.

Goldstein, S., 1971, The role of DNA repair in ageing of cultured fibroblasts from xeroderma pigmentosum and normals, *Proc. Soc. Exp. Biol. Med.* 137:730-731.

Goldstein, S., and Singal, D.P., 1974, Alteration of fibroblast gene products *in vitro* from a subject with Werner's syndrome, *Nature* 251:719-721.

Gordon, P., 1974, Free radicals and the ageing process, *in* "Theoretical Aspects of Ageing" (M. Rockstein, M.L. Sussman, and J. Chesky, eds.), pp. 61-82, Academic Press, New York.

Goth, R., and Pajewsky, M.F., 1974, Persistence of O-6-ethylguanine in rat-brain DNA: correlation with nervous system-specific carcinogenesis by ethylnitrosourea, *Proc. Nat. Acad. Sci. USA* 71:639-643.

Green, M.M., 1973, Some observations and comments on mutable and mutator genes in Drosophila, *Genetics* 73:187-194.

Griggs, H.G., and Bender, M.A., Photo-reactivation of ultraviolet-induced chromosomal aberrations, *Science* 179:86-87.

Habazin, V., and Han, A., 1970, Ultraviolet-light-induced DNA-to-protein cross-linking in HeLa cells, *Int. J. Radiat. Biol.* 17:569-575.

Hahn, G., King, D., and Young, S., 1971, Quantitative changes in unscheduled DNA synthesis in rat muscle cells after differentiation, *Nature N. Biol.* 230:242-244.

Harris, M., 1973, Anomalous patterns of mutation in cultured mammalian cells, *Genetics* 73(Supplement):181-185.

Harris, R.J.C., 1970, Cancer and the environment, *Int. J. Environ. Studies* 1:59-65.

Hart, R.W., and Trosko, J.E., 1975, DNA repair processes in mammals, *in* "Interdisciplinary Topics in Gerontology" (in press).

Hayflick, L., 1965, The limited in vitro lifetime of human diploid cell strains, *Exp. Cell Res.* 37:614-636.

Hecht, F., Koler, R., Rigas, D., Dahnke, G., Case, M., Tisdale, V., and Miller, R., 1966, Leukemia and lymphocytes in ataxia-telangiectasia, *Lancet* 2:1193.

Hellman, K.B., Haynes, K., and Bockstahler, L.E., 1974, Radiation-enhanced survival of a human virus in normal and malignant rat cells, *Proc. Soc. Exp. Biol. Med.* 145:255-262.

Hennings, H., Michael, D., and Patterson, E., 1973, Enhancement of

skin tumorigenesis by a single application of croton oil before
     or soon after initiation by urethan, *Cancer Res.* 33:3130-3134.
Heston, W.E., 1974, Genetics of cancer, *J. Heredity* 65:262-272.
Hewish, D., and Burgoyne, L., 1973, Chromatin sub-structure. The
     digestion of chromatin DNA at regularly spaced sites by a
     nuclear deoxyribonuclease, *Biochem. Biophys. Res. Commun.* 52:
     504-510.
Higurashi, M., and Conen, P.E., 1973, *In vitro* chromosomal radio-
     sensitivity in chromosomal breakage syndromes, *Cancer* 32:380-
     383.
Higurashi, M., Tamura, T., and Nakatake, T., 1973, Cytogenetic
     observations in cultured lymphocytes from patients with Down's
     syndrome and measles, *Pediat. Res.* 7:582-587.
Hill, R., 1958, A radiation-sensitive mutant of *E. coli*, *Biochim.*
     Biophys. Acta 30:636-637.
Hollaender, A., ed., 1971, "Chemical Mutagens," Vol. 1 and 2, Plenum
     Press, New York.
Hollaender, A., ed., 1973, "Chemical Mutagens," Vol. 3, Plenum Press,
     New York.
Holliday, R., 1972, Ageing in human fibroblasts in culture: studies
     on enzyme and mutation, *Humangenetik* 16:83-86.
Holliday, R., Porterfield, J.S., and Gibbs, D.D., 1974, Premature
     ageing and occurrance of altered enzyme in Werner's syndrome
     fibroblasts, *Nature* 248:762-763.
Holliday, R., and Tarrant, G.M., 1972, Altering enzymes in ageing
     human fibroblasts, *Nature* 238:26-30.
Holmberg, M., and Jonasson, J., 1973, Preferential location of x-ray
     induced chromosome breakage in the R-bands of human chromosomes,
     Hereditas 74:57-68.
Horikawa, M., Nikaido, O., and Sugahara, T., 1968, Dark reactivation
     of damage induced by ultraviolet light in mammalian cells *in*
     vitro, *Nature* 218:489-491.
Huang, A., Kremer, W., Laszlo, J., and Setlow, R.B., 1972, DNA
     repair in human leukaemic lymphocytes, *Nature N. Biol.* 240:
     114-115.
Humphrey, R.M., Sedita, B.A., and Meyn, R.E., 1970, Recovery of
     Chinese hamster cells from ultraviolet irradiation damages,
     Int. J. Radiat. Biol. 18:61-69.
Iversen, O.H., and Evensen, A., 1962, Experimental skin carcinogen-
     esis in mice, *Acta Pathol. Microbiol. Scand. Suppl.* 156:95-143.
Kao, F.T., and Puck, T.T., 1969, Genetics of mutagenesis by physi-
     cal and chemical agents, *J. Cell Physiol.* 74:245-258.
Kao, F.T., and Puck, T.T., 1972, Genetics of somatic mammalian
     cells: demonstration of a human esterase activator gene
     linked to the ade B gene, *Proc. Nat. Acad. Sci. USA* 69:3273-
     3277.
Kaplan, R.W., 1972, Evolutionary adjustment of spontaneous mutation
     rates, *Humangenetik* 16:39-42.
Karran, P., and Omerod, M.G., 1973, Is the ability to repair damage
     to DNA related to the proliferative capacity of a cell? The

rejoining of x-ray produced strand breaks, *Biochim. Biophys. Acta* 299:54-64.

Kato, H., 1974, Photoreactivation of sister chromatid exchanges induced by ultraviolet irradiations, *Nature* 249:552-553.

Kellermann, G., Luyten-Kellermann, M., and Shaw, C.R., 1973, Genetic variation of arylhydrocarbon hydroxylase in human lymphocytes, *Am. J. Human Genet.* 25:327-331.

Kihlman, B.A., 1971, Molecular mechanisms of chromosome breakage and rejoining, *Adv. Cell Med. Biol.* 1:59-107.

Kihlman, B.A., Sturelin, S., Hartley-Asp, B., and Nilsson, K., 1973, Caffeine, caffeine derivatives and chromosomal aberrations, *Mutat. Res.* 17:271-275.

Klein, G., 1972, Herpesviruses and oncogenesis, *Proc. Nat. Acad. Sci. USA* 69:1056-1064.

Klimek, M., 1966, Thymidine dimerization in L-strain mammalian cells after irradiation with ultraviolet light and search for repair mechanisms, *Photochem. Photobiol.* 5:603-607.

Kohn, R.R., 1971, Effects of antioxidants on life-span of C57BL mice, *J. Gerontol.* 26:378-380.

Koller, P.C., 1972, "The Role of Chromosomes in Cancer Biology," Springer-Verlag, Berlin.

Kondo, S., 1974, Evidence that mutations are induced by errors in repair and replication, *Genetics* 73:109-122.

Kouri, R.E., Ratrie, H., and Whitmire, C.E., 1974, Genetic control of susceptibility to 3-methylcholanthrene-induced subcutaneous sarcomas, *Int. J. Cancer* 13:714-720.

Kuhlmann, W., Fromme, H.-G., Geege, E.M., and Ostertag, W., 1968, The mutagenic action of caffeine in higher organisms, *Cancer Res.* 28:2375-2389.

Lehmann, A.R., 1972, Post replication repair of DNA in ultraviolet-irradiated mammalian cells, *J. Mol. Biol.* 66:319-337.

Lehmann, A.R., 1974, Post replication repair of DNA in mammalian cells, *Life Sci.* 15:2005-2016.

Lehmann, A.R., Kirk-Bell, S., Arlett, C.F., Patterson, M.C., Lohman, P.H.M., DeWoerd-Kastelein, E.A., and Bootsma, E.A., 1975, Xeroderma pigmentosum cells with normal levels of excision repair have a defect in DNA synthesis after UV-irradiation, *Proc. Nat. Acad. Sci. USA* 72:219-223.

Lett, J.T., Klucis, E.S., and Sun, C., 1970, On the size of DNA in the mammalian chromosome structural subunits, *Biophys. J.* 10:277-292.

Lett, J.T., and Sun, C., 1970, The production of strand breaks in mammalian DNA by x-rays; at different stages of the cell cycle, *Radiat. Res.* 44:771-787.

Lieberman, M.W., and Poirier, M.C., 1974, Intragenomal distribution of DNA repair synthesis: repair in satellite and mainband DNA in cultured mouse cells, *Proc. Nat. Acad. Sci. USA* 71:2461-2465.

Lumb, J.R., Sideropoulos, A.S., and Shankel, D.M., 1968, Inhibition of dark repair of ultraviolet damage in DNA by caffeine and 8-chloro caffeine, kinetics of inhibition, *Mol. Gen. Genet.*

102:108-111.

Lynch, H.T., and Kaplan, A.R., 1974, Cancer genetic problems: host-environmental considerations, *Immunol. of Cancer Progr. Exp. Tumor Res.* 19:332-352.

Lytle, C.D., Benane, S.G., and Bockstahler, L.E., 1974, Ultraviolet-enhanced reactivation of Herpes virus in human tumor cells, *Photochem. Photobiol.* 20:91-94.

Malling, H.V., and Chu, E.H.Y., 1974, Development of mutational model systems for the study of carcinogenesis, *in* "Model Studies in Chemical Carcinogenesis" (P.O.P. Ts'o and J.A. Di Poalo, eds.), pp. 545-563, Marcel Dekker, Inc., New York.

Markert, C.L., 1968, Neoplasia: a disease of cell differentiation, *Cancer Res.* 28:1908-1914.

McClintock, B., 1951, Chromosome organization and genetic expression, *Cold Spring Harbor Symp. Quant. Biol.* 16:13-47.

Meltz, M.L., and Painter, R.B., 1973, Distribution of repair replication in the HeLa cell genome, *Int. J. Radiat. Biol.* 23:637-640.

Mezger-Freed, L., 1974, An analysis of survival in haploid and diploid cell cultures after exposure to ICR acridine half-mustard compounds mutagenic for bacteria, *Proc. Nat. Acad. Sci. USA* 71:4416-4420.

Miller, E.C., and Miller, J.A., 1971, The mutagenicity of chemical carcinogens: correlations, problems and interpretations, *in* "Chemical Mutagens-Principles and Methods for Their Detection" (A. Hollaender, ed.), Vol. 1, pp. 83-119, Plenum Press, New York.

Modak, I.P., and Price, G.B., 1971, Exogenous DNA polymerase-catalysed incorporation of deoxyribonucleotide monophosphates in nuclei of fixed mouse brain cells, *Exp. Cell Res.* 65:289-298.

Mohn, G., and Wurgler, F.E., 1972, Mutator genes in different species, *Humangenetik* 16:49-58.

Neel, J.V., 1971, The detection of increased mutation rates in human populations, *Persp. Biol. Med.* 14:522-537.

O'Brien, R.L., Poon, P., Kline, E., and Parker, J.W., 1971, Susceptibility of chromosomes from patients with Down's syndrome to 7,12-dimethyl-benz(a)anthracene-induced aberrations *in vitro*, *Int. J. Cancer* 8:202-210.

Orgel, L.E., 1963, The maintenance of the accuracy of protein synthesis and its relevance to ageing, *Proc. Nat. Acad. Sci. USA* 49:517-521.

Orgel, L.E., 1973, Ageing of clones of mammalian cells, *Nature* 243:441-445.

Painter, R.B., 1974, DNA damage and repair in eukaryotic cells, *Genetics* 78:139-148.

Painter, R.B., Clarkson, J.M., and Young, B.R., 1973, Ultraviolet-induced repair replication in ageing diploid human cells (WI-38), *Radiat. Res.* 56:560-564.

Parrington, J.M., Delhanty, J.D., and Baden, H.P., 1971, Unscheduled

DNA synthesis, UV-induced chromosome aberrations and SV40 transformation in cultured cells from xeroderma pigmentosum, *Annu.
Hum. Genet.* 35:149-160.

Passarge, E., 1972, Spontaneous chromosomal instability, *Humangenetik*
16:151-157.

Paul, D., and Hecker, E., 1969, On the biochemical mechanism of
tumorigenesis in mouse skin. II. Early effects on the biosynthesis of nucleic acids induced by initiating doses of
DMBA and promoting doses of phorbol-12,13-diester TPA, *Z.
Krebsforsch* 73:149-163.

Penn, I., 1974, Occurrence of cancer in immune deficiencies, *Cancer*
34:858-866.

Penn, I., and Starzl, T.E., 1972, Malignant tumors arising de novo
in immunosuppressed organ transplant recipients, *Transplana-
tion* 14:407-417.

Peterson, A.R., Bertram, J.S., and Heidelberger, C., 1974, Cell
cycle dependency of DNA damage and repair in transformable
mouse fibroblast treated with N-methyl-N'-nitro-N-nitroso-
guanidine, *Cancer Res.* 34:1600-1607.

Petes, T.D., Farber, R.A., Tarrant, G.M., and Holliday, R., 1974,
Altering rate of DNA replication in ageing human fibroblast
cultures, *Nature* 251:434-436.

Poon, P.K., Parker, J.W., and O'Brien, R.L., 1974, Defect in DNA
repair in Fanconi's anemia, *Abstr. Proc. 65th Amer. Assoc.
Cancer Res.* 15:19.

Potter, V.R., 1972, Abnormal growth--the challenge of diversity,
in "Challenging Biological Problems," (J.A. Behnke, ed.), pp.
44-61, Oxford University Press, New York.

Potter, V.R., 1973, Biochemistry of cancer, *in* "Cancer Medicine"
(J. Holland and E. Frei, eds.), pp. 178-192, Lea and Febiger,
Philadelphia.

Price, G.B., Modak, S.P., and Makinodan, T., 1971, Age-associated
changes in the DNA of mouse tissue, *Science* 171:917-920.

Propping, P., 1972, Comparison of point mutation rates in different
species with human mutation rates, *Humangenetik* 16:43-48.

Raick, A.N., 1973, Ultrastructural, histological, and biochemical
alterations produced by 12-0-tetradecanoyl-phorbol-13-acetate
on mouse epidermis and their relevance to skin tumor promotion, *Cancer Res.* 33:269-286.

Rasmussen, R.E., and Painter, R.B., 1964, Evidence for repair of
ultraviolet damaged deoxyribonucleic acid in cultured mammalian
cells, *Nature* 203:1360-1362.

Regan, J.D., and Setlow, R.B., 1974, Two forms of repair in the DNA
of human cells damaged by chemical carcinogens and mutagens,
Cancer Res. 34:3318-3325.

Regan, J.D., and Setlow, R.B., 1974, DNA repair in human progeroid
cells, *Biochem. Biophys. Res. Commun.* 59:858-864.

Regan, J.D., Trosko, J.E., and Carrier, W.L., 1968, Evidence for
excision of ultraviolet induced pyrimidine dimers from the
DNA of human cells *in vitro, Biophys. J.* 8:319-325.

Roberts, J.J., and Sturrock, J., 1973, Enhancement by caffeine of N-methyl-N-nitrosourea-induced mutations and chromosome aberrations in Chinese hamster cells, *Mutat. Res.* 20:243-255.

Roman, C.S., and Bobrow, M., 1973, The sites of radiation induced-breakage in human lymphocyte chromosomes determined by quinacrine fluorescence, *Mutat. Res.* 18:325-331.

Rothwell, K., 1974, Dose-related inhibition of chemical carcinogenesis in mouse skin by caffeine, *Nature* 252:69-70.

Ryser, H.J.-P., 1971, Chemical carcinogenesis, *N. Eng. J. Med.* 285: 721-734.

Sasaki, M.S., 1973, DNA repair capacity and susceptibility to chromosome breakage in xeroderma pigmentosum cells, *Mutat. Res.* 20:291-293.

Sasaki, M.D., 1973, DNA repair capacity and susceptibility to chromosome breakage in xerodermia pigmentosum cells, *Mutat. Res.* 20:291-293.

Sasaki, M.S., and Tonomura, A., 1973, A high susceptibility of Fanconi's anemia to chromosome breakage by DNA cross-linking agents, *Cancer Res.* 33:1829-1836.

Satoh, T., and Yamamoto, N., 1972, Repair mechanism in Sendai virus carrying HeLa cells after damage by 4-hydroxyamino-quinoline 1-oxide, *Cancer Res.* 32:440-443.

Schneider, J., and Weiss, M., 1971, Expression of differentiated functions in hepatoma cell hybrids. I. Tyrosine aminotransferase in hepatoma-fibroblast hybrids, *Proc. Nat. Acad. Sci. USA* 68:127-131.

Scudiero, D., and Strauss, B., 1974, Accumulation of single-stranded regions in DNA and the block to replication in human cell line alkylated with methyl methane sulfonate, *J. Mol. Biol.* 83:17-34.

Secher, D.S., Cotton, R.G., and Milstein, C., 1973, Spontaneous mutation in tissue culture-chemical nature of variant immunoglobulin from mutant clones of MOPC 21, *Fed. Eur. Biochem. Soc. Lett.* 37:311-316.

Setlow, J.K., 1966, Photoreactivation, *Radiat. Res.* 6:141-155.

Setlow, R.B., and Carrier, W.L., 1964, The disappearance of thymine dimers from DNA: an error correcting mechanism, *Proc. Nat. Acad. Sci. USA* 51:226-231.

Setlow, R.B., and Regan, J.D., 1972, Defective repair of N-acetoxy-2-acetylaminofluorene-induced lesions in the DNA of xeroderma cells, *Biochem. Biophys. Res. Commun.* 46:1019-1024.

Setlow, R.B., Regan, J.D., and Carrier, W.L., 1972, Different levels of excision repair in mammalian cell lines, *Abstr. 16th Annu. Biophys. Soc. Meetings,* Toronto, Canada.

Setlow, R.B., Regan, J.D., German, J., and Carrier, W.L., 1969, Evidence that xeroderma pigmentosum cells do not perform the first step in the repair of ultraviolet damage to the DNA, *Proc. Nat. Acad. Sci. USA* 64:1035-1041.

Shamberger, R., Baughman, F.F., Kalchert, S.L., Willis, C.E., and Hoffman, G.C., 1973, Carcingen-induced chromosomal breakage decreased by antioxidants, *Proc. Nat. Acad. Sci. USA* 70:1461-

1463.

Sharp, J., Capecchi, N., and Capecchi, M., 1973, Altered enzymes in drug-resistant variants of mammalian tissue culture cells, *Proc. Nat. Acad. Sci. USA* 70:3145-3149.

Shows, T.B., and Ruddle, F.H., 1968, Function of the lactate dehydrogenase B gene in mouse erythrocytes: evidence for control by a regulatory gene, *Proc. Nat. Acad. Sci. USA* 61:574-581.

Silverman, B., and Mirsky, A., 1973, Accessibility of DNA in chromatin to DNA polymerase and RNA polymerase, *Proc. Nat. Acad. Sci. USA* 70:1326-1330.

Sinex, F.M., 1974, The mutation theory of ageing, *in* "Theoretical Aspects of Ageing" (M. Rockstein, M.L. Sussman, and J. Chesky, eds.), pp. 23-32, Academic Press, New York.

Sirover, M.A., and Loeb, L.A., 1974, Erroneous base-pairing induced by a chemical carcinogen during DNA synthesis, *Nature* 252:414-416.

Sivak, A., and Van Durren, B.L., 1971, Cellular interactions of phorbol myristate acetate in tumor promotion, *Chem. Biol. Interactions* 3:401-411.

Smith, K.C., 1975, The radiation-induced addition of proteins and other molecules to nucleic acids, *in* "Photochemistry and Photobiology of Nucleic Acids" (S.Y. Wang, ed.), Academic Press, New York (in press).

Stein, G.S., Spelsberg, T.C., and Kleinsmith, L.J., 1974, Nonhistone chromosomal proteins and gene regulation, *Science* 183:817-824.

Steward, D.L., and Humphrey, R.M., 1966, Induction of thymine dimers in synchronized populations of Chinese hamster cells, *Nature* 212:298-300.

Stich, H.F., San, R.H.C., and Kawazoe, Y., 1971, DNA repair synthesis in mammalian cells exposed to a series of onocogenic and non-oncogenic derivatives of 4-nitroquinoline 1-oxide, *Nature* 229:416-419.

Stich, H.F., Stich, W., and Lam, P., 1974, Susceptibility of xeroderma pigmentosum cells to chromosome breakage by adenovirus type 12, *Nature* 250:599-601.

Stockdale, F., 1971, DNA synthesis in differentiating skeletal muscle cells: initiation by ultraviolet light, *Science* 171:1145-1147.

Strauss, B., Coyle, M., McMahon, M., Kato, K., and Dolyniuk, M., 1972, DNA synthesis, repaired chromosome breaks in eukaryotic cells, *in* "Molecular and Cellular Repair Processes" (R. Beers, Jr., R. Herriott, and R.C. Tighman, eds.), pp. 111-124.

Sun, N.C., Chang, C.C., and Chu, E.H.Y., 1974, Chromosome assignment of the same human gene for galactose-1-phosphate uridyltransferase, *Proc. Nat. Acad. Sci. USA* 71:404-407.

Sun, N.C., Chang, C.C., and Chu, E.H.Y., 1975, Mutant hamster cells exhibiting a pleiotropic effect on carbohydrate metabolism, *Proc. Nat. Acad. Sci. USA* 72:469-473.

Sutherland, B.M., Rice, M., and Wagner, E.K., 1975, Xeroderma pigmentosum cells contain low levels of photoreactivating enzyme,

Proc. Nat. Acad. Sci. USA 72:103-107.

Sutherland, E.W., and Rall, T.W., 1958, Fractionation and characterization of a cyclic adenine ribonucleoside formed by tissue particles, *J. Biol. Chem.* 232:1077-1091.

Szilard, L., 1959, On the nature of the ageing process, *Proc. Nat. Acad. Sci. USA* 45:30-45.

Teebor, G., Duker, N., Raucan, S., and Zachary, K., 1973, Inhibition of thymine dimer excision by the phorbol ester, phorbol myristate acetate, *Biochem. Biophys. Res. Commun.* 50:66-70.

Temin, H.M., 1971, The protovirus hypothesis: speculations on the significance of RNA-directed DNA synthesis for normal development and carcinogenesis, *J. Nat. Cancer Inst.* 46:iii-vii.

Temin, H.M., 1974, On the origin of the genes for neoplasia: G.H.A. Clowes Memorial Lecture, *Cancer Res.* 34:2835-2841.

Terzi, M., 1974, Chromosomal variation and the origin of drug-resistant mutants, *Proc. Nat. Acad. Sci. USA* 71:5027-5031.

Thompson, L.H., Harkins, J.L., and Stanners, C.P., 1973, A mammalian cell mutant with a temperature-sensitive leucyl-transfer RNA synthetase, *Proc. Nat. Acad. Sci. USA* 70:3094-3098.

Todd, P., Coohill, T.P., Hellewell, A.B., and Mahoney, J.A., 1969, Post-irradiation properties of cultured Chinese hamster cells exposed to ultraviolet light, *Radiat. Res.* 38:321-339.

Trosko, J.E., and Chu, E.H.Y., 1973, Inhibition of repair of UV-damaged DNA by caffeine and mutation induction in Chinese hamster cells, *Chem.-Biol. Inter.* 6:317-332.

Trosko, J.E., and Chu, E.H.Y., 1975, The role of DNA repair and somatic mutation in carcinogenesis, *in* "Advances in Cancer Research" (S. Weinhouse, ed.), pp. 391-425, Academic Press, New York.

Trosko, J.E., Chu, E.H.Y., and Carrier, W.L., 1965, The induction of thymine dimers in ultraviolet irradiated mammalian cells, *Radiat. Res.* 24:667-672.

Trosko, J.E., Frank, P., Chu, E.H.Y., and Becker, J., 1973, Caffeine inhibition of post replication repair of N-acetoxy-2-acetyl-amino-fluorene damaged DNA in Chinese hamster cells, *Cancer Res.* 33:2444-2449.

Trosko, J.E., and Hart, R., 1975, DNA mutation frequencies in mammals, *in* "Interdisciplinary Topics in Gerontology" (in press).

Trosko, J.E., Yager, J.D., Bowden, G.T., and Butcher, F.R., 1975, The effects of several croton oil constituents on two types of DNA repair and cyclic nucleotide levels in mammalian cells *in vitro, Chem.-Biol. Inter.* 11:191-205.

Verly, W.G., Gossard, F., and Crine, P., 1974, *In vitro* repair of apurinic sites in DNA, *Proc. Nat. Acad. Sci. USA* 71:2273-2275.

Von Borstel, R.C., 1969, On the origin of spontaneous mutations, *Jap. J. Genet.* 44:102-105.

Walker, J.G., and Reid, B.D., 1971, Caffeine potentiation of lethal action of alkylating agents on L-cells, *Mutat. Res.* 12:101-104.

Walters, R.A., Gurley, L.R., and Tobey, R.A., 1974, Effects of caffeine on radiation-induced phenomena associated with cell-cycle traverse of mammalian cells, *Biophys. J.* 14:99-118.

Wattenberg, L.W., 1973, Inhibition of chemical carcinogen-induced pulmonary neoplasm by butylated hydroxyaniosole, *J. Nat. Cancer Inst.* 50:1541-1544.

Weber, A., 1968, The mechanism of the action of caffeine on sarco-plasmic reticulum, *J. Gen. Physiol.* 52:760-772.

Weksler, M.E., and Hutteroth, T.H., 1974, Impaired lymphocyte function in aged humans, *J. Clinical Invest.* 53:99-104.

Wheeler, K.T., and Lett, J.T., 1972, Formation and rejoining of DNA strand breaks in irradiated neurons: *in vivo, Radiat. Res.* 52:59-67.

Wheeler, K.T., Sheridan, R.E., Pantler, E.L., and Lett, J.T., 1973, *In vivo* restitution of the DNA structure in gamma irradiated rabbit retinas, *Radiat. Res.* 53:414-427.

Wilkins, R.J., 1973, DNA repair: a simple enzymatic assay for human cells, *Int. J. Radiat. Biol.* 24:609-613.

Wilkins, R.J., and Hart, R.W., 1974, Preferential DNA repair in human cells, *Nature* 247:35-36.

Wilkinson, R., Kiefer, J., and Nias, A.H.W., 1970, Effects of post-treatment with caffeine on the sensitivity to ultraviolet light irradiation of two lines of HeLa cells, *Mutat. Res.* 10:67-72.

Witkin, E., 1947, Mutations in *Escherichia coli* induced by chemical agents, *Cold Spring Harbor Symp. Quant. Biol.* 12:256-269.

Witkin, E., 1969, Ultraviolet-induced mutation and DNA repair, *Annu. Rev. Genet.* 3:525-552.

Witkin, E., 1975, Relationships between repair, mutagenesis and survival, *in* "Molecular Mechanisms for the Repair of DNA" (P.C. Hanawalt and R.B. Setlow, eds.), Plenum Press, New York (in press).

Wolff, S., Bodycote, J., and Painter, R.B., 1974, Sister chromatid exchanges induced in Chinese hamster cells by UV-irradiation of different stages of the cell cycle: the necessity for cells to pass through S, *Mutat. Res.* 25:73-81.

Yielding, K.L., 1974, A model for ageing based on differential repair of somatic mutational damage, *Persp. Biol. Med.* 17:201-208.

Young, D., 1971, The susceptibility to SV_{40} virus transformation of fibroblasts obtained from patients with Down's syndrome, *Eur. J. Cancer* 7:337-339.

Zajdela, F., and Latarjet, R., 1973, Effet inhibiteur de la cafeine sur l'induction de cancers cutanes par les rayons ultraviolet chez la souris, *C.R. Acad. Sci. Paris* Series D. 277:1073-1076.

Zamenhof, S., 1967, Nucleic acids and mutability, *Prog. Nucl. Acid Res.* 6:1-38.

CROSS-LINKAGE HYPOTHESIS OF AGING: DNA ADDUCTS IN CHROMATIN AS A PRIMARY AGING PROCESS

Richard G. Cutler

Institute for Molecular Biology, The University of Texas

at Dallas, P.O. Box 688, Richardson, Texas 75080

1. INTRODUCTION

There is now substantial evidence which points to the occurrence and biological importance of the formation of protein and
other adducts to DNA after ultraviolet or ionizing radiation of
cells (Smith, 1975a). Many of the reactive cross-linking agents
formed on the irradiation of cells (e.g., free radicals and their
derivatives) are thought to exist naturally within a cell but at a
much lower concentration. In addition, there exist naturally within the cell many non-radical chemical agents such as the aldehydes
which could also cross-link macromolecules (Harman, 1962; Bjorksten,
1962, 1974; Sinex, 1964). The possible parallel between radiation
and naturally induced DNA adducts appears sufficiently great to
warrant serious consideration of the natural occurrence of DNA
adducts as an important primary aging process. The objective of
this paper is to review the concept of primary aging processes and
the cross-linkage hypothesis of aging and to present the major
evidence indicating the natural accumulation of DNA adducts in the
chromatin of mammalian species with increasing age.

1.1. Survival and Lifespan

The length of life characteristic of a given mammalian species
is usually determined by a percent survival curve. Figure 1 illustrates a typical percent survival curve for U.S. white males from
1939 to 1941. The decrease in percent survival represents actual
deaths occurring with respect to a given population size. The slope
of the curve does not correspond to the aging rate of the population or an individual, as is frequently thought (Maynard Smith,
1966). The rate of reaching a certain critical level of dysfunction leading soon to death is represented closely by the force of
mortality function (indicated by the percent mortality rate curve
in Fig. 1), which rapidly increases after 30 to 40 years. The
percent survival curve can be described mathematically by the
Gompertz function R_M:

$$\frac{dN}{dt} = -NR_M \quad \text{and} \quad R_M = R_0 e^{\propto t}$$

where N is the number of living individuals in a population and
R_0 and $\propto$ are constants defining the survival curve and maximum
lifespan potential.

An important characteristic of percent survival curves for a
given species is the maximum lifespan recorded when the percent
survival approaches zero. For man this occurs at approximately
100 years (Acsadi and Nemeskeri, 1970). The maximum lifespan
recorded for most animal species has been found to remain essentially unchanged over a wide range of hazardous living conditions.

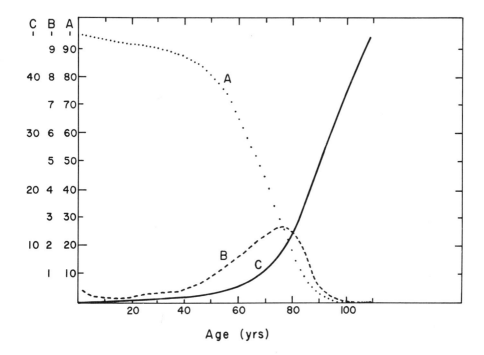

Fig. 1. Three different presentations of the same mortality data of U.S. white males, 1939-1941. (A) percent survivorship vs. age; (B) percent of original population dying/yr vs. age; (C) percent mortality rate (Gompertz function) vs. age (redrawn from Strehler, 1962).

This is illustrated for man in Fig. 2. What has changed with improved living conditions and medical care is the mean or 50% survival of the population. The constancy of the maximum lifespan potential of man and other mammalian species, in spite of substantially improved living conditions and medical care, has led to the concept that a species' characteristic aging rate (which is considered to be approximately inversely proportional to maximum lifespan) is governed more by basic intrinsic biological factors. The maximum lifespan of man (or the average aging rate) is therefore thought to have remained essentially constant over the past 45,000 years (back to *Homo neanderthalensis europaeus*). However, man's earlier ancestors are likely to have had a much faster aging rate. For example, the hominid species living about 3 to 4 million years ago, *Australopithecus africanus*, probably had a maximum lifespan potential of about 50 years, which is similar to the chimpanzee (Cutler, 1975a, b).

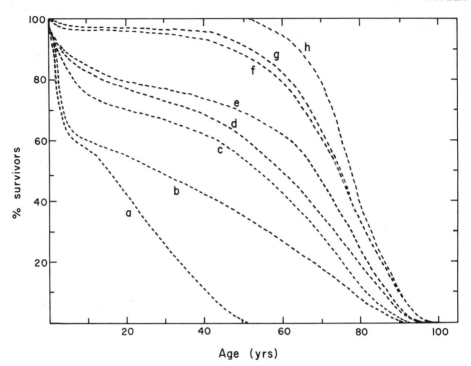

Fig. 2. Percent survival curves for man indicating the effects of living under different environmental hazardous conditions. (a) Hominid species, *Australopithecus africanus*, existing 3 to 4 × 10⁶ years ago; (b) Mexico, 1930; (c) England and Wales, 1891-1900; (d) U.S. all whites, 1900-02; (e) Italy, 1930-32; (f) U.S. all whites, 1959-61; (g) England and Wales, 1965-67; (h) 'theoretical' limit of biological longevity (redrawn from Comfort, 1974).

Different mammalian species have characteristic and different maximum lifespans (Biol. Data Book, 1972; Jones, 1968). This fact is clearly evident when comparing the maximum lifespans recorded for a number of different primate species (Table 1), where a range of about 12-fold is found (Cutler, 1975b). These values were attained under favorable captivity conditions that are expected to provide a reasonable estimate of a species' maximum lifespan potential. However, it is frequently questioned whether many estimates of maximum lifespan may be in error because of the small number of animals that are frequently used for this determination. A certain degree of uncertainty does exist, but it can be shown that the estimates rapidly approach the true maximum lifespan of a species with only a low number of animals and that a substantial increase in number of animals used results in only a small correction (Sacher, 1975). It is therefore considered reasonable to

Table 1.   Maximum Lifespans Recorded for Primates in Captivity
(From Cutler, 1975b)

SUPERFAMILY Family *Genus and species*	Common name	Maximum lifespan (years)
TUPAIOIDEA		
Tupaiidae		
Urogale everette	Philippine tree shrew	7
LORISOIDEA		
Lorisodae		
Nycticebus coucang	Bengal loris	13
Galagidae		
Galago senegalensis	galago	25
LEMUROIDEA		
Daubentoniidae		
Daubentonia madagascariensis	aye-ayes	23
Lemuridae		
Lemur macaco fulvus	lemur	31
CEBOIDEA		
Callithricidae		
Leontocebus rosalia	golden marmoset	15
Cebidae		
Pithecia pithecia	white-masked saki	14
Ateles paniscus	spider monkey	24
Cebus capucinus	capuchin	40
CERCOPITHECOIDEA		
Cercopithecidae		
Cynopithecus niger	Celebes crested macaque	18
Macaca mulatta	rhesus macaque	29
Papio porcarius	baboon	45
HOMINOIDEA		
Hylobatidae		
Hylobates lar	gibbon	32
Pongidae		
Gorilla gorilla	gorilla	40
Pan troglodytes	chimpanzee	45
Pongo pygmaeus	orangutan	50
Hominidae		
Homo sapiens	man	95

conclude that a wide range of maximum lifespan exists between different mammalian species (even between very closely related species) and that the differences in these values reflect their natural intrinsic differences in aging rate.

1.2. Aging Pathology

The aging process can be measured more accurately by determining the actual time-dependent loss of physiological functions
and the onset frequencies of diseases of the population, as compared to observing the time-dependent frequency of death. These
measurements are usually taken from a cross-section of the population at different ages. For man, after the age of about 30 years
there is a steady loss in the maximum capacity of most physiological
functions, a loss in general health, overall vigor and a general
decline in the feeling of well-being. Some examples of such
decline in the maximum capacity of physiological function are
shown in Fig. 3. Accompanying these declines in physiological function is an age-dependent increase in onset frequency of many different identifiable diseases. A well-known age-dependent disease
is cancer, and some examples illustrating this are shown in Fig. 4.

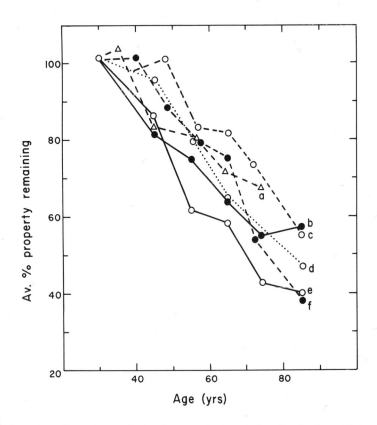

Fig. 3. Age-dependent loss of physiological functions (maximum capacities) in man. Level at age 30 years is assigned a value
of 100%. (a) cardiac index; (b) viral capacity; (c) standard

(Fig. 3, cont.) glomerular filtration rate (inulin); (d) standard renal plasma flow (diodrast); (e) maximum breathing capacity; (f) standard renal plasma flow [modified by Kohn (1971a) from B.L. Strehler, 1960].

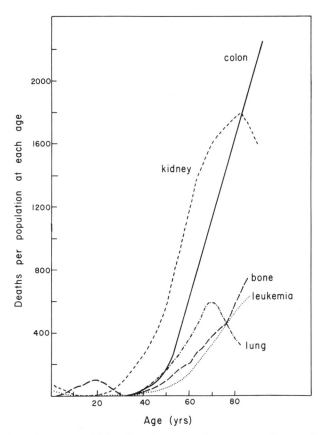

Fig. 4. Age-specific death rate for several neoplasms: colon, lung and leukemia (per 10^6 people); bone and kidney (per 10^7 people) (redrawn from Kohn, 1971a).

　　　There are only a few major disease processes that are now identified as being the major causes of death in man. As a consequence, much medical research has been focused on obtaining an understanding of these disease processes. However, the importance of these diseases to the overall health and longevity of the general population is frequently over-emphasized and the importance of the general aging process ignored. For example, estimates have been made of the amount of additional lifespan gained if the present major causes of death in man were now completely eliminated.

These estimates are shown in Table 2 and clearly show that only a small fraction of additional lifespan is gained. Moreover, the elimination of these specific diseases is not likely to extend general health (e.g., prevention of the age-dependent atrophy of muscle and nervous tissue or the loss of mental functions). The reason why is simply that these and other specific disease processes only represent the peaks of the more general submerged iceberg of age-dependent dysfunctions that are steadily accumulating as a function of age within the organism. The elimination of one disease process would immediately uncover another disease process, and so forth. It is therefore apparent that the elimination of these specific diseases, even if successful, will not result in a uniform maintenance of health, which is necessary for a more useful and enjoyable lifespan. A more general approach to the maintenance of health is necessary. This goal is a primary objective of some of the investigation now being carried out in gerontological research in the biological sciences.

Table 2.   Gain in Expectancy of Life at Birth and at Age 65 Due to Elimination of Various Causes of Death*

Cause of death	Gain in expectation of life (years) if cause was eliminated	
	At birth	At age 65
Major cardiovascular-renal diseases	10.9	10.0
Heart disease	5.9	4.9
Vascular diseases affecting central nervous system	1.3	1.2
Malignant neoplasms	2.3	1.2
Accidents other than by motor vehicles	0.6	0.1
Motor vehicle accidents	0.6	0.1
Influenza and pneumonia	0.5	0.2
Infectious diseases (excluding tuberculosis)	0.2	0.1
Diabetes mellitus	0.2	0.2
Tuberculosis	0.1	0.0

*(From Life tables published by the National Center of Health Statistics, USPHS and U.S. Bureau of the Census, "Some Demographic Aspects of Aging in the United States," February 1973.)

2. THE HYPOTHESIS OF PRIMARY AGING PROCESSES

Two approaches can be taken towards the goal of human health maintenance. The first is the usual compartmentalized approach where specific diseases are studied (e.g., cardiovascular-renal, malignant neoplasms). The second approach is represented by a study of primary disease processes which may underlie many different specific disease processes as observed at the organismic level and, more importantly, the many age-related losses of function that occur which are not associated with a specific disease process but nevertheless result in a progressive decline in general health. Many dysfunctions in man and other mammals appear to be more frequent and severe with increasing age of the organism. The primary disease processes underlying these dysfunctions are termed primary aging processes. The basic concept of primary aging processes is the hypothesis that many of the age-dependent dysfunctions at the phenotypic level are part of a highly complex and interdependent process which is initiated or caused by fewer and less complicated dysfunctions at a more fundamental level. This concept is illustrated in Fig. 5, showing a model of non-primary and primary aging processes. An important feature of the hypothesis of primary aging processes is the optimistic prediction that an understanding and eventual control of many different and very complex dysfunctions may be more readily obtained by a search for a few primary aging processes (Cutler, 1974, 1975a, b).

Support for the concept that primary aging processes can lead to complex phenotypic aging effects is obtained by the complexity of the physiological changes that are characteristic of many inherited genetic diseases. About 500 different genetic diseases are known for man (McKusick, 1971). In many of these a slight alteration in the genome gives rise to a complex expression of dysfunctions at the phenotypic level. Many of these dysfunctions are similar to natural aging processes. A few genetic diseases, such as progeria and Werner's syndrome are known to result in many of the naturally occurring aging processes and to produce the appearance of an accelerated aging process (Goldstein and Moerman, 1975; Goldstein *et al.*, 1975). Because genetic diseases are similar in their physiological effects to the many normally occurring age-dependent disease processes, then this suggests that the genome may be a primary aging target.

3. THE UNIFIED HYPOTHESIS OF AGING PROCESSES IN MAMMALS

The different mammalian species have many common aspects in their biological composition, physiological function and aging processes (Cutler, 1972, 1974, 1975a, b). These are (1) common structural genes. This similarity is particularly evident among the different primate species. Most differences between mammalian

Phenotypic Aging

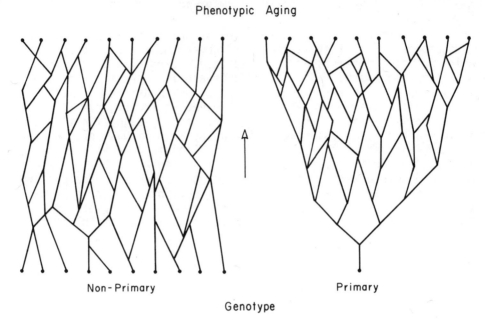

Non-Primary   Primary

Genotype

Fig. 5. Primary and non-primary aging models. These two
models illustrate two extreme cases of the flow of biochemical
interactions arising at the genotypic level on up to the expression
as phenotypic aging processes. In the non-primary aging model, an
equal and/or a greater number of causes at the genotypic level are
involved in producing a similar number of dysfunctions at the
phenotypic level. In this model the complexity of the biochemical
processes involved (including all their interactions with one
another) is not decreased through the identification of "causes
and effects" proceeding from the phenotypic to the genotypic
levels. In the primary aging model, although the complexity at
the phenotypic level is equal to the non-primary aging model, the
identification of "cause and effects" proceeding from the phenotypic level shows a decrease in complexity. Few primary causes
are responsible for the expression of many phenotypic aging processes
even though these aging processes are completely inter-related
(Cutler, unpublished).

species have now been suggested to be primarily in the regulation
of common structural genes (King and Wilson, 1975), (2) common biochemistry and physiology. This is expected if most structural and
regulatory genes are common, and (3) common specific diseases and
age-dependent dysfunctions. This is also expected if biological
composition and physiological functions are common.

It also appears that not only are age-dependent specific diseases and other dysfunctions common to different mammalian species but also, when examined on a normalized fraction-of-maximum-lifespan basis, they occur in a similar temporal pattern. This suggests that different mammalian species age qualitatively in a similar manner but at different overall rates, depending on the maximum lifespan of the species. All mammals may therefore have common aging processes which are regulated by common anti-aging or life maintenance processes, the extent of which determines the species' characteristic aging rate. These observations have led to a unified hypothesis of aging processes in mammals (Cutler, 1972, 1974).

4. GENETIC COMPLEXITY OF AGING IN MAMMALS

An important problem in gerontological research is the genetic complexity of the processes which govern the rate of aging in the different mammalian species. Although it is generally agreed that aging rate is genetically controlled, the complexity of the genetic processes involved is not known. The concept of primary aging processes suggests that the complexity of the key aging processes involved may be less at the cellular than at the organismic level and that, as a consequence, few anti-aging processes may be necessary to regulate most of the aging processes of a mammal. An estimate of the general complexity and/or number of genes involved in regulating aging rate in mammals can be obtained by determining the maximum rate longevity has evolved with respect to the actual frequency of gene or protein evolution (Cutler, 1975a, b; Sacher, 1975). For example, it is found that man's maximum lifespan has approximately doubled (from 50 to 100 years) over the past 3 to 2 million years (Fig. 6). It has also been demonstrated that man and chimpanzee, who have diverged from a common ancestor about 1.5 million years ago, essentially are identical at the structural gene level (King and Wilson, 1975).

These types of data can be used to estimate the amount of lifespan which has increased in the past with reference to the total number of nucleic acid base or amino acid substitutions taking place. It was found that only a small fraction of the genome is likely to be involved in governing the aging processes of mammals in a uniform manner (Cutler, 1975a, b). These anti-aging processes appear likely to be of a regulatory nature, involving the regulation of pre-existing genes and not the evolution of new structural genes.

The unified hypothesis of aging processes in mammals suggests that a comparison between closely related species having significantly different maximum lifespan potentials will be a valuable approach in determining the key differences between species which

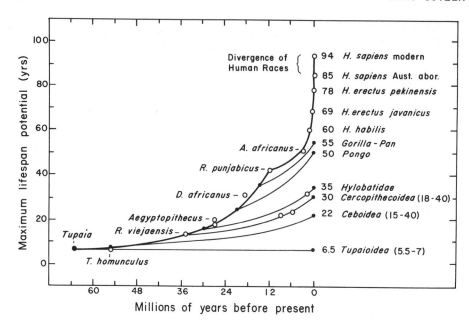

Fig. 6. Evolution of maximum lifespan potential along the
ancestral-descendant sequence of the Anthropoidea-like primates
leading to the appearance of the hominid species and eventually
to modern man. Estimates of maximum lifespan potential were
based on fossil evidence of cranial capacity and body weight
determinations. Maximum lifespan is seen to steadily increase at
an increasing rate, beginning with the origin of the primate species
about 60 million years ago. A maximum rate of increase in maximum
lifespan potential of 14 years per 10^5 years is predicted to have
occurred near the appearance of *H. erectus pekinensis*. During this
time interval, only about 0.5% of the functional genes ($\sim$200 genes)
are estimated to have received one or more adaptive base substitutions (From Cutler, 1975b).

are involved in governing aging rate and in evaluating the biological significance of potential primary aging processes. The value
of this latter approach in evaluating the biological significance
of possible important age-related changes can be illustrated by
the following examples.

No significant correlation between the aging rates of different mammalian species and the age-dependent change in collagen
cross-linkage has been found (Takacs and Verzar, 1968; Deyl *et al.*,
1971). The available data indicates that the degree of collagen
cross-linkage in similar tissues in two different mammalian species
of the same chronological age is similar even if their aging rates

are significantly different. However, many different types of
collagen need to be studied before a more final conclusion can be
made. There is also little correlation between aging rate and
body temperature in mammalian species. On the other hand, significant correlations of aging rate with specific metabolic rate
(Sacher, 1959, 1975) and with the extent of ultraviolet (UV)
radiation repair processes (Hart and Setlow, 1974) have been
noted.

The biological significance of *in vitro* aging of tissue culture cells as a useful model for *in vivo* aging processes can also
be evaluated by comparing the maximum doubling potentials of
tissue culture cells taken from species with different aging rates.
Although some correlation does exist (Hayflick, 1974), recent
comparisons with different mammalian species have now questioned
the value of this *in vitro* aging model (Stanley *et al.*, 1975).

5. THE CROSS-LINKAGE HYPOTHESIS OF AGING

5.1. The Hypothesis

The cross-linkage hypothesis of aging represents a primary
aging process. The basic hypothesis is very general and states
that an age-dependent accumulation of cross-links occurs throughout an organism, both inter- and intracellularly (Bjorksten, 1962,
1969, 1974; Sinex, 1964, 1974). Although many of the cross-links
formed are likely to be removed by repair or normal turnover
processes of the organism, they could accumulate by a certain
fraction of cross-linked macromolecules and/or structures being
resistant to these removal processes. The cross-linkage of inter-
and intracellular structures can theoretically produce a wide
range of damaging effects. The cross-linkage of extracellular
tissues such as collagen and elastin and the possible resulting
pathology has been studied most thoroughly. The presence and
biological effects of cross-linkage within the cell has not been
studied as intensely and is just beginning to attract interest.

The basis of the cross-linkage hypothesis is the natural
presence of a wide variety of cross-linking agents (Harman, 1962;
Slater, 1972; Bjorksten, 1974; Gordon, 1974). These agents are
the various free radicals and other chemical cross-linking agents,
such as the aldehydes. The presence of these cross-linking agents
would in many cases be expected to initiate much more damage than
is actually found, and it is therefore likely that an organism
has evolved many different types of protective and repair processes
to prevent or remove cross-linkage damage (Slater, 1972; Demopoulos,
1973a, b; Sheldrake, 1974).

Another important feature of the cross-linkage hypothesis is
the potential amplification effect of one cross-linkage being able
to inactivate two large macromolecules. For example, the irreversible cross-linkage of one or a few molecules to a chromosome may
be sufficient to completely inactivate a critical gene and to kill
the cell.

The cross-linkage hypothesis not only involves large molecules
but also includes the cross-linkage of small molecules to one
another or to macromolecules or cellular structures. The many
small molecules within a cell such as amino acids or nucleic acid
bases could, on activation, co-valently link to a large variety of
cellular constituents. Thus, the large number of different DNA
adducts found after irradiation are included as potential types of
damage which might accumulate as a function of increasing age
within an organism (Smith, 1975a, b).

The cross-linkage hypothesis of aging clearly has the potential of being an important primary aging process. The problem now
rests in determining the extent of their presence, their biological
significance, and the corresponding protective and repair processes
that may be involved. The approach taken in these investigations
will likely follow the path taken by radiation and photobiologists
in their study of the presence, biological significance and the
protection and repair processes of the cross-linkage damage formed
by radiation.

5.2. The Free Radical-Induced Cross-Linkage Reaction

The natural occurrence of free radicals within the cell is
considered to be an important source of cross-linking agents. In
this sense, the free radical and the cross-linkage hypotheses are
similar (Harman, 1956, 1962, 1969), the only difference being that
free radicals may cause other types of damage in addition to cross-
linking reactions. The free radical is defined as any chemical
species having an odd number of electrons and has a characteristic
high reactivity that can give rise to a wide variety of different
products. Although it has been difficult to determine the various
types of free radicals that may exist in a cell and their concentrations, it is now generally believed that their presence is in
sufficient quantity to warrant the serious consideration of harmful free radical side reactions (Pryor, 1970, 1971, 1973; Slater,
1972; Gordon, 1974).

Theoretically there are many ways by which free radicals could
be generated in a cell and an even larger number of possible reactions that could follow. Free radicals are known to be associated
with mitochondria and other energy-generating reactions present in
the cell (Packer *et al.*, 1967). However, these reactions are

fairly well contained or compartmentalized, and it is the "free" radical that is of most concern. The free radicals that are likely to be of the most damaging type are those free to diffuse throughout the cell. Many of these radicals are probably initiated by oxygen. For example, a wide variety of hydroperoxides can be formed by molecular-induced homolysis:

$$R-H + O_2 \rightarrow R \cdot + HOO \cdot$$

These reactions can be catalyzed by metals such as copper. Redox reactions of the peroxides also produce free radicals, as:

$$Fe^{++} + ROOH \rightarrow Fe^{+++} + RO \cdot + HO^-$$

where the presence of transition metals is important in catalyzing their decomposition.

5.3. Lipid Peroxidation

Free radicals are able to induce a chemical reaction in unsaturated fatty acids known as lipid peroxidation. The importance of this reaction is in the destruction of normal biological structures in the cell whose function depends on the presence of unsaturated lipids and in the generation of the long-lived radical products which can initiate cross-linkage reactions (Barber and Bernheim, 1967; Dormandy, 1969; Kawashima, 1970; Tappel, 1965, 1972, 1973; Slater, 1972). In addition, malonaldehyde, which is produced as a by-product of lipid peroxidation, might also be an important cross-linkage reagent. Chio and Tappel (1969a, b) have shown the inactivation of several enzymes by this reagent.

Evidence for the lipid peroxidation reaction has been obtained from the detection of fluorescent products (Strehler, 1964; Chio and Tappel, 1969a, b; Zeman, 1971; Tappel et al., 1973; Adhikari and Tappel, 1975) and by the thiobarbituric acid test (TBA) (Barber and Bernheim, 1967). Strong support for in vivo lipid peroxidation has recently been obtained from the detection of conjugated diens (di Luzio, 1973) and malonaldehyde (Tappel, 1973). In addition, ethane evolution in whole animals has been indirectly correlated with lipid peroxidation occurring in vivo (Riely et al., 1974). There is therefore good evidence now that lipid peroxidation does occur in vivo, although this conclusion in the past had been quite controversial (Green, 1972; Lucy, 1972). The combination of oxygen, metals and unsaturated fatty acids, which are common constituents in a cell, has emerged as a primary source for free radical production. These free radicals could then lead to damaging cross-linking reactions.

5.4. Free Radical Pathology

A number of specific disease processes have recently been
associated with the occurrence of free radicals (Slater, 1972;
Demopoulos, 1973a, b). For example, age-dependent loss of muscle
strength (Kaldor and Min, 1975), liver injury (di Luzio, 1973),
and the Batten-Vogt syndrome (Zeman, 1971) have been associated
with the possible occurrence of free radical damage. In addition,
high reactivity of membranes containing unsaturated fatty acids are
likely to generate a complex dysfunctional state of the cell and
organism (Packer *et al.*, 1967; Sheldrake, 1974) where changes in
membrane structure of the cell would affect a cell's ability to
react properly to hormone stimulation (Roth and Adelman, 1973).
This idea is supported by the age-dependent alteration in hormone-
induced enzymes and DNA synthesis (Adelman, 1972) and by the alteration of glucocortical binding to membranes (Roth and Adelman, 1973;
Roth, 1974, 1975).

5.5. Cross-Linkage of Collagen

The early work of Verzar (1963) indicated that certain types
of collagen are probably becoming more cross-linked with increasing
age in a number of different animal species. These results have
stimulated considerable interest and research to investigate the
possible biological role collagen cross-linkage may play in the
aging process (Kohn, 1963, 1971a; Hall, 1968, 1969; Bailey, 1969;
Bailey *et al.*, 1974; Vogel, 1973; Tanzer, 1973). From these
studies, a number of serious questions have been raised concerning
the biological significance of collagen cross-linkage to aging
(Jackson, 1973). One of the major criticisms is that there is
little evidence of any significant physico-chemical changes in
collagen in the aging phase of the lifespan. Most of the changes
appear to take place during development and maturation, and these
changes are thought to be essential for proper function of the
tissues. This criticism is further supported by the apparent lack
of any correlation between the cross-linkage rate of collagen-
containing tissues and the aging rate of different mammalian species
(Takacs and Verzar, 1968; Deyl *et al.*, 1971). For example, animals
with different aging rates appear to have the same degree of cross-
linkage in collagen at the same chronological age. Further work
on this comparative approach to the study of collagen cross-linkage
needs to be done before it can be ruled out as not being biologically
significant to aging.

5.6. Control of Free Radical Reactions

The natural presence of potentially harmful cross-linking
agents in the cell suggests that a number of different protective

and/or repair processes related to the presence of the agent are likely to be found in the organism. This possibility has led to the investigation of natural processes which might have evolved to control free radical reactions. The separation or compartmentalization of critical structures that are sensitive to free radicals from the rest of the cell, such as the isolation of chromatin by the nuclear membrane or the separation of reactions generating free radicals such as in mitochondria, are possible examples of cellular morphology used for controlling harmful free radical reactions. Other types of control mechanisms involving membrane structure have also been proposed (Demopoulos, 1973a, b). Direct removal of free radical-generating agents, such as provided by superoxide dismutase in removing the superoxide radical, may also serve as an important mechanism for the control of free radicals in the cell (Yamanaka and Deamer, 1974). Other types of chemical control of free radicals that may be operating in an organism are metal chelators, antioxidants and free radical scavengers.

A number of chemical agents involving the possible protective and/or control of free radicals have been used to study their effects on the aging processes (Tappel, 1965, 1968; Tappel *et al.*, 1973; Harman, 1969; Bender *et al.*, 1970; Kohn, 1971b; Epstein and Gershon, 1972; Milvy, 1973; Comfort, 1974). One of the most widely studied agents used is vitamin E. The biological role of vitamin E has not yet been established (Green, 1972), but because of its known antioxidant properties it has been suggested to be an important natural antioxidant agent by protecting unsaturated lipids from peroxidation and by terminating the propagation reaction of free radicals during lipid peroxidation (Tappel, 1972; Nair and Kayden, 1972; Hoffer and Roy, 1975). Substantial lifespan extension has been reported with vitamin E in nematodes (Epstein and Gershon, 1972) and in human tissue culture cells (Packer and Smith, 1974). However, it is interesting that prevention of malignant transformation in mammalian cells during prolonged culture *in vitro* can be accomplished by introducing a higher oxygen tension in the culture medium by the addition of 1% oxyhemoglobin and not by removing oxygen (Goldblatt and Freedman, 1974).

The extension of lifespan by other antioxidants or free radical scavengers in laboratory animals has also been reported (Harman, 1961, 1968, 1969, 1971, 1972a, b; Comfort, 1974), but in many cases no change has been found (Kohn, 1971b). In addition, a number of different free radical inhibitors and antioxidants (including vitamin E), when fed to mice, were found not to affect the age-dependent rate of increase of chromosomal aberration frequency in liver (Harman *et al.*, 1970). Many studies on the effects of antioxidants on the lifespan of an animal have been complicated by (1) the necessity to differentiate between lifespan extension produced by the drug and by calorie-restricted feeding (Ross, 1961), where some antioxidants have been shown to substantially

reduce food intake and (2) by the possible prevention of accumulation of toxic products in food due to the presence of antioxidants.
It is also necessary to differentiate between an extension of the
50% mean lifespan, which seems to appear more frequently in these
studies, from an extension of maximum lifespan or a decrease in
aging rate, which is of more biological significance. One of the
more impressive studies in this respect is the increase in maximum
lifespan of mice obtained by the continuous feeding of 0.5% W/W
ethoxyquin in their diet (Comfort, 1974). This result is shown in
Fig. 7. The agent is an antioxidant and increased maximum lifespan
by 15-20%. Little change in weight was evident compared to controls,
so the possible effects of restricted-calorie diet appears small.

On evaluating the overall results obtained by antioxidant and
free radical scavenger feeding of animals, it appears that some bene-
fit is being achieved in terms of prevention of disease and general
extension of lifespan. These results strongly support the presence
of naturally-occurring cross-linking reactions in the cell which are
importantly related to the aging process.

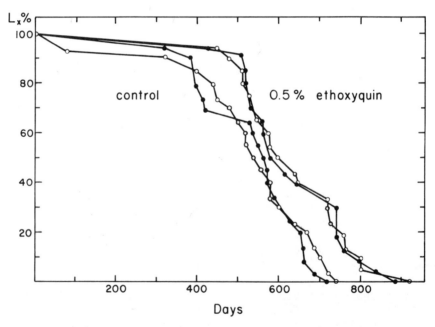

Fig. 7. Effect of the antioxidant, ethoxyquin, on the survival
of C3H mice. Mice were fed *ad libitum* their normal diet with 0.5%
ethoxyquin (W/W). Maximum lifespan of controls are 711 days for males
($\bullet$) and 722 days for females (o); for ethoxyquin-fed mice, 887 days
for males ($\bullet$) and 907 days for females (o). This represents a 25%
increase in maximum lifespan (Redrawn from Comfort, 1974).

6. RADIATION-INDUCED ALTERATION OF MAMMALIAN CHROMATIN

Support for the presence and biological importance of naturally-occurring cross-linking reactions in an organism to age-related pathology has been (1) the presence of naturally-occurring cross-linking agents in the cell; most studies have been concerned with free radicals, but it should be clear that other chemical cross-linking agents also exist in the cell which are normal by-products of metabolism (e.g., aldehydes) or activated metabolites (Heidelberger, This Volume), (2) the presence of free radicals that are propagated by lipid peroxidation, (3) the correlation between the presence of free radical reactions and a number of pathological conditions such as liver injury and the degeneration of muscle tissue, and (4) the extension of general health and lifespan by the feeding of antioxidants and/or free radical inhibitors to animals or to cells in a tissue culture. With this information as a background, we now turn our attention to what structure(s) in the organism may be the most sensitive target to cross-linking.

Although cross-linkage of collagen does occur with increasing age, it appears that this change may not be of biological significance to the organism. In addition, the cross-linkage of cellular constituents that are consistantly turning over, as in membranes and mitochondria, would not be expected to be as significant as in structures showing less turnover. Cross-linking reactions are also probably involved with the accumulation of age-pigments in the cell (Strehler, 1964). These age-pigments appear to have little biological significance and probably reflect the more general occurrence of cross-linking reactions taking place in the cell which are not visible.

A target which could potentially be very sensitive to cross-linkage is chromatin, particularly in postmitotic cells. For some time chromatin has been considered an important target for radiation. The normal continuous production of free radicals in a cell, plus other types of cross-linking agents, could result in producing similar damage and biological effects as a continuous low-energy radiation exposure. Because of this analogy, it is of interest to review what has been found to be the primary target in irradiated cells and the type of damage produced.

Radiation-induced DNA adducts in the genome of prokaryotic cells and chromatin adducts in eukaryotic cells have been suggested (Smith, 1975a) by the correlation found between increased radiation dosage and (1) reduced extractability of protein-free DNA, (2) altered template capacity of chromatin, and (3) the identification of specific DNA adducts. The biological significance of these DNA adducts is indicated by a correlation found between cell killing efficiency and the amount of DNA adducts formed. Thus, an important target in radiation killing of cells appears to be the chromatin

of the cell, and an important type of damage is the chromatin adduct.
Some of the major data supporting these conclusions for mammalian
cells will be briefly reviewed for their comparison to natural age-
related changes in chromatin (See also Todd and Han, This Volume;
Yamamoto, This Volume).

6.1. Extractability of DNA from Chromatin

Habazin and Han (1970), using UV irradiated Hela cells, found
a decrease in extractability of DNA from chromatin with increased
dosage. This effect was twice as large at 0° as at 22°C. At 22°C,
with a dosage of 50 ergs/mm^2, approximately 5% of the DNA was found
to be associated with cross-linked DNA-protein complexes but only
0.1% of the thymine was converted to thymine dimers. This difference in yield of cross-linked DNA-to-thymine dimers suggests that
DNA adduct formation may be the more important radiation-induced
lethal lesion in the cell under these conditions. When synchronized
Hela cells were irradiated with UV light, the extractability of
DNA was found to decrease significantly during the S-phase of the
cell cycle (Han *et al.*, 1975). During the S-phase about 22% of
the DNA was found to be associated with DNA-protein complexes after
an exposure of 250 ergs/mm^2. The S-phase of the cell cycle is also
known to be the most sensitive to cell killing.

Whole-body gamma-radiation of rats decreases the amount of
extractable DNA from liver with increasing dosage (Ivannik and
Ryabchenko, 1969) and *in vitro*-radiation of chromatin preparations
of calf thymus with either UV or gamma-radiation also results in a
decrease in extractability of DNA with increasing dosage (Sklobovskaya and Ryabchenko, 1970). UV irradiation of kidney cells in
tissue cultures containing 5-bromouracil was also found to decrease
the amount of extractable DNA, as compared to DNA not containing
this analogue. This result correlates with the increased killing
of the cells found when the DNA contains 5-bromouracil (Smets and
Cornelis, 1971).

6.2. Template Capacity of Chromatin and DNA

Weiss and Wheeler (1964) found that gamma-irradiation of calf
thymus chromatin *in vitro* altered its template capacity. They
found a decrease in template capacity on increasing dosage (up to
24 krads), followed by an increase in template capacity back up to
the control value (at 30 krads) and on to 130% of the control value
at 72 krads. Pure DNA, however, showed a continuous decrease in
template capacity on increased radiation dosage. A continuous
decrease in template capacity was also found for pure DNA with
increasing dosage of X-rays (Zimmerman *et al.*, 1964). In contrast
to the biphasic template capacity found by Weiss and Wheeler for

the *in vitro*-radiated chromatin, Lloyd *et al.* (1967) reported a continuous decrease in template capacity with increasing amounts of gamma-radiation.

A study of template capacity after *in vivo*-irradiation was made by Zimmerman *et al.* (1972) with guinea pig skin cells. They found evidence for an increased fraction of stable DNA-protein adducts and a general decrease in template capacity with increased radiation dosage. The presence of calcium ions appears to be an important factor in the changes observed in template capacity of chromatin after radiation. Yoshii *et al.* (1974) reported that, with increasing exposures of chromatin *in vitro* without Ca^{++} to radiation, an initial increase was found, followed by a decrease, in template capacity. However, in the presence of Ca^{++}, the initial increase was much less, and the general repression of template capacity was enhanced.

The decrease in template capacity obtained with the *in vitro*-irradiation of protein-free DNA preparations (Weiss and Wheeler, 1964; Zimmerman *et al.*, 1964; Hagen *et al.*, 1969, 1970) appears to be the result of a decrease in size of the RNA synthesized, with the number of initiating sites for RNA polymerase remaining constant (Hagen *et al.*, 1969, 1970). The changes observed in irradiated chromatin are more complex and are likely to involve both a decrease in RNA size and a mixture of repression and derepression of protein-covered DNA (Umansky *et al.*, 1974).

The cross-linkage of histones to DNA in *in vitro*-radiation of chromatin has been reported (Schott and Shetlar, 1974), indicating that the lysine and arginine residues of the histones are reactive. Another amino acid found to cross-link with DNA is tryptophan (Schott and Shetlar, 1974; Smith, 1975a), and it is interesting that this amino acid is absent from the histone proteins. This might be another example of a protective process which has evolved to minimize cross-linking reactions in chromatin.

It is also of interest to consider the possible importance played by the histones in protecting DNA from cross-linkage agents. For example, Roti *et al.* (1974) have found that chromosomal proteins effectively protect the thymine residues from indirect effects of radiation (e.g., by OH· radicals formed by water radiolysis). However, some areas of the chromatin appear to have stretches of uncovered DNA, and it may be these areas that are most reactive to cross-linkage formations with neighboring proteins or other constituents in the environment of the cell chromatin.

Oxygen has also been reported to affect chromatin template capacity without radiation exposure. Harman (1967) has reported that chromatin in an oxygen-saturated solution showed a decrease in template capacity of from 15 to 50%, compared to a similar chromatin preparation in a nitrogen-saturated solution.

In summary, it appears that chromatin irradiated with UV or ionizing radiation *in vivo* or *in vitro* accumulates protein and other DNA adducts. These DNA adducts decrease the extractability of DNA and alter template capacity. The major effect on template capacity appears to be a general repression of template capacity, accompanied by a decrease in length of the RNA molecules being synthesized. The increase in the amount of cross-linkage of chromatin occurring during the S-phase of the cell division cycle correlates well with increased killing of the cells and strongly suggests that the DNA adducts formed are of biological significance, perhaps more than the formation of thymine dimers. The apparent slow removal of DNA adducts after radiation also suggests the importance of this type of damage to the cell.

If similar alterations of chromatin are occurring in non-irradiated cells by the free radicals or other cross-linking agents that are natural by-products of metabolism, then the same processes effective in repairing radiation-induced damage would be expected to be equally effective in repairing non-radiation-produced damage. This idea has received support by the correlation found between aging rate and the extent of UV repair (Hart and Setlow, 1974); and it may be that the major role played by the DNA repair process is in the removal of damage produced by internal and not external agents (Burnet, 1974; Yielding, 1974; Hart and Trosko, 1975; Trosko and Hart, 1975; Hart, This Volume).

7. AGE-INDUCED ALTERATION OF MAMMALIAN CHROMATIN

An investigation designed to detect the presence and possible biological significance of DNA adducts in chromatin as a function of age has not yet been reported. However, a number of studies have been reported on the age-dependent changes in the physico-chemical, template capacity, and transcription properties of chromatin which may be related to the accumulation of DNA adducts.

7.1. Chromosomal Aberration Frequencies

A well-known age-dependent observation is the increased frequency of abnormal births with the increasing age of the mother (Miner, 1954). Some of the most studied cases are those associated with Down's syndrome (Penrose, 1954). This and many similar genetic diseases are related to an abnormal number of chromosomes in the cell or to some type of chromosomal aberration. The age-dependent frequency of these diseases suggests that irreversible damage has been accumulating in the chromosomes of the ova.

A significant age dependent increase in chromosomal aberrations has been found in liver cells of mouse, hamster, guinea pig and dog (Crowley and Curtis, 1963; Curtis et al., 1966; Curtis and Miller, 1971; Brooks et al., 1973). A very interesting aspect of these studies is that the rate of increase in chromosomal aberration frequency is nearly proportional to the aging rate of the animal. Although it is not known why there is an increased frequency of birth defects and/or chromosomal aberration frequencies with increased age of the mother, these results strongly suggest that some type of age-dependent chromosomal alteration is occurring. The correlation of radiation damage with chromosomal aberration frequency suggests that formation of cross-linkages may be involved (Bender et al., 1974).

7.2.   Changes in DNA

An age-dependent increase in the number of DNA breaks per genome has been reported in rats by Massie et al. (1972), using a viscosity technique to detect changes in DNA molecular weight. Modak and Price (1971) and Price et al. (1971) have detected an increase in DNA breaks with increased age in mice by determining the number of free DNA ends available in situ for priming DNA synthesis. The size of DNA from the internal granular layer of neurons in the cerebellum (a fully-differentiated non-dividing population of cells) was determined by alkaline sucrose density gradient sedimentation analysis in Beagle dogs as a function of age (Wheeler and Lett, 1974). They also found evidence for a decrease in size of the extracted DNA as a function of increasing age.

The increase in DNA breaks might be related to direct action of free radicals or even to the thermohydrolysis of DNA phospho-diester bonds (Eigner et al., 1961). The absence of repair of these breaks may be due to interference caused by cross-linked protein. It could also be due to an age-related decrease in repair enzymes (Epstein et al., 1973), but this was not found by Wheeler and Lett (1974). Although these results suggest that an actual increase in number of DNA breaks occurs with increasing age, other interpretations of the data are possible. More extensive studies using the advanced techniques recently developed by radiation biol- ogists for detecting breaks in DNA (as illustrated by the Wheeler and Lett investigation) need to be conducted.

Modification of DNA may be involved in the programming of gene expression, and some interesting models have recently been proposed on how this might be accomplished (Holliday and Pugh, 1975). It is of interest in this respect that the amount of 5-methylcytosine in DNA has been found to vary between the different tissues of the rat and to change significantly on hormone administration (Vanyushin

et al., 1973). Moreover, the amount of 5-methylcytosine in the DNA
of brain, heart, and spleen was found to decrease throughout the
lifespan of the rat, including the aging phase. Thus, even after
sexual maturation, where most developmental and other processes
are apparently complete, the modification of DNA is still taking
place. This result raises the possibility that such post-develop-
mental changes in DNA might be caused by an alteration of the
chromatin and/or by an alteration of the normal DNA modification
enzymes. An observation that may be related to such an age-dependent alteration of chromatin is that the replication rate of DNA
apparently decreases with increasing passage number of WI-38 cells
(Petes *et al.*, 1974). The presence of DNA-protein cross-links in
chromatin might be related to these results.

7.3. Changes in Chromatin Proteins

A number of studies have been reported on the physicochemical
properties of chromatin protein as a function of age (von Hahn,
1970a, b; Price and Makinodan, 1973). Unfortunately, most of these
studies used different methods, tissues, and animals and as a result
there is little agreement as to what if any changes exist. O'Meara
and Herrmann (1972) reported an increase in the amount of histones,
a decrease in the amount of non-histones and an overall slight
increase in total chromatin proteins in mouse liver with increasing
age. Pyhtila and Sherman (1968a, b) also found a small increase
in total chromatin proteins in calf thymus tissue with increasing
age and a decrease in the amount of the F_3 histone (III) component.
Von Hahn *et al.* (1969) found a decreasing ratio of histone proteins, $F_3 + F_{2a1} + F_{2a2}/F_1 + F_{2b}$, with increasing age in rat liver.
However, Zhelabovskaya and Berdyshev (1972) found that the amount
of histone proteins remained constant, the amount of non-histone
proteins decreased, and that the total chromatin proteins decreased
as a function of age for rat liver. And a recent and careful study
by Carter and Chae (1975), using the urea high-resolution polyacrylamide gel electrophoresis system of Panyim and Chalkley (1969),
found no apparent age-related change in the proportion of any histone fraction of mouse and rat liver chromatin.

The chromatin proteins also appear to be undergoing some
chemical modification as a function of age. Ryan and Cristofalo
(1972) have reported a decrease in the rate of histone acetylation
with increasing passage number in WI-38 cells. In contrast to
this *in vitro* aging tissue culture study, Liew and Gornall (1975)
have reported a higher rate of acetylation of liver nuclear proteins of mice with increasing age but no difference in the rate of
phosphorylation. These studies further showed that the F_3 histone
protein was acetylated at a rate of 129% and the F_{2a1} histone protein to 112% of the value found for young mice. Acetylation of
phenol-soluble nuclear acidic proteins was also found to increase

to 250% and phosphorylation to 138%, as compared to young mice, as
a function of increasing age.

These age-related modifications of chromatin protein could
confuse a study designed to detect DNA adducts using the methods
of extractability, thermal stability, and template capacity measurements. The biological significance of such chromatin modifications
is not known and could reflect a more general alteration accumulating in the chromatin.

7.4. Extractability of Chromatin Proteins

Early evidence for the formation of DNA-protein cross-links
in cells after exposure to radiation was the decrease found in the
extractability of protein-free DNA (Smith, 1975a). On reviewing
the literature on the extractability of DNA in non-irradiated
mammalian cells, a similar decrease in extractability of protein-
free DNA was found to occur as a function of increasing age of the
animal.

During the early developmental stages of DNA extraction procedures, there always appeared to be a certain fraction of residue
protein in the DNA preparation that proved impossible to remove
completely. Using rat liver from undefined age animals, Kirby
(1958, 1967) showed that the amount of residue protein depended
upon the type and amount of salt used during the extraction procedure. He found that p-aminosalicylate, which has the ability to
complex with metals in addition to interacting with protein,
was the most successful in reducing the amount of residue protein
from several percent to only a few tenths of a percent of protein.
Leveson and Peacocke (1966) also reported that the amount of residue protein in rat liver (also from animals of unidentified age)
could be further reduced to a few tenths of a percent by the use
of mixtures of p-aminosalicylate, 2 M NaCl, and 4 M urea. These
results suggest that various types of bonds are involved within
the residue protein, such as chelation, electrostatic, hydrophobic,
and hydrogen bonding, and that covalent bonds were not involved for
most of the residue proteins. However, in all of these studies
there was still left a small fraction (0.1-0.5%) of residue protein
after these extensive deproteinization procedures.

Utilizing the Kirby extraction procedure (with p-aminosalicylate
and phenol) Salser and Balis (1967) investigated the amino acid
composition of the residue protein complex as a function of different growth conditions in bacteria (Salser and Balis, 1969), in
tumors (Salser and Balis, 1968), and as a function of age and sex
(Salser and Balis, 1972). In their age-related studies they
investigated the amino acid residue composition (in terms of acid,
neutral and basic amino acids) in liver, kidney, spleen, and

intestine of rats over an age-range of from early weanlings to 30 months. Their results showed a unique distribution of residue amino acids as a function of tissue and age. There was no apparent general pattern in the total amount of acid, neutral, or basic amino acids as a function of age. A significant increase in neutral amino acids and a decrease in acid and basic amino acids were found as a function of increased age in liver; but kidney, spleen and intestine showed different patterns of change. These results indicate that different cells may develop different mechanisms and/or responses to the aging process that are reflected by the changes in the amino acid composition of the residue proteins in the DNA of the chromatin. Although the amino acids may be cross-linked to DNA, there is clearly no general increase in this type of DNA adduct with increasing age.

A decrease in the extractability of chromatin proteins as a function of increasing age of an animal has been found. Such changes can apparently occur at an early age, as indicated by the study of Bojanovic *et al.* (1970) where histones were found to be more difficult to extract from rat thymus chromatin with 50 mM HCl as age increased from 10 to 75 days. A further decrease in extractability was found in much older animals. Amici *et al.* (1974) reported a continuous decrease in the amount of extractable hepatic DNA from rats between ages 2-24 months. A decrease in extractability of chromatin proteins with increasing ionic strength of salt as a function of increasing age has also been reported. O'Meara and Herrmann (1972) determined the amount of chromatin protein removed from mouse liver chromatin as a function of increasing age by NaCl extraction in solutions varying from 0.01 M to 2.0 M. These results are shown in Fig. 8 and indicate that higher ionic strengths of NaCl were required for the older chromatin preparations to remove the same amount of chromatin proteins.

A more detailed study of the age-dependent extractability of chromatin protein with increasing salt concentrations was made by Berdyshev and Zhelabovskaya (1972) with rat liver. These data are shown in Table 3 for histones and Table 4 for non-histone proteins. The histone proteins are clearly seen to be more resistant to salt extraction in the older chromatin preparations. It is also important to note that at 2.5 M NaCl, the oldest chromatin preparation (30 months) still has a 0.048% residue of protein; whereas in the younger groups no detectable residue of protein was found. The age-dependent salt extractability for the non-histones is more complicated. For the histones at zero molar salt extraction, approximately equal amounts of histones for all age-groups were found; but for the non-histones at zero molar salt, a reduction in amount of non-histones was found with increasing age. The non-histones that do remain on the older chromatin preparation, however, are more resistant to further salt extraction at higher ionic strength.

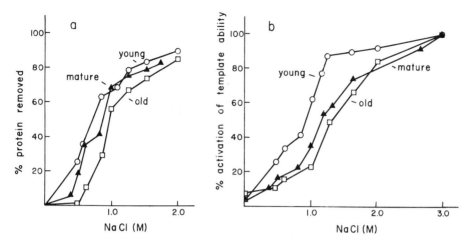

Fig. 8.   Extractability of protein from chromatin as a function of age and NaCl concentration in C57BL/6 mouse liver. (a)
percent total chromatin protein removed, (b) percent activation of
template activity (Redrawn from O'Meara and Herrmann, 1972).

7.5.   Thermal Stability of Chromatin

Thermal stability of chromatin is a sensitive measurement for
many different types of structural changes (Ansevin and Brown,
1971; Ansevin *et al.*, 1971; Li and Bonner, 1971; Li *et al.*, 1973;
Wilhelm *et al.*, 1974) and has been used to detect possible age-
dependent alterations. A general review of the early work on the
age-dependent changes in thermal stability of chromatin was made
by von Hahn (1970a, b). Most of these early studies were made on
cow thymus between ages 8 weeks and 10 years. It is therefore
important to note that the maximum lifespan of the cow, *Bos taurus*,
is about 30 years. These studies may then represent developmental
changes. However, it is also possible to argue that the thymus
gland ages unusually rapidly compared to the rest of the animal.

Thymus chromatin preparations from young calf (8 weeks) and
cow (10 years) were extracted and purified, giving DNA preparations
with about 2% residue protein (von Hahn, 1963, 1964; Pyhtila and
Sherman, 1968a, b). In a low ionic strength solution (0.0025 M
$NaNO_3$), the older DNA preparations gave a 3°C higher thermal
stability. No difference in thermal stability was found at higher
ionic strength solutions (0.01 M $NaNO_3$) or when the amount of
residue protein was lowered to about 0.3%.

DNA preparations from rat liver of ages 3 to 26 months gave a
similar age-dependent increase in thermal stability (von Hahn and

Table 3. Amount of Histone Protein Removed from Liver Chromatin as a Function of Age and Deproteinization by NaCl Solutions (Adapted from Zhelabovskaya and Berdyshev, 1972)

Conc. NaCl (M)	1 month		3 months		12 months		30 months	
	Histones DNA	% histone eliminated	Histones DNA	% histone eliminated	Histones DNA	% histone eliminated	Histones DNA	% histone eliminated
0	1.120	0	1.100	0	1.122	0	1.138	0
0.6	0.600	16	0.564	22	0.550	23	0.578	23
1.25	0.176	13	0.190	11	0.174	11	0.291	3
2.5	0.000	0	0.000	0	0.000	0	0.048	6

Table 4. Amount of Acidic Protein Removed from Liver Chromatin as a Function of Age and Deproteinization by NaCl Solutions (Adapted from Zhelabovskaya and Berdyshev, 1972)

Conc. NaCl (M)	1 month		3 months		12 months		30 months	
	Acid proteins DNA	% acid protein eliminated	Acid proteins DNA	% acid protein eliminated	Acid proteins DNA	% acid protein eliminated	Acid proteins DNA	% acid protein eliminated
0	0.780	0	0.600	0	0.522	0	0.400	0
0.6	0.350	20	0.330	11	0.317	9	0.253	10
1.25	0.328	1	0.320	0	0.300	1	0.244	0
2.5	0.180	7	0.176	5	0.190	5	0.217	0

Fritz, 1966). In preparations with about 1 to 1.5% residue protein, an increase in thermal stability of 8°C was found in a solution of 0.0025 M NaCl. As before, no change in thermal stability was found in a solution of 0.01 or 0.9 M NaCl. Thermal stability of DNA preparations from livers of 2 month and 10 month old mice in 0.005 M NaCl solution were studied by Russell *et al.* (1970). DNA prepared by the Marmur method showed no difference in thermal stability between young and old mice. This DNA contained about 3% protein for both ages. However, DNA extracted by the Kay-Simons-Dounce method, which contained about 9% protein for both ages, showed both an increased thermal stability and a decreased percent hyperchromicity for the old DNA preparation.

The age-dependent thermal stability studies of whole chromatin preparations from mouse brain by Kurtz and Sinex (1967) and Kurtz *et al.* (1974) show both possible developmental and aging components. These results are shown in Fig. 9. In these studies (in contrast to the work reported by von Hahn and other workers) whole chromatin preparations were used, not DNA containing resistant proteins which was obtained after a certain type of purification procedure. Thermal stability was measured in a solution of 0.0025 M NaCl and was found to steadily decline from about 80° to 72°C during the first year of life of the mouse. This change corresponds to a decrease in protein-to-DNA ratio or percent protein. However, after one year of age, thermal stability is found to increase, reaching a value of 82.4°C at 30 months of age. Again, this increase corresponds to a similar increase in the protein-to-DNA ratio or total percent protein found in the chromatin preparation. These data indicate the importance of considering the age of an animal when any study of chromatin is being made.

There is no clear explanation for this age-dependent biphasic change in the amount of chromatin proteins and the corresponding change in thermal stability. However, the change seen up to one year of age may be related to a changing cell population in the brain, such as in the ratio of neuron-to-glia cells (Timeras, 1972; Vernadakis, 1975) or to changes in genetic expression of the cells in mouse brain during this period. On the other hand, the increase in thermal stability occurring during the latter stages of life is more likely to represent a non-developmental aging-type of change that may involve cross-linkage.

A similar biphasic change as a function of age in rat brain chromatin protein has been reported by Biessmann and Rajewsky (1975). Measuring total protein content of chromatin, they found a value of 2.15 ±0.22 mg protein/mg DNA for fetal brain (18th day of gestation), which increased to 2.8 ±0.24 at age 10 days and then decreased to 2.16 ±0.23 for the mature adult. They also found a decrease in total protein content of rat liver chromatin

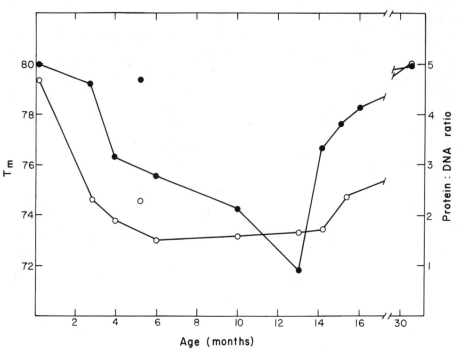

Fig. 9. Thermal stability of whole chromatin preparations from mouse brain (C57BL/6) as a function of age. Tm (●) and protein:DNA ratio (W/W) (o) (Redrawn from Kurtz and Sinex, 1967).

from a value of 2.18 ±0.10 for 10-day old to 1.81 ±0.27 for the adult. Because histone content of the chromatin is not expected to change as a function of age, the higher protein content of brain chromatin is thought to correspond to an increase in template activity (Grouse *et al.*, 1972). For liver, this would correspond to a general repression in transcription activity after the age of 10 days. Significant quantitative and qualitative differences were also observed in the non-histone banding patterns on urea polyacrylamide gel electrophoresis as a function of age.

Berdyshev and Zhelabovskaya (1972) have found an increase in thermal stability of whole chromatin as a function of increased age in the liver of rats. These results are shown in Table 5. Thermal stability was measured as a function of increasing ionic strength for two ages (1 and 30 months). An increase of 14°C was found in the thermal stability for the older animal chromatin preparation in zero ionic strength solution. This difference decreased to 7°C at 2.5 M NaCl, where only a few percent of residue non-histone remain on the DNA.

Table 5. Melting Temperature of Liver Chromatin from Young and
Old Rats as a Function of Deproteinization by NaCl Solutions
(Adapted from Berdyshev and Zhelabovskaya, 1972)

Conc. NaCl (M)	T_m, °C	
	1 month	30 months
0	70	84
0.6	62	76
1.25	52	67
2.5	51	58

From these studies it appears that for chromatin preparations
from mammals in general, a decrease in extractability of chromatin
proteins and an increase in thermal stability occur with increasing
age. It is therefore of importance to observe if similar chromatin
changes are found in the *in vitro* aging of cells. Thermal stabilities of purified DNA and whole chromatin preparations of human
WI-38 cells in 0.0025 M salt solutions were studied by Comings and
Vance (1971) as a function of passage number. They found no
detectable change in the thermal stabilities of either the DNA or
chromatin. This indicates that the mechanism of *in vitro* aging
may be fundamentally different from normal *in vivo* cellular aging
processes.

It is also of interest to note the effect of 5-bromouracil
(BrUra)-substituted DNA on the thermal stability of chromatin. In
mammalian cells, BrUra substitution is known to affect states of
differentiation and to increase sensitivity of the cells to UV
radiation (Smith, 1975a). David *et al.* (1974) have reported that
replacement of thymine by BrUra in DNA leads to an increase in
thermal stability of chromatin from hepatoma tissue culture cells
or from embryonic rat pancreatic tissue culture cells without
radiation exposure. These results suggest that regulatory proteins may have an increase in binding affinity to BrUra-DNA and,
as such, may increase the probability for the formation of DNA
cross-linkage. Tighter binding or cross-linking of chromatin
proteins may therefore lead to alterations in the differentiated
state of the cell, which is similar to many age-dependent cellular
changes.

7.6. Template Capacity of Chromatin

Chromatin template capacity is a measurement of the rate of RNA synthesis obtained under saturation conditions of RNA polymerase using chromatin as the source of template. Usually, a non-homologous RNA polymerase is used, such as from *E. coli*. The measurement is thought to reflect the accessibility of the DNA to the RNA polymerase and therefore the amount and degree of binding of chromatin proteins. A review of the earlier work on chromatin template capacity as a function of age has been made by von Hahn (1970a, b), Price and Makinodan (1973), and Stein and Stein (1975). A number of different methods, tissues, and animals were used. Unfortunately, as with the thermal stability measurements, this results in some conflict as to what the age-dependent changes are (if any) in chromatin template capacity.

Pyhtila and Sherman (1968a, b) measured chromatin template capacity of chromatin extracted from beef thymus of ages 8 weeks and over 10 years and found a 25% decrease in the older chromatin preparation but no age-dependent change with the purified DNA preparations. These results correspond to an increase in thermal stability of the older chromatin preparations.

A more detailed study of chromatin template capacity was reported by Berdyshev and Zhelabovskaya (1972) for rat liver. The results of this study are shown in Table 6. At a zero molar concentration of NaCl, a significant age-related decrease in template capacity was found. The lower value found for the older chromatin is maintained with increasing molarity of NaCl until the two preparations become equal at 2.5 M NaCl. This result is similar to the lower template capacity found for mouse liver preparations at increasing ionic strength (see Fig. 8) reported by O'Meara and Herrmann (1972).

Table 6. Liver Chromatin Template Capacity in Rats as A Function of Age and Deproteinization by NaCl Solutions (Adapted from Berdyshev and Zhelabovskaya, 1972)

Conc. NaCl (M)	Template Activity			
	1 month	2 months	12 months	30 months
0	14.4 ± 1.3	12.3 ± 0.9	12.0 ± 1.0	8.7 ± 1.4
0.6	42.0 ± 3.1	40.0 ± 2.9	39.4 ± 3.2	26.2 ± 2.5
1.25	90.6 ± 3.3	85.0 ± 3.2	85.0 ± 3.6	54.5 ± 3.8
2.5	100	100	100	100

Template activity in rat brain and liver chromatin as a function of age has been studied by Bondy and Roberts (1967, 1968,
1969, 1970) and Roberts (1973). In these studies, chromatin was
isolated from liver and different areas of the brain and template
activity measured. Areas of the brain were cerebral cortex,
cerebellum, thalamus-hypothalamus, hindbrain-medulla, as well as
the whole brain. The overall result from fetal (age 5 days pre-
natal) to adult (6 weeks) was a general repression of template
activity of about two-fold. These changes are probably developmental and represent an overall progressive restriction of RNA
synthesis from different areas of the chromatin in both liver and
brain tissues.

In contrast to these studies, Samis *et al.* (1968) and Samis
and Wulf (1969) found no change in template capacity of chromatin
in rat liver as a function of age (from 206 to 965 days of age).
In addition, they found no change in protein content of chromatin
as a function of age. Similarly, Shirey and Sobel (1972) found
no changes in the polyacrylamide gel electrophoresis patterns of
histone and non-histone proteins from the chromatin of heart
muscle of young, mature and old dogs. Moreover, they found no
change in the ratio of total chromatin protein-to-DNA and no
change in template capacity as a function of age.

Chromatin template capacity in rat submandibular gland and
liver in 2 and 12 month old rats were studied by Stein *et al.*
(1973). These results are of interest in showing that an increase
in template capacity of over two-fold was found for the submandibular gland with no significant change for liver. However, the
maximum lifespan of the rat is about 4 years, and it was therefore
not possible to differentiate between possible developmental and
aging changes.

Developmental patterns of template capacity could result in
either a repression or a derepression of activity, although a
repression would be expected for most phases of development until
sexual maturation is reached. A repression of the chromatin, where
the repressed state remains stable (as in postmitotic cells), might
result in an increased probability for cross-linkage to occur.
These cross links may further repress the genome and perhaps more
importantly prevent the derepression of needed genes which may be
required by the organism during stress, regeneration or healing
processes, or during serious illness.

Changes in chromatin template capacity were also investigated
in *in vitro*-aged tissue culture cells. Courtois (1974) studied
chromatin preparations from cultured chick fibroblast cells as a
function of passage number. Some differences were found in the
radioactivity labeling profiles of the histone and non-histone
proteins in polyacrylamide gel electrophoretic analysis, but

essentially no differences were found in the circular dichroism patterns or in template capacity of the chromatin as a function of passage number. Similarly, Stein and Stein (1975) have found no significant differences in template capacity of chromatin from both *in vitro* and *in vivo* transcription studies of human WI-38 cells as a function of passage number. These negative results, in addition to those reported by Comings and Vance (1971) on chromatin thermal stability and the poor correlation found between doubling capacity and the donor species' aging rate (Stanley *et al.*, 1975), further support the view that *in vitro*-aged tissue culture cells may age by a different mechanism, as compared to normal *in vivo*-aged postmitotic cells.

7.7. Qualitative Changes in Transcription Activity

A more sensitive measurement of genetic activity of chromatin than thermal stability or template capacity measurements is the determination of the percent of DNA being transcribed and of the qualitative changes that may occur in the population of RNA species being synthesized. These studies were made for both reiterated and unique DNA sequences in both brain and liver tissues as a function of age in mouse (Cutler, 1975d). Although similar results were obtained for both reiterated and unique DNA sequences, the results for unique DNA are considered more reliable because of the higher DNA/RNA hybridization specificities achieved. These results are shown in Table 7, showing the percent unique DNA transcribed. For liver, a general repression in the concentration of the number of different types of RNA sequences is found. This is shown by the percent hybridization decreasing from a value of about 8% in 15-day old embryos to about 4% at 746 days of age. This change is illustrated in Fig. 10 to point out that most of the repression occurs during the first 120 days of life. For brain, an early depression is found instead of an early repression. In this case, percent hybridization increases from 6.1% for 15-day old embryos to 12.2% for animals of 120 days of age. From this value, there is a steady decrease in percent hybridization, reaching about 6% in the oldest animals, which is approximately what was found in the embryonic brain.

In terms of the percent of DNA being transcribed, the derepression found for chromatin from mouse brain may be a developmental change similar to the derepression of template activity reported by Stein *et al.* (1973) for the submandibular gland. In addition, the biphasic change in percent hybridization corresponds closely to the biphasic change in thermal stability found in mouse brain that was reported by Kurtz and Sinex (1967) and Kurtz *et al.* (1974). The repression of liver chromatin during the first 120 days may also be mainly a developmental rather than an aging change. However, the general repression of genetic activity for both brain

Table 7. Percent Unique DNA Sequences Transcribed (From Cutler, 1975d)

Age (days)	Percent hybridization*		Percent transcription**		Thermal stability of hybrid (T_m °C)	
	Liver	Brain	Liver	Brain	Liver	Brain
Embryo (15 days)	8.0	6.1	26.7	20.4	80.5	79.1
48	6.3	7.7	21.0	25.6	82.1	81.6
120	5.1	12.2	17.0	40.6	81.0	82.3
550	4.3	8.6	14.3	28.8	79.8	82.7
746	3.6	6.0	12.0	20.0	79.3	82.1

*Percent hybridization is defined as maximum g RNA per g DNA × 10^2 capable of hybridization.
**Percent transcription is based on 60% DNA being unique and only one complementary DNA strand being transcribed.

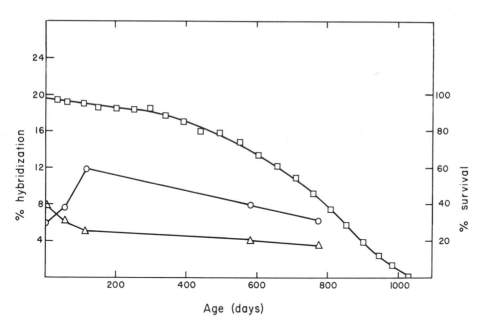

Fig. 10. Percent hybridization of unique DNA sequences using nuclear RNA extracted from liver (△) and brain (o) as a function of age of the C57BL/6 mouse. Assuming single-stranded DNA transcription, the percent transcription activity would be twice the values shown. Percent survival of mouse colony (□) is shown for reference (From Cutler, 1975d).

and liver tissues after maturation (120 days) may be a true aging
change. This repression correlates well with the findings of
Zhelabovskaya and Berdyshev (1972) in terms of an increased ratio
of histone-to- non-histone protein, an increase in thermal stability
of the chromatin, and a decrease in template capacity of the chromatin and may reflect an accumulation of cross-linkage in the chromatin.

The pattern and complexity of RNA sequences involved in the
age-related derepression and repression of chromatin was studied
by measuring the percent hybridization obtained after mixing equal
portions of RNA samples obtained from different tissues and/or ages.
Results of these experiments are shown in Table 8 and indicate that
the increase in percent hybridization represents the derepression
of different DNA sequences and not more of the same type. Similarly,
the decrease found in percent hybridization represents a repression
of the same sequences that were derepressed at an early age. There
is very little if any simultaneous derepression and repression of
different DNA sequences occurring after the age of 120 days.

An important feature of these studies is that the RNA species
used in these hybridization tests were synthesized *in vivo* and not
by *in vitro* transcription. This method has important advantages as
well as disadvantages. The major advantage is the avoidance of
possible artifacts characteristic of *in vitro* chromatin studies,
such as damage to the chromatin during preparation or the use of
non-homologous RNA polymerase. The disadvantage is in the possibility of selective loss of RNA sequences during extraction and purification. This may be caused by age-dependent changes in nuclease
activity or perhaps even more likely an age-dependent change in
nuclear membrane permeability to RNA. Therefore, additional confirmation of these results will be necessary using other methods,
as for example the use of different RNA extraction techniques or
the *in vitro* chromatin transcription technique.

Table 8. Resultant Percent Hybridization of Mixed RNA Samples to
Unique DNA Sequences (Adapted from Cutler, 1975d)

RNA mixture	Individual percent hybridization	Resultant percent hybridization
Liver: 48 day + 746 day	6.3 + 3.6	7.1
Brain: embryo (15 day) + 120 day	6.1 + 12.2	12.2
Brain: 120 day + 746 day	12.2 + 6.0	12.7
Liver + Brain: 48 day + 48 day	6.3 + 7.7	13.1
Liver + Brain: 746 day + 746 day	3.6 + 6.0	6.2

If these age-related changes are confirmed by further studies, they would have some interesting implications to the control of gene expression and to the possible functional role of the RNA being synthesized. For example, the general repression of the DNA in liver and the derepression of DNA in brain found to occur up to 120 days could be thought of as due to normal gene control mechanisms. The difficulty with this explanation is in the general magnitude found for the age-related change in genome expression. If these changes in percent hybridization correspond to changes in structural genes of an average molecular weight (1000 nucleotide pairs per gene), then 1% hybridization is equivalent to 27,500 genes (assuming only one strand of the DNA is transcribed). Thus, an increase in percent hybridization for the brain from 6.1 to 12.2% represents an increase of 6.1%, or the additional synthesis of 167,750 different proteins. This value could be lowered by half by assuming a 50% loss of RNA during the maturation of heterogeneous RNA to mRNA.

The increase in percent hybridization for brain may not all be represented in new proteins and could instead be involved only in RNA synthesis. The possible correlation of the increase in percent hybridization in brain with increased learning ability and/or memory is of interest. In this respect, the following decrease in percent hybridization may be related to the animal's mental decline in memory capacity and/or functions. However, this explanation cannot apply to liver, where a general repression from 8 to 3.6%, or a difference of about 4%, was found. This corresponds to a decrease in expression of about 110,000 genes. It is difficult to believe that the aging of the liver would correspond to a loss in function or expression of 100,000 different proteins, particularly when liver appears to be able to synthesize all the required proteins even in old age (Finch, 1969; Adelman, 1972).

7.8. Evolutionary RNA and Protein

One possible explanation for the ability of a tissue to remain essentially unchanged in biological function yet to undergo approximately a 50% repression of genetic activity is to predict that much of the DNA that is transcribed is not functional. If we assume that the mouse is not evolutionarily static, then the evolution of new proteins (either enzymatic, structural, or regulatory) requires the synthesis of at least some non-functional proteins to be "tried-out". Thus, in the same sense, where evolutionary DNA has been predicted to exist (Ohno, 1970; Britten and Davidson, 1971), it would also be necessary to predict the existance of evolutionary RNA and protein. If these genes are somehow repressed (as the result of some type of aging process), then no loss of function in the cell would result. The dramatic increase and decline of percent transcription in the brain and the steady decline of percent transcription in the liver might therefore represent, in part, the change in expression of these evolutionary DNA sequences. This process could be the result of a random repression, perhaps caused by increased cross-linkage of chromatin proteins. A few cells receiving a repression in critical genes would die, thus accounting for the observed loss of some liver and brain cells with increasing age. However, this fraction would be small if only about 0.5% of the genome were functional.

However, the genomes of different cells are transcribed to different degrees (all at extraordinarily high levels in relation to the number of gene equivalents), and brain cells have a percent transcription level which is approximately two to three-fold higher than most other mammalian cells. The overall rate of evolution of a certain function is likely to be proportional to the number of different possibilities that are "tried out" per unit time interval. Thus, if in the past a high evolutionary rate for the brain during evolution of the different mammalian species has proved advantageous (and there is evidence for this: Cutler, 1975b, c), then a more rapid evolution of the brain could be achieved over that of other tissues or organs by the derepression of most of the evolutionary DNA sequences in that organ. In this manner, evolutionary rate can be directed away from cell types that have proven best to remain stable and directed toward those cell types where changes in the past have proven most advantageous. In this model, natural selection operates on the derepression of selected areas of the chromatin in certain cells without prior evidence for the presence of a specific advantageous gene which may be expressed by this process in the mature individual.

8.   SUMMARY AND CONCLUSIONS

The processes of biological aging are known to follow a characteristic pattern in different mammalian species and to proceed at a rate inversely proportional to their maximum lifespan potential. These aging processes are known to result in a progressive loss of most physiological functions and in an increase in onset frequency of many diseases. However, almost nothing is known about the molecular basis or the genetic complexity of the aging process.

The genetic and biochemical complexities of the aging process are usually considered to be very large, yet relatively few aging processes might underlie many of the age-related diseases. Some of the age-related dysfunctions observed at the phenotypic level might be the result of complex processes, but having a common target or mechanism of action. These common targets or mechanisms of action could then be subject to less complex controls or "aging rate pace-setters" which are able to govern their rate of expression. This idea is represented by the "primary aging hypothesis" and has far-reaching implications to the health-related sciences by suggesting a more general approach towards the goal of maintaining human health.

The cross-linkage hypothesis of aging represents a primary aging process and is based on the large number of different cross-linking agents that exist naturally in an organism. Most work in the past on evaluating the possible occurrence and biological significance of the cross-linkage hypothesis of aging has concentrated on cellular and extra-cellular constituents not directly involved with the information transfer system of the cell (e.g., collagen or the formation of age-pigments). Some positive correlations of increased cross-linkage with age have been reported, but the biological significance is questionable. On the other hand, the age-dependent formation of cross-links in structures involved with information transfer processes in the cell has received little attention. One of the most sensitive targets in this area to cross-linkage or more generally to the formation of DNA adducts is chromatin.

A parallel in the physico-chemical and functional properties of chromatin has been found between cells after radiation exposure and with non-irradiated cells as a function of age. Radiation and chemical-induced cross-linking between the various constituents of chromatin has been suggested by (1) reduced extractability of protein-free DNA, (2) altered template capacity of chromatin, and (3) the identification of specific DNA adduct products. The biological significance of such DNA adducts is suggested by the positive correlation of effectiveness of cell killing and DNA adducts formed. Similar age-dependent changes have been found in chromatin. These are: (1) a decrease in extractability of protein-free DNA, (2) an increase in thermal stability of chromatin, and (3) an alteration of template capacity and percent transcription of chromatin. The biological significance of these changes to aging has not been determined but is suggested by the correlation found by Hart and Setlow (1974) between the extent of excision repair of UV radiation-induced DNA damage and aging rate for a number of different mammalian species.

This parallel in radiation and natural age-induced changes in chromatin suggests that some of the age-dependent chromatin changes may involve the natural accumulation of DNA adducts. An age-dependent accumulation of DNA adducts in chromatin may be occurring which acts as a primary aging process in mammalian species. The removal of some of these DNA adducts may be occurring by the same repair processes that are capable of removing radiation-induced damage. A more systematic study of these possibilities should be undertaken.

Acknowledgments. I would like to acknowledge support from the

Biomedical Sciences Support Grant RR-07133 from the General Research
Support Branch, Division of Research Resources, N.I.H., the Yarbo-
rough and Associates Research Fund, and the Glenn Foundation for
Medical Research.

References

Acsadi, G., and Nemeskeri, J., 1970, "History of Human Lifespan
    and Mortality," Akademiai Kiado, Budapest.
Adelman, R.C., 1972, Age-dependent control of enzyme adaptation,
        in "Advances in Gerontological Research" Vol. 4 (B.L. Strehler,
        ed.), pp. 1-23, Academic Press, New York.
Adhikari, H.R., and Tappel, A.L., 1975, Fluorescent products from
        irradiated amino acids and proteins, *Radiat. Res.* 61:177-183.
Ambe, K.S., and Tappel, A.L., 1961, Oxidative damage to amino acids,
        peptides and proteins by radiation, *J. Food Sci.* 26:448-451.
Amici, D., Gianfranceschi, G.L., Marsili, G., and Michetti, L.,
        1974, Young and old rats. ATP, alkaline phosphatase, choles-
        terol and protein levels in the blood; DNA and RNA contents
        of the liver. Regulation by an aqueous thymus extract,
        Experientia 30:633-635.
Ansevin, A.T., and Brown, B.W., 1971, Specificity in the associa-
        tion of histones with deoxyribonucleic acid. Evidence from
        derivative thermal denaturation profiles, *Biochemistry* 7:1133-
        1142.
Ansevin, A.T., Hnilica, L.S., Spelsberg, T.C., and Kehm, S.L.,
        1971, Structure studies on chromatin and nucleohistones.
        Thermal denaturation profiles recorded in the presence of urea,
        Biochemistry 10:4793-4803.
Ansevin, A.T., Macdonald, K.K., Smith, C.E., and Hnilica, L.S.,
        1975, Mechanisms of chromatin template activation. Physical
        evidence for destabilization of nucleoproteins by polyanions,
        J. Biol. Chem. 250:281-289.
Bailey, A.J., 1969, The stabilization of the intermolecular cross-
        links of collagen with ageing, *Gerontologia* 15:65-76.
Bailey, A.J., Robins, S.P., and Balian, G., 1974, Biological signi-
        ficance of the intermolecular crosslinks of collagen, *Nature*
        251:105-109.
Barber, A.A., and Bernheim, F., 1967, Lipid peroxidation, its
        measurement, occurrence, and significance in animal tissues,
        in "Advances in Gerontological Research" Vol. 2 (B.L. Strehler,
        ed.), pp. 355-403, Academic Press, New York.
Bender, A.D., Kormendy, C.G., and Powell, R., 1970, Pharmacological
        control of aging, *Exp. Gerontol.* 5:97-129.
Bender, M.A., Griggs, H.G., and Bedford, J.S., 1974, Mechanisms of
        chromosomal aberration production III. Chemicals and ionizing
        radiation, *Mutat. Res.* 23:197-212.

Berdyshev, G.D., and Zhelabovskaya, S.M., 1972, Composition, template
    properties and thermostability of liver chromatin from rats of
    various age at deproteinization by NaCl solutions, *Exp. Gerontol.*
    7:321-330.
Biessmann, H., and Rajewsky, M.F., 1975, Nuclear protein patterns
    in developing an adult brain and in ethylnitrosourea-induced
    neuroectodermal tumours of the rat, *J. Neurochem.* 24:387-393.
Biology Data Book. Vol. 1, 1972, (P. Altman and D. Dittmer, eds.),
    p. 229, Fed. Am. Soc. Exp. Biol.
Bjorksten, J., 1962, Aging: present status of our chemical know-
    ledge, *J. Am. Geriat. Soc.* 10:125-139.
Bjorksten, J., 1969, Theories, *in* "Aging Life Processes" (S. Baker-
    man, ed.), pp. 147-179, C.C. Thomas Pub., Springfield, Illinois.
Bjorksten, J., 1974, Crosslinkage and the aging process, *in* "Theore-
    tical Aspects of Aging" (M. Rockstein, ed.), pp. 43-59,
    Academic Press, New York.
Bojanovic, J.J., Jevtovic, A.D., Pantic, V.S., Dugandzic, S.M.,
    and Jovanovic, D.S., 1970, Thymus nucleoproteins. Thymus
    histones in young and adult rats, *Gerontologia* 16:304-312.
Bondy, S.C., and Roberts, S., 1967, Messenger ribonucleic acid of
    cerebral nuclei, *Biochem. J.* 105:1111-1117.
Bondy, S.C., and Roberts, S., 1968, Hybridizable ribonucleic acid
    of rat brain, *Biochem. J.* 109:533-541.
Bondy, S.C., and Roberts, S., 1969, Developmental and regional
    variations in ribonucleic acid and synthesis on cerebral
    chromatin, *Biochem. J.* 115:341-349.
Bondy, S.C., and Roberts, S., 1970, Histone-acetylating enzyme of
    brain, *Biochem. J.* 119:665-672.
Britten, R., and Davidson, E., 1971, Repetitive and nonrepetitive
    DNA sequences and a speculation of the origins of evolutionary
    novelty, *Quart. Rev. Biol.* 46:111-133.
Brooks, A.L., Mead, D.K., and Peters, R.F., 1973, Effect of aging
    on the frequency of metaphase chromosome aberrations in the
    liver of the Chinese hamster, *J. Gerontol.* 28:452-454.
Burnet, M., 1974, "Intrinsic Mutagenesis: A Genetic Approach to
    Ageing," J. Wiley, New York.
Carter, D.B., and Chae, C., 1975, Composition of liver histones in
    aging rat and mouse, *J. Gerontol.* 30:28-32.
Chio, K.S., and Tappel, A.L., 1969a, Synthesis and characterization
    of the fluorescent products derived from malonaldehyde and
    amino acids, *Biochemistry* 8:2821-2827.
Chio, K.S., and Tappel, A.L., 1969b, Inactivation of ribonuclease
    and other enzymes by peroxidizing lipids and by malonaldehyde,
    Biochemistry 8:2827-2832.
Comfort, A., 1974, The position of aging studies, *Mech. Ageing
    Develop.* 3:1-31.
Comings, D.E., and Vance, C.K., 1971, Thermal denaturation of DNA
    and chromatin of early and late passage human fibroblasts,
    Gerontologia 17:116-121.

Courtois, Y.G.C., 1974, Chromatin modification of chick embryo cells during *in vitro* senescence, *Mech. Ageing Develop.* 3:51-63.

Crowley, C., and Curtis, H.J., 1963, The development of somatic mutations in mice with age, *Proc. Nat. Acad. Sci. USA* 49:626-628.

Curtis, H.J., Leith, J., and Tilley, J., 1966, Chromosome aberrations in liver cells of dogs of different ages, *J. Gerontol.* 21:268-270.

Curtis, H.J., and Miller, K., 1971, Chromosome aberrations in liver cells of guinea pigs, *J. Gerontol.* 26:292-293.

Cutler, R.G., 1972, Transcription of reiterated DNA sequence classes throughout the lifespan of the mouse, *in* "Advances in Gerontological Research" Vol. 4 (B.L. Strehler, ed.), pp. 219-321, Academic Press, New York.

Cutler, R.G., 1974, Redundancy of information content in the genome of mammalian species as a protective mechanism determining aging rate, *Mech. Ageing Develop.* 2:381-408.

Cutler, R.G., 1975a, Evolution of human longevity and the genetic complexity governing aging rate, *Proc. Nat. Acad. Sci. USA* (in press).

Cutler, R.G., 1975b, Evolution of longevity in mammals. I. Primates, *J. Human Evol.* (in press).

Cutler, R.G., 1975c, Evolution of longevity in mammals. II. Ungulates and carnivores, *J. Human Evol.* (in press).

Cutler, R.G., 1975d, Transcription of unique and reiterated DNA sequences in mouse liver and brain tissues as a function of age, *Exp. Gerontol.* 10:37-60.

David, J., Gordon, J.S., and Rutter, W.J., 1974, Increased thermal stability of chromatin containing 5-bromodeoxyuridine-substituted DNA, *Proc. Nat. Acad. Sci. USA* 71:2808-2812.

Demopoulos, H.B., 1973a, The basis of free radical pathology, *Fed. Proc.* 32:1859-1861.

Demopoulos, H.B., 1973b, Control of free radicals in biological systems, *Fed. Proc.* 32:1903-1908.

Deyl, Z., Juricova, M., Rosmus, J., and Adam, M., 1971, Aging of the connective tissue: collage cross linking in animals of different species and equal ages, *Exp. Gerontol.* 6:227-233.

di Luzio, N.R., 1973, Antioxidants, lipid peroxidation and chemical-induced liver injury, *Fed. Proc.* 32:1875-1881.

Dormandy, T.L., 1969, Biological rancidification, *Lancet*, Sept. 27:684-688.

Ebbesen, P., 1974, Aging increases susceptibility of mouse skin to DMBA carcinogenesis independent of general immune status, *Science* 183:217-218.

Eigner, J., Boedtker, H., and Michaels, G., 1961, The thermal degradation of nucleic acids, *Biochim. Biophys. Acta* 51:165-168.

Epstein, J., and Gershon, D., 1972, Studies on ageing in nematodes. IV. The effect of antioxidants on cellular damage and life span, *Mech. Ageing Develop.* 1:257-264.

Epstein, J., Himmelhock, S., and Gershon, D., 1972, Studies on ageing in nematodes. III. Electronmicroscopical studies on age-associated cellular damage, *Mech. Ageing Develop.* 1:245-255.

Epstein, J., Williams, J.R., and Little, J.B., 1973, Deficient DNA repair in human progeroid cells, *Proc. Nat. Acad. Sci. USA* 70:977-981.

Finch, C.E., 1969, "Cellular Activities During Ageing in Mammals," MSS Inform. Corp., New York.

Goldblatt, H., and Friedman, L., 1974, Prevention of malignant change in mammalian cells during prolonged culture *in vitro*, *Proc. Nat. Acad. Sci. USA* 71:1780-1782.

Goldstein, S., and Moerman, E.J., 1975, Defective proteins in normal and abnormal human fibroblasts during aging *in vitro*, *Gerontologia* (in press).

Goldstein, S., Niewiarowski, S., and Singal, D.P., 1975, Pathological implications of cell aging *in vitro*, *Fed. Proc.* 34:56-63.

Gordon, P., 1974, Free radicals and the aging process, *in* "Theoretical Aspects of Aging" (M. Rockstein, ed.), pp. 61-81, Academic Press, New York.

Green, J., 1972, Vitamin E and the biological antioxidant theory, *Annu. New York Acad. Sci.* 203:29-44.

Grouse, L., Chilton, M., and McCarthy, B.J., 1972, Hybridization of RNA with unique sequences of mouse DNA, *Biochemistry* 11:798-805.

Habazin, V., and Han, A., 1970, Ultra-violet-light-induced DNA-to-protein cross-linking in Hela cells, *Int. J. Radiat. Biol.* 17:569-575.

Hagen, U., Ullrich, M., and Jung, H., 1969, Transcription on irradiated DNA, *Int. J. Radiat. Biol.* 16:597-601.

Hagen, U., Ullrich, M., Petersen, E.E., Werner, E., and Kroger, H., 1970, Enzymatic RNA synthesis on irradiated DNA, *Biochim. Biophys. Acta* 199:115-125.

Hahn, H.P. von, 1963, Age-dependent thermal denaturation and viscosity of crude and purified DNA prepared from bovine thymus, *Gerontologia* 8:123-131.

Hahn, H.P. von, 1964, Age-related alterations in the structure of DNA. II. The role of histones, *Gerontologia* 10:174-182.

Hahn, H.P. von, 1970a, The regulation of protein synthesis in the ageing cell, *Exp. Gerontol.* 5:323-334.

Hahn, H.P. von, 1970b, Structural and functional changes in nucleoprotein during the ageing of the cell, *Gerontologia* 16:116-128.

Hahn, H.P. von, and Fritz, E., 1966, Age-related alterations in the structure of DNA. III. Thermal stability of rat liver DNA, related to age, histone content and ionic strength, *Gerontologia* 12:237-250.

Hahn, H.P. von, Miller, J., and Eichhorn, G.L., 1969, Age-related alterations in the structure of nucleoprotein. IV. Changes in the composition of whole histone from rat liver, *Gerontologia* 15:293-301.

Hall, D.A., 1968, The ageing of connective tissue, *Exp. Gerontol.* 3:77-89.

Hall, D.A., 1969, Connective tissues, *in* "Aging Life Processes" (S. Bakerman, ed.), pp. 79-122, C.C. Thomas, Pub., Springfield, Ill.

Han, A., Korbelik, M., and Ban, J., 1975, DNA-to-protein cross-linking in synchronized Hela cells exposed to ultra-violet light, *Int. J. Radiat. Biol.* 27:63-74.

Harman, D., 1956, Aging: a theory based on free radical and radiation chemistry, *J. Gerontol.* 11:298-300.

Harman, D., 1961, Prolongation of the normal lifespan and inhibition of spontaneous cancer by antioxidants, *J. Gerontol.* 16:247-254.

Harman, D., 1962, Role of free radicals in mutation, cancer, aging and the maintenance of life, *Radiat. Res.* 16:753-763.

Harman, D., 1967, Chromatin template capacity: effect of oxygen, abstract, *The Gerontologist*: Part II, 7:29.

Harman, D., 1968, Free radical theory of aging: effect of free radical reaction inhibitors on the mortality rate of male LAF_1 mice, *J. Gerontol.* 23:476-482.

Harman, D., 1969, Prolongation of life: role of free radical reactions in aging, *J. Am. Geriat. Soc.* 17:721-734.

Harman, D., 1971, Free radical theory of aging: effect of the amount and degree of unsaturation of dietary fat on mortality rate, *J. Gerontol.* 26:451-457.

Harman, D., 1972a, Free radical theory of aging: dietary implications, *Am. J. Clin. Nutri.* 25:839-843.

Harman, D., 1972b, Increasing the healthy life span, *Acta Geront. Belg.* 10:83-88.

Harman, D., Curtis, H.J., and Tilley, J., 1970, Chromosomal aberrations in liver cells of mice fed free radical reaction inhibitors, *J. Gerontol.* 25:17-19.

Hart, R.W., and Setlow, R.B., 1974, Correlation between deoxyribonucleic acid excision repair and lifespan in a number of mammalian species, *Proc. Nat. Acad. Sci. USA* 71:2169-2173.

Hart, R.W., and Trosko, J.E., 1975, DNA repair processes in mammals, *Gerontologia* (in press).

Hayflick, L., 1974, Cytogerontology, *in* "Theoretical Aspects of Aging" (M. Rockstein, ed.), pp. 83-103, Academic Press, New York.

Hjelm, R.P., and Huang, R.C.C., 1974, The role of histones in the conformation of DNA in chromatin as studied by circular dichroism, *Biochemistry* 13:5275-5283.

Hoffer, A., and Roy, R.M., 1975, Vitamin E decreases erythrocyte fragility after whole-body irradiation, *Radiat. Res.* 61:439-443.

Holliday, R., and Pugh, J.E., 1975, DNA modification mechanisms and gene activity during development, *Science* 187:226-232.

Ivannik, B.P., and Ryabchenko, N.I., 1969, Some physicochemical changes in DNA isolated from the organs of irradiated rats, *Radiobiologiya* 9:7-14.

Jackson, D.S., 1973, Some properties of the cross-linking theory of ageing of collagen, *in* "Connective Tissue and Aging" (H.G. Vogel, ed.), pp. 191-194, Excerpta Medica, Amsterdam.

Jones, M.L., 1968, Longevity of primates in captivity, *International Zoo Yearbook* 8:183-192.

Kaldor, G., and Min, B.K., 1975, Enzymatic studies on the skeletal myosin A and actomyosin of aging rats, *Fed. Proc.* 34:191-194.

Kawashima, S., 1970, The possible role of lipoperoxide in aging, *Nagoya J. Med. Sci.* 32:303-326.

King, M., and Wilson, A.C., 1975, Evolution at two levels in humans and chimpanzees, *Science* 188:107-116.

Kirby, K.S., 1958, Preparation of some deoxyribonucleic acid-protein complexes from rat-liver homogenates, *Biochem. J.* 70:260-265.

Kirby, K.S., 1967, Isolation of deoxyribonucleic acid from mammalian tissues, *Biochem. J.* 104:254-257.

Kohn, R.R., 1963, Human aging and disease, *J. Chron. Dis.* 16:5-21.

Kohn, R.R., 1971a, "Principles of Mammalian Aging," Prentice-Hall, Englewood Cliffs, New Jersey.

Kohn, R.R., 1971b, Effect of antioxidants on life-span of C57BL mice, *J. Gerontol.* 26:378-380.

Kurtz, D.I., Russell, A.P., and Sinex, F.M., 1974, Multiple peaks in the derivative melting curve of chromatin from animals of varying age, *Mech. Ageing Develop.* 3:37-49.

Kurtz, D.I., and Sinex, F.M., 1967, Age related differences in the association of brain DNA and nuclear protein, *Biochim. Biophys. Acta* 145:840-842.

Leveson, J.E., and Peacocke, A.R., 1966, Studies of a complex of deoxyribonucleic acid with non-histone protein, *Biochim. Biophys. Acta* 123:329-336.

Li, H.J., and Bonner, J., 1971, Interactions of histone half-molecules with deoxyribonucleic acid, *Biochemistry* 10:1461-1470.

Li, H.J., Chang, C., and Weiskopf, M., 1973, Helix-coil transition in nucleoprotein-chromatin structure, *Biochemistry* 12:1763-1772.

Liew, C.C., and Gornall, A.G., 1975, Covalent modification of nuclear proteins during aging, *Fed. Proc.* 34:186-187.

Lloyd, P.H., Nicholson, B.H., and Peacocke, A.R., 1967, The effects of γ-irradiation on the priming by deoxyribonucleohistone of ribonucleic acid polymerase, *Biochem. J.* 104:999-1003.

Lucy, J.A., 1972, Functional and structural aspects of biological membranes: a suggested structural role for vitamin E in the control of membrane permeability and stability, *Annu. New York Acad. Sci.* 203:4-11.

Massie, H.R., Baird, M.B., Nicolosi, R.J., and Samis, H.V., 1972, Changes in the structure of rat liver DNA in relation to age, *Arch. Biochem. Biophys.* 153:736-741.

Maynard Smith, J., 1966, Theories of aging, *in* "Topics in the Biology of Aging," (P.L. Krohn, ed.), pp. 1-27, J. Wiley and Sons, New York.

McKusick, V.A., 1971, "Mendelian Inheritance in Man," Johns Hopkins Press, Baltimore, Maryland.

Milvy, P., 1973, Control of free radical mechanisms in nucleic acid systems: studies in radioprotection and radiosensitivity, *Fed. Proc.* 32:1895-1902.

Miner, R.W., 1954, "Parental age and characteristics of the off-spring, *Annu. New York Acad. Sci.* 57:451-462.

Modak, S.P., and Price, G.B., 1971, Exogenous DNA polymerase-cata-lyzed incorporation of deoxyribonucleotide monophosphates in nuclei of fixed mouse brain cells. Changes associated with age and x-irradiation, *Exp. Cell Res.* 65:289-296.

Nair, P.P., and Kayden, H.J., eds., 1972, "Vitamin E and Its Role in Cellular Metabolism," *Annu. New York Acad. Sci.*, Vol. 23.

Ohno, S., 1970, "Evolution by Gene Duplication," Springer Verlag, Heidelberg.

O'Meara, A.R., and Herrmann, R.L., 1972, A modified mouse liver chromatin preparation displaying age-related differences in salt dissociation and template ability, *Biochim. Biophys. Acta* 269:419-427.

Packer, L., Deamer, D.W., and Heath, R.L., 1967, Regulation and deterioration of structure in membranes, *in* "Advances in Gerontological Research" (B.L. Strehler, ed.), pp. 77-120, Academic Press, New York.

Packer, L., and Smith, J.R., 1974, Extension of the lifespan of cultured normal human diploid cells by vitamin E, *Proc. Nat. Acad. Sci. USA* 71:4763-4767.

Panyim, S., and Chalkley, R., 1969, High resolution acrylamide gel electrophoresis of histones, *Arch. Biochem. Biophys.* 130:337-346.

Penrose, L.S., 1954, Mongolism idiocy (mongolism) and maternal age, *Annu. New York Acad. Sci.* 57:494-502.

Petes, T.D., Farber, R.A., Tarrant, G.M., and Holliday, R., 1974, Altered role of DNA replication in ageing human fibroblast cultures, *Nature* 251:434-436.

Price, G.B., and Makinodan, T., 1973, Aging: alteration of DNA-protein information, *Gerontologia* 19:58-70.

Price, G.B., Modak, S.P., and Makinodan, T., 1971, Age-associated changes in the DNA of mouse tissue, *Science* 171:917-920.

Pryor, W.A., 1970, Free radicals in biological systems, *Scien. Amer.* 223:70-83.

Pryor, W.A., 1971, Free radical pathology, *Chem. Eng. News* 49:34-51.

Pryor, W.A., 1973, Free radical reactions and their importance in biochemical systems, *Fed. Proc.* 32:1862-1869.

Pyhtila, M.J., and Sherman, F.G., 1968a, Age-associated studies on
    thermal stability and template effectiveness of DNA and nucleo-
    proteins from beef thymus, *Biochem. Biophys. Res. Commun.* 31:
    340-344.
Pyhtila, M.J., and Sherman, F.G., 1968b, Studies on the histones
    and DNA of calf and old cow thymus, *J. Gerontol.* 23:450-453.
Riely, C.A., Cohen, G., and Lieberman, M., 1974, Ethane evolution:
    A new index of lipid peroxidation, *Science* 183:208-210.
Roberts, S., 1973, Alterations in cerebral protein. Synthesizing
    systems during maturation, *in* "Neurobiological Aspects of
    Maturation and Aging," (D.H. Ford, ed.), pp. 277-292, Elsevier
    Pub. Co., New York.
Ross, M., 1961, Length of life and nutrition in the rat, *J. Nutrit.*
    75:197-210.
Roth, G.S., 1974, Age-related changes in specific glucocorticoid
    binding by steroid-responsive tissues of rats, *Endocrinology*
    94:82-90.
Roth, G.S., 1975, Age-related changes in glucocorticoid binding by
    rat splenic leukocytes: possible cause of altered adaptive
    responsiveness, *Fed. Proc.* 34:183-185.
Roth, G.S., and Adelman, R.C., 1973, Possible changes in tissue
    sensitivity in the age-dependent stimulation of DNA synthesis
    in vivo, *J. Gerontol.* 28:298-301.
Roti, J.L., Stein, G.S., and Cerutti, P.A., 1974, Reactivity of
    thymine to x-rays in Hela chromatin and nucleoprotein prepara-
    tions, *Biochemistry* 13:1900-1905.
Russell, A.P., Dowling, L.E., and Herrmann, R.L., 1970, Age-related
    differences in mouse liver DNA melting and hydroxylapatite
    fractionation, *Gerontologia* 16:159-171.
Ryan, J.M., and Cristofalo, V.J., 1972, Histone acetylation during
    aging of human cells in culture, *Biochem. Biophys. Res. Commun.*
    48:735-742.
Sacher, G., 1959, Relation of lifespan to brain weight and body
    weight in mammals, *in* "Ciba Found. Colloquium on Aging," Vol.
    5, pp. 115-141, Churchill, London.
Sacher, G., 1975, Maturation and longevity in relation to cranial
    capacity in hominid evolution, *in* "Antecedents of Man and
    After. Vol 1, Primates: Functional Morphology and Evolution,"
    Mouton, The Hague (in press).
Salser, J.S., and Balis, M.E., 1967, Investigations on amino acids
    bound to DNA, *Biochim. Biophys. Acta* 149:220-227.
Salser, J.S., and Balis, M.E., 1968, Amino acids associated with
    DNA of tumors, *Cancer Res.* 28:595-600.
Salser, J.S., and Balis, M.E., 1969, The effect of growth conditions
    on amino acids bound to deoxyribonucleic acid, *J. Biol. Chem.*
    244:822-828.
Salser, J.S., and Balis, M.E., 1972, Alterations in deoxyribonucleic
    acid-bound amino acids with age and sex, *J. Gerontol.* 27:1-9.

Samis, H.V., Poccia, D.L., and Wulf, V.J., 1968, The effect of salt
    extraction and heat-denaturation on the behavior of rat liver
    chromatin, *Biochim. Biophys. Acta* 166:410-418.
Samis, H.V., and Wulf, V.J., 1969, The template activity of rat
    liver chromatin, *Exp. Gerontol.* 4:111-117.
Schott, H.N., and Shetlar, M.D., 1974, Photochemical addition of
    amino acids to thymine, *Biochem. Biophys. Res. Commun.* 59:
    1112-1116.
Sheldrake, A.R., 1974, The ageing, growth and death of cells, *Nature*
    250:381-385.
Shirey, T.L., and Sobel, H., 1972, Compositional and transcriptional
    properties of chromatins isolated from cardiac muscles of young-
    mature and old dogs, *Exp. Gerontol.* 7:15-29.
Sinex, F.M., 1964, Cross-linkage and ageing, *in* "Advances in
    Gerontological Research," Vol. 1 (B.L. Strehler, ed.), pp.
    165-180, Academic Press, New York.
Sinex, F.M., 1974, The mutation theory of aging, *in* "Theoretical
    Aspects of Aging" (M. Rockstein, ed.), pp. 23-31, Academic
    Press, New York.
Sklobovskaya, M.V., and Ryabchenko, N.N., 1970, Reduction of the
    yield of DNA in the deproteinization of UV or gamma-irradiated
    solutions of deoxyribonucleoprotein I. Dependence of the mag-
    nitude of the effect on the completeness of the complexation
    of DNA with protein, *Radiobiologiya* 10:18-24.
Slater, T.F., 1972, "Free Radical Mechanisms in Tissue Culture,"
    Pion Ltd., London.
Smets, L.A., and Cornelis, J.J., 1971, Repairable and irrepairable
    damage in 5-bromouracil-substituted DNA exposed to ultra-
    violet radiation, *Int. J. Radiat. Biol.* 19:445-457.
Smith, K.C., 1975a, The radiation-induced addition of proteins and
    other molecules to nucleic acids, *in* "Photochemistry and
    Photobiology of Nucleic Acids," (S.Y. Wang, ed.), pp.
    Academic Press, New York.
Smith, K.C., 1975b, Chemical adducts to DNA: their importance to
    the genetic alteration theory of aging, *Gerontologia* (in press).
Stanley, J.F., Pye, D., and MacGregor, A., 1975, Comparison of
    doubling numbers attained by cultured animal cells with life
    spans of species, *Nature* 255:158-159.
Stein, G.S., and Stein, J.L., 1975, *In vitro* studies of transcrip-
    tion as a function of age in mammalian cells, *Gerontologia*
    (in press).
Stein, G.S., Wang, P.L., and Adelman, R.C., 1973, Age-dependent
    changes in the structure and function of mammalian chromatin.
    I. Variations in chromatin template activity, *Exp. Gerontol.*
    8:123-133.
Strehler, B.L., ed., 1960, "The Biology of Aging," A.I.B.S. Pub.
    No. 6, p. 23, Waverly Press, Baltimore.
Strehler, B.L., 1962, "Time, Cells, and Aging," Academic Press,
    New York.

Strehler, B.L., 1964, On the histochemistry and ultrastructure of age pigment, *in* "Advances in Gerontological Research," Vol. 1 (B.L. Strehler, ed.), pp. 343-384, Academic Press, New York.

Strehler, B.L., 1975, Implications of aging research for society, *Fed. Proc.* 34:5-8.

Takacs, I., and Verzar, F., 1968, Macromolecular aging of collagen. I. Experiments *in vivo* and *in vitro* with different animal races, *Gerontologia* 14:15-23.

Tanzer, M.L., 1973, Cross-linking of collagen, *Science* 180:561-566.

Tappel, A.L., 1965, Free-radical lipid peroxidation damage and its inhibition by vitamin E and selenium, *Fed. Proc.* 24:73-78.

Tappel, A.L., 1968, Will antioxidant nutrients slow aging processes? *Geriatrics* 23:97-105.

Tappel, A.L., 1972, Vitamin E and free radical peroxidation of lipids, *Annu. New York Acad. Sci.* 203:12-28.

Tappel, A.L., 1973, Lipid peroxidation damage to cell components, *Fed. Proc.* 32:1870-1874.

Tappel, A.L., Fletcher, B., and Deamer, D., 1973, Effect of antioxidants and nutrients on lipid peroxidation fluorescent products and aging parameters in the mouse, *J. Gerontol.* 28:415-424.

Timiras, P.S., ed., 1972, "Developmental Physiology and Aging," Macmillan Co., New York.

Trosko, J.E., and Hart, R.W., 1975, DNA mutation frequencies in mammals, *Gerontologia* (in press).

Umansky, S.R., Korol, B.A., Runova, Y.N., and Tokarskaya, V.I., 1974, Possible mechanisms for radiation disturbance of transcription, *Int. J. Radiat. Biol.* 25:31-41.

Vanyushin, B.F., Nemerovsky, L.E., Klimenko, V.V., Vasiliev, V.K., and Belozersky, A.N., 1973, The 5-methylcytosine in DNA of rats. Tissue and age specificity and the changes induced by hydrocortisone and other agents, *Gerontologia* 19:138-152.

Vernadakis, A., 1975, Neuronal-glia interactions during development and aging, *Fed. Proc.* 34:89-95.

Verzar, F., 1963, The aging of collagen, *Scien. Amer.* 208:104-114.

Vogel, H.G., ed., 1973, "Connective Tissue and Aging," Excerpta Medica, Amsterdam.

Weiss, J.J., and Wheeler, C.M., 1964, Effect of γ-radiation on deoxynucleoprotein acting as a primer in RNA synthesis, *Nature* 203:291-292.

Wheeler, K.T., and Lett, J.T., 1974, On the possibility that DNA repair is related to age in non-dividing cells, *Proc. Nat. Acad. Sci. USA* 71:1862-1865.

Wilhelm, F.X., de Murcia, G.M., Champagne, M.H., and Daune, M.P., 1974, Conformational changes of histones and DNA during the thermal denaturation of nucleoprotein, *Eur. J. Biochem.* 45:431-443.

Wolpert, L., and Lewis, J.H., 1975, Towards a theory of development, *Fed. Proc.* 34:14-20.

Yamanaka, N., and Deamer, D., 1974, Superoxide dismutase activity
    in WI-38 cell cultures: Effects of age, trypsinization and
    SV-40 transformation, *Physiol. Chem. Physics* 6:95-106.
Yielding, K.L., 1974, A model for aging based on differential repair
    of somatic mutational damage, *Persp. Biol. Med.* 17:201-208.
Yoshii, G., Juwabara, M., and Hayashi, M., 1974, Irradiation effects
    on deoxyribonucleoprotein in the presence of Ca ion, abstr.
    A-3-3, *Radiat. Res.* 59:7.
Zeman, W., 1971, The neuronal ceroid-lipofuscinoses-Batten-Vogt
    syndrome: A model for human aging? *in* "Advances in Gerontolo-
    gical Research," (B.L. Strehler, ed.), pp. 147-170, Academic
    Press, New York.
Zhelabovskaya, S.M., and Berdyshev, G.D., 1972, Composition, template
    activity and thermostability of the liver chromatin in rats of
    various ages, *Exp. Gerontol.* 7:313-320.
Zimmerman, E., Pathak, M.A., and Kornhauser, A., 1972, The *in vivo*
    effect of UV irradiation on epidermal chromatin, abstr.,
    Clin. Res. 20:420.
Zimmerman, F., Kroger, H., Hagen, U., and Kech, K., 1964, The effect
    of x-irradiation on the priming ability of DNA in the RNA poly-
    merase system, *Biochim. Biophys. Acta* 87:160-162.

DOSE, DOSE RATE, RADIATION QUALITY, AND HOST FACTORS

FOR RADIATION-INDUCED LIFE SHORTENING

George A. Sacher

Division of Biological and Medical Research

Argonne National Laboratory, Argonne, Illinois 60439

1. INTRODUCTION

This paper reviews the effects of ionizing radiations on disease incidence and life shortening in experimental animals, with the aim of establishing a phenomenological model of the dose and time kinetics for the production of late radiation damage. Aspects of this problem have been discussed previously (Sacher, 1956a). At that time, mammalian cellular radiology had barely begun its dramatic development, and there were no experimental data against which to test the hypothesis adopted then, that the phenomena of radiation life shortening are due to chromosome breakage and rejoining. This hypothesis was stated most explicitly by Muller (1950), but it was also implicit in the discussion of lethal effects in cells by Lea (1947), and in a real sense it was a development that epitomized the classical period of radiation genetics.

493

Less than two decades later, the picture has changed completely. The phenomenology of radiation lethality and molecular damage and repair in mammalian cells is now so complex that it is difficult to perceive even the outlines of a satisfactory theory of radiation lethality in cells (Elkind and Whitmore, 1967). Knowledge about radiation life shortening has also increased in the intervening two decades, but the remarkable fact is that the additional information continues to fit and reinforce the phenomenological model developed 20 years earlier, so that no substantial changes in the model are required. This quantitative simplicity and consistency of the late effects of radiations assumes greater importance in relation to the great complexity of acute radiation effects on cells, so the view adopted in the present paper is that the hypothesis of chromosome aberrations continues to deserve first consideration in the search for a cellular-molecular basis for late radiation effects.

2.   METHODS

The data discussed here were obtained from three experimental radiation procedures--single exposure, fractionated exposure to fixed total dose, and daily exposure for the duration of life. The delivery time for individual fractions, or protraction time, is an additional exposure parameter. Experiments using time-dependent exposure rates, such as exponential decrease, are not considered.

The endpoint used is the time to death of the animal. Age-specific death rates, Ω_x are calculated by the formula (Sacher, 1966)

$$\Omega_{x+h/2} = h^{-1}(\ln L_x - \ln L_{x+h}) \tag{1}$$

where L_x is the number living at age x and h is the length of the interval over which the rate is calculated.

The logarithm of Ω_x plotted *versus* age is called the Gompertz function, and denoted $G(x)$.

Sacher (1956a) and Sacher and Trucco (1962) developed a mathematical theory of mortality as a stochastic transition process, in which it is shown that $G(x)$ is approximately a linear measure of the *physiological state* of a homogeneous population. On the basis of this theory, the relation of the logarithm of the rate of mortality to time can be interpreted--even when it is not linear with time--as representing the temporal variation of physiological state arising from natural aging processes or from tissue injury processes by external agents. The Gompertz functions for natural aging of adult mammals--and many other metazoan forms also--are usually straight lines, indicating that the molecular aging process proceeds at a uniform rate throughout adult life. For example, populations of seven species of captive rodents undergoing natural aging have been shown experimentally (Sacher and Staffeldt, 1972) to yield a linear relation of log Ω_x to age,

$$G(x) = \ln \Omega_0 + \tau^{-1}x \qquad (2)$$

where Ω_0 is the intercept of the Gompertz line at age zero, and τ^{-1} is the rate of aging, so 0.693τ is the (constant) time for the death rate to increase by a factor of 2, also called the doubling time, T_d. There is need for a generalized interpretation of mortality processes such as that provided by the Gompertz function, $G(x)$, in experimental gerontology and toxicology, because it is a matter of common observation that some physico-chemical aging and tissue injury processes are nonlinear functions of time. However, with few exceptions, the experimental data to be discussed here obey the linear relation of Eq. (2).

Life table analysis of the experimental data is not always possible, either because samples are too small or because the data are published in an inadequate summary fashion. In such cases, the after-expectation of life is used as a measure of the displacement of the basic Gompertz equation parameter. The life expectation, E_x, for a mortality process obeying the Gompertz equation is (Sacher, 1960)

$$E_x = \tau \exp(\Omega_0\tau e^{x/\tau})[-Ei(-\Omega_0\tau e^{x/\tau})] \qquad (3)$$

where $-Ei(-z)$, the exponential integral for argument z, is a trans-cendental function that has been tabulated (W.P.A., 1940). Only two special cases of Eq. (3) need be used here. When Ω_0 is small enough so that $\Omega_0\tau \ll 1$, the after-expectation from time zero, E_0, has the approximate form

$$E_0 = -\tau(\ln \Omega_0\tau + 0.577) \qquad (4)$$

This approximation is accurate for control or treated populations starting from young adult ages. For duration-of-life (D.o.L.) exposure, the effects on Ω_0 are secondary, and the cumulative irreparable damage is measured by the displacement of the Gompertz slope, τ^{-1}. In this case, the mean radiation-specific death rate, estimated as $M_R^{-1} - M_O^{-1}$, where M_R is the mean after-survival time of the group given daily dose R, and M_O is the mean after-survival of the control group, is very nearly proportional to the displacement of the slope, $\Delta\tau^{-1} = \tau_R^{-1} - \tau_0^{-1}$.

Experimental data for mice, rats, guinea pigs, and dogs are examined, but there is no attempt to make comparisons to man because it has not yet been possible for me to analyze the data for the Japanese atomic bomb survivors or other human populations by the

actuarial methods used here for the experimental animal data. Data
on the effects of X-rays, gamma rays, and fast neutrons are analyzed,
but the data are not sufficient to justify analysis in terms of
quantitative linear energy transfer (LET) values, so the discussion
of LET effects is confined to qualitative comparisons between fast
neutrons as high-LET radiations and X-rays or gamma rays as low-LET
radiations.

3. EXPERIMENTAL FINDINGS

3.1. Single Dose

The first major epidemiological experiment on the effects of
single radiation exposures on the survival of mice was carried out
by Upton *et al.* (1960) on mice exposed to the radiations from an
experimental thermonuclear detonation (project Greenhouse). The
radiation spectrum was essentially high-energy gamma rays. There
were eight radiation dose levels with 440 mice at each, plus 620
controls. Age-specific death rates, Ω in Eq. (1), are plotted
for each dose level and controls on a logarithmic scale against
time. The resulting Gompertz function diagram is seen in Fig. 1
to be a family of parallel straight lines. There is an upward
displacement of the Gompertz lines for the exposed groups, and the
displaced curves do not depart significantly from parallelism with
the controls (Sacher, 1956a). This is characteristic for mammals
after single exposures (Sacher, 1956a, 1966). Figure 2 gives the
relation of the displacement from control, $\Delta G(D)$, to dose for the
male and female LAF$_1$ mice, based on the data published by Furth
et al. (1954). The data for the two sexes are fitted with a
quadratic function of dose with identical coefficients for the
first and second power terms for the two sexes, but the $\Delta G(D)$ function for the female mouse requires an additional additive constant
(Sacher, 1956a). This constant term arises from the fact that the
adult female mouse ovary is uniquely radiosensitive, and is steril-
ized by a dose of about 100 rads (Lindop *et al.*, 1966), so that
the dose-response function of female mice given doses above 100
rads has a dose-independent term that represents the attainment
of a saturation level of increased mortality arising from the
disturbed endocrine function in the radiation-sterilized female
mouse.

Lindop and Rotblat (1961) reported a linear relation of life
shortening to dose for the SAS-4 mouse, with no sex difference.
These mice, an inbred substrain of the *A* strain, were exposed at
age 30 days to pulsed 15 MeV X-rays from a linear accelerator.
The reasons for the linear dose response and the lack of sex difference in this experiment are not known, but it may be significant that the mice were exposed before sexual maturity, at the age

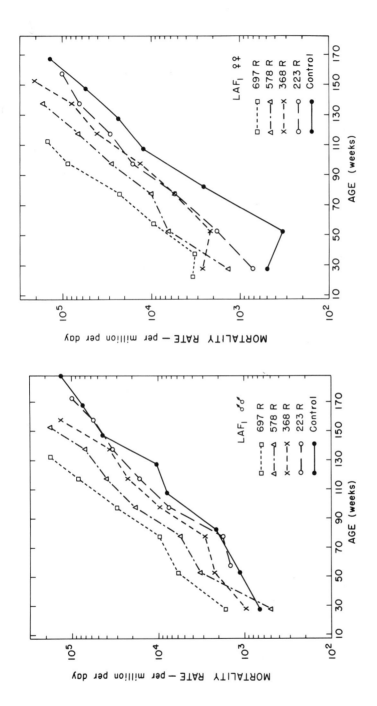

Fig. 1. Logarithm of age-specific mortality rate from all causes *versus* age (Gompertz function diagram) for LAF$_1$ male and female mice given single brief exposures to gamma rays from a nuclear device (project Greenhouse), and their specific controls. Ages at exposure were 6 to 12 weeks (From Upton *et al.*, 1960).

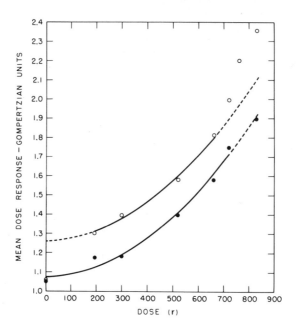

Fig. 2. Dose-effect relations for excess mortality of LAF_1 male (lower line) and female (upper line) mice exposed to gamma rays from a nuclear detonation (project Greenhouse). Data of Furth *et al.* (1954). Effect measured by the mean displacement of Gompertz function for treated groups from control. All parameters were calculated by a nonorthogonal analysis of variance. The smooth curves were fitted to the data by least squares, subject to the constraint that the coefficients for dose and dose-squared are the same for the two sexes. The dose-effect relation for males is $\Delta G(D) = 56 \cdot 10^{-6}D + 1.15 \cdot 10^{-6}D^2$. The zero-dose intercept for females is $\Delta G(O) = 0.21$ (Sacher, 1956a).

at which sensitivity to acute killing and life shortening is greater than at any other postnatal age. Such a phenomenon is known at the cellular level, for cells in culture tend to show survival curves with decreased extrapolation number when they are unusually sensitive to ionizing radiations (Elkind and Whitmore, 1967). There is also variability in the amount of excess female mortality when irradiation is delivered after sexual maturity (see below).

The effects of brief and protracted doses of gamma rays and fast neutrons on the survival and tumor incidence of male and female RFM mice and BALB/c mice are being investigated by Storer and colleagues at the Oak Ridge National Laboratory. Interim results (Storer *et al.*, 1973, 1974) indicate that the saturating component of excess female mortality is identifiable in the groups given brief single gamma ray exposures, and that the saturation dose is less than 100 R. The dependence of life shortening on dose is quadratic for both the saturating female-specific mortality and the major mortality component for mice given brief single gamma ray exposures.

In an experiment in progress at the Argonne National Laboratory to evaluate the influence of fractionation and protraction on the late effects of fast neutrons and gamma rays (the JANUS program), male and female B6CF$_1$ mice were given single gamma ray exposures of 90, 268, or 788 rads, and fast neutron doses of 20, 80, or 240 rads. The life shortening by gamma rays is a linear function of dose, and the life shortening function for fast neutrons is negatively accelerated (Ainsworth *et al.*, 1974, 1976; Fig. 3). The effectiveness of gamma rays relative to fast neutrons (the reciprocal of the conventional RBE) increases as a linear function of gamma ray dose. An excess of sensitivity of females over males is present for both gamma rays and fast neutrons, but is smaller than the sex difference in the experiments of Sacher (1956a), Upton *et al.* (1960), or Storer *et al.* (1973, 1974). The incidence of ovarian and mammary tumors in the irradiated and control mice in the JANUS program is low. This is consistent with the observed small sex difference in survival, for Grahn (1960) has shown that the amount of excess female-specific mortality in six inbred or F$_1$ hybrid mouse genotypes has a high positive correlation with the ovarian tumor incidence. However, the B6CF$_1$ hybrid, which has a low ovarian tumor incidence in the JANUS experiment, had the highest ovarian tumor incidence, and the largest excess of female life shortening, in Grahn's (1960) experiment. It must be concluded that the variation in the amount of excess tumor incidence among populations of irradiated female mice is in part due to an unknown environmental factor, such as the presence or absence of a virus.

Noonan *et al.* (1951) found an accelerated dose-effect relation for reduction of mean after-survival time in male and female Wistar rats exposed to X rays. Life shortening has been estimated for dogs exposed to X rays and guinea pigs exposed to single doses of gamma rays (Sacher, 1966), but the data are not sufficient for an estimate of the dose dependence.

The results of these experiments are not completely consistent, and bear out the generalization that it is difficult to reproduce any kind of end point produced by brief single exposures. However, the following characteristics are demonstrable.

i. There is a quadratic dependence of life shortening on dose of low-LET radiations in a majority of the epidemiological studies surveyed (Sacher, 1956a; Upton *et al.*, 1960; Storer *et al.*, 1974; Noonan *et al.*, 1951).

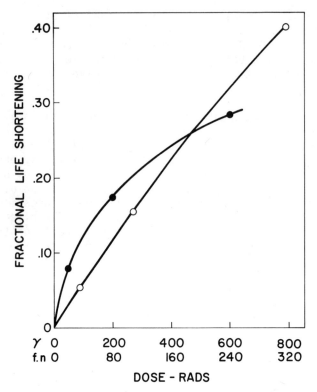

Fig. 3. Dose-effect relation for B6CF$_1$ mice, sexes combined, given single doses of ^{60}Co gamma rays (open circles) or fast neutrons (solid circles). Effect plotted as percent decrease of after-expectation of life from control at the age at exposure, $\Delta E/E_O$ (Data of Ainsworth et $al.$, 1976).

ii. Two major investigations (Lindop and Rotblat, 1961; Ainsworth et $al.$, 1976) show a first-power relation of life shortening to dose for low-LET radiations, but it can be concluded on the basis of the data of Ainsworth et $al.$ (1976) that even in these cases the quadratic dependence for low-LET radiations holds, for in the JANUS experiment the effectiveness of gamma rays relative to fast neutrons increases as a function of dose, consistent with a quadratic relation of gamma dose to fast neutron dose. These results of Ainsworth et $al.$ (1976) require the conclusion that tissue injury by low-LET radiations obeys quadratic dose kinetics, but that there is in addition a nonlinear decelerating relation of life shortening to injury in their experimental conditions. The reason for the variability in the relation between tissue injury and morbidity remains to be clarified.

iii. A female-specific component of mortality that is virtually
dose-independent at doses above 100 R of gamma rays is
present in four experiments (Sacher, 1956a; Grahn, 1960;
Upton *et al.*, 1960; Storer *et al.*, 1974), but the size of
the component varies between mouse genotypes (Grahn, 1960),
is greatly reduced in magnitude in one experiment (Ainsworth *et al.*, 1976), and is absent in another (Lindop and
Rotblat, 1961). The amount of female-specific radiation
mortality is correlated with incidence of ovarian tumors,
but the ovarian tumor incidence is governed by environmental as well as genetic factors.

3.2. Duration-of-Life Exposure

Unlike single-dose late effects, which are somewhat variable
and difficult to reproduce, the life shortening produced by D.o.L.
irradiation is highly reproducible, for it has been found to have
the same mathematical form in every one of 14 species that have
been tested, ranging from radioresistant to extremely radiosensitive (Sacher, Staffeldt, and Tyler, work in progress). The major
feature of the increase of mortality produced by D.o.L. exposure
is an increase of the slope of the Gompertz relation (Fig. 4;
Brues and Sacher, 1952; Sacher, 1956; Grahn, 1970). The increase
of Gompertz slope in irradiated groups is consistent with the
hypothesis that irreparable injury is additive (cf. Fig. 1), so
the difference in slope between irradiated and control groups is
used as the measure of the cumulative irreparable tissue lesion
produced by D.o.L. exposure. Figure 4 gives the relation of
Gompertz slope increment to daily dose on logarithmic coordinates
for two hybrid mice, the LAF_1 and the $B6CF_1$ (Sacher, 1973; Sacher
and Grahn, 1964; Grahn, 1970). At daily doses below 125 R/day the
function has a well defined branch on which Gompertz slope varies
as the square of the daily dose. This trend is superseded, at a
daily dose below 24 R/day, by a branch on which Gompertz slope
varies as the first power of the daily dose. The rate-squared
branch has by now been observed in either inbred, F_1, or F_2 hybrid
laboratory mouse populations, and in 14 other species, including
rodents, ungulates, and carnivores (Sacher and Tyler, 1972). The
branch of unit slope has thus far been observed only for rats and
mice (see below).

In most studies on species other than the laboratory mouse,
sample sizes are not large enough to allow the estimation of
Gompertz slopes, so the mean radiation-specific mortality rate is
used instead (see Methods). This substitution is permissible
because mean mortality rates and Gompertz function slopes are
very nearly proportional for populations that have linear Gompertz

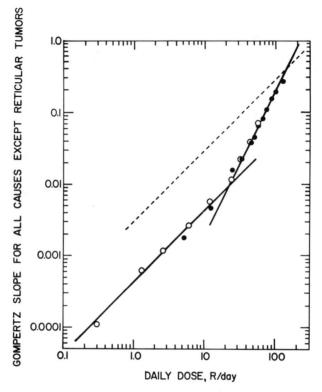

Fig. 4.   Increase of slope of Gompertz function over control for LAF$_1$ mice (solid circles; Sacher and Grahn, 1964) and B6CF$_1$ mice (open circles; Grahn, 1960) given D.o.L. exposure to ^{60}Co gamma rays.   The fitted line for daily fast neutron exposure (Evans, 1948; Henshaw *et al.*, 1947) is also shown (dashed line).

functions (Sacher, 1960).   Figure 5 gives the relation of radiation-specific mortality rate to daily dose for three species--mouse, dog, and guinea pig--that have a wide range of radiosensitivities.   This figure illustrates another feature of the radiation lethality produced by D.o.L. exposure.   At sufficiently high daily doses, all species tested roll off the rate-squared trend, and as daily dose increases, the slope of the dose-effect function decreases toward unity.   It should be noted that the relationship at high daily doses and short survival times is complex and is better analyzed by means of a different mathematical model (Sacher, 1956b; Sacher and Grahn, 1964).

It can be seen in Fig. 5 that the species vary in sensitivity by about a factor of two on the high-dose branch, but that the spread in sensitivities increases to as much as a factor of 10 on

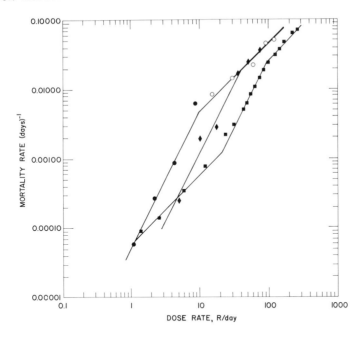

Fig. 5. Relation of mean radiation-specific mortality rate to daily dose for LAF$_1$ and B6CF$_1$ hybrid mice, dogs, and guinea pigs given D.o.L. exposure to gamma rays (From Norris *et al.*, 1976).

the rate-squared branch. However, at sufficiently low daily doses the sequence of species sensitivities is radically changed, because the mouse branch of unit slope cuts across the continuing rate-squared decreasing trends for the dog and guinea pig.

The low-dose branch of unit slope has also been estimated by Boche (1954) for rats given brief daily exposure to 10 R/day or less of supervoltage X-rays and by Lorenz *et al.* (1954) for LAF mice exposed to radium gamma rays at daily doses up to 8.8 R/day. In these cases, the transition to the second-power trend can be inferred to occur above 10 R/day. The dog (Norris *et al.*, 1976) and the guinea pig (Lorenz *et al.*, 1954; Rust *et al.*, 1966), have been investigated at daily doses of 5 R/day or less without as yet giving evidence of a branch of unit slope. A major experiment is now under way in which beagles will be given D.o.L. exposure at daily doses down to 0.5 rad/day, with the specific purpose of looking for a transition from the rate-squared branch to a branch of unit slope (Norris *et al.*, 1976).

The effectiveness per rad for life shortening in mice given D.o.L. exposure to gamma rays and fast neutrons, which is given by

the slope of the dose-effect function, is graphed in Fig. 6. For
^{60}Co gamma rays, it is constant on the low-dose branch, increases
as the first power of the daily dose on the intermediate branch,
and rolls off toward a constant value at very high daily dosages.

Two investigations of life shortening by D.o.L. exposure to
fast neutrons were conducted by Henshaw *et al.* (1947), using nuclear
reactor fast neutrons, and Evans (1948), using cyclotron neutrons.
These two independent investigations gave the same result, which is
that the relation of radiation-specific mortality rate to daily
dose has a slope that is not significantly different from unity
(Sacher, 1973) over the range of daily doses and survival times
for which the gamma ray response is a 3-step function. The effectiveness per rad for fast neutrons is, therefore, constant over
this entire range (Fig. 6). Its absolute value can only be estimated approximately because modern methods of absolute fast neutron
dosimetry had not yet been developed when these experiments were
carried out, but that has no effect on the value of these data in
establishing the shape of the effectiveness function for fast neutrons. The fast neutron data in Fig. 6 were scaled relative to
the gamma ray data by introducing the results of Ainsworth *et al.*
(1976), who gave B6CF$_1$ mice 36 rads/day of gamma rays or 3.6 rads/
day of fast neutrons and found an RBE very near to 10.

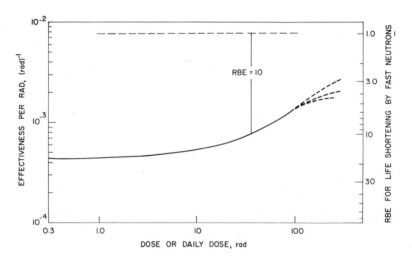

Fig. 6. Effectiveness functions for mice given daily duration-
of-life exposure to gamma rays and fast neutrons. Gamma ray data of
Grahn (1960) and Sacher and Grahn (1964), and fast neutron data of
Evans (1948) and Henshaw *et al.* (1947), as presented in Fig. 4
(Sacher, 1973). Scaling factor for effectiveness of fast neutrons
from the data of Ainsworth *et al.* (1974, 1976) for mice given weekly
fractions of 35.7 rad gamma rays and 3.3 rad fast neutrons. The
RBE scale on the right hand ordinate indicates that as dose decreases
the RBE approaches a limiting value of 18.

Since the effectiveness per rad of fast neutrons for D.o.L. exposure is constant, the effectiveness function for gamma rays is proportional to the reciprocal of the RBE (relative biological effectiveness) of fast neutrons relative to gamma rays. Therefore, Fig. 6 is the most direct evidence we have that the RBE for life shortening in mice by fast neutrons does not increase indefinitely, but instead approaches a constant value of 18 at low doses. However, such a limiting RBE cannot yet be estimated for dogs or guinea pigs.

Although the existence of a branch of constant effectiveness at low doses is known only for mouse and rat, the prudent course at this time is to postulate that there is a low-dose branch of constant effectiveness for low-LET radiation in every species. We must intensify our efforts to estimate the low-dose effectiveness parameter for at least a few species that are longer-lived than the mouse and rat, so that we can arrive at an estimate of its magnitude for man. In addition to the effort currently under way using the beagle dog (Norris *et al.*, 1976), another experiment will begin soon in the JANUS program, using the white-footed mouse, *Peromyscus leucopus*, a small rodent that has an 8-year lifespan as compared to the 3-year span of the laboratory mouse, but has acute and chronic radiosensitivity parameters similar to those for laboratory mice (Sacher and Staffeldt, 1973).

3.3. Fractionated Exposure

Brues and Sacher (1952) and Sacher (1960) exposed CF#1 female mice to X rays in six fractionation patterns, as specified in the legend to Fig. 8. Life tables were computed for the major neoplastic and non-neoplastic causes of death. Thymic lymphoma has a wave of increased incidence in the first year after exposure, and fractionation of the dose over a 12-day period is more effective than a single exposure for induction of lymphoma (Fig. 7). Increased effectiveness of fractionated exposure for lymphoma induction was observed independently by Kaplan and Brown (1952), who kept the number of exposure fractions constant and varied the interval between fractions. Total exposure time is a common factor between the two experiments, and hence is probably significant, along with the fractionation interval, for the production of a maximal fractionation effect in lymphoma induction. Other tumor types and non-neoplastic diseases typically show an increase of rate of incidence at all ages after exposure (Upton, 1961; Upton *et al.*, 1963).

The Gompertz function for all causes of death except thymic lymphoma is displaced upward parallel to the control by all patterns of fractionated exposure if exposure is completed before the onset of senescent mortality (Sacher, 1956), so the mean upward

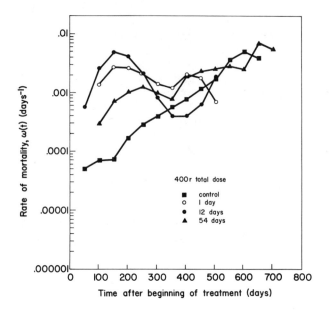

Fig. 7. Age-specific rates of incidence of thymic lymphoma
in CF#1 female mice given 400 R in 1, 10, or 40 fractions on a
schedule of 5 fractions per week. Mortality rates calculated by
Eq. (1).

displacement of the Gompertz function, $\Delta G(D)$, is a valid measure
of the amount of non-recovering injury produced by fractionated
exposure. Figure 8 gives $\Delta G(D)$ *versus* D for the six fractionation
conditions. The response is an accelerated function of dose, with
the curvature of the function decreasing as the number of fractions
and the total exposure time increases. The increment of $\Delta G(D)$ for
mammary tumor incidence in female CF#1 mice is constant, independent of dose and fractionation, in all treatment groups, consistent
with what was said above about a dose-independent component of
increased incidence of diseases of the reproductive system in
female mice given single doses greater than 100 R. It was therefore necessary to add an intercept parameter for the dose-independent sensitivity component of female mice, of about the same magnitude as the dose-independent sex difference observed for LAF_1 mice
given single exposures in the study by Upton *et al.* (1960).

A study of the effects of fractionation and protraction was
carried out by Noble *et al.* (1957, 1959a, b), using an F_2 hybrid
mouse. In one experiment they varied the fractionation interval,
keeping total dose and total elapsed time constant. Under these
conditions, with a total dose of 532 R of gamma rays given in 54
days at intervals of 1, 3, or 9 days, the Gompertz functions were

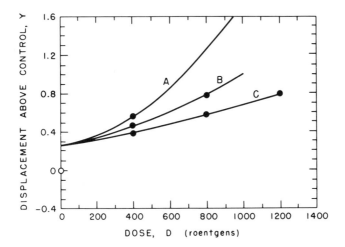

Fig. 8. The dose-effect relationship for CF#1 female mice
given single or fractionated exposures to X-rays. Effect estimated
as mean displacement of Gompertz function of treated groups from
controls. Exposure conditions are: single dose of 400 R; 400 and
800 R delivered in 10 fractions over 12 days; 400, 800, and 1200 R
delivered in 40 fractions over 54 days. Displacements calculated
by a nonorthogonal analysis of variance (From Sacher, 1956a).

displaced upward parallel to controls, and the effectiveness for
life shortening increased as dose per fraction increased from 10 R
to 30 R to 90 R.

Noble *et al.* (1959a) also compared the effects of fractionated
fast neutron and gamma ray exposures on the survival of male LAF_1
mice. The reduction of life expectation, ΔE, produced by gamma
rays in treatment groups given fractionated exposure for 18 or 54
days was a quadratic function of dose

$$\Delta E = 4.5 - 2.4 \cdot 10^{-3}D - 2.6 \cdot 10^{-6}D^2 \qquad (5)$$

while the life shortening by fast neutrons in similarly fractionated
treatments, was linear with dose

$$\Delta E = 8.0 - 31 \cdot 10^{-3}D \qquad (6)$$

Ainsworth *et al.* (1976), in the work in progress on the late
effects of fast neutrons and gamma rays on mice, observed that
fractionated fast neutron exposures are slightly more effective
than single doses for life shortening and for the induction of
lethal pulmonary tumors, and that delivery of 240 rad in 6 monthly
exposures decreases the life shortening effectiveness by 7 per cent

as compared to the same dose delivered in 24 weekly fractions.

4.   A PHENOMENOLOGICAL MODEL FOR THE FRACTIONATION AND QUALITY EFFECTS

The important feature of life shortening by low-LET radiations brought out by the fractionation studies is the existence of a time constant for the accumulation of the life-shortening lesion: a dose given over a period of several days or more is less effective for shortening life than the same dose given in a single brief exposure.   This was denied by Blair (1952, 1956), but the accumulated evidence for such an effect is now overwhelming.   This can be summarized by the somewhat paradoxical statement that there is a repair rate operating in the accumulation of the irreparable component of tissue injury.

Moreover, since the results of the D.o.L. survival studies on many species uniformly show that the mortality rate varies precisely as the square of the daily dose, we are obliged to consider the specific hypothesis that two latent injury events are involved in producing the dose-dependent component of irreparable injury.

In this section a phenomenological model of cellular radiation damage is developed that accounts for the quantitative characteristics of radiation life shortening brought out in Section 3.

The properties of radiation life shortening can be deduced from a mathematical model based on the following postulates:

   i.   Latent injury events are produced independently by low-LET radiation at a rate proportional to the instantaneous dose rate, and are distributed at random in the target regions of cells;

  ii.   Each latent event is repaired according to a characteristic function of time;

 iii.   Two injury events present simultaneously in the same target region can interact to produce a permanent cellular lesion.

The rate of production of permanent injury, x, then has the form

$$dx/dt = mR(t)\int_0^t R(\tau)\phi(t-\tau)d\tau, \qquad\qquad \tau \leq t \qquad\qquad (7)$$

in which

x is the amount of irreparable cell injury,
$R(t)$ is the dose rate at time t, $t \geq 0$,

$\phi(t-\tau)$ is the probability that a latent injury event occurring at time $0 \le \tau < t$ will be still unrepaired at time t.

It is postulated in addition that:

iv. A component of permanent cellular injury is produced in a single step at a rate k, proportional to the first power of the dose rate.

The complete expression for permanent tissue injury accumulation due to both single- and dual-event mechanisms is

$$dx/dt = kR(t) + mR(t)\int_0^t R(\tau)\phi(t-\tau)d\tau \qquad (8)$$

There is also an incidence of latent injury events at a rate, ρ, independent of radiation dose, produced by other environmental factors (Brewen and Preston, 1974), or by intrinsic replication errors. This leads to a modification of Eq. (8)

$$dx/dt = kR(t) + m[\rho + R(t)]\int_0^t [\rho + R(\tau)]\phi(t-\tau)d\tau \qquad (9)$$

The interaction between radiation-induced and other latent injury events gives rise to a term for first-power dependence of manifest injury on radiation dose which is indistinguishable from the term for the direct first-power production of permanent injury. Discrimination between the k-type and the ρ-type of first-power late effect terms is a matter of great importance for the evaluation of the effects of environmental radiations and other environmental factors on man.

In what follows, it will be assumed that the repair function, $\phi(t-\tau)$ obeys first-order chemical kinetics

$$\phi(t-\tau) = e^{-(t-\tau)/\Theta} \qquad (10)$$

where Θ is the mean recovery time. For the case of continuous exposure at constant rate R, Eq. (8) then becomes

$$dx/dt = kR + mR^2\Theta(1-e^{-t/\Theta}) \qquad (11)$$

and the solution is

$$x = kRt + mR^2\Theta[t-\Theta(1-e^{-t/\Theta})] \qquad (12)$$

The effects of brief single doses can be evaluated by making t small, $t << \Theta$, so that Eq. (12) becomes

$$x = kD + mD^2/2 \qquad (13)$$

where $D = Rt$.

In the D.o.L. exposure condition, irradiation continues to death, which is postulated to occur at a constant level of injury, so we introduce the assumption that for each R the lethal end point is reached at the time, T, when x reaches a critical value which can be assumed to be equal to unity

$$1 = kRT + mR^2\Theta[T-\Theta(1-e^{-T/\Theta})] \qquad (14)$$

Eq. (14) gives the entire range of the three-branched D.o.L. survival relation. In the limit for very long survival times, $T \gg \Theta$, Eq. (14) reduces to

$$T^{-1} = kR + m\Theta R^2 \qquad (15)$$

Here T^{-1} is the mean mortality rate in the absence of other causes of death, and it can therefore be equated to the mean radiation-specific death rate. The first- and second-power trends at low and medium daily doses (Fig. 4) are accounted for by Eq. (15). At very low survival times, $T \ll \Theta$, we may expand the exponential term in Eq. (11) and integrate to find

$$x = kRT + mR^2T^2/2 \qquad (16)$$

The term in the first power of T is negligible, so setting $x = 1$ and solving for T^{-1} yields

$$T^{-1} = R(m/2)^{\frac{1}{2}} \qquad (17)$$

Equation (17) shows that the life shortening relation for D.o.L. exposure rolls off from the second-power trend to a first-power trend at sufficiently high daily doses. However, this simple model is not adequate for the analysis of the lethality produced by D.o.L. exposure at very high daily dosages. The model employed by Sacher (1954; Sacher and Grahn, 1964) is more appropriate for these conditions, but it is not relevant to our present purposes.

The mathematical analysis of fractionation effects will be considered for the case of n brief equal fractions, spaced at equal interval h. The amount of permanent injury accumulated at the completion of such a series of treatment is

$$x = kD + m(2n^2)^{-1}D^2[n + (n-1)e^{-\Theta h} + (n-2)e^{-2\Theta h} + \dots + e^{-(n-1)\Theta h}] \qquad (18)$$

If $\Theta h \gg 1$, the exponential terms vanish, so the fractions do not interact, and the bracketed function in Eq. (18) reduces to the first term, which is the sum of the effects of the doses given separately,

$$x = kD + m(2n)^{-1}D^2 \tag{19}$$

If the total dose is fixed and the number of fractions varies, a more convenient form is

$$x = kD(1 + mD_f/2k) \tag{20}$$

where D_f is dose per fraction, equal to D/n.

The time constant, Θ, that is needed to account for the time-dependence of the accumulation of permanent injury produced by fractionated exposure has a numerical value of 5 days in Sacher's (1956a) fractionation experiment. An experiment is in progress at Argonne National Laboratory on the comparison of fractionation and protraction effects produced by fast neutrons and gamma rays (Ainsworth *et al.*, 1976). Definitive analysis of the data is not yet possible, but a preliminary analysis indicates that the time constant, Θ, for repair of the latent lesion in this experiment can be tentatively bounded between 3 and 10 days.

5.   IMPLICATIONS FOR THE CELLULAR LESION

The foregoing brief examination of the dose- and time-kinetics for the production of irreparable tissue injury suffices to show that the data of late radiation damage can be accounted for by a consistent phenomenological model. The important inferences deducible from the model are: (1) an important component of late effect arises from an interaction between two injury events, and (2) this interaction has a time constant on the order of several days.

The existence of a time constant of this magnitude may also be inferred from the data of radiation therapy. Cohen and Scott (1968) have carried out a theoretical analysis of the effects of fractionated exposure in radiotherapy, and show that the existance of an optimum fractionation schedule for tumor therapy depends on a difference in the growth constants of the normal and tumor tissues.

The reciprocal growth rates for normal tissues range from about one day to many months (Fry and Reiskin, 1972), so they are of the correct magnitude, but there remains the question of the mechanism whereby the growth rate of tissue cells is implicated in the accumulation of irreparable damage in tissues. The large variation of species sensitivity to D.o.L. exposure (Fig. 5) presents a favorable situation for examination of that relationship.

The fact that irreparable radiation damage induced by D.o.L. exposure to gamma rays accumulates almost exactly as the square of the daily dose (Fig. 4, 5) is a finding of great importance for future work on the underlying cellular lesion, because it requires us to seek an explanation of the late effect lesion in terms of a two-event process. This highly specific dose-dependence cannot be predicted from current knowledge about the effects of ionizing radiations on cultured mammalian cells, for cell survival curves vary in shape, and the extrapolation numbers for low-LET exposures show a wide range of variation above and below 2.0 (Elkind and Whitmore, 1967). Cohen (1971) developed a mathematical model for estimating the effects of fractionated exposures on healthy and tumorous tissues, based on the postulate that the cell parameters estimated by *in vitro* assay procedures carry over to the late responses of tissues given fractionated exposures *in situ*. That may indeed be true for a similar end point, such as the killing of tumor cells, but in view of the results reported here the possibility arises that for the kinds of tissue damage that arise from non-lethal changes in surviving cells the multiplicity parameter has a more restricted range than those estimated for cell killing *in vitro*.

The greatly strengthened evidence for a strict dependence of effect on the square of the dose or fraction makes it obligatory to give continued consideration to the hypothesis that late effects are primarily a consequence of chromosome rearrangements. A mathematical analysis of chromosome damage and cell lethality now in progress (Sacher, 1973; Sacher, Gabriel and Tyler, 1974) is yielding interesting new results that account quantitatively for the effects of D.o.L. exposure to low-LET radiations, and therefore support the hypothesis that late radiation damage is chromosomal.

6. SUMMARY

The salient phenomena of life shortening in mammals due to ionizing radiations can be summarized as follows:

  i.   Actuarial analysis of the effects of single exposure and lifetime exposure to gamma rays and fast neutrons leads to the conclusion that radiation injury does not "accelerate" the aging process, but rather is superimposed additively on the aging injury, which continues to accumulate much as it does in the untreated population.

  ii. Ionizing radiation leaves a residue of irreparable tissue damage, so that each increment of dose causes a permanent increase by a constant factor in the death rate.

  iii. The life shortening, for mice and rats given single doses of low-LET radiation, estimated either by the decrease of life expectation, $\Delta E(D)$, or by the increase of Gompertz function intercept, $\Delta G(D)$, is a quadratic function of dose.

iv. In mammals given daily duration-of-life exposure to low-LET radiations the increase of Gompertz function slope or increase of mean radiation-specific mortality rate is proportional to the daily dose at low daily doses, then shifts to the square of daily dose at higher daily doses, and decreases again toward a first-power dependence on daily dose for daily doses in the range of hundreds of rad/day. This means that the effectiveness per rad is constant at low daily doses, increases over an intermediate range, then approaches constancy again at very high daily doses.

v. The effectiveness per rad for fast neutrons is almost constant, but has a weak dependence on dose and fractionation.

vi. The effectiveness per rad for life shortening by fractionated exposures to a fixed total dose of low-LET radiation decreases with increase in the number of fractions, or interval between fractions, or total elapsed exposure time.

These phenomena can be accounted for by a simple and consistent mathematical model. It is noteworthy that the kinetics of life shortening consistently show a dependence of effect on the square of the dose, whereas the data on killing of cultured mammalian cells show a considerably greater degree of variability in dose-dependence. The reason for this difference is not known, but the facts justify serious consideration for the hypothesis that the quadratic dose dependence for irreparable injury arises from chromosome aberrations.

Acknowledgment. Work supported by the U.S. Energy Research and Development Administration.

References

Ainsworth, E.J., Fry, R.J.M., Grahn, D., Williamson, F.S., Brennan, P.C., Stearner, S.P., Carrano, A.V., and Rust, J.H., 1974, Late effects of neutron or gamma irradiation, *in* "Biological Effects of Neutron Irradiation," pp. 359-379, IAEA-SM-179/1, International Atomic Energy Agency, Vienna.
Ainsworth, E.J., Fry, R.J.M., Brennan, P.C., Stearner, S.P., Rust, J.H., Lombard, L.S., and Williamson, F.S., 1976, Life shortening, neoplasia, and systemic injuries in mice after single or fractionated doses of neutron or gamma irradiation, *in* "Proceedings of the International Symposium on Biological Effects of Low Level Radiation Pertinent to Protection of Man and His Environment," Chicago, November, 1975 (to be published).
Blair, H.A., 1952, A formulation of the injury, life span, dose

relations for ionizing radiations. I. Application to the
mouse, University of Rochester Atomic Energy Project Report
No. UR-206, Rochester, New York.

Blair, H.A., 1956, Data pertaining to shortening of life span by
ionizing radiation, University of Rochester Atomic Energy
Project Report No. UR-442, Rochester, New York.

Boche, R.D., 1954, Effects of chronic exposure to X radiation on
growth and survival, *in* "Biological Effects of External
Radiation" (H.A. Blair, ed.), pp. 220-252, McGraw-Hill, New
York.

Brewen, J.G., and Preston, R.J., 1974, Cytogenetic effects of
environmental mutagens in mammalian cells and the extrapolation to man, *Mutat. Res.* 26:297-305.

Brues, A.M., and Sacher, G.A., 1952, Analysis of mammalian radia-
tion injury and lethality, *in* "Symposium on Radiobiology"
(J.J. Nickson, ed.), pp. 441-465, John Wiley and Sons, New
York.

Cohen, L., 1971, A cell population kinetic model for fractionated
radiation therapy. I. Normal tissues, *Radiology* 101:419-427.

Cohen, L., and Scott, M.J., 1968, Fractionation procedures in radiation therapy: A computerized approach to evaluation, *Brit. J.
Radiol.* 41:529-533.

Elkind, M.M., and Whitmore, G.F., 1967, "The Radiobiology of Cultured Mammalian Cells," Gordon and Breach, New York.

Evans, T.C., 1948, Effects of small daily doses of fast neutrons
on mice, *Radiology* 50:811-833.

Fry, R.J.M., and Reiskin, A., 1972, Tissue growth and renewal:
Mammals, *in* "Biology Data Book" (P.L. Altman and D. Dittmer,
eds.), 2nd edition, Vol. 1, pp. 95-115, Federation of American
Societies for Experimental Biology, Bethesda, Maryland.

Furth, J., Upton, A.C., Christenberry, K.W., Benedict, W.H., and
Moshman, J., 1954, Some late effects in mice of ionizing radiation from an experimental nuclear detonation, *Radiology* 63:
562-570.

Grahn, D., 1960, Genetic control of physiological processes: The
genetics of radiation toxicity in animals, *in* "Symposium on
Radioisotopes in the Biosphere" (R.S. Caldecott and L.A.
Snyder, eds.), pp. 181-200, The Center for Continuation
Study, University of Minnesota, Minneapolis, Minnesota.

Grahn, D., 1970, Biological effects of protracted low dose radiation exposure of man and animals, *in* "Late Effects of Radiation" (R.J.M. Fry, D. Grahn, M.L. Griem, and J.H. Rust, eds.),
pp. 101-136, Taylor and Francis, London.

Henshaw, P.S., Riley, E.F., and Stapleton, G.E., 1947, The biologic
effects of pile radiations, *Radiology* 49:349-360.

Kaplan, H.S., and Brown, M.B., 1952, A quantitative dose-response
study of lymphoid tumor development in irradiated C57 black
mice, *J. Nat. Cancer Inst.* 13:185-208.

Lea, D.E., 1947, Actions of Radiations on Living Cells, 416 pp.,
First Edition, Cambridge, The University Press.

Lindop, P.J., and Rotblat, J., 1961, Long-term effects of a single
     whole-body exposure of mice to ionizing radiations. I. Life
     shortening, *Proc. Roy. Soc. (London)* Ser. B 154:332-349.
Lindop, P.J., Rotblat, J., and Vatistas, S., 1966, The effect of
     age and hypoxia on the long-term response of the ovary to
     radiation, *in* "Radiation and Ageing" Proceedings of a Collo-
     quium held in Semmering, Austria, June 23-24, 1966" (P.J.
     Lindop and G.A. Sacher, eds.), pp. 307-324, Taylor and Francis,
     London.
Lorenz, E., Jacobson, L.O., Heston, W.E., Shimkin, M., Eschenbrenner,
     A.B., Deringer, M.K., Doniger, J., and Schweisthal, R., 1954,
     Effects of long-continued total-body gamma irradiation on mice,
     guinea pigs, and rabbits. III. Effects on life span, weight,
     blood picture, and carcinogenesis and the role of the intensity
     of radiation, *in* "Biological Effects of External X and Gamma
     Radiation" (R.E. Zirkle, ed.), National Nuclear Energy Series,
     Div. IV, Vol. 22B, pp. 24-148, McGraw-Hill, New York.
Muller, H.J., 1950, Some present problems in the genetic effects
     of radiation, *J. Cell Comp. Physiol.* 35:Suppl. 1, 9-70.
Noble, J.F., Hasegawa, A.T., Hallesy, D.W., Landahl, H.D., and Doull,
     J., 1957, The influence of exposure to low levels of gamma and
     fast neutron irradiation on the lifespan of mice, University
     of Chicago USAF Radiation Laboratory Quarterly Progress Report
     23:78-96.
Noble, J.F., Hasegawa, A.T., Landahl, H.D., and Doull, J., 1959a,
     The influence of exposure to low levels of gamma and fast
     neutron irradiation on the life span of mice. I. Current
     status of chronic gamma and fast neutron irradiation studies,
     University of Chicago USAF Radiation Laboratory Quarterly
     Progress Report 31:54-62.
Noble, J.F., Hasegawa, A.T., Landahl, H.D., and Doull, J., 1959b,
     The influence of exposure to low levels of gamma and fast
     neutron irradiation on the life span of mice. III. The
     survival time of mice exposed to radiation at various doses
     and exposure patterns for prolonged periods early in life,
     University of Chicago USAF Radiation Laboratory Quarterly
     Progress Report 31:78-91.
Noonan, T., Van Slyke, F., and Hursh, J., 1951, Effect of single
     doses of X-ray on the survival of rats, The University of
     Rochester Atomic Energy Project Report UR-161.
Norris, W.P., Tyler, S.A., and Sacher, G.A., 1976, An interspecies
     comparison of the response of mice and dogs to continuous
     ^{60}Co γ-irradiation, *in* "Proceedings of I.A.E.A. Symposium on
     Biological Effects of Low Level Radiation Pertinent to Pro-
     tection of Man and His Environment," Chicago, November, 1975
     (to be published).
Rust, J.H., Robertson, R.J., Staffeldt, E.F., Sacher, G.A., Grahn,
     D., and Fry, R.J.M., 1966, Effects of lifetime periodic gamma-
     ray exposure on the survival and pathology of guinea pigs, *in*
     "Radiation and Ageing: Proceedings of a Colloquium held in

Semmering, Austria, June 23-24, 1966" (P.J. Lindop and G.A. Sacher, eds.), pp. 217-244, Taylor and Francis, London.

Sacher, G.A., 1956a, On the statistical nature of mortality, with especial reference to chronic radiation mortality, *Radiology* 67:250-257.

Sacher, G.A., 1956b, Survival of mice under duration-of-life exposure to X-rays at various rates, *in* "Biological Effects of External X and Gamma Radiation" (R.E. Zirkle, ed.), Part 2, TID-5220, Ch. 24, pp. 435-453, Department of Commerce, Office of Technical Services, Washington, D.C.

Sacher, G.A., 1959, Reparable and irreparable injury. A survey of the position in experiment and theory, *in* "Radiation Biology and Medicine" (W. Claus, ed.), Ch. 12, pp. 283-313, Addison-Wesley, Reading, Mass.

Sacher, G.A., 1960, Problems in the extrapolation of long term effects from animals to man, *in* "The Delayed Effects of Whole-Body Radiation" (B.B. Watson, ed.), pp. 31-40, The Johns Hopkins Press, Baltimore, Md.

Sacher, G.A., 1966, The Gompertz transformation in the study of the injury-mortality relationship: Application to late radiation effects and aging, *in* "Radiation and Ageing: Proceedings of a Colloquium held in Semmering, Austria, June 23-24, 1966" (P.J. Lindop and G.A. Sacher, eds.), pp. 411-441, Taylor and Francis, London.

Sacher, G.A., 1973, Dose dependence for life shortening by X-rays, gamma rays and fast neutrons, *in* "Advances in Radiation Research, Biology and Medicine: Proceedings of the Fourth International Congress of Radiation Research, Evian, France, June 29-July 4, 1970" (J.P. Duplan and A. Chapiro, eds.), Vol. 3, pp. 1425-1432, Gordon and Breach, New York.

Sacher, G.A., Gabriel, M., and Tyler, S.A., 1974, Markov chain model for chromosome aberrations and cell lethality (abstract), *Radiat. Res.* 59:296-297.

Sacher, G.A., and Grahn, D., 1964, Survival of mice under duration-of-life exposure to gamma rays. I. The dosage-survival relation and the lethality function, *J. Nat. Cancer Inst.* 32:277-321.

Sacher, G.A., and Staffeldt, E., 1972, Life tables of seven species of laboratory-reared rodents, *Gerontologist* 12(3 Part II):39 (abstract).

Sacher, G.A., and Staffeldt, E., 1973, Species differences of rodents to life shortening by chronic gamma irradiation, *in* Proceedings Third National Symposium on Radioecology, Oak Ridge, Tennessee, May 10-12, 1971" (D.J. Nelson, ed.), U.S.A.E.C. Report No. Conf. 710501-P1, pp. 1042-1047.

Sacher, G.A., and Trucco, E., 1962, A theory of the improved performance and survival produced by small doses of radiations and other poisons, *in* "Biological Aspects of Aging: Proceedings of the Fifth International Congress of Gerontology, San Francisco, August, 1960" (N.W. Shock, ed.), pp. 244-251, Columbia

University Press, New York.

Sacher, G.A., and Tyler, S.A., 1972, Dose dependence for life short-
     ening in mammals exposed to gamma rays, X-rays or fast neutrons
     (abstract), *Radiat. Res.* 51:477.

Storer, J.B., Cosgrove, G.E., Darden, E.B., Jr., Jernigan, M.C.,
     Klima, W.C., Satterfield, L.C., Swann, H.C., and Yuhas, J.M.,
     1973, Late somatic effects of low doses of gamma rays, Oak
     Ridge National Laboratory, Biology Division Annual Progress
     Report, ORNL-4915, October, p. 141.

Storer, J.B., Cosgrove, G.E., Darden, E.B., Jr., Serrano, L.J.,
     Jernigan, M.C., Klima, W.C., Satterfield, C., Swann, H.C.,
     and Martin, F.S., 1974, Late somatic effects of ionizing
     radiation in mice as a function of dose, dose rate, and
     radiation quality, Oak Ridge National Laboratory, Biology
     Division Annual Progress Report, ORNL-4993, November, pp. 149-
     150.

Upton, A.C., 1961, The dose-response relation in radiation-induced
     cancer, *Cancer Res.* 21:717-729.

Upton, A.C., Kastenbaum, M.A., and Conklin, J.W., 1963, Age-specific
     death rates of mice exposed to ionizing radiation and radio-
     mimetic agents, *in* "Symposium on Cellular Basis and Aetiology
     of Late Somatic Effects of Ionizing Radiations" (R.J.C. Harris,
     ed.), pp. 285-294, Academic Press, New York.

Upton, A.C., Kimball, A.W., Furth, J., Christenberry, K.W., and
     Benedict, W.H., 1960, Some delayed effects of atomic-bomb
     radiations in mice, *Cancer Res.* 20(8, Part 2):1-60.

W.P.A., 1940, Tables of sine, cosine and exponential integrals,
     2 Vols., Department of Commerce, Washington, D.C.

PROTECTION OF ENVIRONMENTALLY STRESSED HUMAN CELLS IN CULTURE WITH THE FREE RADICAL SCAVENGER, dl-α-TOCOPHEROL

Lester Packer

Membrane Bioenergetics Group, Lawrence Berkeley Laboratory, and the Department of Physiology-Anatomy, University of California, Berkeley, California 94720

1. INTRODUCTION

Like others, we are interested in the extent to which the lifespan of normal human (WI-38) cells in culture (Hayflick, 1965) is a genetically-determined or environmentally-limited phenomenon. Our approach to this problem stems from our long standing interest in the area of biological oxidation and bioenergetics, and the work of Tappel's laboratory (Tappel, 1962, 1973) which led us to consider that the free-radical mediated damage (Harman, 1956) might be amenable for investigation in human cells in culture using free-radical scavengers. In particular, that free-radical damage to membranes containing biological oxidation catalysts (Packer *et al.*, 1967) or environmentally-induced free-radicals might be important in limiting the lifespan of WI-38 cells.

A scheme for free-radical damage is shown in Fig. 1. Induced damage may arise as by photosensitized reactions which lead to singlet oxygen formation initiating free-radicals or may occur by hydrogen abstraction via electron transport catalysts in membranes, leading to hydroperoxides, breakdown products, polymerization and other protein adducts, in a chain reaction leading to the inactivation of enzymes (Tappel, 1973; Packer *et al.*, 1967; Bindra, 1974). A naturally occurring antioxidant, which partitions into membranes and which tends to break this chain of events, is dl-α-tocopherol or vitamin E. In Fig. 2, this substance is depicted in a bilayer of phospholipids to act by quenching free-radicals, itself becoming a free-radical, but in this case, a more stable radical is formed.

2. VITAMIN E RADICALS IN MEMBRANES

Vitamin E may partition into a membrane by intercollating with the hydrocarbon tails of the phospholipids perhaps as shown in Fig. 3. Model building studies (Lucy, 1972) tend to suggest that vitamin E lies next to the arachidonic acid, the 20:4 unsaturated fatty acid of membrane phospholipids. The charged portion of the molecule on the chromanol ring probably partitions at the polar hydrocarbon interface. The role of vitamin E as an antioxidant has been well established. In animals, many different reactions

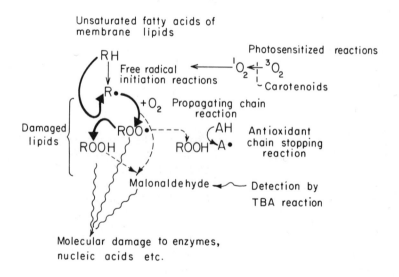

Fig. 1. Scheme for environmental and metabolically induced free-radical mediated oxidation of lipids.

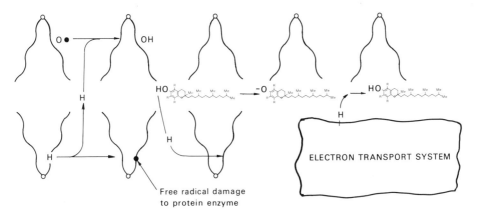

Fig. 2.   Diagram illustrating free-radical chain terminating
properties of dl-α-tocopherol (vitamin E) in a membrane.

are affected by the presence or absence of vitamin E, yet looking
at its molecular structure it is not immediately apparent how it
can exert all these different affects.   This suggests that it may
have some sort of structural effect at the membrane level (Lucy,
1972; Molenaar *et al.*, 1972) in addition to antioxidant activity.
Some of the approaches we are pursuing are: a) to synthesize a
spin labeled vitamin E and examine its orientation in the membrane
(Dr. R. Mehlhorn); b) to investigate how vitamin E partitions in
the membrane (Dr. A. Quintanilha); c) to generate electrolytically
the semiquinone forms of vitamin E and to investigate the hyperfine splittings in EPR spectra (Dr. G. Case).   The EPR spectra
suggest that the free-radicals are distributed not only over the
chromanol ring, but may extend into 2-3 methylene groups of the
hydrocarbon tail; d) to incorporate vitamin E into liposomes and
then to generate free-radicals of vitamin E with ultraviolet
irradiation (Michaelis and Wollman, 1950).   Such preparations were
then treated with various rare earth ions like lanthanum or
gadolinium, neither of which penetrate liposome vesicles. La^{+3}
is diamagnetic, hence it would not alter the EPR spectrum, but Gd^{+3}
is paramagnetic and could cause exchange broadening of the spectrum
if it can approach near to the unpaired electron of the chromanol
ring; but this was not found.   Hence these results thus far suggest
that in this model system the unpaired electron is probably distributed in an inaccessible region of the hydrocarbon domain of the
membrane.

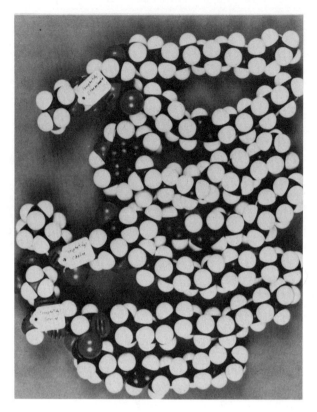

Fig. 3. Proposed partitioning of dl-α-tocopherol in the bilamelar structure of membrane phospholipids. Shown are three membrane phospholipids and vitamin E (unlabeled). The chromanol ring is presumed to be oriented with the charged hydroxyl group at the polar hydrocarbon interface. The hydrocarbon tail extends into the interior of the phospholipid bilayer parallel to fatty acid hydrocarbon tails.

3. CELL PROLIFERATION STUDIES - LONG-TERM STUDIES IN THE CULTURE ENVIRONMENT

About two years ago Dr. J. Smith and I began to study the effect of vitamin E on the growth of WI-38 cells. Initially we found it to be highly toxic to cell growth. We were then dispensing it into the medium in alcohol solution. When the amounts were lowered, toxicity was apparent only after several population doublings. When the alcohol was eliminated and dl-α-tocopherol was blended into the serum, toxicity was eliminated. A series of six independent experiments (shown in Fig. 4) were performed in which a marked extension in the lifespan of WI-38 cells was found

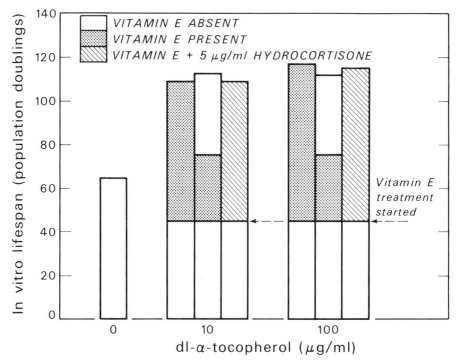

Fig. 4. Summary of a series of six experiments with WI-38 human cells showing extension of lifespan in the presence of vitamin E (Packer and Smith, 1974).

(Packer and Smith, 1974). Cells exposed to vitamin E did not show marked changes in the pattern of the growth. For example, as seen in Fig. 5, when three times the amount was blended into the culture medium as used in the long-term experiments, there was a slight lag before growth commenced, but the cells grew at the same rate and reached the same saturation density as in the absence of vitamin E. Various other parameters were investigated. There was no evidence of SV-40 tumor antigen, and also the cultures were mycoplasma free. The morphology of passage 93 cells were like young cells; also the karyotype was normal. The progressive accumulation of autofluorescent material in WI-38 cells in long-term culture (Packer and Smith, 1974; Deamer and Gonzales, 1974) was virtually absent in cells beyond passage 90. Deamer and Gonzales (1974) found, by autoradiographic techniques with [H³]thymidine incorporation, that those cells in the population having high levels of this fluorescent material are precisely the cells of the population which are incapable of DNA synthesis. Dr. J. Smith and I decided that if the cells reached the 100th population doubling level and their karyotype and other control parameters were normal, we would

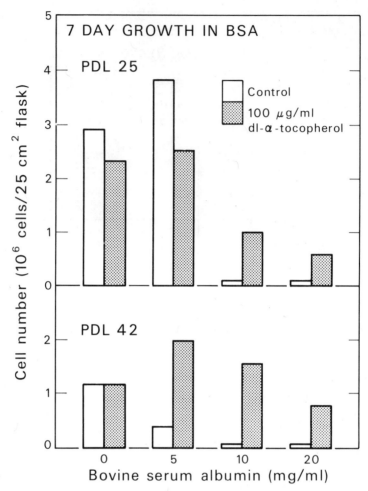

Fig. 5. Synergistic effects of bovine serum albumin and dl-α-tocopherol in stimulating growth of young and old human WI-38 cells in culture. PDL = population doubling level (after J. Smith and L. Packer).

report our results (Packer and Smith, 1974). Subsequently, the cells ceased to divide somewhere between 110 and 118 population doublings as shown in a summary of this series of experiments (Fig. 4). Cells grown in the presence of 100 µg of vitamin E/ml were capable of a few more population doubling levels than cells cultivated in the presence of 10 µg/ml.

Initially, when these results were observed, we were surprised because, on the basis of population doubling rate at the 100th population doubling level, it appeared that they would have continued growing in culture for a very long time. There was no evidence that the cells were reaching the senescent stage (phase III). However, we then recognized that the end of this experiment was a "blessing in disguise," because it answered the important question: Had the cells become transformed? Virus transformed WI-38 cells in the same culture environment proliferate indefinitely (but manifest an abnormal karyotype including polyploidy). Although the karyotypic analysis performed tended to rule out this possibility, it was still possible that negative results might not suffice. Examination of our protocols showed that the original lot of serum (lot #1023) was exhausted at about the 100th population doubling level, and it became necessary to continue growing the cells on another lot of serum (lot #4041). It was not anticipated that this series of experiments would last 1.2 years. It appears that changing the lot of serum had the effect of essentially placing the cells into phase III and cell division ceased. Thus, the action of dl-α-tocopherol in this system is probably synergistic with a particular lot of serum.

It is known that vitamin E and unsaturated fatty acids, especially arachidonic acid, parallel one another in terms of their requirements for human nutrition. So we became interested in testing the fatty acid composition of serum being used in these and other growth experiments. Furthermore, the only other direct affect of vitamin E on human cells is the hemolytic anemias to which certain children are susceptible. When the unsaturated fatty acids like arachidonic acid are lowered and the vitamin E levels of the diet are increased, this disease is corrected (Brin et al., 1974). Indeed, the biological test used for vitamin E-deficiency is the induction of erythrocyte hemolysis.

Therefore, analyses of several different sera were performed by gas-liquid chromatography techniques. Data on fatty acid composition is shown in Table 1. One point of interest was that the growth-promoting serum (lot #1023) had the lowest concentration of arachidonic acid. Another lot of serum (lot #4041) was the most toxic and had the highest arachidonic acid levels. There wasn't much difference in the total amount of the fatty acids present. Such data for the distribution of fatty acids shown here is similar to what has been reported by other laboratories (Kritchevsky and Howard, 1970). Another finding of interest (not shown in Table 1) is that the free fatty acid content of the long-life promoting serum (lot #1023) was about one half that of the toxic serum (lot #4041) that caused the cells after the 100th population doubling level to go into senescence.

This finding caused us to reflect further, as for several years our laboratory has been trying to extend the "shelf-life" of isolated organelles like mitochondria and chloroplasts *in vitro,*

Table 1. Analyses of the Fatty Acid Composition of Several Lots of Fetal Calf Serum used for Growth Experiments with WI-38 Cells

| | PERCENT TOTAL FATTY ACID | | | |
| | Serum lot no. | | | |
FATTY ACID	1023	2343	5542	4014C
14:0	1.8	1.7	1.3	1.6
14:0	—	—	—	2.9
16:0	19.7	24.9	22.4	20.8
16:1	11.2	9.0	8.3	10.3
iso 16:1	1.4	0.9	0.8	0.8
17:0	1.3	1.1	1.3	1.3
18:0	15.7	15.0	17.7	11.7
18:1	32.2	31.6	33.2	34.4
18:2	8.0	5.4	5.5	4.7
20:4	7.0	7.6	8.1	10.8
22:0	1.6	1.2	1.4	0.8
Total fatty acid (μg/ml serum)	372	318	331	320

i.e., how long can isolated organelles maintain function *in vitro*? Recently, our laboratory reported (Takaoki *et al.*, 1974) that chloroplasts could be kept functioning with respect to energy dependent light and/or electron transport-dependent proton gradients for 45 days if the stock chloroplast suspension was kept in the presence of a radical scavenger (butylated hydroxytoluene) and bovine serum albumin (BSA) as a scavenger for free fatty acids. Numerous investigators have noted during storage of organelles a low level of phospholipase activity releases free fatty acids from membrane phospholipids, and free fatty acids are known to be very damaging to membrane structure and function. In fact, Todaro and Green (1964) reported that normal human fibroblasts in culture could be cultivated to 100 population doublings if the culture medium was supplemented with high levels of BSA. This observation has been "lying in the closet" for a long time, and appears on the basis of our current studies to warrant reinvestigation. Hence, we decided to initiate experiments on the effects of BSA on WI-38 cell proliferation.

It can be seen in Fig. 5 that a stimulation of growth occurs in young cells with some levels of BSA, but this is not observed in older cells unless vitamin E is also present. BSA may be providing a vehicle for scavenging the fatty acids, or may permit better exchange of the vitamin E into cells. It may be that several other reports of protein factors stimulating the growth of cells in culture may act in a similar way. When we know more about such factors we may be able to cultivate WI-38 and other cells in long-term culture on a more routine basis than is possible at present. The experiments described here and those proposed above should further elucidate the conditions required for long-term culture.

In Fig. 6 an experiment is shown where we had been nursing cells along on a lot of serum (lot #4144) which is toxic, the cells were then transferred to lot #2343 and eventually to yet a new lot of serum (lot #5542). Eventually cells in the presence of vitamin E began to grow. It could be that the presence of vitamin E may "tip the balance," in terms of the ability of the cells to survive exposure to toxic sera enabling a sub-population to develop which eventually can grow out.

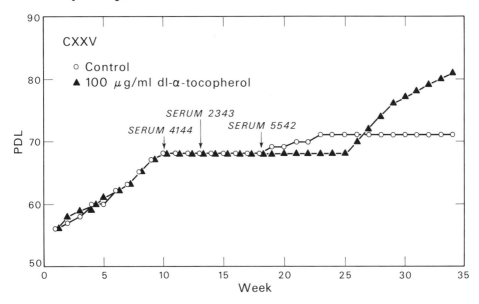

Fig. 6. Dependence of dl-α-tocopherol stimulation of human WI-38 cell growth in the presence of different lots of sera (L. Packer and J. Smith, unpublished results).

The levels of vitamin E in fetal calf serum are normally about 1 μg/ml. This is 10 times less than that in human plasma. Its supplementation into the medium can effectively prevent the oxidation of WI-38 cell lipids. Table 2 shows data for malondialdehyde formation in sonicated cells. Malondialdehyde formation is inhibited when cells are grown in the presence of solubilized preparations of tocopherol acetate (gift of Hoffman-La Roche, Nutley, N.J.); the presence of an esterase in WI-38 cells renders this form biologically active. Also, the dl-α-tocopherol which is blended into the medium at concentrations >10 μg/ml virtually eliminates

Table 2. Affect of Vitamin E on Malondialdehyde Formation and
WI-38 Cells

| dl-α-tocopherol in growth medium (μg/ml) | Solubilized | | Blended |
	dl-α-tocopherol acetate	dl-α-tocopherol	dl-α-tocopherol
5	87 ±5	96 ±1	
10	97 ±1	99 ±1	90
50	98 ±1	97 ±1	95
100	95 ±0.5	94 ±3	98 ±1

Sonicated WI-38 cells, 1 mg protein/ml
Incubated 2 hrs at 37°C in 0.05 M phosphate buffer, pH 7.0
plus 0.2 mg/ml ascorbic acid, 10 μg/ml FeCl$_2$

the oxidation of WI-38 cell lipids. Hence vitamin E, insofar as
its antioxidant function toward lipids is concerned, seems effective under the conditions of our experiments.

4. GROWTH AND PROTECTION OF ENVIRONMENTALLY STRESSED WI-38 CELLS

In a given environment, cells suffer a certain amount of
damage. If the rate at which the damage accumulates exceeds the
rate at which the cell's genetic potential can correct it by
division or biosynthesis, then the damage should accumulate. We
should essentially clog the works much as in glycogen storage
diseases (Hers and Hoof, 1973) when a genetic defect of a hydrolytic enzyme decreases the time scale of the accumulation of an
insoluble, indigestible, intracellular material which eventually
destroys human cells. To evaluate the importance of environmental
factors in limiting the lifespan of WI-38 cells, we are investigating the effects of several different types of environmental
and/or nutritional stresses. These are: starvation, the effects
of gaseous substances (such as oxygen and other gaseous pollutants)
and riboflavin photosensitized damage. In each case we are evaluating the protective effects of dl-α-tocopherol in protecting
WI-38 cells from lethal effects.

4.1. Senescence of Nonmitotic Low Serum Starved Cells

The result of starvation in 0.1% serum is shown in Fig. 7
(D.W. Deamer, collaboration). After 7 weeks, cells maintained in

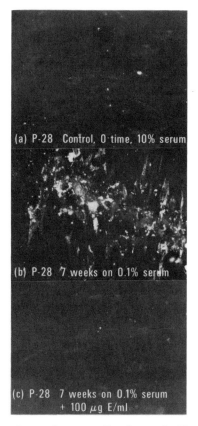

(a) P-28 Control, 0 time, 10% serum

(b) P-28 7 weeks on 0.1% serum

(c) P-28 7 weeks on 0.1% serum
          + 100 μg E/ml

Fig. 7. Prevention of accumulation of fluorescent damage
material in low serum starved human WI-38 cells. Confluent cultures of cells were kept in 0.1% serum for a 7 week interval in
the absence and presence of vitamin E (courtesy Dr. David W.
Deamer).

the presence of low serum show appreciable accumulation of autofluorescent material. The cells appear like senescent cells
characteristic of phase III. However, cells kept for 7 weeks in
the presence of the low serum plus vitamin E do not show this
accumulation; they are "clean." They look just like cells in
young cultures or cells in our long-term cultures supplemented
with vitamin E and examined at passage 93 (Packer and Smith, 1974).
Indeed, qualitatively they look "cleaner" than early passage controls. As mentioned above, the presence of high levels of this
material in WI-38 cells is directly correlated with the inability
of individual cells of the population to synthesize DNA. Although
these findings do not prove that progressive accumulation of autofluorescent material kills WI-38 cells, it does provide

circumstantial evidence of it.

4.2. Oxygen Toxicity (J. Smith, K. Collier, collaboration)

Cells that had reached confluency were exposed to various oxygen tensions in the presence of increasing amounts of dl-α-tocopherol in the medium. Protection against the toxic effects of oxygen is afforded by the presence of dl-α-tocopherol. A linear increase in the number of viable cells is found as the vitamin is increased from 10 to 100 μg/ml for cells exposed to 50% oxygen (Fig. 8).

In other experiments with confluent cultures exposed to oxygen and treated with vitamin E, we have observed in the range from 40%

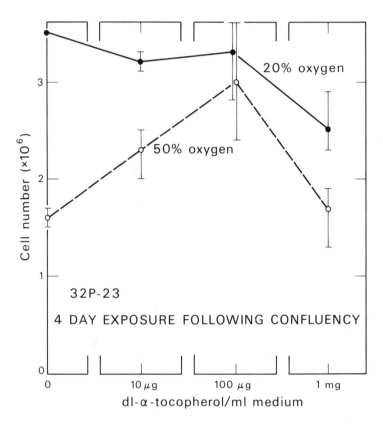

Fig. 8. Tocopherol protection from oxygen toxicity in actively growing cultured human cells (J. Smith and L. Packer, unpublished results). In oxygen toxicity experiments we have found that the percent attachment of the cells to the growing surface is affected by the oxygen tension; hence, the data were corrected for the percent attached cells.

to 60% oxygen, that partial protection from the damaging effects of oxygen are afforded by vitamin E (Fig. 9). However, at oxygen concentrations above 50%, the effectiveness of vitamin E falls off. We have observed this with either confluent cultures or actively growing cells exposed to various concentrations of oxygen in the absence and presence of vitamin E.

Vitamin E does not afford complete protection against oxygen toxicity. However, this seems reasonable since it is well known that the sensitivity of animals to ionizing radiation damage is increased by the presence of oxygen (Scott and Revesz, 1974). Oxygen toxicity likely involves the aqueous as well as hydrophobic regions within the cell. Since vitamin E partitions in hydrophobic regions mainly in cellular membranes, it would not be expected to act as effectively as a radical scavenger in aqueous regions. These results are also consistent with animal studies showing that hyperbaric oxygen toxicity can be partially protected with vitamin E (Menzel *et al.*, 1972).

4.3. Riboflavin Photosensitized Damage (O. Pereira, 1975)

In this type of stress, photosensitized damage was induced by adding riboflavin to the culture medium and later exposing the cells to visible light. Riboflavin acts as a photosensitizer to

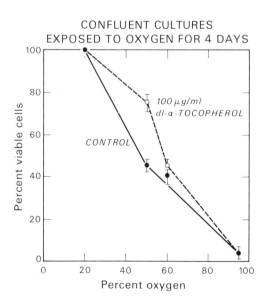

Fig. 9. Vitamin E dependent protection against oxygen toxicity in confluent human cells (J. Smith and L. Packer, unpublished results).

generate singlet oxygen according to the scheme shown in Fig. 1 (Krinsky *et al.*, 1974). Since flavin enzymes generally are in membranes, riboflavin may serve as a convenient photosensitizer for membrane damage. In a model system composed of linolenic acid and riboflavin, production of malondialdehyde occurs when the system is illuminated with visible light in the region where flavin absorbs.

In WI-38 cells as the concentration of riboflavin in the medium is increased, progressively more killing occurs. About 90% of the cells are killed by the riboflavin at 1 μg/ml. In the series of experiments shown in Fig. 10, it is seen that young cells exposed to increasing light doses (in the presence of about 0.1 μg/ml of riboflavin) are more susceptible than the older cells in the population. Thus, the cells capabable of growing more rapidly are more susceptible to being damaged (as in the case with ionizing radiation).

Both young and old cells were analyzed with regard to protection from this type of damage by dl-α-tocopherol (Fig. 11A-B). Complete protection from this type of damage is obtained if 100 μg/ml of vitamin E is present during growth prior to exposure of the cells to a visible light dose sufficient to kill about 50% of the control cells. It is presumed that both riboflavin and tocopherol probably partition into the membranes. Hence, this type of environmental stress probably involves a membrane-damage/membrane-protection situation, which may account for the remarkable ability of vitamin E to protect cells from this kind of damage.

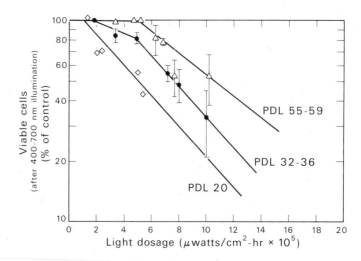

Fig. 10. Riboflavin photosensitized damage to early, middle, and late passage human cells in culture (O. Pereira, J. Smith, and L. Packer, unpublished results).

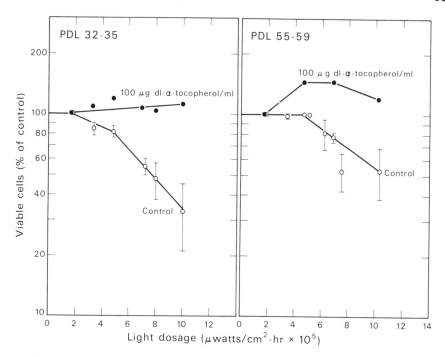

Fig. 11. Protection by tocopherol from riboflavin photosensitized damage to human cells in culture. A. Young or early passage cells (PDL 32-35). B. Old or late passage cells (PDL 55-59) (O. Pereira, J. Smith, and L. Packer, unpublished results).

5. CONCLUDING REMARKS

Our investigations show that free-radical mediated oxidative damage of membrane lipids may be averted by the naturally-occurring free-radical scavenger, vitamin E, and may increase the potential of WI-38 cells growing in culture to proliferate both under conditions of "normal aging" obtained in the *in vitro* culture environment and upon exposure to certain types of environmentally-induced damage. The WI-38 normal diploid cell seems to be an excellent test system in which to evaluate constraints which environmental factors have upon limiting life of human cells. Further investigations to determine which factors in the environment need to be manipulated to prevent or reduce the free-radical damage are required to identify where and how the damage arises and how we can prevent it in human cells. Until we can optimize many of the environmental factors that affect cell viability, we cannot assign a precise lifespan to different types of cells *in vitro* because the full genetic potential of cells will not be expressed unless they are cultured in an optimum environment.

References

Bindra, J.S., 1974, Anti-aging drugs, *Annu. Rep. Med. Chem.* 9:214-221.

Brin, M., Horn, L.R., and Barker, M.O., 1974, Relationship between fatty acid composition of erythrocytes and susceptibility to vitamin E deficiency, *Amer. J. Clin. Nut.* 27:945-951.

Deamer, D.W., and Gonzales, J., 1974, Autofluorescent structures in cultured WI-38 cells, *Arch. Biochem. Biophys.* 165:421-426.

Harman, D., 1956, Aging: A theory based on free radical and radiation chemistry, *J. Gerontol.* 16:247-254.

Hayflick, L., 1965, The limited *in vitro* lifetime of human diploid cell strains, *Exp. Cell Res.* 37:614-636.

Hers, H.G., and Hoof, F.V., 1973, Genetic abnormalities of lysosomes, *in* "Lysosomes in Biology and Pathology" (J.T. Dingle and H.B. Fell, eds.), Vol. 2, pp. 19-40, American Elsevier, New York.

Krinsky, N.I., Bymun, E.N., and Packer, L., 1974, Retention of K^+ gradients in imidoester cross-linked erythrocyte membranes, *Arch. Biochem. Biophys.* 160:90-99.

Kritchevsky, D., and Howard, B.V., 1970, Lipid metabolism in human diploid cells, *in* "Aging in Cell and Tissue Culture" (E. Holeckva and V.J. Cristofalo, eds.), pp. 57-82, Plenum Press, New York.

Lucy, J.A., 1972, Functional and structural aspects of biological membranes: A suggested structural role for vitamin E in the control of membrane permeability and stability, *Annu. N.Y. Acad. Sci.* 203:4-11.

Menzel, D.B., Roehm, N.J., and Lee, S.E., 1972, Vitamin E: The biological and environmental antioxidant, *J. Agr. Food Chem.* 20:481-486.

Michaelis, L., and Wollman, S.H., 1950, Free radicals derived from tocopherol and related substances, *Biochim. Biophys. Acta* 4:156-159.

Molenaar, I., Vos, J., and Hommes, F.A., 1972, Effect of vitamin E deficiency on cellular membranes, *in* "Vitamins and Hormones" (R.S. Harris, E. Dicfalusy, P.L. Munson, and J. Glover, eds.), Vol. 30, pp. 45-82, Academic Press, New York.

Packer, L., Deamer, D.W., and Heath, R.L., 1967, Regulation and deterioration of structure in membranes, *in* "Advances in Gerontological Research" (B.L. Strehler, ed.), pp. 23-64, Academic Press, New York.

Packer, L., and Smith, J., 1974, Extension of the lifespan of cultured normal human diploid cells by vitamin E, *Proc. Nat. Acad. Sci. USA* 71:4763-4767.

Pereira, O., 1975, Riboflavin sensitized visible light effects on human diploid fibroblasts in culture, Thesis, UC Berkeley.

Scott, O.C.A., and Revesz, L., 1974, Oxygen effects in radiobiology, *in* "Molecular Oxygen in Biology" (O. Hayaishi, ed.), pp. 137-161, North-Holland Publishing Company, Amsterdam.

Takaoki, T., Torres-Pereira, J., and Packer, L., 1974, Factors
    affecting the stability of chloroplast membranes *in vitro,*
    Biochim. Biophys. Acta 352:260-267.
Tappel, A.L., 1962, Vitamin E as the biological lipid antioxidant,
    in "Vitamins and Hormones" (R.S. Harris and I.G. Wools, eds.),
    Vol. 20, pp. 493-510, Academic Press, New York.
Tappel, A.L., 1973, Lipid peroxidation damage to cell components,
    Fed. Proc. 32:1870-1874.
Todaro, G.J., and Green, H., 1964, Serum albumin supplemented
    medium for long-term cultivation of mammalian fibroblast
    strains, *Proc. Soc. Exp. Biol. Med.* 116:688-692.

ROLE OF DNA REPAIR IN AGING

Ronald W. Hart

Department of Radiology, The Ohio State University

Hospitals (N-212), 410 West 10th Avenue, Columbus,

Ohio 43210

1. INTRODUCTION

Aging--which appears to be the most pervasive degenerative
process occurring in the higher animals--is of such general

occurrence and characterized by such a diversity of clinically and
biochemically defined changes that a specific definition, other
than a general loss of the capacity of an organism or cell to function at a level previously characterized as normal, is the only
definition presently agreed upon by all gerontobiologists. Due to
the generalized nature of the aging process, it is reasonable to
assume that if any single molecular target for the aging phenomenon
does exist, it must be related not only to age-related diseases,
but also play a central role in several cellular processes.

Maximum lifespan within the placental mammals varies by approximately 50-fold (Comfort, 1964). The level of environmental insult
to which animals are exposed in the natural environment varies by
less than 10-fold (Comfort, 1964). These small variations in the
environment appear to have only a minimal effect on the maximum
achievable lifespan (Comfort, 1964). When different mammalian
species are compared on a fraction-of-maximum lifespan basis, most
of the age-related changes observed appear to occur at similar
times in the life of an animal (Berg and Simms, 1960; Bourlière,
1962; Burch, 1968). Likewise the decline in "normal" physiological
and biochemical processes occurs at an equivalent rate when maximum
lifespans within the placental mammals is normalized (Gitman, 1967;
Engel and Larsson, 1968; Finch, 1971; Shock, 1971). The time of
onset of various degenerative diseases and loss of immune function
and wound-healing capacity also progress at similar rates in different mammalian species (Engel and Larsson, 1968; Makinodan *et al.*,
1971; Shock, 1971).

The placental mammals are all characterized by similar morphological, physiological, and biochemical procedures and yet differ
significantly in maximum lifespan achieved (Simpson, 1953; Anfinsen,
1961; Simpson, 1961; Andrew, 1968). Even within a relatively closely
associated family such as the primates, lifespans vary by more than
20-fold (Cutler, 1975). Since the primates are a recent evolutionary
occurrence, it would appear that whatever governs the lifespan of a
species must be able to be modified over a relatively short period
of time without qualitatively altering the phenotypic manifesta-
tions of the aging process. The existence of clinically defined
human syndromes (i.e., progeria, Werner's syndrome, etc.) predisposed toward accelerated aging suggests a role for DNA in aging
(Hart and Trosko, 1975; Trosko and Hart, 1975). The observation
that agents which damage DNA (i.e., X-irradiation, UV light and
alkylating agents) uniformally shorten the lifespan of cells *in
vitro*, and in the case of two of these agents *in vivo*, further
supports the involvement of DNA (Van Cleave, 1969). The wide
variation in lifespan of related rodent species and influence of
single gene mutations on longevity indicates that only a few genes
may determine the rate of aging within the mammals and thus their
total lifespan (Sacher, 1972, This Volume).

The fidelity of newly synthesized proteins is an indirect reflection of the fidelity of the genetic material. The proportion of defective proteins synthesized to normal proteins increases with age (Holliday and Lewis, 1970; Holliday and Tarrant, 1972; Lewis and Tarrant, 1972; Gershon and Gershon, 1973a, b; Zeelon *et al.*, 1973). Longer-lived mammals apparently have evolved a mechanism to prevent or retard the production or occurrence of defective proteins since the rate of occurrence is lower in these species than in the shorter-lived species (Cutler, 1974). The production of defective proteins may arise for several reasons, one of which is a defective template. A single template error occurring in the transcribable regions of the cellular genome will be reflected and amplified in macromolecular synthesis. The type and severity of the error will be dependent upon its location in the DNA and the excess redundancy coding for that particular gene function (Orgel, 1970; Lewis, 1972).

2. DNA DAMAGE AND ITS REPAIR

2.1. DNA as a Primary Target

Cellular DNA is characterized as a large (2×10^{11} daltons), unique information-containing macromolecule generally composed of four bases which code in various sequences for all other molecular constituents of the cell. In a differentiated cell the genetic information normally available for transcription varies with the state of differentiation, age of the cell, tissue of origin, stage of the cell cycle, and the environmental milieu surrounding the cell (Trosko and Hart, 1975). It is reasonable to assume that the accumulation of damage within cellular DNA will result in various alterations in genetic function.

Numerous physical and chemical agents normally found in the environment produce DNA damage. Studies on microorganisms and mammalian cells have shown that such damage results in change of physiological processes such as growth, division, transcription of DNA, cell death, mutation, and induction of cellular transformation (Setlow, 1968; Rauth, 1970; Smith, 1971; Cerutti, 1974; Lehmann, 1974; Hart and Trosko, 1975). The ability of the cells composing an organism to repair various forms of genetic damage is proportional to the sensitivity of the system to the deleterious effects of an environmental agent producing DNA damage (Cleaver, 1968; Setlow and Setlow, 1972; Trosko and Hart, 1975).

Since (1) a large fraction of cellular DNA is present in unique sequences; (2) information for RNA, protein, and lipid synthesis is read from DNA; and (3) the physiological changes in cells by one of the environmental agents--UV radiation--has in microorganisms been identified with specific alteration in DNA, it is a reasonable assumption that damage to the DNA of mammalian cells is the important macromolecular change resulting from the action of physical and chemical agents. Hence, the physiological responses characterizing the aging process will be thought of as the result of changes to DNA and the persistence of these changes. If the changes are repaired rapidly compared to the times for transcription and replication, they will have little biological significance.

2.2. Unrepaired DNA Damage as the Primary Lesion

It is obvious that accumulated DNA damage in and of itself is insufficient as an explanation of the aging process. Therefore, it is a reasonable hypothesis that the aging process is a sequence of events involving the induction of DNA damage and its subsequent manifestation at the physiological level. Under this hypothesis, the rate-modifying factors for the expression of such damage are assumed to be the ability of the system to repair DNA damage and the redundancy of genetic information within the system. Since there are many unique sequences of genetic information within DNA, it is a reasonable assumption that for these regions the fidelity of DNA transcription would be directly related to the repair capacity of the system for damage occurring within these unique sequences; whereas the complete fidelity of physiological functions controlled by redundant information would be proportional to the extent of excess information for that function and the capacity of the system to repair damage to that information.

The majority of the genetic information in a differentiated cell is normally non-transcribable (Cutler, 1974). Most mammalian systems do not show total repair of DNA damage and the fraction of damage repaired decreases as the amount of insult to DNA increases (Hart and Setlow, 1974). Preferential repair of DNA damage in non-chromatin-bound DNA following UV irradiation has been demonstrated in human fibroblast cultures *in vitro* (Wilkins and Hart, 1974). When previously UV irradiated cells are exposed to a high salt solution and the number of endonuclease-sensitive regions remaining are determined, a significant fraction appear to remain unrepaired in the chromatin-bound regions even several days after UV treatment. Thus, even if the rate of occurrence of random DNA damage is constant and the fraction of new damage accumulates at a constant rate over the lifespan of an animal, it would be expected that there would occur a preferential increase in the amount of distortion of the DNA helix in the chromatin-bound regions of the DNA.

At the functional level, unrepaired or incorrectly repaired DNA damage can be reflected in (1) transcription of erroneous mRNA; (2) synthesis of non-functional enzymes; (3) cessation of transcription; or (4) gene de-repression (Trosko and Chang, This Volume;

Trosko and Hart, 1975). In any system where repair of DNA is incomplete and damage thus accumulates with time, the results of these
functional alterations would also be expected to increase. When
the amount of damage a system can tolerate is exceeded, system
malfunction and death ensue. Assuming that the tolerance levels
for DNA damage are equal across the placental mammals, differences
in the extent of DNA repair for different species or tissues will
result in different lifespans. If these circumstances were indeed
the case, death might appear to be programmed due to the random
nature of occurrence within a large macromolecule consisting of
numerous small targets.

3. DNA REPAIR PROCESSES

3.1. Forms of Repair

Repair is a general term which in its simplicity is often
misleading. There are at least three general types of repair of
DNA damage in mammalian cells: (1) excision or pre-replication
repair; (2) strand break repair; and (3) post-replication repair
(Painter, 1970a, b; Strauss, 1974; Hart and Trosko, 1975). A
fourth form of repair recently found to be active in mammalian
systems (enzymatic photoreactivation) is specific for the monomerization of UV-induced cyclobutane dimers (Cook, 1967; Sutherland,
1974; Sutherland *et al.*, 1974, 1975). Each of these repair systems,
except for perhaps the latter, appears to have many subcomponents
which may be specific for the repair of particular forms of DNA
damage. It is expected that the importance of a given repair
deficiency will be related to: (1) the frequency of exposure of
an organism to an agent producing genetic damage repaired by that
repair system; (2) the location of the damage within the DNA; (3)
the cell type affected; and (4) the importance of unrepaired damage
of that form in the aging process. The determination of whether
or not DNA plays a role in the aging process must, therefore, involve
an examination of a number of repair processes and their efficiency
in various species and tissues following exposure to a variety of
environmental agents known to shorten lifespan, produce genetic
damage, or inhibit the repair of such damage within the organism.

3.2. Excision Repair

In its most general form, excision repair involves the removal
of damaged parental DNA by a complex of enzymes. It is the best
understood of the various repair processes and presently the most
extensively studied (Cerutti, 1974; Hart and Trosko, 1975). The
first step in the excision repair sequence--nicking of the damaged
DNA strand--proceeds by endonuclease attack near the damage. *In*

vitro studies indicate that there are endonucleases for specific
forms of DNA damage--pyrimidine dimers, interstrand cross-links,
depurinations, debrominations of BrdUrd, and other base damage
resulting from ionizing radiation or chemical treatment (Cerutti,
1974). Therefore, although excision repair is functional for DNA
damage induced by both physical (e.g., heat, UV and γ-radiation)
and chemical (e.g., N-acetoxy-acetylaminofluorene, BrdUrd, and
MNNG) agents, it is possible that an organism may be proficient in
one form of DNA excision repair and deficient in another. The
sensitivity of an organism or tissue to an environmental agent
producing DNA damage will be proportional to its exposure to the
agent and its ability to repair the genetic damage induced by the
agent. Thus, a repair deficiency may not be important to the aging
process unless the organism is exposed to agents producing that
form of damage and the damage accumulates with time of exposure.

3.2.1. *Measurement of Excision Repair.* Excision repair may
be measured by the (1) removal of known lesions, such as UV-induced
pyrimidine dimers (Setlow and Carrier, 1964); (2) production of
single-strand breaks after treatment with one of a number of exogenous repair endonucleases (e.g., UV-endonuclease, γ-endonuclease
or chemical endonuclease) (Ganesan, 1973; Van Lancker and Tomura,
1974; Wilkins and Hart, 1974); or (3) measurements of repair synthesis following excision (Painter and Cleaver, 1969; Regan *et al.*,
1971; Hart and Setlow, 1974). At the single-cell stage, repair
synthesis is equated with unscheduled DNA synthesis--the incorporation of radioactive precursors into DNA during non-S periods or
into cells whose normal semi-conservative DNA synthesis has been
inhibited by hydroxyurea (Painter and Cleaver, 1969). Some of the
repair enzymes from bacteria, such as incising endonucleases (the
first enzymes in the sequence of excision steps) have been purified
(Kaplan *et al.*, 1969; Carrier and Setlow, 1970; Ganesan, 1973).
They represent reagents that detect lesions in DNA. Such endonucleases *in vitro* make strand breaks near lesions and, for known
lesions such as pyrimidine dimers, the number of strand breaks is
approximately equal to the number of lesions (Carrier and Setlow,
1970). Thus, even though the chemical nature of a lesion may not
be known, endonuclease might be used to determine the number of
lesions.

3.2.2. *Excision Repair Capacity as a Function of Age.* Recently
several reports on excision repair as a function of age in human
fibroblast cultures have appeared. The results can be classified
into three general categories: those showing either (1) little or
no significant alteration in excision capacity (Painter *et al.*,
1973; Clarkson and Painter, 1974); (2) those reporting a gradual
decline in excision repair starting in late phase III cultures (Hart
and Setlow, 1975a); or (3) a total turning off of excision in late
phase III cultures (Mattern and Cerutti, 1975). Since the same
cell line (WI-38) was used in each of the above determinations, an

apparent conflict in results exists. This might, however, be
explained by the fact that each investigator used different techniques in the analysis of the DNA repair processes.

Goldstein originally observed that only in the last subpassage
did primary human fibroblast cultures have, on the average, somewhat less unscheduled DNA synthesis after UV-irradiation (Goldstein, 1971). Similarly, Painter and co-workers in a series of
papers reported that they could demonstrate a decline in repair
replication, following treatment with a number of agents only in
the last subpassage of WI-38 cultures (Painter *et al.*, 1973; Clarkson and Painter, 1974). Hart and Setlow (1975a, b), however,
demonstrated, using a double labeled autoradiographic procedure,
that in late phase III, unscheduled DNA synthesis gradually decreases
at a rate slightly less than that for scheduled DNA synthesis in
WI-38 cultures. With the resultant being three distinct populations
of cells: (1) those able to perform both scheduled and repair synthesis normally; (2) those unable to perform either form of DNA
synthesis; and (3) those able to perform repair synthesis but not
unscheduled DNA synthesis following UV irradiation (Hart and Setlow,
1975a, b). The proportion of cells unable to perform unscheduled
DNA synthesis gradually increases with age of the culture beginning
in mid-phase III and continues until death of the culture six to
eight generations later. Recently it has been reported (Mattern
and Cerutti, 1975) that senescent WI-38 cells lose their capacity
for excision of γ-ray induced thymine damage in mid-phase III cultures. The loss of excision repair capacity in this case appears
to be more precipitous than the loss of semi-conservative DNA
synthesis previously reported in the WI-38 system (Cristofalo and
Sharf, 1973).

The cause for the apparent discrepancy between these laboratories is unknown. However, regardless of its basis none of these
present observations are able to discern the cause and effect relationship between unrepaired DNA damage and cellular aging *in vitro*.
In all cases DNA excision repair does not vary significantly until
mid or late phase III in WI-38 cells. Since many enzymatic and
physiological properties of cells are known to change with age,
both *in vitro* and *in vivo* (Cutler, 1974), it is at best tenuous
to speculate that a decline in DNA repair of whatever form is the
causal event in cellular aging. Likewise, it would be premature
to draw from these limited observations the conclusions that either
all tissues maintain a constant or near constant rate of all forms
of repair throughout their lifespan or that accumulation of DNA
damage is unimportant in the aging process.

3.2.3. *Lifespan-related Excision Repair*. Numerous laboratories have measured the repair of UV-induced DNA damage in different tissues derived from a number of placental mammals by a
variety of different techniques (Setlow, 1968; Painter, 1970a, b;

Regan and Setlow, 1973; Hart and Setlow, 1974; Hart and Setlow, 1975a). It has been assumed that though the techniques employed measure different parameters, they give similar estimates (Painter and Cleaver, 1969; Setlow *et al.*, 1972). This may not be a valid assumption, however, since these studies have not all been performed in the same laboratory, under identical conditions, with the same cell type in which the adduct may be directly and specifically modified. The possible presence of enzymatic photoreactivation in human cells may present an opportunity for such a direct comparison in a mammalian system (Sutherland, 1975).

Until such a comprehensive evaluation is performed, any comparison of excision repair capacity between tissue and species can only be qualitative at best. Normal human cells derived from either dermal, lung, or lymphoid tissues appear to be extremely proficient at dimer removal with approximately 75 to 85% of all dimers removed following a fluence of 20 J/m^2 of UV light (254 nm) (Cleaver and Trosko, 1970; Regan *et al.*, 1971; Setlow *et al.*, 1972; Trosko and Hart, 1975). Dermal fibroblast cultures derived from cows are only slightly less proficient in UV-induced excision repair than man (Cleaver *et al.*, 1972; Hart and Setlow, 1974). In hamster fibroblast cultures dimer excision is barely detectable and is not detectable at all in mouse cells (Painter and Cleaver, 1969; Rauth, 1970). These studies imply that, when removal of one of the major photoproducts induced by UV light (the pyrimidine dimers) is directly measured by the same technique in fibroblast cultures derived from a number of placental mammals with different lifespans and frequencies of spontaneous tumor induction (Hart *et al.*, 1975; Trosko and Hart, 1975), a variation in excision repair does exist. Other perhaps more sensitive techniques clearly indicate that mouse cells do carry out some excision and that hamster cells carry out more than mouse cells *in vitro* (Painter and Cleaver, 1969; Setlow *et al.*, 1971) when tissues are derived from adults or neonates. Previous controversy concerning variations in excision between species has been somewhat resolved by recent data showing that mouse embryos up to day nineteen appear to have a much higher excision capacity than tissue derived from either newborn or adult donors (Ben-Ishai and Peleq, 1974). When tissue is subpassaged three or more times, excision capacity declines to a level characteristic of the adult tissue (Ben-Ishai and Peleq, 1974). These few data indicating a possible correlation between the extent of excision repair and lifespan in adult tissue led to a more critical evaluation of this correlation (Hart and Setlow, 1974). Since past estimates of the magnitude of repair depended not only on the species (Painter and Cleaver, 1969; Setlow *et al.*, 1972; Fox and Fox, 1973) but on the state of differentiation of particular cell types (Hahn *et al.*, 1971) and tissues (Ben-Ishai and Peleq, 1974), they minimized these variables by using one technique on one cell type (primary fibroblasts) of similar gerontological ages. The correlation observed between both the rate and extent of unscheduled

DNA synthesis and lifespan of the species examined correlated well
except for a slight variation in hamster fibroblast tissue. Additional studies in the same laboratory have subsequently shown that
other species--including the field mouse, Syrian hamster, dog and
cat also follow this same correlation (Hart *et al.*, unpublished
data). Recent work by Cutler (1974) suggests that the primates,
due to their rapid rate of evolution of lifespan might form an ideal
closely related group of species on which to continue these studies.
Additional work being performed on related murine species with
different lifespans will also aid in determination of the validity
of the correlation between excision and lifespan (Hart and Sacher,
unpublished data).

Any interpretation of these results with regard to the aging
process must be made cautiously since it must first make the
assumption that UV light is a reasonable model insult producing
forms of DNA damage similar to those induced by numerous other
agents to which cells composing the interior portions of the body
are exposed. Cerutti has proposed that specific endonucleases
exist for recognition of specific sizes of alterations in the DNA
helix (Cerutti, 1974), suggesting that the pyrimidine dimer may
be only one of several forms of DNA lesions recognized by the same
repair endonuclease. Van Lancker's studies with isolated repair
endonuclease from rat liver homogenates further substantiate the
possibility of size specific endonucleases (Van Lancker and Tomura,
1972, 1974). While appealing, several factors might well invali-
date the correlation between excision repair and lifespan, for
example: (1) UV light readily penetrates the surrounding histone
coating of DNA whereas environmental chemical agents may have difficulty doing so before reacting with some other cellular constituents; (2) the UV exposures used in these experiments are generally
above the lethal dose and given in a short time whereas in the natural environment chemical and physical insults are delivered at
a much slower rate and at a non-lethal level; (3) thymidine pool
sizes or total content of DNA may vary between species and be
related to the lifespan of the species, thus modifying either the
rate of repair or the number of damaged sites per cell and (4)
at present no uniform correlation between the lifespan shortening
effects of UV light and tissue repair capacity has been reported.
Nevertheless, since UV light does seem to induce accelerated aging
in skin tissue (Johnson *et al.*, 1968) and repair of damage induced
by it seems to be similar to that for damage induced by a number
of chemical agents, it seems to represent, at this time, a reasonable tool for such studies when the proper constraints are made in
interpretation.

3.2.4. *Speculations as to the Mode of Action of Unrepaired
DNA Lesions of the Cyclobutane Dimer Form.* The different extents
of excision repair in dermal fibroblast tissues derived from species
exhibiting different lifespans implies that species proficient in

excision repair remove more damage than those deficient in repair.
Thus, though the total amount of damage accumulated over the lifespan of different species might be similar over a fixed period of
time, a repair-deficient species such as mouse might be expected to
accumulate in its cellular DNA more damage per unit length per unit
time than a longer-lived species such as the field mouse or man.
If a more rapid accumulation of errors did result, a more rapid
deterioration of the fidelity of transcription and translation
would be expected and could account for a shortened lifespan (Orgel,
1963).   The effectiveness of any given error would be dependent
upon several factors including: (1) the excess redundancy of information for a given function; (2) the location of the error in
transcribable or non-transcribable regions of the cellular DNA;
(3) the function of the region in which the error occurred; and
(4) the relationship of the tissue to normal body function and its
rate of turnover. Thus, if an error occurs in a low redundancy
gene coding for a major function in a post-mitotic tissue, it is
a reasonable assumption that at least part of the tissue's normal
function would be interfered with. Preferential repair of UV-
induced DNA damage in non-chromatin-bound regions of cellular DNA
has been reported to occur in human fibroblast cultures (Wilkins
and Hart, 1974). Lesions remain in the chromatin-bound fractions
of DNA for at least 196 h following exposure to UV light and presumably remain permanently. The number of endonuclease sensitive
sites observed in these studies in both chromatin and non-chromatin
bound regions of the DNA are approximately equivalent to the theoretical number of pyrimidine dimers induced in the DNA at the
fluences given. Witkin (1974, 1975) has reported that in *E. coli*
unrepaired UV-induced cyclobutane-type pyrimidine dimers result
in de-repression of specific gene products of λ integrated phage
and further that this derepression is photoreactivable. In mammalian cells, UV light and certain steroids such as 17-β-estradiol
act synergistically to induce expression of normally non-expressible
regions of cellular DNA (Trosko and Chang, This Volume). Similarly,
one explanation of the differential of effects of various chemical
carcinogens on the enhancement of SV40-induced transformation may
relate to the differential effects of these agents on cellular DNA
(Yohn *et al.*, 1975). In these studies, agents producing single-
strand breaks enhance transformation only when added prior to SV40
infection whereas those agents producing DNA damage repaired by a
process similar to that for the repair of UV-induced DNA damage
preferentially enhance transformation when applied following SV40
infection. In all cases non-carcinogenic analogs of these compounds
neither produced DNA damage nor enhanced viral transformation and
neither the carcinogenic agent nor its non-carcinogenic analog
modified viral absorption. One possible explanation for these
results would be that while agents producing single-strand breaks
enhanced viral insertion by producing additional sites for such
insertions, those producing certain sized alterations in the
helixical structure of DNA--similar to that produced by the

cyclobutane-type pyrimidine dimer--led to viral expression.

Though admittedly speculative, it is possible that when damage to cellular DNA is not recognized, a de-repression or repression of genetic information might occur. If the cell affected is not post-mitotic and semi-conservative DNA synthesis ensues prior to excision, then recent data suggests that the action of the post-replication repair system might result in a permanent mutation or de-repression (Trosko and Hart, 1975). Obviously, effective excision repair is not the only repair mechanism determining genetic fidelity or lifespan. Many other molecular, cellular, and physiological repair and maintenance systems must be involved (Strehler, 1962; Price and Makinodan, 1973; Yielding, 1974; Hart and Trosko, 1975; Trosko and Hart, 1975). In addition, other correlations between lifespan and various physiological parameters (such as specific metabolic rate, body weight, deep body temperature, brain weight) have yet to be related to the correlations observed at the molecular level (Sacher, 1959, 1972, This Volume). Nevertheless, there does seem to be both an intuitive and scientific impetus toward the assumption that the maintenance of genetic fidelity is of importance in determining the rate at which the aging process proceeds.

3.3. Other Repair Processes

3.3.1. *Accumulation of Alkali Labile Sites*. Strand break repair is usually studied after single-strand breaks are introduced into DNA by supralethal doses of ionizing radiation (Setlow and Setlow, 1972). Various radiomimetic chemical agents also induce single- and double-strand breaks in cellular DNA at more biologically significant doses (Hart *et al.*, 1975). The strand break repair process is a rapid one and in bacteria and possibly in mammalian systems, it seems to have several components (Town *et al.*, 1971; Lindahl and Nyberg, 1972). The specific steps involved in this repair process are not clear but may relate to both the direct induction of DNA strand breaks as well as alkaline labile sites (Strauss, 1974; Cerutti, 1974; Hart and Trosko, 1975; Howland *et al.*, 1975) which break upon exposure of cellular DNA to alkali.

Several experiments have evaluated the accumulation of this form of damage in the DNA of older cells and to the question of the existence and efficiency of repair systems in such older cells. When tissues from aging mice are measured autoradiographically for the ability of the DNA to act as a primer for *in vitro* nucleotide incorporation catalyzed by calf thymus polymerase, an increase with age of the cell is observed (Modak and Price, 1971; Price *et al.*, 1971). Since single-strand breaks are known to act as initiating centers for the *in vitro* enzymatic synthesis of DNA, these observations were interpreted as indicating that DNA from

older cells contain relatively large numbers of such breaks compared
to younger cells, and that these breaks accumulate with age. Supporting evidence for this interpretation came from several experiments on the measurement of alkaline labile bonds (single-strand
breaks) in the DNA of old and young cells. Not only did the DNA
of chick red cells have more breaks than that from lymphocytes,
but the DNA of young red cells had fewer breaks than old ones
(Karran and Ormerod, 1973). Older cells were also not as proficient
as younger cells in the repair of breaks introduced by γ-irradia-
tion. Chick red cells did not repair such damage, and old rat
muscle cells not only had more alkaline labile sites than young
rat muscle cells but also did not repair damage as well as the
younger cells (Karran and Ormerod, 1973). In the case of neural
cells from the dog (Wheeler and Lett, 1972) or retinal cells from
the rabbit (Wheeler *et al.*, 1973) repair of ionizing radiation-
induced breaks seems comparable to that of dividing fibroblast
tissues yet the number of accumulated alkaline labile sites in
old neural cells seems greater than in either old fibroblast cells
or younger neural cells. It thus appears to be a reasonable asser-
tion that alkaline labile sites accumulate with age in a number of
post-mitotic tissues and at a more rapid rate than in mitotic
tissues.

3.3.2. *Age-Related Species Variation in Repair of Ionizing
Radiation-Induced DNA Damage.* Only a few studies have been reported
on the comparative ability of similar tissues derived from different species to repair γ-radiation-induced DNA damage. Of these
studies most were related to either cell survival or division suppression rather than aging. The most inclusive study thus far
performed (Shaeffer and Merz, 1972) indicated no causal relationship between X-ray-induced unscheduled DNA synthesis, possibly
an indirect measurement of strand break repair (Cerutti, 1974), and
cell recovery. Unscheduled DNA synthesis following X-irradiation
does, however, correspond to chromosome number but possibly not to
total DNA content. No direct correlation between lifespan and
repair could be drawn from this data for several reasons: (1) the
studies were performed primarily on transformed cell lines rather
than primaries; (2) the lines chosen for study represent only a
total of four species, and (3) no attempt to measure rate or
extent of single-strand breaks compared to X-ray-induced unscheduled
DNA synthesis was attempted. Thus, presently no direct data exist
comparing the ability of organisms to perform single-strand break
repair or γ-ray-induced unscheduled DNA synthesis with lifespan.

3.3.3. *Comparative Tissue and Age-Related Repair of Ionizing
Radiation-Induced DNA Damage.* Recently it has been demonstrated
that cultures derived from individuals afflicted with progeria are
defective in strand break repair (Epstein *et al.*, 1973). Other
investigators however, using the same or similar cell systems, have
been unable to repeat this observation (Regan and Setlow, 1974).

No satisfactory explanation for these differences presently exists. Similar conflicts exist in the literature concerning the ability of older cells to perform unscheduled DNA synthesis or strand break repair (Clarkson and Painter, 1974; Williams and Little, 1975; Hart and Setlow, 1974; Regan and Setlow, 1974; Mattern and Cerutti, 1975), following various doses of ionizing radiation. Thus, at this time no direct relationship between the ability of cells to perform DNA strand break repair and age *in vitro* can realistically be made.

Variations in the ability of different histologically discernible tissue types in 12- to 15-day-old hamster cell cultures to perform strand break repair have been reported (Williams and Little, 1975). Similar confirming observations have been made in chick red cells which appear to have more repair capacity than chick lymphocytes (Karran and Ormerod, 1973). However, repair of ionizing radiation-induced breaks in dividing fibroblasts and neural cells from the dog seem comparable to one another (Wheeler and Lett, 1972), as does strand break repair in dog neural cells (Wheeler and Lett, 1972) and retinal cells from the rabbit (Karran and Ormerod, 1973).

Presently there would seem to be an urgent need for similar comparative studies performed both between species and tissues. Of the various repair processes known for the numerous forms of DNA damage that may be induced by both physical and chemical agents normally occurring in the environment, only excision repair and strand break repair have been extensively studied and then only following the induction of DNA damage by either UV light or ionizing radiation. Thus, it would appear that a great deal more study needs to be performed before a conclusion can be reached as to the role of DNA repair in the aging process. Indeed, at this time it would be premature to infer that DNA repair in and of itself is a primary determinant of lifespan, much less to state that any single repair process is of more significance than any other.

4. SUMMARY

It is often advantageous to have a working hypothesis to structure experiments around, as long as it is recognized that the only value of a hypothesis is its ability to be tested. With this in mind, in the summary I have attempted to compile the present information into a possible series of events which might lead to cellular dysfunction and ultimately cell death, as well as to summarize the various observations presented in the text.

Physical and chemical agents damage DNA *in vivo*. These agents produce changes in various physiological processes, including growth, division, transcription of DNA, cell death, mutation, and induction of cellular transformation. Since DNA is the largest target, containing unique sequences and the information coding for other macromolecules, it is a reasonable assumption that damage to DNA of mammalian cells is an important macromolecular change resulting from the action of physical and chemical agents. Most of the age-related physiological responses could be thought of as the result of changes in DNA and the persistence of these changes.

Therefore, it is our working hypothesis that the aging process is a sequence of events involving the induction of DNA damage and its subsequent manifestation at the physiological level. The rate-modifying factors for the expression of such damage are assumed to be the ability of the system to repair DNA damage and the redundancy of genetic information within the system. Since there are many unique sequences of genetic information within DNA, it is a reasonable assumption that for these regions the fidelity of DNA transcription would be directly related to the repair capacity of the system for damage occurring within these unique sequences; whereas the complete fidelity of physiological functions controlled by redundant information would be proportional to the extent of excess information for that function and the capacity of the system to repair damage to that information.

At the functional level, unrepaired or incorrectly repaired DNA damage can be reflected in: (1) transcription of erroneous mRNA; (2) synthesis of non-functional enzymes; (3) cessation of transcription; or (4) gene derepression. In any system where repair of DNA is incomplete and damage thus accumulates with time, the results of these functional alterations would also be expected to increase. When the amount of damage a system can tolerate is exceeded, system malfunction and death ensue. Assuming that the tolerance levels for DNA damage are equal for the placental mammals, differences in the extent of DNA repair for different species or tissues will result in different lifespans. If these circumstances were indeed the case, death might appear to be programmed. However, we emphasize that relations among repair capacity, accumulation of DNA damage, and aging are mostly hypothetical.

Nevertheless, we hypothesize that the aging process represents the manifestation of a series of events involving: (1) the induction of numerous forms of DNA damage by various physical and chemical agents; (2) its accumulation with time within the genetic material at rates which are constant over the lifespan of the species but differ between species; and (3) the subsequent manifestation of these genetic alterations in various forms of cellular (e.g., decreased rates of semi-conservative DNA synthesis, increased cell cycle times, formation of erroneous mRNA and its products) and whole animal (e.g., decreased immunofunction, neural degeneration, organ atrophy, and altered hormonal secretion) dysfunction. Thus, we feel that while free radical formation, DNA cross-link production, alterations in the immune system, DNA transcription, or membrane function are important in the aging process, these are separately or together insufficient to completely explain the aging process. In addition, two other processes must play a significant role in the aging process, namely, the redundancy of genetic information for vital functions within the system, and the ability of the system to maintain genetic fidelity via enzymatic repair systems. Alterations in either one or both of these systems would be expected to extensively modify life expectancy.

Acknowledgments. The research of the author was supported by NCI Grant No. CA 17917-01 and a University General Research Support Grant No. 7452. I would like also to acknowledge the critical and invaluable help of Ms. Gibson and Callahan in the editing, typing and review of this manuscript.

References

Andrew, W., 1968, "The Fine Structure and Histochemical Changes in Ageing," Academic Press, New York.

Anfinsen, C., 1961, "The Molecular Basis of Evolution," Wiley, New York.

Ben-Ishai, R., and Peleq, L., 1974, Excision repair in primary mouse embryo cells and its decline in progressive passages and established cell lines, Abstr. ICN-UCLA Winter Conf. on Molecular Mechanisms for the Repair of DNA, Squaw Valley, California, Feb. 24-March 1, 1974.

Berq, B., and Simms, H., 1960, Nutrition and longevity in the rat. II. Longevity and onset of disease with different levels of food intake, *Nutrition* 71:255-263.

Bourlière, F., 1962, Comparative longevity of higher vertebrates, *in* "Biological Aspects of Aging" (N. Shock, ed.), p. 3, Columbia Univ. Press, New York.

Burch, P., 1968, "An Inquiry Concerning Growth, Disease and Ageing," Oliver and Boyd, Edinburgh.

Carrier, W.L., and Setlow, R.B., 1970, Endonuclease from *Micrococcus luteus* which has activity toward ultraviolet irradiated deoxyribonucleic acid: purification and properties, *J. Bacteriol.* 102:178-186.

Cerutti, P.A., 1974, Minireview: excision repair of DNA base damage, *Life Sci.* 15:1567-1575.

Clarkson, J.M., and Painter, R.B., 1974, Repair of X-ray damage in aging WI-38 cells, *Mutat. Res.* 23:107-112.

Cleaver, J.E., 1968, Defective repair replication of DNA in xeroderma pigmentosum, *Nature* 218:652-656.

Cleaver, J.E., Thomas, G.H., Trosko, J.E., and Lett, J.T., 1972, Excision repair (dimer excision, strand breakage and repair replication) in primary cultures of eukaryotic (bovine) cells, *Exp. Cell Res.* 74:67-80.

Cleaver, J.E., and Trosko, J.E., 1970, Absence of excision of ultra-violet-induced cyclobutane dimers in xeroderma pigmentosum, *Photochem. Photobiol.* 11:547-550.

Comfort, A., 1964, "Ageing, the Biology of Senescence," Holt, Rinehart & Wilson, New York.

Cook, G.S., 1970, Photoreactivation in animal cells, *Photophysiology* 5:191-233.

Cristofalo, V.J., and Sharf, B.B., 1973, Cellular senescence and DNA synthesis. Thymidine incorporation as a measure of population age in human diploid cells, *Exp. Cell Res.* 76:419-427.

Cutler, R.G., 1974, Redundancy of information content in the genome of mammalian species as a protective mechanism determining aging rate, *Mech. Ageing Develop.* 2:381-408.

Cutler, R.G., 1975, Evolution of longevity in mammals. I. Primates, *J. Human Evolution* (in press).

Engel, A., and Larsson, T., 1968, Cancer and Aging, Thule Intern. Symp., Norcliska Bakhandelns Forlaq, Stockholm, pp. 48-71.

Epstein, J., Williams, J.R., and Little, J.B., 1973, Deficient DNA repair in human progeroid cells, *Proc. Nat. Acad. Sci. USA* 70:977-981.

Finch, C., 1971, Comparative biology of senescence; evolutionary and developmental considerations, *in* "Animal Models for Biomedical Research IV," Nat. Acad. Sci. USA, pp. 47-53, Washington, D.C.

Fox, M., and Fox, B.W., 1973, Repair replication after UV-irradiation in rodent cell lines of different sensitivity, *Int. J. Radiat. Biol.* 23:359-376.

Freeman, J.T., 1967, Endocrinology in geriatrics: historical background, *in* "Endocrines and Aging" (L. Gitman, ed.), C.C. Thomas, Springfield, Illinois.

Ganesan, A.K., 1973, Post-replication repair in UV-irradiated *Bacillus subtilis, Biophys. Soc. Abstr.* 13:116a.

Gershon, H., and Gershon, D., 1973a, Altered enzymes in senescent organisms; mouse muscle; aldolase, *Mech. Ageing Develop.* 2:33-41.

Gershon, H., and Gershon, D., 1973b, Inactive enzyme molecules in ageing mice; liver aldolase, *Proc. Nat. Acad. Sci. USA* 70:909-913.

Goldstein, S., 1971, The role of DNA repair in aging of cultured fibroblasts from xeroderma pigmentosum and normals, *Proc. Soc. Exp. Biol. Med.* 137:730-734.

Hahn, G.M., King, D., and Yang, S.-J., 1971, Quantitative changes in unscheduled DNA synthesis in rat muscle cells after differentiation, *Nature New Biol.* 230:242-244.

Hart, R.W., Gibson, R.E., Chapman, J.D., Reuvers, A.P., Sinha, B.K., Griffith, R.K., and Witiak, D.T., 1975, A radioprotective stereostructure-activity study of *cis-* and *trans*-2-mercaptocyclobutylamine analogs and homologs of 2-mercaptoethylamine (MEA), *J. Med. Chem.* 18:323-331.

Hart, R.W., and Setlow, R.B., 1974, Correlation between deoxyribo-
    nucleic acid excision repair and lifespan in a number of
    mammalian species, *Proc. Nat. Acad. Sci. USA* 71:2169-2173.
Hart, R.W., and Setlow, R.B., 1975a, DNA repair in late-passage
    human cells, *Mech. Ageing Develop.* (in press).
Hart, R.W., and Setlow, R.B., 1975b, Role of DNA repair in aging,
    in "Molecular Mechanisms for the Repair of DNA" (P.C. Hanawalt
    and R.B. Setlow, eds.), Plenum Press, New York (in press).
Hart, R.W., Setlow, R.B., Gibson, R.E., and Hoskins, T.L., 1975,
    DNA repair: a possible control mechanism for cellular aging,
    Abstr. for "10th Int. Cong. on Gerontol.," Jerusalem,
    Israel.
Hart, R.W., and Trosko, J.E., 1975, DNA repair processes in mammals,
    Gerontologia (in press).
Holliday, R., and Tarrant, G.M., 1972, Altered enzymes in ageing
    human fibroblasts, *Nature* 238:26-30.
Howland, G.P., Hart, R.W., and Yette, M., 1975, Repair of DNA
    strand breaks after gamma-irradiation of protoplasts isolated
    from cultured wild carrot cells, *Mutat. Res.* 27:81-87.
Johnson, B.E., Daniels, F., Jr., and Magnus, I.A., 1968, Chronic
    effects of ultraviolet radiation in human skin, *Photophysiology*
    4:139-202.
Kaplan, J.C., Kushner, S.R., and Grossman, L., 1969, Enzymatic repair
    of DNA. I. Purification of two enzymes involved in the exci-
    sion of thymine dimers from ultraviolet-irradiated DNA, *Proc.
    Nat. Acad. Sci. USA* 63:144-151.
Karran, P., and Ormerod, M.G., 1973, Is the ability to repair
    damage to DNA related to the proliferative capacity of a
    cell? The rejoining of X-ray produced strand breaks,
    Biochim. Biophys. Acta 299:54-64.
Lehmann, A.R., 1974, Minireview: post-replication of DNA in mamma-
    lian cells, *Life Sci.* 15:2005-2016.
Lewis, C.M., 1972, Protein turnover in relation to Orgel's error
    theory of ageing, *Mech. Ageing Develop.* 1:43-52.
Lewis, C.M., and Holliday, R., 1970, Mistranslation and ageing in
    Neurospora, Nature 228:877-880.
Lewis, C.M., and Tarrant, G.M., 1972, Error theory and ageing in
    human diploid fibroblasts, *Nature* 239:316-318.
Lindahl, T., and Nyberg, B., 1972, Rate of depurination of native
    deoxyribonucleic acid, *Biochemistry* 11:3610-3618.
Makinodan, T., Perkins, E., and Chen, M., 1971, Immunologic acti-
    vity of the aged, *Adv. Gerontol. Res.* 3:171-178.
Mattern, M.R., and Cerutti, P.A., 1975, Age-dependent excision
    repair of damaged thymine from γ-irradiated DNA by isolated
    nuclei from human fibroblasts, *Nature* 254:450-452.
Modak, S.P., and Price, G.B., 1971, Exogenous DNA polymerase-
    catalyzed incorporation of deoxyribonucleotide monophosphate
    in nuclei of fixed mouse brain cells, *Exp. Cell Res.* 65:289-
    296.

Orgel, L., 1963, The maintenance of the accuracy of protein syn-
    thesis and its relevance to aging, *Proc. Nat. Acad. Sci. USA*
    49:517-521.
Painter, R.B., 1970a, The action of ultraviolet light on mammalian
    cells, *Photophysiology* 5:169-189.
Painter, R.B., 1970b, Non-conservative replication of damaged DNA
    in mammalian cells, *in* "Genetic Concepts and Neoplasia,"
    pp. 593-603, Williams and Wilkins, Baltimore.
Painter, R.B., Clarkson, J.M., and Young, B.R., 1973, Ultraviolet-
    induced repair replication in aging diploid human cells
    (WI-38), *Radiat. Res.* 56:560-564.
Painter, R.B., and Cleaver, J.E., 1969, Repair replication, unsched-
    uled DNA synthesis, and the repair of mammalian DNA, *Radiat.
    Res.* 37:451-466.
Price, G.B., and Makinodan, T., 1973, Aging: alteration of DNA
    protein information, *Gerontologia* 19:58-70.
Price, G.B., and Modak, S.P., and Makinodan, T., 1971, Age-associ-
    ated changes in the DNA of mouse tissue, *Science* 171:917-920.
Rauth, A.M., 1970, DNA repair processes in mammals, *Current Topics
    in Radiat. Res. Quart.* 6:193-245.
Regan, J.D., and Setlow, R.B., 1973, Repair of chemical damage to
    human DNA, *in* "Chemical Mutagens" (A. Hollaender, ed.), pp.
    151-170, Plenum Press, New York.
Regan, J.D., and Setlow, R.B., 1974, DNA repair in human progeroid
    cells, *Biochem. Biophys. Res. Commun.* 59:858-864.
Regan, J.D., Setlow, R.B., and Ley, R.D., 1971, Normal and defec-
    tive repair of damaged DNA in human cells: a sensitive assay
    utilizing the photolysis of bromodeoxyuridine, *Proc. Nat. Acad.
    Sci. USA* 68:708-712.
Sacher, G., 1959, Relation of lifespan to brain weight and body
    weight in mammals, *Ageing-Methodology of the Study of Ageing,
    Ciba Collog. on Ageing* 15:115-126.
Sacher, G., 1972, Genetic and evolutionary factors in the ageing
    of short and long lived myomorph rodents, *in* "9th Intern.
    Cong. Gerontol." Kiev, pp. 374-375.
Setlow, R.B., 1968, The photochemistry, photobiology and repair of
    polynucleotides, *Progr. Nucleic Acid Res. Mol. Biol.* 8:257-294.
Setlow, R.B., and Carrier, W.L., 1964, The disappearance of thymine
    dimers from DNA: An error correcting mechanism, *Proc. Nat.
    Acad. Sci. USA* 51:226-231.
Setlow, R.B., Regan, J.D., and Carrier, W.L., 1972, Different levels
    of excision repair in mammalian cell lines, *Biophys. Soc. Abstr.*
    12:19a.
Setlow, R.B., and Setlow, J.K., 1972, Effects of radiation on poly-
    nucleotides, *Annu. Rev. Biophys. Bioeng.* 1:293-346.
Sheaffer, J., and Merz, T., 1971, Unscheduled DNA synthesis and
    cellular recovery in various mammalian cell lines, *in* "Mole-
    cular and Cellular Repair Process - Vth Internatl. Symp. on
    Mol. Biol.," (June, 1971), pp. 174-181, Johns Hopkins Univ.
    Press, Baltimore.

Shock, N., 1961, Physiological aspects of ageing in man, *Annu. Rev. Physiol.* 23:97-122.

Simpson, G., 1953, "The Major Features of Evolution," Columbia Univ. Press, New York.

Simpson, G., 1961, "Principles of Animal Taxonomy," Columbia Univ. Press, New York.

Smith, K.C., 1971, The roles of genetic recombination and DNA polymerase in the repair of damaged DNA, *Photophysiology* 6:209-278.

Strauss, B.S., 1974, Minireview: Repair of DNA in mammalian cells, *Life Sci.* 15:1685-1693.

Strehler, B.L., 1962, "Time, Cells, and Aging," Academic Press, New York.

Sutherland, B.M., 1974, Photoreactivating enzyme from human leukocytes, *Nature* 248:109-112.

Sutherland, B.M., Rice, M., and Wagner, E.K., 1975, Xeroderma pigmentosum cells contain low levels of photoreactivating enzyme, *Proc. Nat. Acad. Sci. USA* 72:103-107.

Sutherland, B.M., Runge, P., and Sutherland, J.C., 1974, DNA photoreactivating enzyme from placental mammals; origin and characteristics, *Biochemistry* 13:4710-4714.

Town, C.D., Smith, K.C., and Kaplan, H.S., 1971, DNA polymerase required for rapid repair of X-ray-induced DNA strand breaks *in vitro, Science* 172:851-854.

Trosko, J.E., and Hart, R.W., 1975, DNA mutation frequencies in mammals, *Gerontologia* (in press).

Van Cleave, C.D., 1969, Late Somatic Effects of Ionizing Radiation, U.S.A.E.C. Publication.

Van Lancker, J.L., and Tomura, T., 1972, A mammalian DNA repair endonuclease, *Proc. Amer. Assoc. Cancer Res.* 13:112.

Van Lancker, J.L., and Tomura, T., 1974, Purification and some properties of a mammalian repair endonuclease, *Biochim. Biophys. Acta* 353:99-114.

Wheeler, K.T., and Lett, J.T., 1972, Formation and rejoining of DNA strand breaks in irradiated neurons *in vivo. Radiat. Res.* 52:59-67.

Wheeler, K.T., Sheridan, R.E., Pautler, E.L., and Lett, J.T., 1973, *In vivo* restitution of the DNA structure in gamma-irradiated rabbit retinas, *Radiat. Res.* 53:414-427.

Wilkins, R.J., and Hart, R.W., 1974, Preferential DNA repair in human cells, *Nature* 247:35-36.

Williams, J.R., and Little, J.B., 1975, Correlation of DNA repair and *in vitro* growth potential in hamster embryo cells, Abstr. "23rd Annu. Meeting Radiat. Res. Soc.," (May, 1975), p. 30, Miami Beach, Florida.

Witkin, E.M., 1974, Thermal enhancement of ultraviolet mutability in a *tif*-1 *uvrA* derivative of *E. coli* B/r: evidence that ultraviolet mutagenesis depends upon an inducible function, *Proc. Nat. Acad. Sci. USA* 71:1930-1934.

Witkin, E.M., 1975, Relationship between repair, mutagenesis and
    survival, *in* "Molecular Mechanisms for the Repair of DNA"
    (P.C. Hanawalt and R.B. Setlow, eds.), Plenum Press, New
    York (in press).
Yielding, K.L., 1974, A model for ageing based on differential
    repair of somatic mutational damage, *Persp. Biol. Med.* 17:
    201-208.
Yohn, D.S., Blakeslee, J.R., Milo, G.E., and Hart, R.W., 1975,
    Promotion of chemical-viral transformation of human fibro-
    blasts by 17-β-estradiol, an inhibitor of excision DNA
    repair, Abstr. Int. Symp. on "Protein and Other Adducts to
    DNA: Their Significance to Aging, Carcinogenesis and
    Radiation Biology," Williamsburg, Virginia, May 2-6, 1975.
Zeelon, P., Gershon, H., and Gershon, D., 1973, Inactive enzymes
    molecules in Aging Organisms: nematode fructose-1,6,-diphos-
    phate aldolase, *Biochemistry* 12:1743-1750.

557